CARDIOVASCULAR PHARMACOTHERAPEUTICS

Companion Handbook

NOTICE

Medicine is an ever-changing science. As new research and clinical experience broaden our knowledge, changes in treatment and drug therapy are required. The editors and the publisher of this work have checked with sources believed to be reliable in their efforts to provide information that is complete and generally in accord with the standards accepted at the time of publication. However, in view of the possibility of human error or changes in medical sciences, neither the editors nor the publisher nor any other party who has been involved in the preparation or publication of this work warrants that the information contained herein is in every respect accurate or complete, and they are not responsible for any errors or omissions or for the results obtained from use of such information. Readers are encouraged to confirm the information contained herein with other sources. For example and in particular, readers are advised to check the product information sheet included in the package of each drug they plan to administer to be certain that the information contained in this book is accurate and that changes have not been made in the recommended dose or in the contraindications for administration. This recommendation is of particular importance in connection with new or infrequently used drugs.

CARDIOVASCULAR PHARMACOTHERAPEUTICS Companion Handbook

WILLIAM H. FRISHMAN, M.D.
Professor and Chairman, Dept. of Medicine
Professor of Pharmacology
New York Medical College
Chief of Medicine
Westchester Medical Center
Valhalla, New York

EDMUND H. SONNENBLICK, M.D.
Safra Distinguished Professor of Medicine
Department of Medicine, Division of Cardiology
Albert Einstein College of Medicine
Bronx, New York

McGRAW-HILL

Health Professions Division
New York St. Louis San Francisco Aukland Bogotá
Caracas Lisbon London Madrid Mexico City Milan
Montreal New Delhi Paris San Juan Singapore
Sydney Tokyo Toronto

McGraw-Hill

A Division of The ***McGraw·Hill*** *Companies*

CARDIOVASCULAR PHARMACOTHERAPEUTICS COMPANION HANDBOOK

234567890 DOCDOC 99

ISBN 0-07-022488-9

This book was set in Times Roman by Better Graphics, Inc.
The editors were Joseph Hefta and Pamela Touboul.
The production supervisor was Richard C. Ruzycka.
The cover was designed by Robert Freese.
The index was prepared by Jerry Ralya.
R.R. Donnelley & Sons Company was printer and binder.

Library of Congress Cataloging-in-Publication Data

Cardiovascular pharmacotherapeutics, companion handbook / edited by William H. Frishman, Edmund H. Sonnenblick.
p. cm.
Companion v. to: Cardiovascular pharmacotherapeutics. c1997
Includes bibliographical references and index.
ISBN: 0-07-022488-9. — ISBN: 0-07-022488-9
1. Cardiovascular agents—Handbooks, manuals, etc.
I. Frishman, William H., 1946– . II. Sonnenblick, Edmund H., 1932– . III. Cardiovascular pharmacotherapeutics.
[DNLM: 1. Cardiovascular Agents—pharmacology handbooks.
2. Cardiovascular Diseases—drug therapy handbooks.
3. Cardiovascular System—drug effects handbooks. QV 39 C26772 1998]
RM345.C3768 1998
615′.71—dc21
DNLM/DLC
for Library of Congress 98-9637
CIP

CONTENTS

Contributors ***vii***
Preface ***xi***

1 Basic Principles of Clinical Pharmacology Relevant to Cardiology **1**
Walter G. Levine

2 Alpha- and Beta-Adrenergic Blocking Drugs **23**
William H. Frishman

3 Parasympathetic Drugs **65**
B. Robert Meyer

4 Calcium Channel Blockers **73**
William H. Frishman

5 Drugs That Affect the Renin-Angiotensin System **107**
Michael C. Ruddy, John B. Kostis, William H. Frishman

6 Diuretic Therapy in Cardiovascular Disease **152**
Michelle Mokrzycki, Praveen Tamirisa, William H. Frishman

7 Magnesium, Potassium, and Calcium as Potential Cardiovascular Disease Therapies **175**
William H. Frishman, Erdal Cavusoglu, Joel Zonszein

8 Digitalis Preparations and Other Inotropic Agents **188**
Edmund H. Sonnenblick, Thierry H. LeJemtel, William H. Frishman

9 The Organic Nitrates and Nitroprusside **203**
Jonathan Abrams

10 Antiadrenergic Drugs with Central Action, Ganglionic Blockers, and Neuron Depletors **220**
Lawrence R. Krakoff

11 Nonspecific Antihypertensive Vasodilators **228**
Lawrence R. Krakoff

12 Antiarrhythmic Drugs **234**
Scott E. Hessen, Eric L. Michelson, William H. Frishman

13 Antiplatelet and Other Anthithrombotic Drugs **292**
William H. Frishman, Michael D. Klein, Ira Blaufarb, Bryan Burns

14 Thrombolytic Agents **324**
Robert Forman, William H. Frishman, Brian Strizik

15 Lipid-Lowering Drugs **346**
William H. Frishman, Peter Zimetbaum

16 Combination Drug Therapy in Hypertension **391**
Michael A. Weber, Benjamin E. Zola, Joel M. Neutel

17 Selective Dopamine Receptor Agonists; Fenoldopam **411**
William H. Frishman, Hilary Hotchkiss

18 Prostacyclin in Cardiovascular Disease **419**
William H. Frishman, Andrew N. Fink, Arif Ahmad

SPECIAL TOPICS SECTION

19 Use of Pharmaceuticals in Noninvasive Cardiovascular Diagnosis **427**
Jay S. Meisner, Jamshid Shirani, Joel A. Strom, William H. Frishman

20 Drug Therapy of Orthostatic Hypotension and Vasovagal Syncope **443**
William H. Frishman, Tracy Shevell

21 Drug Treatment of Infective Endocarditis **453**
Mark H. Goldberger, Gary E. Kalkut, Joseph N. Cosico William H. Frishman

22 Cardiovascular Drug Interactions **479**
Lionel H. Opie

APPENDICES

Appendix 1: Pharmacokinetic Properties of Approved Cardiovascular Drugs 506
Sylvia Thomas, Angela Cheng, William H. Frishman

Appendix 2: Therapeutic Use of Available Cardiovascular Drugs 540
William H. Frishman, Adam J. Spiegel, Angela Cheng, Sylvia Thomas

Appendix 3: Use of Cardiovascular Drugs in Special Populations 651
William H. Frishman, Angela Cheng

Index 687

CONTRIBUTORS*

Jonathan Abrams, M.D. (9), Division of Cardiology, Department of Medicine, University of New Mexico School of Medicine, Albuquerque, New Mexico

Arif Ahmad, M.D. (18), Department of Medicine, St. Barnabas Hospital, Cornell University Medical College, New York, New York

Ira Blaufarb, M.D. (13), Division of Cardiology, Department of Medicine, Albert Einstein College of Medicine, Bronx, New York

Bryan Burns, M.D. (13), Department of Medicine, New York Hospital, Cornell Medical Center, New York, New York

Erdal Cavusoglu, M.D. (7), Division of Cardiology, Department of Medicine, Bronx VA Medical Center, Mount Sinai School of Medicine, New York, New York

Angela Cheng, Pharm.D. (Appendices 1, 2), Department of Pharmacy, Montefiore Medical Center, Bronx, New York

Joseph Cosico RN, MA, CCRN (21), Division of Cardiology, Montefiore Medical Center, Bronx, New York

Andrew N. Fink, M.D. (18), Department of Medicine, Jacobi Hospital Center, Albert Einstein College of Medicine, Bronx, New York

Robert Forman, M.D. (14), Division of Cardiology, Department of Medicine, Montefiore Medical Center, Albert Einstein College of Medicine, Bronx, New York

William H. Frishman, M.D. (2, 4–8, 12–15, 17–21, Appendices 1, 2), Department of Medicine, New York Medical College, Westchester County Medical Center, Valhalla, New York

Mark H. Goldberger, M.D. (21), Division of Cardiology, Department of Medicine, Montefiore Medical Center, Albert Einstein College of Medicine, Bronx, New York

Scott E. Hessen, M.D. (12), Division of Cardiology, Department of Medicine, Hahnemann University Hospital, Medical College of Pennsylvania-Hahnemann Medical School, Philadelphia, Pennsylvania

*The numbers in parentheses following the contributors' names indicate the chapters written by that contributor.

Hilary Hotchkiss (17), Albert Einstein College of Medicine, Bronx, New York

Gary E. Kalkut, M.D. (21), Division of Infectious Diseases, Department of Medicine, Montefiore Medical Center, Albert Einstein College of Medicine, Bronx, New York

Michael D. Klein, M.D. (13), Division of Cardiology, Department of Medicine, University Hospital, Boston University Medical School of Medicine, Boston, Massachusetts

John B. Kostis, M.D. (5), Department of Medicine, The Robert Wood Johnson School of Medicine, New Brunswick, New Jersey

Lawrence R. Krakoff, M.D. (10, 11), Department of Medicine, Englewood Hospital, Mount Sinai School of Medicine, Englewood, New Jersey

Thierry H. LeJemtel, M.D. (8), Division of Cardiology, Department of Medicine, Montefiore Medical Center, Albert Einstein College of Medicine, Bronx, New York

Walter G. Levine, Ph.D. (1), Department of Molecular Pharmacology, Albert Einstein College of Medicine, Bronx, New York

Jay S. Meisner, M.D., Ph.D. (19), Division of Cardiology, Department of Medicine, Jacobi Hospital Center, Albert Einstein College of Medicine, Bronx, New York

B. Robert Meyer, M.D. (3), Department of Medicine, New York Hospital, Cornell Medical Center, New York, New York

Eric L. Michelson, M.D. (12), Division of Cardiology, Department of Medicine, Hahnemann University Hospital, Medical College of Pennsylvania-Hahnemann Medical School, Philadelphia, Pennsylvania

Michelle Mokrzycki, M.D. (6), Division of Nephrology, Department of Medicine, Jacobi Hospital Center, Albert Einstein College of Medicine, Bronx, New York

Joel M. Neutel, M.D. (16), Orange County Heart Institute and Research Center, UC-Irvine School of Medicine, Orange, California

Lionel Opie, M.D., Ph.D. (22), Heart Research Unit and Hypertension Clinic, University of Cape Town Medical School, Cape Town, South Africa

Michael C. Ruddy, M.D. (5), Division of Hypertension, Department of Medicine, The Robert Wood Johnson School of Medicine, New Brunswick, New Jersey

Tracy Shevell, M.D. (20), Department of Obstetics and Gynecology, Mt. Sinai School of Medicine, New York, New York

Jamshid Shirani, M.D. (19), Division of Cardiology, Department of Medicine, Montefiore Medical Center, Albert Einstein College of Medicine, Bronx, New York

Edmund H. Sonnenblick, M.D. (8), Division of Cardiology, Department of Medicine, Albert Einstein College of Medicine, Bronx, New York

Adam Spiegel, B.S. (Appendix 2), New York College of Osteopathic Medicine, Hempstead, New York

Brian Strizik, M.D. (14), Division of Cardilogy, Department of Medicine, Montefiore Medical Center, Albert Einstein College of Medicine, Bronx, New York

Joel A. Strom, M.D. (19), Division of Cardilogy, Department of Medicine, Montefiore Medical Center, Albert Einstein College of Medicine, Bronx, New York

Praveen Tamirisa, M.D., M.D. (6), Division of Cardiology, Department of Medicine, Barnes-Jewish Hospital Center, Washington University School of Medicine, St. Louis, Missouri

Sylvia Thomas, M.S., RPH. (Appendices 1, 2), Beth Israel North Department of Pharmacy, New York, New York

Michael A. Weber, M.D. (16), Department of Medicine, Brookdale University Hospital Center, State University of New York Health Science Center at Brooklyn, Brooklyn, New York

Peter Zimetbaum, M.D. (15), Division of Cardilogy, Department of Medicine, Beth Israel Hospital, Harvard Medical School, Boston, Massachusetts

Benjamin E. Zola, M.D. (16), Division of Cardiology, Department of Medicine, Brookdale University Hospital Center, State University of New York Science Center, Brooklyn, New York

Joel Zonszein, M.D. (7), Division of Endocrinology, Department of Medicine, Montefiore Medical Center, Albert Einstein College of Medicine, Bronx, New York

[illegible]

[illegible] Medicine, [illegible] Albert Einstein College of Medicine, Bronx, New York

[illegible]

PREFACE

This is the companion handbook to the first edition of *Cardiovascular Pharmacotherapeutics*. The chapters in the handbook were prepared by the authors of the corresponding chapters in the large book. The handbook was designed to provide a consise, portable reference source on cardiovascular drug treatment for physicians and students who cannot always access the larger textbooks. However, it is not intended to replace the more detailed reference sources in cardiology, adult medicine, and pharmacology.

ACKNOWLEDGMENTS

The editors would like to express their gratitude to the authors who contributed to the handbook. We also would like to thank our editoral assistant and secretary, Joanne Cioffi-Pryor, for her expert effort in helping to put both this handbook as well as the textbook together. We are grateful for the efforts of McGraw-Hill and its editorial and production staffs for their hard work in ultimately seeing this project through to its completion. Finally, we would like to acknowledge the support of our families and the encouragement of our students who have always provided the spark.

Chapter 1

Basic Principles of Clinical Pharmacology Relevant to Cardiology

Walter G. Levine

This chapter discusses some of the basic pharmacologic principles that influence the manner by which cardiovascular drugs manifest their pharmacodynamic and pharmacokinetic actions. A discussion of drug receptor pharmacology is followed by a review of drug disposition, drug metabolism, and excretion. In subsequent chapters that discuss different drug classes, these pharmacologic principles are represented relevant to the specific drugs being reviewed.

RECEPTORS

For nearly 100 years, it has been recognized that in order to elicit a response, a drug must interact with a receptor, the interface between drug and body and principal determinant of drug selectivity. The receptor (1) recognizes and binds the drug, (2) undergoes changes in conformation and charge distribution, and (3) transduces information inherent in the drug structure (extracellular signal) into intracellular messages, resulting in a change in cellular function. A receptor may be any functional macromolecule and is often a receptor for endogenous regulatory substances, such as hormones or neurotransmitters.

Nature of Receptors

Receptors typically are proteins, lipoproteins, or glycoproteins, including (1) regulatory proteins, which mediate the action of endogenous substances such as neurotransmitters or hormones, (2) enzymes, which typically are inhibited by drugs, (3) transport proteins such as Na^+/K^+-ATPase, and (4) structural proteins such as tubulin.

1. Gated channels involve synaptic transmitters (e.g., acetylcholine, norepinephrine) and drugs mimicking their action. These receptors regulate ion flow through membranes, altering transmembranal potentials. The well-characterized nicotinic acetylcholine receptor is a protein consisting of five subunits, two of which selectively bind acetylcholine, opening the Na^+ channel through conformational alterations. In the absence of agonist, the channel remains closed. Other drugs, for example, certain anxiolytics, act similarly at GABA-regulated Cl^- channels. The time sequence is extremely fast (milliseconds).
2. G proteins (interact with guanine nucleotides) diffuse within the cell membrane, interacting with more than one receptor. They regulate enzymes, such as adenyl cyclase, or ion channels. Their large number and great diversity may account for drug selectivity in some cases. A

prominent example is the role of a specific G protein in the regulation of muscarinic receptors in cardiac muscle. Activation enhances potassium permeability, causing hyperpolarization and depressed electrical activity.

3. Transmembranal enzymes, for example, protein tyrosine kinases, recognize ligands such as insulin and several growth factors. These bind to an extracellular domain of the receptor and allosterically activate the enzyme site at the cytoplasmic domain, enabling phosphorylation of receptor tyrosines. The signaling process proceeds to phosphorylation of other intracellular proteins, involving serine and threonine as well.

4. With intracellular receptors the lipophilic drug (agonist) permeates the plasma membrane and binds selectively to an intracellular macromolecule. The drug-receptor complex subsequently binds to DNA, modifying gene expression. Response time is slow (up to several hours) and duration of hours or days after disappearance of the drug due to turnover time of the proteins is expressed by the affected gene. The four major classes of receptors are depicted in Fig. 1-1.

Transmembrane signal transduction also involves a number of second messenger systems that respond to receptor activation. These systems include (1) cyclic AMP, formed by the action of ligand-activated adenyl cyclase on ATP. Through activation of selective protein kinases, it mediates numerous hormonal and drug responses. (2) Also included is phosphatidyl inositol hydrolysis by phospholipase C within the cell membrane, yielding water-soluble inositol triphosphate, which enters the cell and releases bound Ca^{2+}, and lipid-soluble diacylglycerol, which remains in the membrane where it activates protein kinase C.

Kinetics of Drug-Receptor Interactions

Drug or agonist interacts with its receptor as follows:

$$A + R \underset{k_2}{\overset{k_1}{\rightleftharpoons}} AR$$

where R = unoccupied receptor
AR = drug/receptor complex

According to the law of mass action, the forward reaction rate is given by $k_1[A][R]$ and the reverse reaction rate by $k_2[AR]$.

The dissociation constant (K_d) $= \dfrac{[A]\,[R]}{[AR]}$ relates to $\dfrac{k_2}{k_1}$

The binding (affinity) constant (K_a) $= \dfrac{1}{K_d}$ relates to $\dfrac{k_1}{k_2}$

Each constant is characteristic of a drug and its receptor.

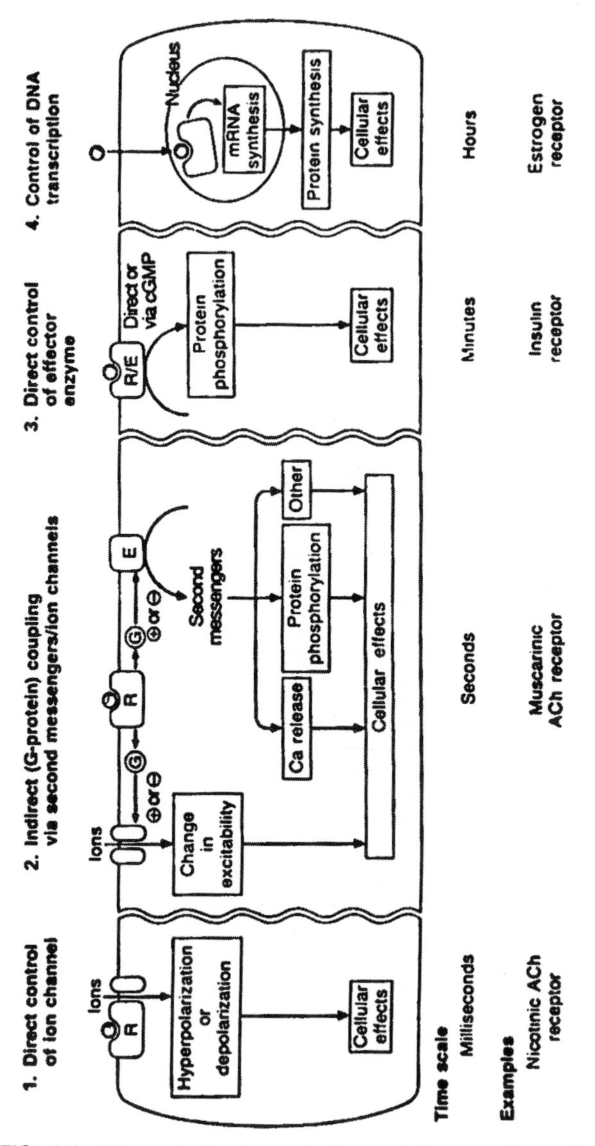

FIG. 1-1 Scheme for the four major types of drug receptors and linkage to their cellular effects. *R* = receptor molecule; *G* = *G* protein; *E* = enzyme.

Drug-receptor interaction may involve any type of bond: van der Waals, ionic, hydrogen, or covalent. The interaction is usually of the weaker, reversible type because covalent binding would effectively destroy receptor function (which may be desirable in the case of an irreversible inhibitor such as the choline esterase inhibitors, echothiophate, and parathione). Affinity for receptors varies considerably in a teleologically satisfactory manner. Postsynaptic receptors have low affinity for endogenous neurotransmitters released in high concentrations into the synaptic cleft. In contrast, intracellular steroid receptors have high affinity for hormones, which are found in the circulation in very low concentration.

Quantitative Considerations

If one measures an effect at varying drug doses (concentrations) and plots the drug response versus the dose, a rectangular hyperbola is obtained (Fig. 1-2*A*). Since quantitative comparisons among drugs and types of receptors are best described in terms of ED_{50} (the dose eliciting 50% maximal response), it is necessary to plot the response versus the log dose. In this way, the ED_{50} can be more accurately determined (Fig. 1-2*B*), since it is found in a relatively linear part of the curve. This relationship is valid when a graded response is discernible.

The log dose-response curve also can be used to distinguish competitive and noncompetitive inhibition, characteristic of many commonly used drugs. *Competitive inhibition* implies that the agonist and antagonist compete for binding at the active site of the receptor (e.g., β-adrenergic blocking drugs are competitive inhibitors at β-adrenergic receptor sites). Binding of the antagonist to the active site induces no biologic response but causes a shift to the right of the log dose-response curve, indicating that more agonist is required to attain a maximal response (Fig. 1-3*A*). A noncompetitive inhibitor, on the other hand, binds at other than the active site, preventing the agonist from inducing a maximal response at any dose (Fig. 1-3*B*). There also may be blockade of an action distal to the active site of the receptor. For example, verapamil and nifedipine are calcium channel blockers and prevent influx of calcium ions, nonspecifically blocking smooth-muscle contraction.

A partial agonist induces a response qualitatively similar to the true agonist but far less than the maximal response. Of critical importance is the lack of full response to the agonist in the presence of the partial agonist, the latter thereby acting as an inhibitor. The nonselective β blocker pindolol exhibits prominent partial agonist activity. The original hope that such a drug would be valuable in cardiac patients with asthma or other lung diseases has not materialized.

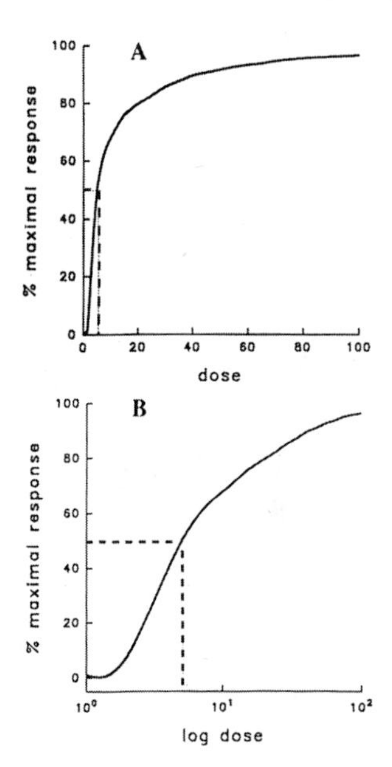

FIG. 1-2 Theoretical dose (concentration)-response curves. (*A*) Arithmetic dose scale. (*B*) Log dose scale. ----------- = determination of 50% effect.

FIG. 1-3 Log dose-response curves illustrating competitive (*A*) and noncompetitive (*B*) antagonism. In *A*, *a* is the curve for agonist alone; *b*, *c*, and *d* are curves obtained in the presence of increasing concentration of a competitive inhibitor. In *B*, *a* is the curve for agonist alone; *b*, *c*, and *d* are the curves obtained in the presence of increasing concentrations of a noncompetitive inhibitor.

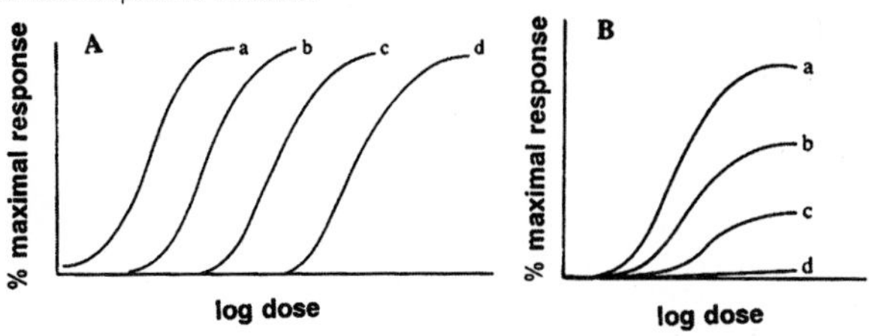

Two fundamental properties of drugs, efficacy (intrinsic activity) and potency, must be distinguished (Fig. 1-4*A*). A partial agonist, unable to elicit a full response, has lower efficacy than does a true agonist. *Efficacy* is actually a property of the drug-receptor complex, since the efficacy of a drug may change from one receptor system to another. *Potency* refers to the concentration or dose of drug required to elicit a standard response. Figure 1-4*B* shows that a series of drugs acting on the same receptor and differing in potency may possess similar efficacy; with increasing dose, each can induce the same maximal response. In Fig. 1-4*C* are log dose-response curves for several agonists with similar potencies but with varying efficacies. Potency is often considered to be a function of the drug-receptor binding constant. Clinically, a drug that undergoes extensive first pass, is rapidly inactivated, or has other impediments to accessing its receptor actually may require a high dose despite demonstration of high receptor affinity in vitro. High potency in itself is not a therapeutic advantage for a drug. The therapeutic index always must be considered. A twofold increase in potency may be accompanied by a similar increase in toxicity, yielding no advantage.

A fundamental tenet in receptor theory is that a receptor must be "occupied" by an agonist to elicit a biologic response, and the biologic response is proportional to the number of receptors occupied. However, the ultimate response, for example, change in blood pressure, renal function, or secretion, may not exhibit a simple proportional relationship owing to the complexity of postreceptor events. The spare receptor theory states that a maximal response may be attained prior to occupancy of all receptors at a particular site. This is strictly a quantitative concept, since the spare (unoccupied) receptors do not differ qualitatively from other receptors at the same site. Spare receptors may represent 10 to 99% of the total and may allow agonists of low affinity to exert a maximal effect.

Modulation of receptor function is seen frequently. Downregulation is the decrease in the number of receptors on chronic exposure to an agonist, resulting in lower sensitivity to the agonist. The receptor number may later normalize. For example, administration of a dobutamine infusion to patients with cardiac failure often leads to loss of efficacy of the drug due to downregulation of myocardial β adrenoceptors. Upregulation was first illustrated by denervation supersensitivity. Sympathetic denervation reduces the amount of neurotransmitter (norepinephrine) to which the postsynaptic adrenoceptor is exposed. Over a period of time, the receptor population increases, resulting in a heightened sensitivity to small doses of agonist. Drug-induced depletion of sympathetic neurotransmitter (reserpine, guanethidine) elicits a similar response. The increase in cardiac β receptors during hyperthyroidism increases the sensitivity of the heart to catecholamines.

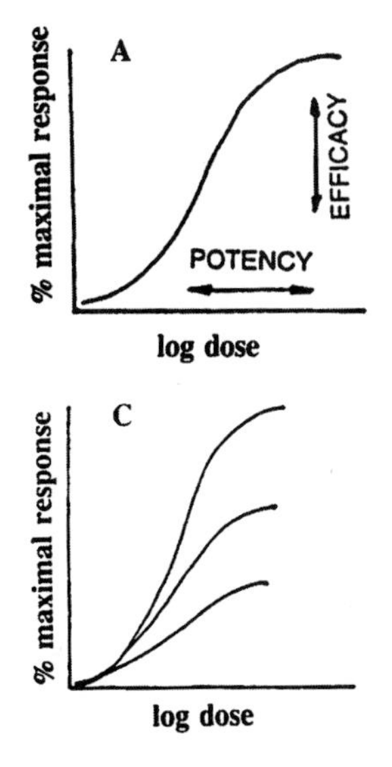

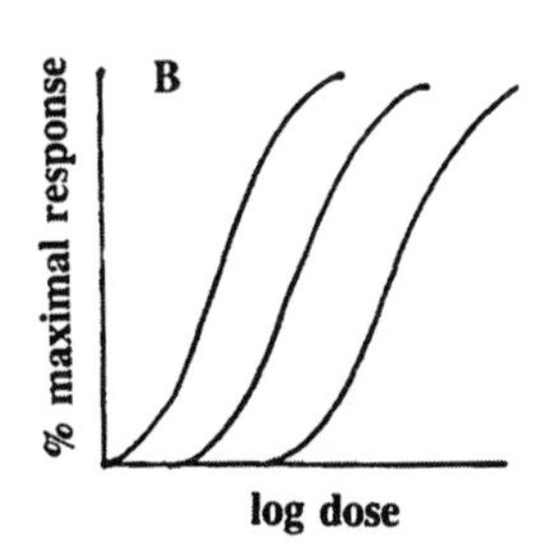

FIG. 1-4 (*A*) Log dose-response curves distinguishing potency from efficacy (intrinsic activity). (*B*) Response to three drugs with similar efficacies but differing in potency. (*C*) Response to three drugs with similar potencies but differing in efficacy. In each case the receptor system is the same.

DRUG DISPOSITION AND PHARMACOKINETICS

Although binding of a drug to its receptor is required for most drug effects, the amount bound is a small fraction of the total within the body. The mechanisms controlling the movement, metabolism, and excretion of total drug within the body are critical. On them depend the dose, route of administration, onset and duration, intensity of effect, frequency of administration, and often, toxic side effects.

Passage of Drugs across Cell Membranes

Movement of nearly all drugs within the body requires transport across cell membranes by filtration (kidney glomerulus), active transport (renal tubules), passive transport, and facilitated diffusion. Most drugs cross most membranes under most conditions by simple diffusion. Therefore, rate and direction of passage depend on (1) concentration gradient across the membrane of unbound drug and (2) lipid solubility of drug. Most drugs, being weak organic bases or acids, will be ionized or un-ionized depending on their p*K* and the pH of their environment. The *un-ionized* form, being more lipid soluble, readily diffuses across the membrane, whereas the *ionized* form is mainly excluded from the membrane. This principle is adhered to most rigidly in the brain, where the tight gap junctions in cerebral capillaries prevent intercellular diffusion of hydrophilic drugs, creating the so-called blood-brain barrier. Drugs having a charge at physiologic pH, for example, terfenidine (Seldane) and neostigmine are generally excluded from the brain. By contrast, in the liver, blood passes through sinusoids that are highly fenestrated, allowing plasma constituents, including charged and noncharged drugs, to pass readily into the interstitial space and have direct contact with the liver cells, where selectivity for drug transport is far less.

Absorption

Absorption of drugs from sites of administration follows the general principles just described. Other factors include solubility, rate of dissolution, concentration at site of absorption, circulation to site of absorption, and area of the absorbing surface.

Routes of Drug Administration

Sublingual route Administration avoids destruction because of the acidic environment of the stomach and bypasses the intestine and liver, avoiding loss through adsorption and enzymic destruction (first-pass effect). It is used for nitroglycerin (angina pectoris), ergotamine (migraine), and certain testosterone preparations (avoids prominent first-pass effects).

Oral route In addition to the convenience of this route, the structure, surface area, and movement of intestines are conducive to absorption, which takes place throughout the gastrointestinal (GI) tract. Rules for passive transport are applicable; pH gradient along the tract influences absorption of drugs with varying p*K*. Aqueous and lipid solubility of drug may be competing factors; that is, a drug may be lipid-soluble, favoring absorption, but so insoluble in water that absorption is very poor or erratic. Rate of absorption is partially regulated by intestinal blood flow, which serves to remove drug from the absorption site, maintaining a high GI tract–blood concentration gradient and gastric emptying time (most drugs are mainly absorbed in the intestine). Absorption varies with pH, presence and nature of food, mental state, GI and other diseases, endocrine status, and drugs that influence GI function.

Drugs may be extensively (high extraction) or minimally (low extraction) cleared from both the portal and systemic circulation by the liver. The extent of removal is referred to as the *extraction ratio*. It follows that the rate of plasma clearance of high-extraction drugs is very sensitive to hepatic blood flow. An increase or decrease in hepatic blood flow will enhance or depress, respectively, drug clearance from the plasma. Conversely, variations in hepatic blood flow have minimal influence on removal of low extraction drugs, since so little is removed per unit time. Diminished hepatic extraction capacity, as seen in severe liver disease and aging, can significantly decrease the first-pass effect and plasma disappearances of high extraction drugs.

Rectal route This route is reserved mainly for infants, cases of persistent vomiting, and the unconscious patient. Absorption follows rules for passive transport but is often less efficient than in other parts of tract. Since blood flow in the lower part of the rectum connects directly with the systemic circulation, portions of rectally administered drugs bypass the first-pass effect.

Pulmonary route The pulmonary route is primarily for gaseous and volatile drugs as well as nicotine and other drugs of abuse, for example, crack cocaine. These are rapidly absorbed because of high lipid solubility, small molecular size, and vast alveolar surface area (approximately 200 m^2).

Transdermal route This route has come into vogue for administration of certain cardiac, central nervous system (CNS), and endocrine drugs for a slow, sustained effect. The large surface area (2 m^2) and blood supply of the skin (30%) are conducive to absorption. Advantages include more stable blood levels, avoidance of first-pass effect, better compliance because frequency of administration is greatly diminished, no injection risks, and elimination of variability in oral absorption. The drug must be relatively potent, that is, effective in low dose, sufficiently lipid and water soluble to penetrate the several layers of the skin, nonirritating, and stable for several days. Drugs administered by the transdermal route include scopolamine, nitrate, clonidine, and estradiol.

Injected drugs This route avoids the first-pass effect. The *intravenous* route allows rapidity of access to the systemic circulation and a degree of accuracy for dosage not possible with other routes. *Intramuscular* and *subcutaneous* routes require absorption into the systemic circulation at rates dependent on lipid solubility of the drug and circulation to the injected area. Epinephrine may be added to a subcutaneous injection to constrict blood vessels and thus retard absorption.

Bioavailability

There are two aspects of this concept: (1) *absolute bioavailability*, the proportion of administered drug gaining access to the systemic circulation after oral compared with intravenous administration, reflecting the first-pass effect, and (2) *relative bioavailability* of different preparations of the same drug.

By plotting plasma concentration versus time, one can calculate the area under the curve (AUC), a measure of bioavailability (Fig. 1-5). The curve also indicates peak plasma levels and time to attain peak levels. Bioequivalent preparation should be identical in each of these parameters. However, considerable variation may be seen among different preparations, reflecting extent and rate of drug release from its dosage form (pill, capsule, etc.) within the GI tract. Factors that may affect bioavailability include conditions within the GI tract, pH, food, disease, other drugs, metabolism, and/or binding within the intestinal wall and liver. Ideally, preparations should be tested for bioavailability under identical conditions in the same subject. The narrower the therapeutic index of a drug, the greater is the concern for variation in bioavailability.

Distribution to Tissues

Vascularity and plasma concentration of drug are the main determinants in tissue distribution. Organs receiving a high blood supply, like

FIG. 1-5 Theoretical plasma levels of drug as a function of time. The curve is used to determine bioavailability, since it illustrates peak concentration, time of peak concentration, and area under the curve (AUC).

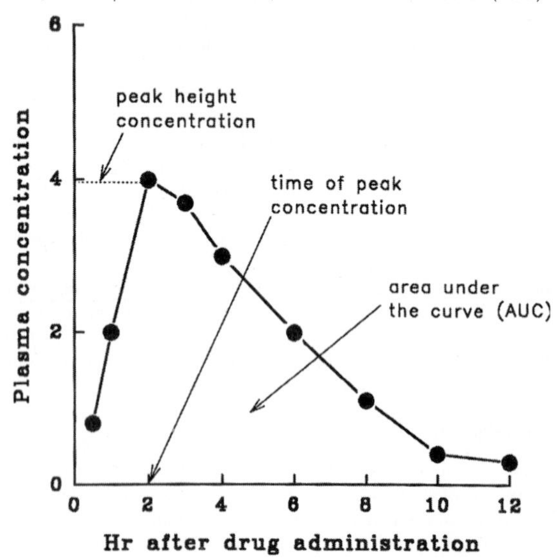

the kidney, brain, and thyroid, are rapidly exposed to drugs, whereas bone and adipose tissue receive only a minor fraction of the dose. High plasma concentrations of drugs result in high tissue levels due to mass action and passive diffusion across cell membranes. Lipid-soluble drugs readily pass the placenta, enabling distribution to and possible action on the developing fetus. Therefore, the use of any drug is not recommended during pregnancy; thiazide diuretics and warfarin, among others, are particularly discouraged. Redistribution of drugs can influence pharmacologic response. For example, it is well established that the actions of benzodiazepines and thiopental are terminated not by metabolism or excretion but by redistribution of the drugs away from the brain.

Site-specific drug delivery would enhance therapeutic effectiveness and limit side and toxic effects. This has been achieved for very few drugs, since normal body mechanisms are generally conducive to wide distribution to sites unrelated to the desired drug receptors. A type of organ targeting is seen with prodrugs such as L-dopa, which is converted to the active form, dopamine, in the CNS, and sulfasalazine, which is converted to the active salicylate by gut bacteria within the lower bowel.

Binding to Plasma Proteins

Most drugs are bound to plasma proteins to some extent. Albumin binds a wide spectrum of drugs, particularly those with acidic and neutral characteristics. Binding is usually nonspecific, although some selective sites are known. Basic drugs also may bind to albumin but mainly to α_1-acid glycoprotein, an acute-phase reactant protein. Lipoproteins also bind some lipophilic and basic compounds. A number of highly specific proteins exist that bind thyroxin, retinal, transcortin, etc., but these are of little consequence for drugs and other xenobiotics.

Binding to plasma proteins is always reversible, and the $t_{1/2}$ of binding and release is exceedingly short (measured in milliseconds). Thus, even in the case of extensive (tight) binding, it is rapidly reversible under physiologic conditions. Since concentration gradients, which determine the rate of passive transport across membranes, are based solely on free drug, it follows that binding to plasma proteins slows the rate of removal of drug from plasma by diminishing the concentration gradient across capillary cell membranes. Thus access to all extravascular sites, receptors, metabolism, storage, and excretion is to a great extent regulated by plasma protein binding. It follows that the half-lives of many drugs correlate with the extent of binding.

Hepatic extraction is sensitive to plasma protein binding. For low-extraction drugs, binding is of considerable importance, whereas hepatic uptake of high-extraction drugs is little influenced by binding.

Active transport is unaffected by plasma protein binding because the concentration gradient of unbound drug across the cell membrane is of little significance. In this case, the protein-bound portion of the drug serves as a readily accessible reservoir owing to rapid reversibility of binding.

Displacement of drugs from binding sites increases the proportion of free drug in the plasma and thus the effective concentration of the drug in extravascular compartments. Similarly, increasing the dose of a drug beyond binding capacity disproportionately increases the unbound fraction within the plasma and may lead to undesired pharmacologic effects. Plasma binding proteins may be decreased in concentration or effectiveness under the following conditions:

Albumin Burns, nephrosis, cystic fibrosis, cirrhosis, inflammation, sepsis, malnutrition, neoplasia, aging, pregnancy, stress, and heart failure. Uremia causes decreased binding of acidic but not basic drugs.

α_1-Acid glycoprotein Aging, oral contraceptives, pregnancy.

The possibility of altered drug disposition should be considered in each case.

Volume of Distribution

Under ideal conditions, drugs are considered to be distributed in one or more of the body fluid compartments. The apparent volume of distribution (Vd) is the body fluid volume that appears to contain the drug.

$$\text{Vd} = \frac{\text{amount of drug in body}}{\text{concentration of drug in blood or plasma}}$$

For example, Vd = plasma volume (e.g., heparin) implies extensive binding of the drug to plasma proteins, with the bulk of the drug remaining in the plasma. Vd = total body water (e.g., phenytoin, diazepam) implies that the drug is evenly distributed throughout the body. However, one should avoid associating Vd values with a specific anatomic compartment because binding at extravascular sites (e.g., procainamide, verapamil, and metoprolol) may significantly affect Vd determinations. Their importance lies in the fact that Vd can vary with age, sex, disease, etc. Thus changes in plasma protein synthesis, skeletal muscle mass, adipose tissue mass, adipose-muscle ratio, and body hydration will be reflected in Vd and may markedly alter therapeutic as well as toxic response to a drug. Values of Vd, if used intelligently, can provide information on body distribution of a drug as well as changes in body water compartments and implications for intensity of effect and rate of elimination.

Half-Life and Clearance

The half-life ($t_{1/2}$) of a drug is the time for the plasma concentration to be decreased by one-half. It is usually independent of route of administration and dose. Assuming equilibration among all body fluid compartments, it theoretically is a true reflection of the $t_{1/2}$ within the total body and correlates closely with duration of action. Half-life is derived from a first-order reaction calculated from a semilog plot of the plasma concentration versus time during the elimination phase that reflects metabolism and excretion of the drug (Fig. 1-6). Linearity of this phase reflects exponential kinetics (first order) in which plasma concentrations of drug do not saturate the rate-limiting step in elimination. The process may be expressed as a rate constant k, the fractional change per unit time. $t_{1/2}$ and k are related by the following equation:

$$t_{1/2} \times k = 0.693(\ln 0.5) \qquad \text{or} \qquad t_{1/2} = \frac{0.693}{k}$$

After oral administration, the initial period is called the *absorption phase*. Here too, $t_{1/2}$ is calculated from the elimination phase. In a few cases (alcohol, phenytoin, high-dose aspirin), the rate-limiting step is

FIG. 1-6 Theoretical plasma disappearance curve for a drug after intravenous or oral administration. During the elimination phase, the straight line obtained from a semilog plot reflects first-order kinetics.

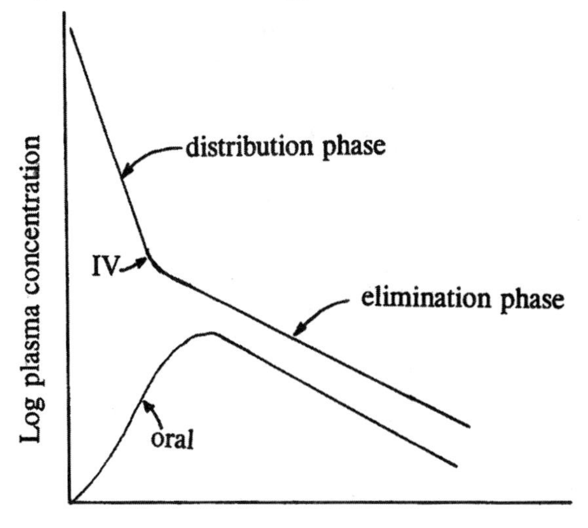

saturated, and the plasma disappearance rate is zero order. For phenytoin, this may lead to difficulty in controlling blood levels to maintain efficacy while avoiding toxicity.

Total body clearance (Cl_T) is an expression of the fluid volume (Vd) cleared per unit time. It is calculated as the product of the elimination rate constant and the volume of distribution.

$$Cl_T = k\text{Vd}$$

It follows that

$$t_{1/2} = \frac{0.693\,\text{Vd}}{\text{Cl}}$$

This concept assumes clearance from a single body-fluid compartment and is the sum of renal and hepatic clearances. Disease states, aging, and other conditions where Vd may be altered would change clearance. Clearance can be used to determine correct dosage when the desired plasma concentration has been predetermined but changes in physiologic parameters governing drug disposition occur, thus altering clearance.

$$\text{Dosage} = \text{Cl} \times C_{ss}$$

where Cl = clearance
C_{ss} = steady-state plasma drug concentration

Dosage, therefore, is a replacement of cleared drug.

Caution Since clearance is calculated from Vd, a theoretical rather than physiologic term, the number derived may itself not be truly physiologic. In therapeutics, it is the change of clearance that is a marker for altered drug disposition.

Steady-State Kinetics

During chronic oral administration of a drug, its steady-state plasma level is not a set concentration but a fluctuating concentration reflecting periodic absorption and continuous removal. When drug administration is begun, in accord with first-order kinetics, the elimination rate gradually increases with increasing plasma levels, and eventually a steady state is attained where input = output. This is the *plateau effect* (Fig. 1-7).

It can be shown that after

one half-life	50% of steady state attained
two half-lives	75% of steady state attained
three half-lives	87.5% of steady state attained
four half-lives	93.75% of steady state attained

The rule of thumb is that steady state is attained in four or five half-lives.

After drug withdrawal, the converse of the plateau effect is seen; that is, plasma levels are reduced by

50% in one half-life
75% in two half-lives
87.5% in three half-lives
93.75% in four half-lives

When long half-life, for example, 14 h, and therapeutic demands preclude waiting four or five half-lives to attain desired plasma concentration of drug, a loading dose (LD) is used, calculated as follows:

$$LD = \frac{Vd \times C}{F}$$

where Vd = apparent volume of distribution
C = desired plasma concentration
F = fraction of oral dose that reaches the systemic circulation (first-pass effect)

FIG. 1-7 Blood level–time profile for a drug, half-life = 4 h, administered every 4 h. The plateau effect determines that 95% of the final mean blood level is attained in four to five half-lives.

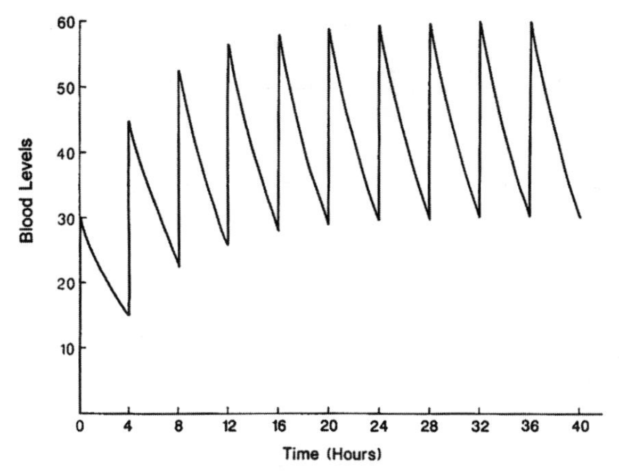

This is based on the need to fill the entire volume of distribution to the desired concentration as rapidly as possible. The dose is limited by toxicity, distribution rate, and other variables.

For a drug given by intravenous infusion,

$$\text{LD} = \text{infusion rate} \times t_{1/2}$$

DRUG METABOLISM (BIOTRANSFORMATION)

Mechanisms and Pathways

Most drugs and other xenobiotics are metabolized prior to excretion. Although most drugs are ultimately converted to inactive products, many are transformed to pharmacologically active metabolites. In some instances, a drug is metabolized via several pathways, some of which represent inactivation, while others represent activation to toxic product(s).

For many drugs, the first step (phase I) is catalyzed by the cytochrome P450 (mixed-function oxidase) system of the endoplasmic reticulum (microsomal fraction). Cytochrome P450 is actually a large family of isozymes, members of which vary with species, gender, and age. Each has its own spectrum of substrates and can be independently influenced by induction and inhibition. The mixed-function oxidase system exists mainly in the liver but has been detected in nonhepatic tissue as well, particularly at other sites of xenobiotic entry, like lung and skin. Total metabolism in these tissues is a fraction of that of the liver. Nevertheless, since environmental chemicals often enter the body through the lungs and skin, these tissues are of considerable importance in their metabolism.

Major phase I pathways, microsomal and nonmicrosomal, include (1) aliphatic and aromatic hydroxylation, (2) *N* dealkylation, (3) *O* dealkylation, (4) sulfoxidation, (5) *N* hydroxylation (commonly associated with toxic activation of aromatic amines, including a number of chemical carcinogens), (6) azo and nitro reduction, (7) *O* methylation, and (8) hydrolysis by plasma esterase.

Conjugation (synthetic) pathways (phase II) often, but not always, follow phase I. They include (1) acylation, a common pathway for aliphatic and aromatic primary amines, (2) glucuronide formation, (3) sulfate formation, and (4) glutathione conjugate formation. Phase II reactions increase drug polarity and charge and thus promote renal excretion (see later).

Glutathione conjugation is a major inactivation mechanism for toxic metabolic intermediates of numerous drugs. For example, in normal dosage, a toxic metabolite of acetaminophen is effectively removed as a glutathione conjugate. In extreme overdose (10 to 15 g), the demand for glutathione exceeds its rate of hepatic biosynthesis, and the accumulation of toxic intermediate leads to liver toxicity and, in rare cases, necrosis and death. Toxicity is treated with acetylcysteine, which serves to restore liver glutathione.

Factors Affecting Drug Metabolism

Species This is a major problem in drug development and research.

Age Few drugs are studied in young children prior to FDA approval, presenting a considerable challenge in the treatment of this population. In the *neonate*, factors affecting drug disposition include prolonged gastric emptying time, fluctuating gastric pH, smaller muscle mass, greater cutaneous absorption of toxic substances (e.g., hexachlorophene), changing body water–fat ratio, less effective plasma protein binding, poor hepatic drug metabolism, and low renal blood flow. Drugs that pass the placenta present problems of disposition to the fetus. The newborn often exhibits a deficiency in glucuronyl transferase, which catalyzes the essential step in bilirubin excretion. If unattended, kernicterus may ensue. The post-neonatal period is also a time of rapid structural and physiologic changes including drug metabolism capacity. Therefore, calculation of dosage based solely on body weight or surface area may not always be appropriate. In the elderly, one sees diminished renal plasma flow and glomerular filtration rate, decreased hepatic phase I but not phase II drug metabolism, diminished Vd due to loss of body water compartment, decreased muscle mass, decreased or increased adipose tissue, and decreased first-pass effect.

Genetic factors Marked differences in drug metabolism rates are often attributable to genetic factors. Approximately half the male population in the United States acetylates aromatic amines such as isoniazid rapidly, and the other half acetylates slowly (Fig. 1-8). The slow acetylator phenotype is inherited as an autosomal recessive trait. Neither slow nor fast acetylation is an advantage, since toxicity of both isoniazid (peripheral neuropathies, preventable by pyridoxine administration) and its acetylated metabolite (hepatic damage) is known. Other affected drugs include procainamide, hydralazine, and sulfasalazine.

A small percentage ($<1\%$) of the population has an abnormal form of plasma pseudoesterase and is unable to hydrolyze succinylcholine at the normal rapid rate, leading to an exaggerated duration of action. Two forms of cytochrome P450 exhibit polymorphism. The phenotypes are slow and rapid metabolizers of many drugs, including debrisoquin, tricyclic antidepressants, phenformin, dextromethorphan, some antiarrhythmic drugs (encainide, flecainide, propafenone, and mexiletine), and several β blockers. Three to ten percent of the population has the slow trait, inherited as autosomal recessive.

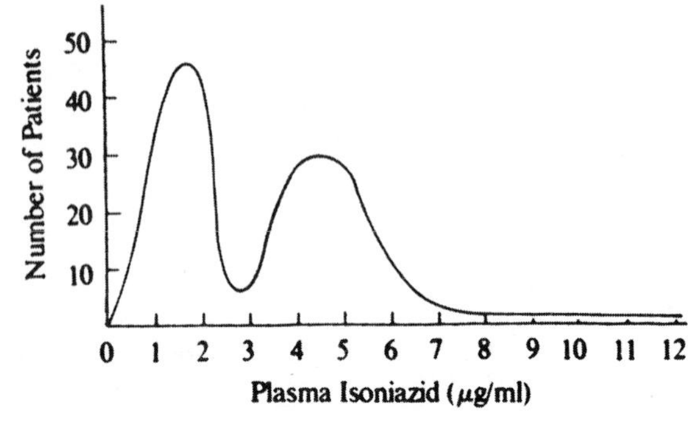

FIG. 1-8 Bimodal distribution of patients into rapid and slow acetylators of isoniazid. Slow acetylators are homozygous for an autosomal recessive gene.

Nutritional and disease states Multiple manifestations of malnutrition may significantly affect drug disposition. These include changes in GI and renal function, body composition (fluids, electrolytes, fat, protein, etc.), hepatic drug metabolism, endocrine function, and immune response. This is most likely among economically depressed populations and in diseases such as cancer, which are often accompanied by malnutrition. Obviously, hepatic or renal disease can have major consequences for drug disposition. Half-lives for many drugs increase in cirrhosis, hepatitis, obstructive jaundice, and nephritis and other types of kidney failure. Liver disease may result in altered hepatic blood flow, decreased extraction, or depressed metabolizing enzymes. Kidney disease may be manifest as altered renal blood flow and depressed glomerular filtration, active transport, or passive reabsorption. In cardiac failure, the decreased blood supply to most organs means delayed and incomplete absorption of drugs. On the other hand, decreased Vd may mean higher plasma drug levels and consequently exaggerated responses to drug.

Induction Chronic exposure to any of a large number of drugs and other environmental chemicals induces the synthesis of selective drug metabolizing enzymes. Typically, cytochrome P450–mediated reactions are induced, but conjugation with glucuronic acid and glutathione also may be affected. The duration of action of some drugs is thereby shortened, their blood levels lowered, and their potency diminished. The half-lives of drugs with low hepatic extraction are mainly affected, whereas drugs not metabolized by these enzymes are not affected. Examples of well-known inducing agents are (1) lipid-soluble drugs such as phenobarbital, phenytoin, rifampicin, and ethanol, (2) glucocorticoids, and (3) environmental pollutants such as benzo(a)pyrene and other polycyclic hydrocarbons formed in cigarette smoke, polychlorinated biphenyls (PCBs), and dioxin. The effect of smoking on plasma drug levels is seen in Fig. 1-9.

Inhibition Inhibition of drug metabolism will have the opposite effect, leading to prolonged half-life and an exaggerated pharmacologic response. Drugs well known for their inhibitory effects include chloramphenicol, cimetidine, allopurinol, and monoamine oxidase inhibitors. Alcohol acutely depresses certain drug metabolism pathways (although chronically it induces) and may lead to enhanced and prolonged effects of other drugs. Erythromycin and ketoconazole block the conversion of terfenadine (Seldane), a prodrug, to its active metabolite. Since the parent compound is arrhythmogenic, serious cardiac toxicity may be seen with such drug combinations. It is suspected that there are many more such inhibitory drugs, but it is difficult to predict, a priori, when inhibition will occur.

Metabolism by Intestinal Microorganisms

The abundant flora of the lower gut include many organisms capable of metabolizing drugs as well as their metabolic derivatives. Since the microflora consist mainly of obligate anaerobes and the gut environment is anaerobic, only pathways not requiring oxygen are seen. These bacteria make a significant contribution to drug metabolism, and suppression of the gut flora by oral antibiotics or other drugs will appreciably alter the fate, and thus the effects, of many other drugs. The various pathways include hydrolysis of glucuronides, sulfates, and amides; dehydroxylation; deamination; and azo and nitro reduction.

Enterohepatic Circulation

Many conjugated drugs are transported into the bile and pass into the intestine. Here, intestinal microorganisms hydrolyze the conjugate (glucuronides in particular), yielding the original, less polar compound, which can then be reabsorbed. This cycle tends to repeat itself and makes a major contribution to maintenance of drugs and certain endogenous compounds within the body. For example, bile salts are 90% recirculated through this mechanism. Suppression of gut bacteria by oral antibiotics will appreciably affect the half-lives, and thus the plasma levels, of compounds that undergo extensive enterohepatic circulation.

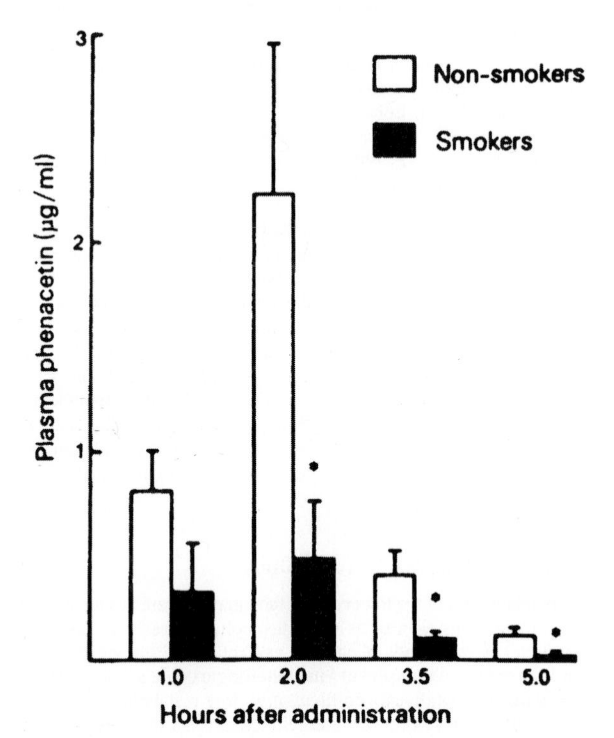

FIG. 1-9 Blood levels of phenacetin in smoking and nonsmoking populations, reflecting the inducing effect of components of cigarette smoke on drug metabolizing enzymes.

EXCRETION

All drugs are ultimately eliminated from the body via one route or another. Elimination rate, as reflected in plasma disappearance rate for most drugs, is generally proportional to the total amount in the body, following first-order kinetics.

1. *Kidney*. The kidney is the major organ of excretion for most drugs and associated metabolites. Its large blood supply (25% of cardiac output) is conducive to efficient excretion. Drugs not bound to plasma proteins are filtered in the glomerulus with nearly 100% efficiency.

Reabsorption within the tubule is mainly by passive diffusion. Thus highly charged drugs (or metabolites) will be poorly reabsorbed and readily excreted. Changes in tubular pH alter excretion rates by influencing the net charge on the compound. Appropriate manipulation of urinary pH is helpful in facilitating excretion in cases of drug overdose. For example, raising the pH increases excretion of phenobarbital, an organic acid, whereas lowering the pH increases excretion of amphetamine, an organic base. Active transport of organic anions and cations takes place in the tubules. Penicillin, a weak organic acid, is actively pumped into the tubule lumen by the tubular anion transport system, an action readily suppressed by an inhibitor of the anion pump, probenacid. Renal failure presents a major therapeutic problem due to accumulation of drug as well as toxic metabolites. Hemodialysis filters out unbound drugs from the plasma, thus assisting clearance.

2. *Biliary excretion.* This is usually reserved for highly polar compounds with a molecular weight greater than 500. Bile empties into the duodenum, and drugs passing via this route are frequently reabsorbed in the intestinal tract (see Enterohepatic Circulation earlier). Unlike with urine, the mechanisms of bile formation and biliary excretion are poorly understood. Biliary secretion is greatly, but not entirely, dependent on bile salt transport. Bile salts may facilitate or inhibit biliary excretion of drugs, depending on the drug and the concentration of bile salts.

3. *Lungs.* These are the excretion route for many general anesthetics and other volatile substances. A clever utilization of the lungs as a route of excretion is the *aminopyrine breath test.* Aminopyrine, labeled with radioactive carbon in its methyl moiety, is administered. It is demethylated by the liver P450 system, ultimately forming radioactive carbon dioxide, which is then collected from the expired air and counted. The amount of radioactivity is a reflection of hepatic drug metabolism and has been used as a noninvasive assessment of liver function, for example, in liver cirrhosis.

4. *Milk.* Considerable concern has been raised regarding drugs in breast milk in view of the increase in the past two decades in the number of nursing mothers affected by p*K* of drug, pH of milk and plasma, binding to plasma and milk proteins, and fat composition of milk. Drugs enter the milk by passive diffusion. The pH of milk (6.5 to 7.0), its varying volume, and its high content of fat globules and unique proteins influence drug secretion, especially for lipid-soluble compounds. Drugs known to be secreted into milk include cardiovascular drugs (hydralazine, digoxin), CNS drugs (caffeine, amitriptyline, primadone, ethosuximide), drugs of abuse (nicotine, narcotics, cocaine), and others (metronidazole, medroxyprogesterone, nor-testosterone). This does not necessarily imply an incompatibility between nursing and taking any of these drugs. However, drugs contraindicated or used with caution dur-

ing lactation include alcohol, amiodarone, atropine, chlorpromazine, cimetidine, cocaine, cyclosporin, doxorubicin, lithium, morphine, nitrorfurantoin, phenytoin, phenindione, salicylates, tetracyclines, and tinidazole. At present, drugs must be evaluated individually when deciding on the safety of nursing infants. Similar considerations are valid for cow's milk, since these animals may be given drugs to increase milk production.

Another route of excretion being developed for noninvasive assessment of blood levels of drugs is saliva. For some drugs, a known equilibrium exists between the plasma and saliva. Although the work is only in its infancy, one can foresee the day when, if plasma levels are required, a patient will simply spit for the doctor rather than being stuck with a needle five or six times.

SUGGESTED READING

Berndt WO, Stitzel RE: Excretion of drugs, in Craig CR, Stitzel RE (eds): *Modern Pharmacology*, 4th ed. Boston, Little, Brown, 1994, chap 5, pp 47–53.

Bourne HR, Roberts JM: Drug receptors and pharmacodynamics, in Katzung BG (ed): *Basic and Clinical Pharmacology*. Norwalk, Conn, Appleton & Lange, 1995, chap 2, pp 9–32.

Correia MA: Drug biotransformation, in Katzung BG (ed): *Basic and Clinical Pharmacology*. Norwalk, Conn, Appleton & Lange 1995, chap 4, pp 48–59.

Fleming WW: Mechanisms of drug action, in Craig CR, Stitzel RE (eds): *Modern Pharmacology*, 4th ed. Boston, Little, Brown, 1994, chap 2, pp 9–18.

Godin DV: Pharmacokinetics: Disposition and metabolism of drugs, in Munson PL, Mueller RA, Breese GR (eds): *Principles of Pharmacology: Basic Concepts and Clinical Applications*. New York, Chapman & Hall, 1995, chap 2, pp 39–84.

Gram TE: Drug absorption and distribution, in Craig CR, Stitzel RE (eds): *Modern Pharmacology*, 4th ed. Boston, Little, Brown, 1994, chap 3, pp 19–32.

Gram TE: Metabolism of drugs, in Craig CR, and Stitzel RE (eds): *Modern Pharmacology*, 4th ed. Boston, Little, Brown, 1994, chap 4, pp 33–46.

Gwilt PR: Pharmacokinetics, in Craig CR, Stitzel RE (eds): *Modern Pharmacology*, 4th ed. Boston, Little, Brown, 1994, chap 6, pp 55–64.

Holford NHG, Benet LZ: Pharmacokinetics and pharmacodynamics: Rational dose selection and the time course of drug action, in Katzung BG (ed): *Basic and Clinical Pharmacology*. Norwalk, Conn, Appleton & Lange, 1995, chap 3, pp 33–47.

Hollenberg MD, Severson DL: Pharmacodynamics: drug receptors and receptors/mechanisms, in Munson PL, Mueller RA, Breese GR (eds): *Principles of Pharmacology: Basic Concepts and Clinical Applications*. New York, Chapman & Hall, 1995, chap 1, pp 7–37.

Levine WG: Basic principles of clinical pharmacology relevant to cardiology, in Frishman WH, Sonnenblick EH (eds): *Cardiovascular Pharmacotherapeutics*. New York, McGraw-Hill, 1997, pp 3–15.

Rang HP, Dale MM, Ritter HM, Gardner P: *Pharmacology*. New York, Churchill-Livingstone, 1995, chaps 1, 2, 4, 42.

Chapter 2 Alpha- and Beta-Adrenergic Blocking Drugs

William H. Frishman

Catecholamines are neurohumoral substances that mediate a variety of physiologic and metabolic activities in humans. The effects of the catecholamines ultimately depend on their chemical interactions with receptors, which are discrete macromolecular structures located on the plasma membrane. Differences in the ability of the various catecholamines to stimulate a number of physiologic processes were the criteria used by Ahlquist in 1948 to separate these receptors into distinct types: α and β adrenergic. Subsequent studies have revealed that β-adrenergic receptors exist as three discrete subtypes called β_1, β_2 and β_3 (Table 2-1). It is now appreciated that there are two subtypes of α receptors, designated α_1 and α_2 (Table 2-1). At least three subtypes of both α_1- and α_2-adrenergic receptors are known, but distinctions in their mechanisms of action and tissue location have not been defined.

This chapter examines the adrenergic receptors and the drugs that can inhibit their function. The rationale for use and clinical experience with α- and β-adrenergic drugs in the treatment of various cardiovascular disorders are also discussed.

ADRENERGIC RECEPTORS: HORMONAL AND DRUG RECEPTORS

The effects of an endogenous hormone or exogenous drug depend ultimately on physiochemical interactions with macromolecular structures of cells called *receptors*. Agonists interact with a receptor and elicit a response; antagonists interact with receptors and prevent the action of agonists.

In the case of catecholamine action, the circulating hormone or drug (*first messenger*) interacts with its specific receptor on the external surface of the target cells. The drug/hormone-receptor complex, mediated by a G protein that is called Gs, activates the enzyme adenyl cyclase on the internal surface of the plasma membrane of the target cell, which accelerates the intracellular formation of cyclic adenosine monophosphate (cyclic AMP). Cyclic AMP–dependent protein kinase (*second messenger*) then stimulates or inhibits various metabolic or physiologic processes. Catecholamine-induced increases in intracellular cyclic AMP are usually associated with stimulation of β-adrenergic receptors, whereas α-adrenergic receptor stimulation is mediated by a G protein known as Gi and is associated with lower concentrations of cyclic AMP and possibly increased amounts of guanosine-3′5′-monophosphate in the cell. These changes may result in the production of opposite physi-

TABLE 2-1 Characteristics of Subtypes of Adrenergic Receptors*

Receptor	Tissue	Response
α_1[†]	Vascular smooth muscle, genitourinary smooth muscle	Contraction
	Liver[‡]	Glycogenolysis; gluconeogenesis
	Heart	Increased contractile force; arrhythmias
α_2[†]	Pancreatic islets (β cells)	Decreased insulin secretion
	Platelets	Aggregation
	Nerve terminals	Decreased release of NE
	Vascular smooth muscle	Contraction
β_1	Heart	Increased force & rate of contraction and AV nodal conduction velocity
	Juxtaglomerular cells	Increased renin secretion
β_2	Smooth muscle (vascular, bronchial, GI, & genitourinary)	Relaxation
	Skeletal muscle	Glycogenolysis; uptake of K^+
	Liver[‡]	Glycogenolysis; gluconeogenesis
β_1[¶]	Adipose tissue	Lipolysis, thermogenesis

*This table provides examples of drugs that act on adrenergic receptors and of the location of subtypes of adrenergic receptors. NE = norepinephrine.

[†]At least three subtypes of each α_1- and α_2-adrenergic receptor are known, but distinction in their mechanism of action and tissue location have not been clearly defined.

[‡]In some species (e.g., rat), metabolic responses in the liver are mediated by α_1-adrenergic receptors, whereas in others (e.g., dog), β_2-adrenergic receptors are predominantly involved. Both types of receptors appear to contribute to responses in human beings.

[¶]Metabolic responses in adipocytes and certain other tissues with atypical pharmacologic characteristics may be mediated by this subtype of receptor. Most β-adrenergic receptor antagonists (including propranolol) do not block these responses.

Source: Adapted from Lefkowitz RJ et al: Neurotransmission: The autonomic and somatic motor nervous system, in *Goodman & Gilman's The Pharmacological Basis of Therapeutics*, 9th ed. New York, McGraw-Hill, 1996, p 125.

ologic effects from catecholamines, depending on what adrenergic receptor system is activated.

Until recently, most research on receptor action bypassed the initial binding step and the intermediate steps and examined either the accumulation of cyclic AMP or the end step, the physiologic effect. Currently, radioactive agonists or antagonists (radioligands) that attach to and label the receptors have been used to study binding and hormone action. The cloning of adrenergic receptors also has revealed important clues about receptor function.

α-ADRENERGIC BLOCKERS

Clinical Pharmacology

When an adrenergic nerve is stimulated, catecholamines are released from their storage granules in the adrenergic neuron, enter the synaptic cleft, and bind to α receptors on the effector cell. A feedback loop exists by which the amount of neurotransmitter released can be regulated; accumulation of catecholamines in the synaptic cleft leads to stimulation of α receptors in the neuronal surface and inhibition of further catecholamine release. Catecholamines from the systemic circulation also can enter the synaptic cleft and bind to presynaptic or postsynaptic receptors.

Initially it was believed that α_1 receptors were limited to postsynaptic sites where they mediated vasoconstriction, whereas the α_2 receptors existed only at the prejunctional nerve terminals and mediated the negative feedback control of norepinephrine release. The availability of compounds with high specificity for either α_1 or α_2 receptors demonstrated that while presynaptic α receptors are almost exclusively of the α_2 subtype, the postsynaptic receptors are made up of comparable numbers of α_1 and α_2 receptors. Stimulation of the postsynaptic α_2 receptors causes vasoconstriction. A functional difference does, however, exist between the two types of postsynaptic receptors. The α_1 receptors appear to exist primarily within the region of the synapse and respond preferentially to neuronally released catecholamine, whereas α_2 receptors are located extrasynaptically and respond preferentially to circulating catecholamines in the plasma.

Drugs having α-adrenergic blocking properties are of several types as follows:

1. Nonselective α blockers having prominent effects on both the α_1 and α_2 receptors (e.g., the older drugs such as phenoxybenzamine and phentolamine). Although virtually all the clinical effects of phenoxybenzamine are explicable in terms of α blockade, this is not the case with phentolamine, which also possesses several other properties, including a direct vasodilator action and sympathomimetic and parasympathomimetic effects.
2. Selective α_1 blockers having little affinity for α_2 receptors (e.g., prazosin, terazosin, doxazosin, and other quinazoline derivatives). Originally introduced as direct-acting vasodilators, it is now clear that these drugs exert their major effect by reversible blockade of postsynaptic α_1 receptors. Other selective α_1 blockers include indoramin,

trimazosin, and urapadil (Table 2-2). Urapadil is of interest because of its other actions, which include stimulation of presynaptic α_2-adrenergic receptors and a central effect.

3. Selective α_2 blockers (e.g., yohimbine). The primary use of these drugs has been as tools in experimental pharmacology. Yohimbine is now marketed in the United States as an oral sympatholytic and mydriatic agent. Male patients with impotence from vascular or diabetic origin or from psychogenic origin have been treated successfully with yohimbine.

4. Blockers that inhibit both α- and β-adrenergic receptors (e.g., carvedilol, labetalol). Carvedilol and labetalol are selective α_1 blockers. Since these agents are much more potent as β blockers than as α blockers, they are discussed in greater detail in the section on β blockers.

5. Agents having α-adrenergic blocking properties but whose major clinical use appears unrelated to these properties (e.g., chlorpromazine, haloperidol, quinidine, bromocriptine, amiodarone, and ketanserin, a selective blocking agent of serotonin$_2$ receptors). It has been demonstrated that verapamil, a calcium channel blocker, also has α-adrenergic blocking properties. Whether this is a particular property of verapamil and its analogues or is common to all calcium channel blockers is not clear. Also to be clarified is whether verapamil-induced α blockade occurs at physiologic plasma levels and helps to mediate the vasodilator properties of the drug.

All the α blockers in clinical use inhibit the postsynaptic α_1 receptor and result in relaxation of vascular smooth muscle and vasodilation. However, the nonselective α blockers also antagonize the presynaptic α_2 receptors, allowing for increased release of neuronal norepinephrine. This results in attenuation of the desired postsynaptic blockade and spillover stimulation of the β receptors and, consequently, in troublesome side effects such as tachycardia and tremulousness and increased renin release. The α_1-selective agents that preserve the α_2-mediated presynaptic feedback loop prevent excessive norepinephrine release and thus avoid these adverse cardiac and systemic effects.

TABLE 2-2 Pharmacokinetics of Selective α_1-Adrenergic Blocking Drugs

Selective α1 blocker	Daily dose, mg	Frequency per day	Bioavailability, % of oral dose	Plasma half-life, h	Urinary excretion, % of oral dose
Doxazosin	1–16	1	65	10–12	NA
Prazosin	2–20	2–3	44–69	2.5–4	10
Terazosin	1–20	1	90	12	39

Source: Adapted from Luther RR: New perspectives on selective α_1 blockade. *Am J Hypertens* 2:731, 1989.

Because of these potent peripheral vasodilatory properties, one would anticipate, however, that even the selective α_1 blockers would induce reflex stimulation of the sympathetic and renin-angiotensin system similar to that seen with other vasodilators such as hydralazine and minoxidil. The explanation for the relative lack of tachycardia and renin release observed after prazosin, terazosin, and doxazosin may, in part, be due to the drugs' combined action of reducing vascular tone in both resistance (arteries) and capacitance (veins) beds. Such a dual action may prevent the marked increases in venous return and cardiac output observed with agents that act more selectively to reduce vascular tone only in the resistance vessels. The lack of tachycardia with prazosin, terazosin, and doxazosin use also has been attributed by some investigators to a significant negative chronotropic action of the drugs independent of their peripheral vascular effects.

Use in Cardiovascular Disorders

Hypertension Increased peripheral vascular resistance is present in the majority of patients with long-standing hypertension. Since dilation of constricted arterioles should result in lowering of elevated blood pressure, interest has focused on the use of α-adrenergic blockers in the medical treatment of systemic hypertension. The experience with nonselective α blockers in the treatment of hypertension, except for pheochromocytoma, was disappointing because of accompanying reflex stimulation of the sympathetic and renin-angiotensin system, resulting in frequent side effects and limited long-term antihypertensive efficacy. However, the selective α_1 blockers prazosin, doxazosin, and terazosin have been shown to be effective antihypertensive agents.

Prazosin, doxazosin, and terazosin decrease blood pressure in both the standing and supine positions, although blood pressure decrements tend to be somewhat greater in the upright position. Because their antihypertensive effect is accompanied by little or no increase in heart rate, plasma renin activity, or circulating catecholamines, prazosin, doxazosin, and terazosin have been found useful as first-step agents in hypertension. Monotherapy with these agents, however, promotes sodium and water retention in some patients, although it is less pronounced than with other vasodilators. The concomitant use of a diuretic prevents fluid retention and in many cases markedly enhances the antihypertensive effect of the drugs. In clinical practice, prazosin, doxazosin, and terazosin have their widest application as adjuncts to one or more established antihypertensive drugs in treating moderate to severe hypertension. Their effects are additive to those of diuretics, β blockers, α-methyldopa, and the direct-acting vasodilators. The drugs cause little change in glomerular filtration rate or renal plasma flow and can be used safely in patients with severe renal hypertension. There is no evidence for attenuation of the antihypertensive effect of prazosin, doxazosin, or terazosin during chronic therapy.

In large comparative clinical trials, the efficacy and safety of α_1 blockers have been well documented. In the TOMHS (Treatment of Mild Hypertension Study), doxazosin 2 mg/day given over 4 years reduced blood pressure as much as agents from other drugs classes. Doxazosin is one of the drugs being used in the Lipid Lowering Treatment to Prevent Heart Attack Trial (ALLHAT), which is comparing various antihypertensive drugs and their effects on coronary morbidity and mortality. In a large Veterans Administration study where more severe hypertensives were studied, prazosin 4 to 20 mg/day given over 1 year had a treatment success rate significantly greater than placebo.

Selective α_1 blockers appear to have neutral or even favorable effects on plasma lipids and lipoproteins when administered to hypertensive patients. Investigators have reported mild reductions in levels of total cholesterol, low-density lipoprotein (LDL) and very-low-density lipoprotein (VLDL) cholesterol, and triglycerides; elevations in levels of high-density lipoprotein (HDL) cholesterol; and insulin sensitivity with prazosin, doxazosin, and terazosin. With long-term use, selective α_1 blockers also appear to decrease left ventricular mass in patients with hypertension and left ventricular hypertrophy.

A number of prazosin, doxazosin, and terazosin analogues have been developed (e.g., trimazosin) that in preliminary clinical trials also have shown promise as antihypertensive agents. Doxazosin and terazosin have a longer duration of action than prazosin and have been shown to produce sustained blood pressure reductions with single daily administration. Indoramin, also a selective α_1 blocker, has been found to be effective in the treatment of systemic hypertension, but it produces many unwanted effects, such as lethargy and impotence, which may limit its clinical value. In contrast to prazosin, the drug appears to have little dilatory effect on the venous circulation. Prazosin, doxazosin, and terazosin are available for clinical use in the United States.

Congestive heart failure α-Adrenergic blocking drugs appear particularly attractive for use in the treatment of heart failure because they hold the possibility of reproducing balanced reductions in resistance and capacitance beds. In fact, phentolamine was one of the earlier vasodilators shown to be effective in the treatment of heart failure. The drug was infused into normotensive patients with persistent left ventricular dysfunction after a myocardial infarction and found to induce a significant fall in systemic vascular resistance accompanied by considerable elevation in cardiac output and a reduction in pulmonary artery pressure. Because of its high cost and the frequent side effects that it produces, especially tachycardia, phentolamine is no longer used in the treatment of heart failure. Oral phenoxybenzamine also has been used as vasodilator therapy in heart failure; like phentolamine, it has been replaced by newer vasodilator agents.

Studies evaluating the acute hemodynamic effects of prazosin in patients with congestive heart failure consistently find significant reductions in systemic and pulmonary vascular resistances and left ventricular filling pressures associated with increases in stroke volume. In most studies there is no change or a decrease in heart rate. The response pattern seen with prazosin is similar to that observed with nitroprusside, with the exception that the heart rate tends to be higher with the use of nitroprusside, and therefore, the observed increases in cardiac output are also higher with the latter agent.

Controversy still exists as to whether the initial clinical and hemodynamic improvements seen with prazosin are sustained during long-term therapy. Whereas some studies have demonstrated continued efficacy of prazosin therapy after chronic use, others have found little hemodynamic difference between prazosin- and placebo-treated patients. Some investigators believe that whatever tolerance to the drug does develop is most likely secondary to activation of counterposing neurohumoral forces; if the dose is raised and the tendency toward sodium and water retention is countered by appropriate increases in diuretic dose, prazosin is likely to remain effective. Others argue that sustained increases in plasma renin activity or plasma catecholamines are not seen during long-term therapy and that tolerance is not prevented or reversed by a diuretic. Some clinical studies suggest that patients with initially high plasma renin activity experience attenuation of beneficial hemodynamic effects more frequently. What appears clear is the need to evaluate patients individually as to the continued efficacy of their prazosin therapy. Whether there are subgroups of patients with heart failure (e.g., those with highly activated sympathetic nervous systems) that are more likely to respond to prazosin or other α blockers remains to be determined.

A multicenter study from the Veterans Administration hospitals has shown that prazosin, when compared with placebo therapy, did not reduce mortality with long-term use in patients with advanced forms of congestive heart failure. In the same study, a favorable effect on mortality was seen with an isosorbide dinitrate–hydralazine combination.

Doxazosin and metoprolol were combined and compared with metoprolol alone in the treatment of patients with chronic heart failure. After 3 months of continuous therapy, both treatment groups showed similar and significant reductions in systemic vascular resistance and heart rate, with significant increases in cardiac index, ejection fraction, and exercise capacity. It was concluded that the combination of doxazosin and metoprolol was no better than metoprolol used alone.

There is increasing evidence that α_1-adrenergic receptors, different from those of other tissues, also exist in the myocardium and that an increase in the force of contraction may be produced by stimulation of these sites. The mechanism of α-adrenergic positive inotropic response is unknown. What the biologic significance of α-adrenergic receptors in cardiac muscle is and whether these receptors play a role in the response to α-blocker therapy in congestive heart failure also remain to be determined.

Use in Other Disorders

Pheochromocytoma α Blockers have been used in the treatment of pheochromocytoma to control the peripheral effects of the excess catecholamines. In fact, intravenous phentolamine was used as a test for this disorder, but the test is now rarely done because of reported cases of cardiovascular collapse and death in patients who exhibited exaggerated sensitivity to the drug. The drug is still rarely used in cases of pheochromocytoma-related hypertensive crisis. However, for long-term therapy, oral phenoxybenzamine is the preferred agent. β-Blocking agents also may be needed in pheochromocytoma for control of tachycardia and arrhythmias. All β blockers, but primarily the nonselective agents, should not be initiated prior to adequate α blockade because severe hypertension may occur as a result of the unopposed α-stimulating activity of the circulating catecholamines.

Shock In shock, hyperactivity of the sympathetic nervous system occurs as a compensatory reflex response to reduced blood pressure. Use of α blockers in shock has been advocated as a means of lowering peripheral vascular resistance and increasing vascular capacitance while not antagonizing the cardiotonic effects of the sympathomimetic amines. Although investigated for many years for the treatment of shock, α-adrenergic blockers are still not approved for this purpose. A prime concern of the use of α blockers in shock is that the rapid drug-induced increase in vascular capacitance may lead to inadequate cardiac filling and profound hypotension, especially in the hypovolemic patient. Adequate amounts of fluid replacement prior to use of an α blocker can minimize this concern.

Pulmonary hypertension The part played by endogenous circulating catecholamines in the maintenance of pulmonary vascular tone appears to be minimal. Studies evaluating the effects of norepinephrine administration on pulmonary vascular resistance have found the drug to have little or no effect. The beneficial effects on the pulmonary circulation that phentolamine and other α blockers have demonstrated in some studies are most likely primarily due to their direct vasodilatory actions rather than to α blockade. Like other vasodilators, in patients with pulmonary hypertension due to fixed anatomic changes, α blockers can produce hemodynamic deterioration secondary to their systemic vasodilatory properties.

Arterioconstriction Oral α-adrenergic blockers can produce subjective and clinical improvement in patients experiencing episodic arterioconstriction (Raynaud's phenomenon). α Blockers also may be of value in the treatment of severe peripheral ischemia caused by an α agonist (e.g., norepinephrine) or ergotamine overdose. In cases of inadvertent infiltration of a norepinephrine infusion, phentolamine can be given intradermally to avoid tissue sloughing.

Benign prostatic obstruction α-Adrenergic receptors have been identified in the bladder neck and prostatic capsule of male patients. In clinical studies, use of α blockers in patients with benign prostatic obstruction has resulted in increased urinary flow rates and reductions in residual volume and obstructive symptoms. The drugs terazosin and doxazosin are both approved as medical therapies for benign prostatic hypertrophy. A new, highly selective α blocker, tamsulosin, is now available. It appears to be as effective as terazosin and doxazosin for prostatic obstruction but appears to have little effect on blood pressure.

Clinical Use and Adverse Effects

Oral phenoxybenzamine has a rapid onset of action, with the maximal effect from a single dose seen in 1 to 2 h. The gastrointestinal (GI) absorption is incomplete, and only 20 to 30% of an oral dose reaches the systemic circulation in active form. The half-life of the drug is 24 h, with the usual dose varying between 20 and 200 mg daily in one or two doses. Intravenous phentolamine is initially started at 0.1 mg/min and is then increased at increments of 0.1 mg/min every 5 to 10 min until the desired hemodynamic effect is reached. The drug has a short duration of action of 3 to 10 min. Little is known about the pharmacokinetics of long-term oral use of phentolamine. The main side effects of the drug include postural hypotension, tachycardia, GI disturbances, and sexual dysfunction. Intravenous infusion of norepinephrine can be used to combat severe hypotensive reactions. Oral phenoxybenzamine is approved for use in pheochromocytoma.

Prazosin is almost completely absorbed following oral administration, with peak plasma levels achieved at 2 to 3 h. The drug is 90% protein bound. Prazosin is extensively metabolized by the liver. The usual half-life of the drug is 2½ to 4 h; in patients with heart failure, the half-life increases to the range of 5 to 7 h.

The major side effect of prazosin is the first-dose phenomenon—severe postural hypotension occasionally associated with syncope seen after the initial dose or after a rapid dose increment. The reason for this phenomenon has not been clearly established but may involve the rapid induction of venous and arteriolar dilatation by a drug that elicits little reflex sympathetic stimulation. It is reported more often when the drug is administered as a tablet rather than as a capsule, possibly related to the variable bioavailability or rates of absorption of the two formulations. (In the United States, the drug is available in capsule form.) The postural hypotension can be minimized if the initial dose of prazosin is not higher than 1 mg and if it is given at bedtime. In treating hypertension, a dose of 2 to 3 mg/day should be maintained for 1 to 2 weeks, followed by a gradual increase in dosage titrated to achieve the desired reductions in pressures, usually up to 20 to 30 mg/day, given in two or three doses. In treating heart failure, larger doses (2 to 7 mg) may be used to initiate therapy in recumbent patients, but the maintenance dose is also usually not more than 30 mg. Higher doses do not seem to produce additional clinical improvement.

Other side effects of prazosin include dizziness, headache, and drowsiness. The drug produces no deleterious effects on the clinical course of diabetes mellitus, chronic obstructive pulmonary disease, renal failure, or gout. It does not adversely affect the lipid profile. Prazosin is presently approved for use in hypertension. Prazosin GITS may soon become available for once-daily use in systemic hypertension. With this formulation, there are narrower peak-to-trough fluctuations in drug plasma levels that may be associated with less postural hypotension.

Terazosin, which has been approved for once-daily use in hypertension, may be associated with a lesser incidence of first-dose postural hypotension than prazosin. The usual recommended dose range is 1 to 5 mg administered once a day; some patients may benefit from doses as high as 20 mg daily or from divided doses.

Doxazosin is also approved as a once-daily therapy for systemic hypertension. The initial dosage of doxazosin is 1 mg once daily. Depending on the patient's standing blood pressure response, the dosage may then be increased to 2 mg and, if necessary, to 4, 8, or 16 mg to achieve the desired reduction in blood pressure. Doses beyond 4 mg increase the likelihood of excessive postural effects including syncope, postural dizziness or vertigo, and postural hypotension.

The α_2 blocker yohimbine, 5.4 mg orally, is used four times daily to treat male impotence. Urologists have used yohimbine for the diagnostic classification of certain cases of male erectile impotence. Increases in heart rate and blood pressure, piloerection, and rhinorrhea are the most common adverse reactions. Yohimbine should not be used with antidepressant drugs.

β-ADRENERGIC BLOCKING DRUGS

β-Adrenergic blocking drugs, which constitute a major pharmacotherapeutic advance, were conceived initially for the treatment of patients with angina pectoris and arrhythmias; however, they also have therapeutic effects in many other clinical disorders, including systemic hypertension, hypertrophic cardiomyopathy, mitral valve prolapse, silent myocardial ischemia, migraine, glaucoma, essential tremor, and thyrotoxicosis. β Blockers have been effective in treating unstable angina and for reducing the risk of cardiovascular mortality and nonfatal reinfarction in patients who have survived an acute myocardial infarction. β Blockade is a potential treatment modality, with and without thrombolytic therapy, for reducing the extent of myocardial injury and mortality during the hyperacute phase of myocardial infarction. Recently, a β blocker was approved for use in patients with mild to moderate congestive heart failure for reducing the progression of disease and reducing mortality.

β-Adrenergic Receptor

Radioligand labeling techniques have greatly aided the investigation of adrenoreceptors, and molecular pharmacologic techniques have positively delineated the β-adrenoceptor structure as a polypeptide with a molecular weight of 67,000.

In contrast to the older concept of adrenoreceptors as static entities in cells that simply serve to initiate the chain of events, newer theories hold that the adrenoceptors are subject to a wide variety of controlling influences that result in dynamic regulation of adrenoceptor sites and/or their sensitivity to catecholamines. Changes in tissue concentration of receptor sites are probably involved in mediating important fluctuations in tissue sensitivity to drug action. These principles may have significant clinical and therapeutic implications. For example, an apparent increase in the number of β adrenoceptors, and thus a supersensitivity to agonists, may be induced by chronic exposure to antagonists. With prolonged adrenoceptor blocker therapy, receptor occupancy by catecholamines can be diminished and the number of available receptors can be increased. When the β-adrenoceptor blocker is withdrawn suddenly, an increased pool of sensitive receptors becomes open to endogenous catecholamine stimulation. The resultant adrenergic stimulation could precipitate unstable angina pectoris and/or a myocardial infarction. The concentration of β adrenoceptors in the membrane of mononuclear cells decreases significantly with age.

Using radioligand techniques, a decrease in β-adrenoceptor sites in the myocardium has been demonstrated in patients with chronic congestive heart failure. An apparent reduction in β adrenoceptors and/or β-adrenoceptor function also has been associated with the development of refractoriness or desensitization to endogenous and exogenous catecholamines, a phenomenon probably caused by the prolonged exposure of these adrenoceptors to high levels of catecholamines. This desensitization phenomenon is caused not by a change in receptor formation or degradation but rather by catecholamine-induced changes in the conformation of the receptor sites, thus rendering them ineffective. β-Adrenoceptor blocking drugs do not induce desensitization or changes in the conformation of receptors but do block the ability of catecholamines to desensitize receptors.

Basic Pharmacologic Differences Among β-Adrenoceptor Blocking Drugs

More than 100 β-adrenoceptor blockers have been synthesized during the past 35 years, and more than 30 are available worldwide for clinical use. Selectivity for two subgroups of the β-adrenoceptor population also has been taken advantage of: β_1 receptors in the heart and β_2 receptors in the peripheral circulation and bronchi. More controversial has been the introduction of β-blocking drugs with α-adrenergic blocking actions, varying amounts of selective and nonselective intrinsic sympathomimetic activity (partial agonist activity), calcium channel blocker activity, and nonspecific membrane-stabilizing effects. There are also pharmacokinetic differences between β-blocking drugs that may be of clinical importance.

Fifteen β-adrenoceptor blockers are now marketed in the United States for cardiovascular disorders: propranolol for angina pectoris, arrhythmias, systemic hypertension, migraine prophylaxis, essential tremor, and hypertrophic cardiomyopathy, and reducing the risk of cardiovascular mortality in survivors of an acute myocardial infarction; nadolol for hypertension and angina pectoris; timolol for hypertension and for reducing the risk of cardiovascular mortality and nonfatal reinfarction in survivors of myocardial infarction and in topical form for glaucoma; atenolol and metoprolol for hypertension and angina and in intravenous and oral formulations for reducing the risk of cardiovascular mortality in survivors of myocardial infarction; penbutolol, bisoprolol, and pindolol for treating hypertension; betaxolol and carteolol for hypertension and in a topical form for glaucoma; acebutolol for hypertension and ventricular arrhythmias; intravenous esmolol for supraventricular arrhythmias; sotalol for ventricular arrhythmias; labetalol for hypertension and in intravenous form for hypertensive emergencies; and carvedilol both for hypertension and for reducing the rate of disease progression and mortality in patients with mild to moderate congestive heart failure. In addition, oxprenolol has been approved for use in hypertension but is not marketed in the United States. Bucindolol is now being evaluated in a clinical trial in patients having moderate to severe congestive heart failure.

Despite the extensive experience with β blockers in clinical practice, there have been no studies suggesting that any of these agents have major advantages or disadvantages in relation to the others for treatment of many cardiovascular diseases. When any available blocker is titrated properly, it can be effective in patients with arrhythmia, hypertension, or angina pectoris. However, one agent may be more effective than others in reducing adverse reactions in some patients and for managing specific situations.

Potency β-Adrenergic receptor blocking drugs are competitive inhibitors of catecholamine binding at β-adrenergic receptor sites. The dose-response curve of the catecholamine is shifted to the right; that is, a given tissue response requires a higher concentration of agonist in the presence of β-blocking drugs. β_1-Blocking potency can be assessed by the inhibition of tachycardia produced by isoproterenol or exercise (the more reliable method in the intact organism); the potency varies from compound to compound (Table 2-3). These differences in potency are of no therapeutic relevance; however, they do explain the different drug

TABLE 2-3 Pharmacodynamic Properties of β-Adrenoceptor Blocking Drugs

Drug	β_1-Blockade potency ratio (propranolol = 1.0)	Relative β_1 selectivity	Intrinsic sympatho-mimetic activity	Membrane-stablizing activity
Acebutolol	0.3	+	+	+
Atenolol	1.0	++	0	0
Betaxolol	1.0	++	0	+
Bisoprolol	10.0	++	0	0
Bucindolol	1.0	0	+	+
Carteolol	10.0	0	+	0
Carvedilol*	10.0	0	0	++
Esmolol	0.02	++	0	0
Labetalol†	0.3	0	+	0
Metroprolol	1.0	++	0	0
Nadolol	1.0	0	0	0
Oxprenolol	0.5–1.0	0	+	+
Penbutolol	1.0	0	+	0
Pindolol	6.0	0	++	+
Propranolol	1.0	0	0	++
Sotalol‡	0.3	0	0	0
Timolol	6.0	0	0	0
Isomer:				
D-propranolol	—	—	—	++

*Carvedilol has additional α_1-adrenergic blocking activity without peripheral β_2 agonism.

†Labetalol has additional α_1-adrenergic blocking activity and direct vasodilatory actions (β_2 agonism).

‡Sotalol has an additional type of antiarrhythmic activity.

Source: Adopted from Frishman WH: *Clinical Pharmacology of the β-Adrenoreceptor Blocking Drugs, 2d ed. Norwalk, CT,* Appleton-Century-Crofts, 1984.

doses needed to achieve effective β-adrenergic blockade when initiating therapy in patients or when switching from one agent to another.

Structure-activity relationships The chemical structures of most β-adrenergic blockers have several features in common with the agonist isoproterenol, an aromatic ring with a substituted ethanolamine side chain linked to it by an $—OCH_2$ group. The β blocker timolol has a catecholamine-mimicking side chain but has a more complex ring.

Most β-blocking drugs exist as pairs of optical isomers and are marketed as racemic mixtures. Almost all the β-blocking activity is found in the negative (−) levorotatory stereoisomer. The two stereoisomers of β-adrenergic blockers are useful for differentiating between the pharmacologic effects of β blockade and membrane-stabilizing activity (possessed by both optical forms). The positive (+) dextrorotatory stereoisomers of β-blocking agents have no apparent clinical value except for D-sotalol, which appears to have type III antiarrhythmic properties. Penbutolol and timolol are marketed only in the L-form. As a result of asymmetric carbon atoms, labetalol has four stereoisomers and carvedilol two. With carvedilol, β-blocking effects are seen in the levorotatory stereoisomer and α-blocking effects in both the levorotatory and dextrorotatory stereoisomers.

Membrane-stabilizing activity At concentrations well above therapeutic levels, certain β blockers have a quinidine-like or local anesthetic membrane-stabilizing effect on the cardiac action potential. This property is exhibited equally by the two stereoisomers of the drug and is unrelated to β-adrenergic blockade and major therapeutic antiarrhythmic actions. There is no evidence that membrane-stabilizing activity is responsible for any direct negative inotropic effect of the β blockers, since drugs with and without this property equally depress left ventricular function. However, membrane-stabilizing activity can manifest itself clinically with massive β-blocker intoxications.

β_1 selectivity β-Adrenoceptor blockers may be classified as selective or nonselective, according to their relative abilities to antagonize the actions of sympathomimetic amines in some tissues at lower doses than those required in other tissues. When used in low doses, β_1-selective blocking agents such as acebutolol, betaxolol, bisoprolol, esmolol, atenolol, and metoprolol inhibit cardiac β_2 receptors but have less influence on bronchial and vascular β adrenoceptors (β_2). In higher doses, however, β_1-selective blocking agents also block β_2 receptors. Accordingly, β_1-selective agents may be safer than nonselective ones in patients with obstructive pulmonary disease, since β_2 receptors remain available to mediate adrenergic bronchodilatation. Even selective β blockers may aggravate bronchospasm in certain patients, so these drugs generally should not be used in patients with bronchospastic disease.

A second theoretical advantage is that unlike nonselective β blockers, β_1-selective blockers in low doses may not block the β_2 receptors that mediate dilatation of arterioles. During infusion of epinephrine, nonselective β blockers can cause a pressor response by blocking β_2-receptor-mediated vasodilatation, since α-adrenergic vasoconstrictor receptors are still operative. Selective β_1 antagonists may not induce this pressor effect in the presence of epinephrine and may lessen the impairment of peripheral blood flow. It is possible that leaving the β_2 receptors unblocked and responsive to epinephrine may be functionally important in some patients with asthma, hypoglycemia, hypertension, or peripheral vascular disease treated with β-adrenergic blocking drugs.

Intrinsic sympathomimetic activity (partial agonist activity) Certain β-adrenoceptor blockers possess intrinsic sympathomimetic activity (ISA, partial agonist activity) at β_1-adrenoceptor sites, β_2-adrenoceptor sites, or both. In a β blocker, this property is identified as a slight cardiac stimulation that can be blocked by propranolol. The β blockers with this property slightly activate the β receptor in addition to preventing the access of natural or synthetic catecholamines to the receptor. Dichloroisoprenaline, the first β-adrenoceptor blocking drug synthesized, exerted such marked partial agonist activity that it was unsuitable for clinical use. However, compounds with less partial agonist activity are effective β-blocking drugs. The partial agonist effects of β-adrenoceptor blocking drugs such as pindolol differ from those of the agonist epinephrine and isoproterenol in that the maximum pharmacologic response that can be obtained is low, although the affinity for the receptor is high. In the treatment of patients with arrhythmias, angina pectoris of effort, and hypertension, drugs with mild to moderate partial agonist activity appear to be as efficacious as are β blockers lacking this property. It is still debated whether the presence of partial agonist activity in a β blocker constitutes an overall advantage or disadvantage in cardiac therapy. Drugs with partial agonist activity cause less slowing of the heart rate at rest than do propranolol and metoprolol, although the increments in heart rate with exercise are similarly blunted. These β-blocking agents reduce peripheral vascular resistance and also may cause less depression or atrioventricular conduction compared with drugs lacking these properties. Some investigators claim that partial agonist activity in a β blocker protects against myocardial depression, adverse lipid changes, bronchial asthma, and peripheral vascular complications, as caused by propranolol. The evidence to support these claims is not conclusive, and more definitive clinical trials are necessary to resolve these issues.

α-adrenergic activity Labetalol is a β blocker with antagonistic properties at both α and β adrenoceptors, and it has direct vasodilator activity. Labetalol has been shown to be 6 to 10 times less potent than phentolamine at α-adrenergic receptors and 1.5 to 4 times less potent than propranolol at β-adrenergic receptors and is itself 4 to 16 times less potent at α than at β adrenoceptors. Like other β blockers, it is useful in the treatment of hypertension and angina pectoris. Unlike most β blockers, however, the additional α-adrenergic blocking actions of labetalol lead to a reduction in peripheral vascular resistance that may maintain cardiac output. Whether concomitant α-adrenergic blocking activity is actually advantageous in a β blocker remains to be determined.

Carvedilol is another β blocker having additional α-blocking activity. Compared with labetalol, carvedilol has a ratio of α_1 to β blockade of 1:10. On a milligram-to-milligram basis, carvedilol is about two to four times more potent than propranolol as a β blocker. In addition, carvedilol has antioxidant and antiproliferative activities. Carvedilol has been used for the treatment of hypertension and angina pectoris and is being evaluated as a treatment for patients with symptomatic heart failure.

Direct vasodilator activity Bucindolol is a nonselective b blocker that also has direct peripheral vasodilatory activity. It is currently undergoing clinical evaluation as a treatment of symptomatic congestive heart failure.

Pharmacokinetics Although the β-adrenergic blocking drugs as a group have similar therapeutic effects, their pharmacokinetic properties are markedly different. Their varied aromatic ring structures lead to differences in completeness of GI absorption, amount of first-pass hepatic metabolism, lipid solubility, protein binding, extent of distribution in the body, penetration into the brain, concentration in the heart, rate of hepatic biotransformation, pharmacologic activity of metabolites, and renal clearance of a drug and its metabolites that may influence the clinical usefulness of these drugs in some patients. The desirable pharmacokinetic characteristics in this group of compounds are a lack of major individual differences in bioavailability and in metabolic clearance of the drug and a rate of removal from active tissue sites that is slow enough to allow longer dosing intervals.

The β blockers can be divided by their pharmacokinetic properties into two broad categories: those eliminated by hepatic metabolism, which tend to have relatively short plasma half-lives, and those eliminated unchanged by the kidney, which tend to have longer half-lives. Propranolol and metoprolol are both lipid soluble, are almost completely absorbed by the small intestine, and are largely metabolized by the liver. They tend to have highly variable bioavailability and relatively short plasma half-lives. A lack of correlation between the duration of clinical pharmacologic effect and plasma half-life may allow these drugs to be administered once or twice daily.

In contrast, agents such as atenolol and nadolol are more water soluble, are incompletely absorbed through the gut, and are eliminated unchanged by the kidney. They tend to have less variable bioavailability in patients with normal renal function, in addition to longer half-lives, allowing one dose a day. The longer half-lives may be useful in patients who find compliance with frequent β-blocker dosing a problem.

Long-acting sustained-release preparations of propranolol and metoprolol are available. Studies have shown that long-acting propranolol and metoprolol can provide a much smoother curve of daily plasma levels than do comparable divided doses of conventional immediate-release formulations.

Ultra-short-acting β blockers are now available and may be useful where a short duration of action is desired (e.g., in patients with questionable congestive heart failure). One of these compounds, esmolol, a β_1-selective drug (see Table 2-3), has been shown to be useful in the treatment of perioperative hypertension and supraventricular tachycardias. The short half-life (approximately 15 min) relates to the rapid metabolism of the drug by blood and hepatic esterases. Metabolism does not seem to be altered by disease states. Currently, a propranolol nasal spray that can provide immediate β blockade is being tested in clinical trials, as well as a new sublingual immediate-release formulation.

The specific pharmacokinetic properties of individual β-adrenergic blockers (first-pass metabolism, active metabolites, lipid solubility, and protein binding) may be clinically important. When drugs with extensive first-pass metabolism are taken by mouth, they undergo so much hepatic biotransformation that relatively little drug reaches the systemic circulation. Depending on the extent of first-pass effect, an oral dose of β blocker must be larger than an intravenous dose to produce the same clinical effects. Some β-adrenergic blockers are transformed into pharmacologically active compounds (acebutolol) rather than inactive metabolites. The total pharmacologic effect therefore depends on the amount of the drug administered and its active metabolites. Characteristics of lipid solubility in a β blocker have been associated with the ability of the drug to concentrate in the brain, and many side effects of these drugs that have not been clearly related to β blockade may result from their actions on the central nervous system (lethargy, mental depression, and hallucinations). It is still not certain, however, whether drugs that are less lipid soluble cause fewer of these adverse reactions.

There are genetic polymorphisms that can influence the metabolism of various β-blocking drugs, which include propranolol, metoprolol, timolol, and carvedilol. A single codon difference of CYP2D6 may explain a significant proportion of interindividual variation of propranolol's pharmacokinetics in Chinese subjects. There is no effect of exercise on propranolol's pharmacokinetics.

Relationship among dose, plasma level, and efficacy Attempts have been made to establish a relation between the oral dose, the plasma level measured by gas chromatography, and the pharmacologic effect of each β-blocking drug. After administration of a certain oral dose, β-blocking drugs that are largely metabolized in the liver show large interindividual variation in circulating plasma levels. Many explanations have been proposed to explain wide individual differences in the relation between plasma concentrations of β blockers and any associated therapeutic effect. First, patients may have different levels of "sympathetic tone" (circulating catecholamines and active β-adrenoceptor binding sites) and may thus require different drug concentrations to achieve adequate β blockade. Second, many β blockers have flat plasma drug level response curves. Third, active drug isomers and active metabolites are not specifically measured in many plasma assays. Fourth, the clinical effect of a drug may last longer than the period suggested by the drug's half-life in plasma, since recycling of the β blocker between receptor site and neuronal nerve endings may occur. Despite the lack of correlation between plasma levels and therapeutic effect, there is some evidence that a relationship does exist between the logarithm of the plasma level and the β-blocking effect (blockade of exercise- or isoproterenol-induced tachycardia). Plasma levels have little to offer as therapeutic guides except for ensuring compliance and for diagnosis of overdose. Pharmacodynamic characteristics and clinical response should be used as guides in determining efficacy.

Clinical Effects and Therapeutic Applications

The therapeutic efficacy and safety of β-adrenoceptor blocking drugs have been well established in patients with angina pectoris, cardiac arrhythmias, and hypertension, as well as for reducing the risk of mortality and possibly nonfatal reinfarction in survivors of acute myocardial infarction. These drugs may be useful as a primary protection against cardiovascular morbidity and mortality in hypertensive patients. The drugs are also used for a multitude of other cardiac (Table 2-4) and noncardiac uses.

Effects on Elevated Systemic Blood Pressure

β-Adrenergic blockers are effective in reducing the blood pressure of many patients with systemic hypertension (Tables 2-5 and 2-6), including elderly patients with isolated systolic hypertension, and were recently cited as first-line treatment by both the Fifth and Sixth Reports of the Joint National Committee on Detection, Evaluation and Treatment of High Blood Pressure (JNCV and VI). However, there is no consensus as to the mechanism(s) by which these drugs lower blood pressure. It is probable that some or all of the following proposed mechanisms play a part. β Blockers without vasodilatory activity appear to be more efficacious in white patients and younger patients than they are in elderly or black patients.

Negative Chronotropic and Inotropic Effects

Slowing of the heart rate and some decrease in myocardial contractility with β blockers lead to a decrease in cardiac output, which in the short and long term may lead to a reduction in blood pressure. It might be expected that these factors would be of particular importance in the treatment of hypertension related to high cardiac output and increased sympathetic tone.

Differences in Effects on Plasma Renin

The relation between the hypotensive action of β-blocking drugs and their ability to reduce plasma renin activity remains controversial. Some β-blocking drugs can antagonize sympathetically mediated renin release, although adrenergic activity is not the only mechanism by which renin release is mediated. Other major determinants are sodium balance, posture, and renal perfusion pressure.

The important question remains whether there is a clinical correlation between the β blocker's effect on the plasma renin activity and the lowering of blood pressure. Investigators have found that "high renin" patients do not respond or may even show a rise in blood pressure and that "normal renin" patients have less predictable responses. In high renin hypertensive patients, it has been suggested that renin may not be the only factor maintaining the high-blood-pressure state. At present, the exact role of renin reduction in blood pressure control is not well defined.

Central Nervous System Effect

There is now good clinical and experimental evidence to suggest that β blockers cross the blood-brain barrier and enter the central nervous system (CNS). Although there is little doubt that β blockers with high lipophilicity (e.g., metoprolol, propranolol) enter the CNS in high concentrations, a direct antihypertensive effect mediated by their presence has not been well defined. Also, β blockers that are less lipid soluble and less likely to concentrate in the brain appear to be as effective in lowering blood pressure as propranolol.

Peripheral Resistance

Nonselective β blockers have no primary action in lowering peripheral resistance and indeed may cause it to rise by leaving the α-stimulatory

TABLE 2-4 Reported Cardiovascular Indications for β-Adrenoceptor Blocking Drugs

Hypertension* (systolic and diastolic)
Isolated systolic hypertension in the elderly
Angina pectoris*
"Silent" myocardial ischemia
Supraventricular arrhythmias*
Ventricular arrhythmias*
Reducing the risk of mortality and reinfarction in survivors of acute myocardial infarction*
Hyperacute phase of myocardial infarction*
Dissection of aorta
Hypertrophic cardiomyopathy*
Reversing left ventricular hypertrophy
Digitalis intoxication
Mitral valve prolapse
QT-interval prolongation syndrome
Tetralogy of Fallot
Mitral stenosis
Congestive cardiomyopathy*
Fetal tachycardia
Neurocirculatory asthenia

*Indications formally approved by the Food and Drug Administration.

TABLE 2-5 Proposed Mechanisms to Explain the Antihypertensive Actions of β Blockers

Reduction in cardiac output
Inhibition of renin
CNS effects
Effects on prejunctional β receptors: reductions in norepinephrine release
Reduction in peripheral vascular resistance
Improvement in vascular compliance
Reduction in vasomotor tone
Reduction in plasma volume
Resetting of baroreceptor levels
Attenuation of pressor response to catecholamines with exercise and stress

Source: From Frishman WH: *Clinical Pharmacology of the β-Adrenoreceptor Blocking Drugs,* 2d ed. Norwalk, CT, Appleton-Century-Crofts, 1984, with permission.

mechanisms unopposed. The vasodilating effect of catecholamines on skeletal muscle blood vessels is β_2-mediated, suggesting possible therapeutic advantages in using β_1-selective blockers, agents with partial agonist activity, and drugs with α-blocking activity. Since β_1 selectivity diminishes as the drug dosage is raised, and since hypertensive patients generally have to be given far larger doses than are required

TABLE 2-6 Pharmacodynamic Properties and Cardiac Effects of β-Adrenoceptor Blockers

Drug	Relative β_1 selectivity*	Partial agonist activity	Membrane stabilizing activity	Resting heart rate	Exercise heart rate	Resting myocardial contractility	Resting blood pressure	Exercise blood pressure	Resting atrioventricular conduction	Antiar-rhythmic effect
Acebutolol	+	+	+	↓↔	↓	↓	↓	↓	↓	+
Atenolol	++	0	0	↓	↓	↓	↓	↓	↓	+
Betaxolol	++	0	+	↓	↓	↓	↓	↓	↓	+
Bisoprolol	++	0	0	↓	↓	↓	↓	↓	↓	+
Bucindolol**	0	0	0	↓↔	↓	↓↔	↓	↓	↓	+
Carteolol	0	+	0	↓↔	↓	↓↔	↓	↓	↓	+
Carvedilol[†]	0	0	++	↓↔	↓	↓↔	↓	↓	↓↔	+
Esmolol	++	0	0	↓	↓	↓	↓	↓	↓	+
Labetalol[‡]	0	+	0	↓↔	↓	↓↔	↓	↓↓	↓↔	+
Metoprolol	++	0	0	↓	↓	↓	↓	↓	↓	+
Nadolol	0	0	0	↓	↓	↓	↓	↓	↓	+
Oxprenolol	0	+	+	↓↔	↓	↓↔	↓	↓	↓↔	+
Penbutolol	0	+	0	↓↔	↓	↓↔	↓	↓	↓↔	+
Pindolol	0	++	0	↓↔	↓	↓↔	↓	↓	↓↔	+
Propranolol	0	0	++	↓	↓	↓	↓	↓	↓	+
Sotalol	0	0	0	↓	↓	↓	↓	↓	↓	+
Timolol	0	0	0	↓	↓	↓	↓	↓	↓	+
Isomer: D-propranolol	0	0	++	↔	↔	↔↓[¶]	↔	↔	↔↓[¶]	+[¶]

[*]β_1 selectivity is seen only with low therapeutic drug concentrations. With higher concentrations, β_1 selectivity is not seen.
[**]Bucindolol has direct peripheral vasodilating activity.
[†]Carvedilol has peripheral vasodilating activity and additional α_1-adrenergic blocking activity.
[‡]Labetalol has additional α_1-adrenergic blocking properties and direct β_2-adrenergic vasodilator activity.
[¶]Effects of D-propranolol with doses in human beings well above the therapeutic level. The isomer also lacks β-blocking activity.
Note: ++ = strong effect; + = modest effect; 0 = absent effect; ↑ = elevation; ↓ = reduction; ↔ = no change.
Source: From Frishman WH: *Clinical Pharmacology of the β-Adrenoreceptor Blocking Drugs,* 2d ed. Norwalk, CT, Appleton-Century-Crofts, 1984, with permission.

simply to block the β_1 receptors alone, β_1 selectivity offers the clinician little, if any, real specific advantage in antihypertensive treatment.

Effects on Prejunctional Receptors

Apart from their effects on postjunctional tissue β receptors, it is believed that blockade of prejunctional β receptors may be involved in the hemodynamic actions of β-blocking drugs. The stimulation of prejunctional α_2 receptors leads to a reduction in the quantity of norepinephrine released by the postganglionic sympathetic fibers. Conversely, stimulation of prejunctional β receptors is followed by an increase in the quantity of norepinephrine released by the postganglionic sympathetic fibers. Blockade of prejunctional β receptors should therefore diminish the amount of norepinephrine released, leading to a weaker stimulation of postjunctional α receptors, an effect that would produce less vasoconstriction. Opinions differ, however, on the contributions of presynaptic β blockade to both a reduction in the peripheral vascular resistance and the antihypertensive effects on β-blocking drugs.

Other Proposed Mechanisms

Less well documented effects of β blockers that may contribute to their antihypertensive actions include favorable effects on arterial compliance, venous tone and plasma volume, membrane-stabilizing activity, and resetting of baroreceptors.

Effects in Angina Pectoris

Ahlquist demonstrated that sympathetic innervation of the heart causes the release of norepinephrine, activating β adrenoreceptors in myocardial cells (see Table 2-6). This adrenergic stimulation causes an increment in heart rate, isometric contractile force, and maximal velocity of muscle fiber shortening, all of which lead to an increase in cardiac work and myocardial oxygen consumption. The decrease in intraventricular pressure and volume caused by the sympathetic-mediated enhancement of cardiac contractility tends, on the other hand, to reduce myocardial oxygen consumption by reducing myocardial wall tension (Laplace's law). Although there is a net increase in myocardial oxygen demand, this is normally balanced by an increase in coronary blood flow. Angina pectoris is believed to occur when oxygen demand exceeds supply, that is, when coronary blood flow is restricted by coronary atherosclerosis. Since the conditions that precipitate anginal attacks (exercise, emotional stress, food, etc.) cause an increase in cardiac sympathetic activity, it might be expected that blockade of cardiac β adrenoreceptors would relieve the anginal symptoms. It is on this basis that the early clinical studies with β-blocking drugs in patients with angina pectoris were initiated.

Three main factors—heart rate, ventricular systolic pressure, and the size of the left ventricle—contribute to the myocardial oxygen requirements of the left ventricle. Of these, heart rate and systolic pressure appear to be important. (The product of heart rate multiplied by the systolic blood pressure is a reliable index to predict the precipitation of angina in a given patient.) However, myocardial contractility may be even more important.

The reduction in heart rate effected by β blockade has two favorable consequences: (1) a decrease in blood pressure, thus reducing myocardial oxygen needs, and (2) a longer diastolic filling time associated with a slower heart rate, allowing for increased coronary perfusion. β Blockade also reduces exercise-induced blood pressure increments, the velocity of cardiac contraction, and oxygen consumption at any patient workload. Pretreatment heart rate variability or low exercise tolerance may predict which patients will respond best to treatment with β blockade. Despite the favorable effects on heart rate, the blunting of myocardial contractility with β blockers also may be the primary mechanism of their antianginal benefit.

Studies in dogs have shown that propranolol causes a decrease in coronary blood flow. However, subsequent experimental animal studies have demonstrated that β-blocking-induced shunting occurs in the coronary circulation, maintaining blood flow to ischemic areas, especially in the subendocardial region. In human beings, concomitantly with the decrease in myocardial oxygen consumption, β blockers can cause a reduction in coronary blood flow and a rise in coronary vascular resistance. On the basis of coronary autoregulation, the overall reduction in myocardial oxygen needs with β blockers may be sufficient cause for this decrease in coronary blood flow.

Virtually all β blockers, whether they have partial agonist activity, α-blocking effects, membrane-stabilizing activity, and general or selective β-blocking properties, produce some degree of increased work capacity without pain in patients with angina pectoris. Therefore, it must be concluded that this results from their common property: blockade of cardiac β receptors. Both D- and L-propranolol have membrane-stabilizing activity, but only L-propranolol has significant β-blocking activity. The racemic mixture (D- and L-propranolol) causes a decrease in both heart rate and force of contraction in dogs, while the D isomer has hardly any effect. In human beings, D-propranolol, which has "membrane" activity but no β-blocking properties, has been found to be ineffective in relieving angina pectoris even at very high doses.

Although exercise tolerance improves with β blockade, the increments in heart rate and blood pressure with exercise are blunted, and the rate-pressure product (systolic blood pressure × heart rate) achieved when pain occurs is lower than that reached during a control run. The depressed pressure-rate product at the onset of pain (about 20% reduction from control) is reported to occur with various β-blocking drugs, probably related to decreased cardiac output. Thus, although there is increased exercise tolerance with β blockade, patients exercise less than might be expected. This also may relate to the action of β blockers in increasing left ventricular size, causing increased left ventricular wall tension and an increase in oxygen consumption at a given blood pressure.

Combined Use of β Blockers with Other Antianginal Therapies in Angina Pectoris

Nitrates Combined therapy with nitrates and β blockers may be more efficacious for the treatment of angina pectoris than the use of either drug alone. The primary effects of β blockers are to cause a reduction in both resting heart rate and the response of heart rate to exercise. Since nitrates produce a reflex increase in heart rate and contractility owing to a reduction in arterial pressure, concomitant β-blocker therapy is extremely effective because it blocks this reflex increment in the heart rate. Similarly, the preservation of diastolic coronary flow with a reduced heart rate will also be beneficial. In patients with a propensity for myocardial failure who may have a slight increase in heart size with the β blockers, the nitrates will counteract this tendency by reducing heart size as a result of its peripheral venodilator effects. During the administration of nitrates, the reflex increase in contractility that is mediated through the sympathetic nervous system is checked by the presence of β blockers. Similarly, the increase in coronary resistance associated with β-blocker administration can be ameliorated by the administration of nitrates.

Calcium-entry blockers Calcium-entry blockers are a group of drugs that block transmembrane calcium currents in vascular smooth muscle to cause arterial vasodilatation. Some calcium-entry blockers (diltiazem, mibefradil, verapamil) also slow the heart rate and reduce atrioventricular (AV) conduction. Combined therapy with β-adrenergic and calcium-entry blockers can provide clinical benefits for patients with angina pectoris who remain symptomatic with either agent used alone. Because adverse cardiovascular effects can occur, however, patients being considered for such treatment must be carefully selected and observed.

Angina at Rest and Vasospastic Angina

Angina pectoris can be caused by multiple mechanisms, including coronary vasospasm, myocardial bridging, and thrombosis, which appear to be responsible for ischemia in a significant proportion of patients with unstable angina and angina at rest. Therefore, β blockers that primarily reduce myocardial oxygen consumption but fail to exert vasodilating effects on coronary vasculature may not be totally effective in patients in whom angina is caused or increased by dynamic alterations in coronary luminal diameter. Despite potential dangers in rest and vasospastic angina, β blockers have been used successfully as monotherapy and in combination with vasodilating agents in many patients.

Electrophysiologic and Antiarrhythmic Effects

Adrenoceptor blocking drugs have two main effects on the electrophysiologic properties of specialized cardiac tissue (Table 2-7). The first effect results from specific blockade of adrenergic stimulation of cardiac pacemaker potentials. In concentrations causing significant inhibition of adrenergic receptors, β blockers produce little change in the transmembrane potentials of cardiac muscle. By competitively inhibiting adrenergic stimulation, however, β blockers decrease the slope of phase 4 depolarization and the spontaneous firing rate of sinus or ectopic pacemakers and thus decrease automaticity. Arrhythmias occurring in the setting of enhanced automaticity, as seen in myocardial infarction, digitalis toxicity, hyperthyroidism, and pheochromocytoma, would therefore be expected to respond well to β blockade.

The second electrophysiologic effect of β blockers involves membrane-stabilizing action, also known as "quinidine-like" or "local anesthetic" action, which is observed only at very high dose levels. This property is unrelated to inhibition of catecholamine action and is possessed equally by both the D and L isomers of the drugs (D isomers have almost no β-blocking activity). Characteristic of this effect is a reduction in the rate of rise of the intracardial action potential without an effect on the spike duration of the resting potential. Associated features include an elevated electric threshold of excitability, a delay in conduc-

TABLE 2-7 Antiarrhythmic Properties of β Blockers

β Blockade
Electrophysiology: depress excitability and conduction
Prevention of ischemia: decreased automaticity, inhibit reentrant mechanisms
Membrane-stabilizing effects
Local anesthetic "quinidine-like" properties: depress excitability, prolong refractory period, delay conduction
Clinically: probably not significant
Special pharmacologic properties
β_1 selectivity, intrinsic sympathomimetic activity (do not appear to contribute to antiarrhythmic effectiveness)

Source: Frishman WH: *Clinical Pharmacology of the β-Adrenoreceptor Blocking Drugs,* 2d ed. Norwalk, CT, Appleton-Century-Crofts, 1984, with permission.

tion velocity, and a significant increase in the effective refractory period. This effect and its attendant changes have been explained by inhibition of the depolarizing inward sodium current. There is a greater antifibrillatory effect when β blockers are combined with some other antiarrhythmics.

Sotalol is unique among the β blockers in that it possesses class III antiarrhythmic properties, causing prolongation of the action potential period and thus delaying repolarization. Clinical studies have verified the efficacy of sotalol in control of arrhythmias, but additional investigation is required to determine whether its class III antiarrhythmic properties contribute significantly to its efficacy as an antiarrhythmic agent. A recent study demonstrated an increased mortality risk with D-sotalol, the stereoisomer with type III antiarrhythmic activity and no β-blocking effect.

The most important mechanism underlying the antiarrhythmic effect of β blockers, with the possible exclusion of sotalol, is believed to be β blockade with resultant inhibition of pacemaker potentials. The contribution of membrane-stabilizing action does not appear to be clinically significant. In vitro experiments with human ventricular muscle have shown that the concentration of propranolol required for membrane stabilizing is 50 to 100 times the concentration that usually is associated with inhibition of exercise-induced tachycardia and at which only β-blocking effects occur. Moreover, D-propranolol, which possesses membrane-stabilizing properties but no β-blocking action, is a weak antiarrhythmic even at high doses, whereas β blockers devoid of membrane-stabilizing action (atenolol, esmolol, metoprolol, nadolol, pindolol, etc.) have been shown to be effective antiarrhythmic drugs. Differences in overall clinical usefulness of β blockers for arrhythmia are related to their other associated pharmacologic properties.

Therapeutic Uses in Cardiac Arrhythmias

β-Adrenergic blocking drugs have become an important treatment modality for various cardiac arrhythmias (Table 2-8). While it has long been believed that β blockers are more effective in treating supraventricular arrhythmias than ventricular arrhythmias, it has only recently been appreciated that this may not be the case. These agents can be quite useful in the treatment of ventricular tachyarrhythmias in the setting of myocardial ischemia, mitral valve prolapse, and other cardiovascular conditions. A high prevalence of antibodies against β_1 and β_2 adrenoceptors has been observed in patients with atrial arrhythmias, ventricular arrhythmias, and conduction disturbances.

Effects in Survivors of Acute Myocardial Infarction

β-Adrenergic blockers have beneficial effects on many determinants of myocardial ischemia (Table 2-9). The results of placebo-controlled,

TABLE 2-8 Effects of β Blockers in Various Arrhythmias

Supraventricular
- Sinus tachycardia: treat underlying disorder; excellent response to β blocker, if need to control rate (e.g., ischemia).
- Atrial fibrillation: β blockers reduce rate, rarely restore sinus rhythm, may be useful in combination with digoxin.
- Atrial flutter: β blockers reduce rate, sometimes restore sinus rhythm.
- Atrial tachycardia: effective in slowing ventricular rate, may restore sinus rhythm; useful in prophylaxis.

Ventricular
- Premature ventricular contractions: good response to β blockers, especially digitalis-induced, exercise (ischemia)-induced, mitral valve prolapse, or hypertrophic cardiomyopathy.
- Ventricular tachycardia: effective as quinidine, most effective in digitalis toxicity or exercise (ischemia)-induced.
- Ventricular fibrillation: electrical defibrillation is treatment of choice. β blockers can be used to prevent recurrence in cases of excess digitalis or sympathomimetic amines; appear to be effective in reducing the incidence of ventricular fibrillation and sudden death after myocardial infarction.

Source: Frishman WH: *Clinical Pharmacology of the β-Adrenoceptor Blocking Drugs*, 2d ed. Norwalk, CT, Appleton-Century-Crofts, 1984, p 100, with permission.

long-term treatment trials with some β-adrenergic blocking drugs in survivors of acute myocardial infarction have demonstrated a favorable effect on total mortality; cardiovascular mortality, including sudden and nonsudden cardiac deaths; and the incidence of nonfatal reinfarction. These beneficial results with β-blocker therapy can be explained by both the antiarrhythmic (see Table 2-9) and the anti-ischemic effects of these drugs. It also has been proposed that β-adrenergic blockers could reduce the risk of atherosclerotic plaque fissure and subsequent throm-

TABLE 2-9 Possible Mechanisms by Which β Blockers Protect the Ischemic Myocardium

- Reduction in myocardial consumption, heart rate, blood pressure, and myocardial contractility
- Augmentation of coronary blood flow, increase in diastolic perfusion time by reducing heart rate, augmentation of collateral blood flow, and redistribution of blood flow to ischemic areas
- Prevention of attenuation of atherosclerotic plaque, rupture, and subsequent coronary thrombosis
- Alterations in myocardial substrate utilization
- Decrease in microvascular damage
- Stabilization of cell and lysosomal membranes
- Shift of oxyhemoglobin dissociation curve to the right
- Inhibition of platelet aggregation

bosis. Two nonselective β blockers, propranolol and timolol, have been approved for reducing the risk of mortality in infarct survivors when started 5 to 28 days after an infarction. Metoprolol and atenolol, two β_1-selective blockers, are approved for the same indication, and both can be used intravenously in the hyperacute phase of a myocardial infarction. β Blockers also have been suggested as a treatment for reducing the extent of myocardial injury and mortality during the hyperacute phase of myocardial infarction, but their exact role in this situation remains unclear. Intravenous and oral atenolol have been shown to be effective in causing a modest reduction in early mortality when given during the hyperacute phase of acute myocardial infarction. Atenolol and metoprolol reduce early infarct mortality by 15%, an effect that may be improved on when β-adrenergic blockade is combined with acute thrombolytic therapy. Metoprolol combined with acute thrombolysis has been evaluated in the TIMI-II study. Despite all the evidence showing that β blockers are beneficial in patients surviving myocardial infarction, they are considerably underused in clinical practice.

"Silent" Myocardial Ischemia

In recent years, investigators have observed that not all myocardial ischemic episodes detected by ECG are associated with detectable symptoms. Positron emission imaging techniques have validated the theory that these silent ischemic episodes are indicative of true myocardial ischemia. Compared with symptomatic ischemia, the prognostic importance of silent myocardial ischemia occurring at rest and/or during exercise has not been determined. β Blockers are as successful in reducing the frequency of silent ischemic episodes detected by ambulatory ECG monitoring as they are in reducing the frequency of painful ischemic events.

Other Cardiovascular Applications

Although β blockers have been studied extensively in patients with angina pectoris, arrhythmias, and hypertension, they also have been shown to be safe and effective in diabetic patients for other cardiovascular conditions (see Table 2-4), some of which are described below.

Hypertrophic cardiomyopathy β-Adrenergic receptor blocking drugs have been proved effective in therapy for patients with hypertrophic cardiomyopathy and idiopathic hypertrophic subaortic stenosis (IHSS). These drugs are useful in controlling the symptoms of dyspnea, angina, and syncope. β Blockers also have been shown to lower the intraventricular pressure gradient both at rest and with exercise.

The outflow pressure gradient is not the only abnormality in hypertrophic cardiomyopathy; more important is the loss of ventricular compliance, which impedes normal left ventricular function. It has been shown by invasive and noninvasive methods that propranolol can improve left ventricular function in this condition. The drug also produces favorable changes in ventricular compliance while it relieves symptoms. Propranolol has been approved for this condition and may be combined with the calcium-entry blocker verapamil in patients who do not respond to the β blocker alone.

The salutary hemodynamic and symptomatic effects produced by propranolol derive from its inhibition of sympathetic stimulation of the heart. There is no evidence that the drug alters the primary cardiomyopathic process; many patients remain in or return to their severely symptomatic state, and some die despite its administration.

Congestive cardiomyopathy The ability of intravenous sympathomimetic amines to affect an acute increase in myocardial contractility through stimulation of the β-adrenergic receptor had prompted the hope that the use of oral catecholamine analogues could provide long-term benefit for patients with severe heart failure. However, recent observations concerning the regulation of the myocardial adrenergic receptor and abnormalities of β-receptor-mediated stimulation of the failing myocardium have caused a critical reappraisal of the scientific validity of sustained β-adrenergic receptor stimulation. New evidence suggests that β-receptor blockade may, when tolerated, have a favorable effect on the underlying cardiomyopathic process.

Enhanced sympathetic activation is seen consistently in patients with congestive heart failure (CHF) and is associated with decreased exercise tolerance, hemodynamic abnormalities, and increased mortality. Increases in sympathetic tone can potentiate the renin-angiotensin system in patients, leading to increased salt and water retention, arterial and venous constriction, and increments in ventricular preload and afterload. Catecholamines in excess can increase heart rate and cause coronary vasoconstriction. They can adversely influence myocardial contractility on the cellular level while causing myocyte hypertrophy and vascular remodeling. Catecholamines can stimulate growth and provoke oxidative stress in terminally differentiated cardiac cells; these two factors can trigger the process of programmed cell death known as *apoptosis*. Finally, they can increase the risk of sudden death in patients with CHF by adversely influencing the electrophysiologic properties of the failing heart.

Controlled trials over the last 20 years with several different β blockers in patients with both ischemic and nonischemic cardiomyopathy have shown that these drugs could improve symptoms, ventricular function, and functional capacity while reducing the need for hospitalization. A series of placebo-controlled clinical trials with the α-β blocker carvedilol showed a mortality benefit in patients with New York Heart Association class II–IV heart failure when the drug was used in addition to diuretics, angiotensin converting enzyme inhibitors, and digoxin. Additional placebo-controlled mortality studies are currently in progress in patients with CHF, evaluating immediate and sustained-release metoprolol, bisoprolol, and the vasodilator β blockers bucindolol and carvedilol.

The mechanisms of benefit with β-blocker use are not known as yet. Possible mechanisms for β-blocker benefit in chronic heart failure are listed in Table 2-10 and include the upregulation of impaired β-receptor expression in the heart and an improvement in impaired baroreceptor functioning, which can inhibit excess sympathetic outflow. It has been suggested that long-term therapy with β blockers improves the left atrial contribution to left ventricular filling.

Mitral valve prolapse This auscultatory complex, characterized by a nonejection systolic click, a late systolic murmur, or a midsystolic click followed by a late systolic murmur, has been studied extensively over the past 15 years. Atypical chest pain, malignant arrhythmias, and nonspecific ST- and T-wave abnormalities have been observed with this condition. By decreasing sympathetic tone, β-adrenergic blockers have been shown to be useful for relieving the chest pains and palpitations that many of these patients experience, and for reducing the incidence of life-threatening arrhythmias and other ECG abnormalities.

TABLE 2-10 Possible Mechanisms by Which β-Adrenergic Blockers Improve Ventricular Function in Chronic Congestive Heart Failure

Upregulation of β receptors
Direct myocardial protective action against catecholamine toxicity
Improved ability of noradrenergic sympathetic nerves to synthesize norepinephrine
Decreased release of norepinephrine from sympathetic nerve endings
Decreased stimulation of other vasoconstrictive systems including renin-angiotensin-aldosterone, vasopressin, and endothelin
Potentiation of kalikrein-kinin system and natural vasodilatation (increase in bradykinin)
Antiarrhythmic effects raising ventricular fibrillation threshold
Protection against catecholamine-induced hypokalemia
Increase in coronary blood flow by reducing heart rate and improving diastolic perfusion time; possible coronary dilatation with vasodilator–β blocker
Restoration of abnormal baroreflex function
Prevention of ventricular muscle hypertrophy and vascular remodeling
Antioxidant effects (carvedilol?)
Shift from free fatty acid to carbohydrate metabolism (improved metabolic efficiency)
Vasodilation (e.g., bucindolol, carvedilol)
Antiapoptosis effect
Modulation of post-receptor inhibitory G-proteins
Improved left atrial contribution to left ventricular filling

Dissecting aneurysms β-Adrenergic blockade plays a major role in the treatment of patients with acute aortic dissection. During the hyperacute phase, β-blocking agents reduce the force and velocity of myocardial contraction (dP/dt) and hence the progression of the dissecting hematoma. Moreover, such administration must be initiated simultaneously with the institution of other antihypertensive therapy that may cause reflex tachycardia and increases in cardiac output, factors that can aggravate the dissection process. Initially, propranolol is administered intravenously to reduce the heart rate to below 60 beats per minute. Once a patient is stabilized and long-term medical management is contemplated, the patient should be maintained on oral β-blocker therapy to prevent recurrence.

It has been demonstrated that long-term β-blocker therapy also may reduce the risk of dissection in patients prone to this complication (e.g., Marfan syndrome). Systolic time intervals are used to assess the adequacy of β blockade in children with Marfan syndrome.

Tetralogy of Fallot By reducing the effects of increased adrenergic tone on the right ventricular infundibulum in tetralogy of Fallot, β blockers have been shown to be useful for the treatment of severe hypoxic spells and hypercyanotic attacks. With chronic use, these drugs also have been shown to prevent prolonged hypoxic spells. These drugs should be looked at only as palliative, and definitive surgical repair of this condition is usually required.

QT-interval prolongation syndrome The syndrome of ECG QT-interval prolongation is usually a congenital condition associated with deafness, syncope, and sudden death. Abnormalities in sympathetic nervous system functioning in the heart have been proposed as explanations for the electrophysiologic aberrations seen in these patients. Propranolol appears to be the most effective drug for treatment of this syndrome. It reduces the frequency of syncopal episodes in most patients and may prevent sudden death. This drug will reduce the ECG QT interval.

Regression of left ventricular hypertrophy Left ventricular hypertrophy induced by systemic hypertension is an independent risk factor for cardiovascular mortality and morbidity. Regression of left ventricular hypertrophy with drug therapy is feasible and may improve patient outcome. β-Adrenergic blockers can cause regression of left ventricular hypertrophy, as determined by echocardiography, with or without an associated reduction in blood pressure.

Syncope Vasovagal syncope is the most common form of syncope observed. Upright tilt table testing with isoproterenol can help differentiate vasovagal syncope from other forms. β Blockers have been shown to be useful for both relieving symptoms and normalizing abnormal tilt table tests in patients with syncope. The mechanism for benefit with β blockers may be an interruption of the Bezold-Jarisch reflex or an enhancement of peripheral vasoconstriction by blockade of β_2-adrenergic receptors.

Noncardiovascular applications

β-Adrenergic receptors are ubiquitous in the human body, and their blockade affects a variety of organ and metabolic systems. Some noncardiovascular uses of β blockers (glaucoma, migraine headache prophylaxis, essential tremor) have been approved by the FDA. The combination of nitrates and β blockers was shown recently to be effective in preventing bleeding from esophageal varices.

Adverse Effects of β Blockers

Evaluation of adverse effects is complex as a result of the use of different definitions of side effects, the kinds of patients studied, study design features, and different methods of ascertaining and reporting adverse side effects from study to study. Overall, the types and frequencies of adverse effects attributed to various β-blocker compounds appear similar. The side effect profiles resemble those seen with concurrent placebo treatments, attesting to the remarkable safety margin of the β blockers.

Adverse effects fall in two categories: (1) those from known pharmacologic consequences of β-adrenoceptor blockade and (2) other reactions apart from β-adrenoceptor blockade.

The first type includes asthma, heart failure, hypoglycemia, bradycardia and heart block, intermittent claudication, and Raynaud's phenomenon. The incidence of these adverse effects varies with the β blocker used.

Side effects of the second category are rare. They include an unusual oculomucocutaneous reaction and the possibility of carcinogenesis.

Adverse Cardiac Effects Related to β-Adrenoceptor Blockade

Congestive Heart Failure Blockade of β receptors may cause congestive heart failure in an enlarged heart with impaired myocardial infarction where excessive sympathetic drive is essential to maintain the myocardium on a compensated Starling curve and where left ventricular stroke volume is restricted and tachycardia is needed to maintain cardiac output.

Thus any β-blocking drug may be associated with the development of heart failure. Furthermore, heart failure also may be augmented by increases in peripheral vascular resistance produced by nonselective agents (e.g., propranolol, timolol, sotalol). It has been claimed that β blockers with intrinsic sympathomimetic activity and α-blocking activity are better in preserving left ventricular function and less likely to precipitate heart failure.

In patients with impaired myocardial function who require β-blocking agents, digitalis and diuretics can be used.

Sinus node dysfunction and AV conduction delay Slowing of the resting heart rate is a normal response to treatment with β-blocking drugs with and without intrinsic sympathomimetic activity. Healthy persons can sustain a heart rate of 40 to 50 beats per minute without disability unless there is clinical evidence of heart failure. Drugs with intrinsic sympathomimetic activity do not lower the resting heart rate to the same degree as propranolol, but all β-blocking drugs are contraindicated (unless an artificial pacemaker is present) in patients with sick sinus syndrome.

If there is a partial or complete atrioventricular (AV) conduction defect, the use of a β-blocking drug may lead to a serious bradyarrhythmia. The risk of AV impairment may be less with β blockers that have intrinsic sympathomimetic activity.

Overdosage Suicide attempts and accidental overdosing with β blockers are being described with increasing frequency. Since β-adrenergic blockers are competitive pharmacologic antagonists, their life-threatening effects (bradycardia, myocardial and ventilatory failure) can be overcome with an immediate infusion of β-agonist agents such as isoproterenol and dobutamine. In situations where catecholamines are not effective, intravenous glucagon, amrinone, or milrinone have been used.

Close monitoring of cardiorespiratory function is necessary for at least 24 h after the patient responds to therapy. Patients who recover usually have no long-term sequelae; however, they should be observed for the cardiac signs of sudden β-blocker withdrawal.

β-adrenoceptor blocker withdrawal After abrupt cessation of chronic β-blocker therapy, exacerbation of angina pectoris and, in some cases, acute myocardial infarction and death have been reported. Observations made in multiple double-blind randomized trials have confirmed the reality of a propranolol withdrawal reaction. The mechanism for this reaction is unclear. There is some evidence that the withdrawal phenomenon may be due to the generation of additional β adrenoceptors during the period of β-adrenoceptor blockade. When the β-adrenoceptor blocker is then withdrawn, the increased β-receptor population readily results in an excessive β-receptor stimulation which is clinically important when the delivery and use of oxygen are finely balanced, as occurs in ischemic heart disease. Other suggested mechanisms for the withdrawal reaction include heightened platelet aggregability, an elevation in thyroid hormone activity, and an increase in circulating catecholamines.

Adverse Noncardiac Side Effects Related to β-Adrenoceptor Blockade

Effect on Ventilatory Function The bronchodilatory effects of catecholamines on the bronchial β_2 adrenoceptors are inhibited by nonselective β blockers (e.g, propranolol, nadolol). β-Blocking compounds with partial agonist activity, β_1 selectivity, and α-adrenergic blocking actions are less likely to increase airways resistance in asthmatics. β_1 Selectivity, however, is not absolute and may be lost with high therapeutic doses, as shown with atenolol and metoprolol. It is possible in treating asthma to use a β_2-selective agonist (such as albuterol) in certain patients with concomitant low-dose β_1-selective blocker treatment. In general, all β blockers should be avoided in patients with bronchospastic disease.

Peripheral vascular effects (raynaud's phenomenon) Cold extremities and absent pulses have been reported more frequently in patients receiving β blockers for hypertension than in those receiving methyldopa. Among the β blockers, the incidence was highest with propranolol and lower with drugs having β_1 selectivity or intrinsic sympathomimetic activity. In some instances, vascular compromise has been severe enough to cause cyanosis and impending gangrene. This is probably due to the reduction in cardiac output and blockade of β_2-adrenoceptor-mediated skeletal muscle vasodilatation, resulting in unopposed β-adrenoceptor vasoconstriction. β-Blocking drugs with β_1 selectivity or partial agonist activity will not affect peripheral vessels to the same degree as does propranolol.

Raynaud's phenomenon is one of the more common side effects of propranolol treatment. It is more troublesome with propranolol than with metoprolol, atenolol, or pindolol, probably because of the β_2-blocking properties of propranolol.

Patients with peripheral vascular disease who suffer from intermittent claudication occasionally report worsening of the claudication when treated with β-blocking drugs. Whether drugs with β_1 selectivity or partial agonist activity can protect against this adverse reaction has not been determined.

Hypoglycemia and hyperglycemia Several authors have described severe hypoglycemic reactions during therapy with β-adrenergic blocking drugs. Some of the patients affected were insulin-dependent diabetics, whereas others were nondiabetic. Studies of resting normal volunteers have demonstrated that propranolol produces no alteration in blood glucose values, although the hyperglycemic response to exercise is blunted.

The enhancement of insulin-induced hypoglycemia and its hemodynamic consequences may be less with β_1-selective agents (where there is no blocking effect on β_2 receptors) and agents with intrinsic sympathomimetic activity (which may stimulate β_2 receptors).

There is also marked diminution in the clinical manifestations of the catecholamine discharge induced by hypoglycemia (tachycardia). These findings suggest that β blockers interfere with compensatory responses to hypoglycemia and can mask certain "warning signs" of this condition. Other hypoglycemic reactions, such as diaphoresis, are not affected by β-adrenergic blockade.

Hyperlipidemia The effects of the various β blockers on plasma lipids and lipoproteins have been described. Nonselective β-blocking agents can raise triglycerides and reduce HDL cholesterol. This effect may not be seen with agents having partial agonism or α-blocking activity.

Central nervous system effects Dreams, hallucinations, insomnia, and depression can occur during therapy with β blockers. These symptoms provide evidence of drug entry into the CNS and may be more common with the highly lipid-soluble β blockers (propranolol, metoprolol), which presumably penetrate the CNS better. It has been claimed that β blockers with less lipid solubility (atenolol, nadolol) cause fewer CNS side effects. This claim is intriguing, but its validity has not been corroborated by other extensive clinical experiences.

Miscellaneous side effects Diarrhea, nausea, gastric pain, constipation, and flatulence have been noted occasionally with all β blockers (2 to 11% of patients). Hematologic reactions are rare. Rare cases of purpura and agranulocytosis have been described with propranolol.

A devastating blood pressure rebound effect has been described in patients who discontinued clonidine while being treated with nonselective β-blocking agents. The mechanism for this may be related to an increase in circulating catecholamines and an increase in peripheral vascular resistance. Whether β_1-selective or partial agonist β blockers have similar effects following clonidine withdrawal has not been determined. This has not been a problem with labetalol.

Adverse Effects Unrelated to β-Adrenoceptor Blockade

Oculomucocutaneous Syndrome A characteristic immune reaction, the oculomucocutaneous syndrome, affecting singly or in combination eyes, mucous and serous membranes, and the skin, often in association with a positive antinuclear factor, has been reported in patients treated with practolol and has led to the curtailment of its clinical use. Close attention has been focused on this syndrome because of fears that other β-adrenoceptor blocking drugs may be associated with this syndrome.

Drug-Drug Interactions

β Blockers are commonly employed, and the list of commonly used drugs with which they interact is extensive (Table 2-11). The majority of the reported interactions have been associated with propranolol, the best studied β blocker, and may not necessarily apply to other drugs in this class.

TABLE 2-11 Drug Interactions That May Occur With β-Adrenoceptor Blocking Drugs

Drug	Pharmacokinetic interactions	Pharmacodynamic interactions	Precautions
Alcohol	Enhanced first-pass hepatic degradation	None	May need increased doses of lipid-soluble agents.
α-Adrenergic blockers		Increased risk for first-dose hypotension	Use with caution.
Aluminum hydroxide gel	Decreased β-blocker absorption	None	Clinical efficacy rarely altered.
Amiodarone	None	Enhanced negative chronotropic activity	Monitor response.
Aminophylline	Mutual inhibition		Observe patient's response.
Ampicillin	Impaired GI absorption leading to decreased β-blocker bioavailability		May need to increase β-blocker dose.
Angiotensin II receptor blockers (losartan)	None	Enhanced blood pressure effects & bronchospasm	Monitor response.
Antidiabetics	Both enhanced & blunted responses seen	None	Monitor for altered diabetic response
ACE inhibitors	None	Enhanced blood pressure effects & bronchospasm	Monitor response.
Calcium	Decreases β-blocker absorption		May need to increase β-blocker dose.
Calcium channel inhibitors	Decreased hepatic clearance of lipid-soluble & water-soluble β blockers; decreased clearance of calcium blockers	Potentiation of AV nodal negative inotropic & hypotensive responses	Avoid use if possible, although few patients show ill effects.

Cimetidine	Decreased hepatic clearance of lipid-soluble β blockers	None	Combination should be used with caution.
Clonidine	None	Nonselective agents exacerbate clonidine withdrawal phenomenon	Use only β_1-selective agents or labetalol.
Diazepam	Diazepam metabolism reduced		Observe patient's response.
Digitalis glycosides	None	Potentiation of brady-cardiac & AV blocks	Observe patient's response; interactions may benefit angina patients with abnormal ventricular function.
Epinephrine	None	Severe hypertension & bradycardia	Administer epinephrine cautiously; cardioselective β blocker may be safer.
Ergot alkaloids	None	Severe hypertension & peripheral artery hyper-perfusion have been seen though β blockers are commonly coadministered	Observe patient's response; few patients show ill effects.
Fluvoxamine	Decreased hepatic clearance of propranolol		Use with caution.
Glucagon	Enhanced clearance of lipid soluble β blockers	None	Monitor for reduced response.
Halofenate			Observe for impaired response to β blockade.

TABLE 2-11 (*continued*)

Drug	Pharmacokinetic interactions	Pharmacodynamic interactions	Precautions
Hydralazine	Decreased hepatic clearance of lipid soluble β blockers	Enhanced hypotensive response	Cautious coadministration.
Indomethacin & ibuprofen	None	Reduced efficacy in treatment of hypertension	Observe patient's response.
Isoproterenol	None	Cancels pharmacologic effect	Avoid concurrent use or choose selective β_1 blocker.
Levodopa		Antagonism of hypotensive & positive inotropic effects of levodopa	Monitor for altered response; interaction may have favorable results.
Lidocaine	Decreased hepatic clearance of lidocaine by lipid-soluble β blockers	Enhanced lidocaine toxicity	Combination should be used with caution; use lower doses of lidocaine.
Methyldopa		Hypertension during stress	Monitor for hypertensive episodes.
Monoamine	Uncertain	Enhanced hypotension	Manufacturer of propranolol considered concurrent use contraindicated.
Nitrates	None	Enhanced hypotension	Monitor response.
Omeprazole	None	None	None
Phenobarbital	Increased hepatic metabolism of β blockers		May need to increase lipid-soluble β-blocker dose.
Phenothiazines	Increased phenothiazine & β-blocker blood levels	Additive hypotensive response	Monitor for altered - response; especially with high doses of phenothiazine.

Phenylpropanolamine		Severe hypertensive reaction	Avoid use, especially in hypertension controlled by both methyldopa & β blockers.
Phenytoin		Additive ventricular depressive effects	Use with caution.
Reserpine		Depression, possible enhanced sensitivity to β-adrenergic blockade	Monitor closely.
Ranitidine	Not marked	None	Observe response.
Smoking	Enhanced first-pass metabolism	None	May need to increase dose of lipid-soluble β blockers.
Sulindac & naproxen	None	None	
Tricyclic antidepressants		Inhibits negative inotropic & chronotropic effects; enhanced hypotension	Use with caution with sotalol because of additive effects on ECG QT interval.
Tubucuraine		Enhanced neuromuscular blockade	Observe response in surgical patients, especially after high doses of propranolol.
Type I antiarrhythmics	Propafenone & quinidine decrease clearance of lipid-soluble β blockers	Disopyramide is a potent negative inotropic & chronotropic agent	Cautious coprescription; use with sotalol can be dangerous because of additive effects on ECG QT interval.
Warfarin	Decreased clearance of warfarin	None	Monitor response.

How to Choose a β Blocker

The various β-blocking compounds given in adequate dosage appear to have comparable antihypertensive, antiarrhythmic, and antianginal effects. Therefore, the β-blocking drug of choice in an individual patient is determined by the pharmacodynamic and pharmacokinetic differences between the drugs, in conjunction with the patient's other medical conditions (Table 2-12).

TABLE 2-12 Clinical Situations That Would Influence the Choice of a β-Blocking Drug

Condition	Choice of β blocker
Asthma, chronic bronchitis with bronchospasm	Avoid all β blockers if possible, but small doses of β_1-selective blockers can be used; β_1 selectivity is lost with higher doses; drugs with partial agonist activity and labetalol with α-adrenergic blocking properties can also be used.
Congestive heart failure	Drugs with partial agonist activity and vasodilatory activity (e.g., carvedilol, labetalol) may have an advantage, although all β blockers should be used with caution.
Angina	In patients with angina at low heart rates, drugs with partial agonist activity are probably contraindicated; patients who have angina at high heart rates but who have resting bradycardia may benefit from a drug with partial agonist activity; in vasospastic angina, labetalol may be useful; other β blockers should be used with caution.
Atrioventricular conduction defects	β blockers are generally contraindicated, but drugs with partial agonist activity and labetalol can be tried with caution.
Bradycardia	β blockers with partial agonist activity and labetalol have less of a pulse-slowing effect and are preferable.
Raynaud's phenomenon, intermittent claudication, cold extremities	β_1-selective blocking agents, labetalol, and agents with partial agonist activity may have an advantage.
Depression	Avoid propranolol; substitute a β blocker with partial agonist activity.
Diabetes mellitus	β_1-selective agents and partial agonist drugs are preferable.
Thyrotoxicosis	All agents will control symptoms, but agents without partial agonist activity are preferred.
Pheochromocytoma	Avoid all β blockers unless an α blocker is given; labetalol may be used as a treatment of choice.

TABLE 2-12 (*continued*)

Condition	Choice of β blocker
Renal failure	Use reduced doses of compounds largely eliminated by renal mechanisms (nadolol, sotalol, and atenolol) and drugs whose bioavailability is increased in uremia (propranolol); also consider possible accumulation of active metabolites (propranolol).
Insulin and sulfonylurea use	There is a danger of hypoglycemia; possibly less using drugs with β_1 selectivity.
Clonidine	Avoid nonselective β blockers; there is a severe rebound effect with clonidine withdrawal.
Oculomucocutaneous syndrome	Stop drug; substitute with any β blocker.
Hyperlipidemia	Avoid nonselective β blockers; use agents with partial agonism or β_1 selectivity, or α-blocking activity

Source: Frishman WR: *Clinical Pharmacology of the β-Adrenoreceptor Blocking Drugs,* 2d ed. Norwalk, CT, Appleton-Century-Crofts, 1984, with permission.

SUGGESTED READINGS

Australia/New Zealand Heart Failure Research Collaborative Group: Randomised, placebo-controlled trial of carvedilol in patients with congestive heart failure due to ischemic heart disease. *Lancet* 349:375,1997.

Bristow MR, Gilbert EM, Abraham WT, et al: Carvedilol produces dose-related improvements in left ventricular function and survival in subjects with chronic heart failure. *Circulation* 94:2807, 1996.

Colucci WS, Packer M, Bristow MR, et al: Carvedilol inhibits clinical progression in patients with mild symptoms of heart failure. *Circulation* 94:2800, 1996.

Frishman WH: *Clinical Pharmacology of the* β*-Adrenoceptor Blocking Drugs*, 2d ed. Norwalk, CT, Appleton-Century-Crofts, 1984.

Frishman WH, Charlap S: α-Adrenergic blockers. *Med Clin North Am* 72:427, 1988.

Frishman WH: *Current Cardiovascular Drugs*. Philadelphia, Current Medicine, 1995, p 88.

Frishman WH: Postinfarctrion survival: Role of β-adrenergic blockade, in Fuster V, Ross R, Topol EJ (eds): *Atherosclerosis and Coronary Artery Disease*. Philadelphia, Lippencott, 1996, pp 1205–1214.

Frishman WH: Secondary prevention of myocardial infarction: The roles of β-adrenergic blockers, calcium-channel blockers, angiotensin converting enzyme inhibitors, and aspirin, in Willich SN, Muller JE (eds): *Triggering of Acute Coronary Syndromes*. The Netherlands, Kluwer Academic Publishers, 1996, p 367.

Frishman WH: Beta-adrenergic blocking drugs and calcium channel blockers, in Alexander RW, Schlant RC, Fuster V (eds): *Hurst's The Heart*, 9th ed. New York, McGraw-Hill, 1998, pp 1583–1618.

Frishman WH: Alpha- and beta-adrenergic blocking drugs, in Parmley WW, Chatterjee K (eds): *Cardiology*. Philadelphia, Lippincott-Raven, 1997.

Frishman WH, Cavusoglu E: β-Adrenergic blockers and their role in the therapy of arrhythmias, in Podrid PJ, Kowey PR (eds): *Cardiac Arrhythmias: Mechanisms, Diagnosis and Management*. Baltimore, Williams & Wilkins, 1995, pp 421–433.

Frishman WH, Charlap S: Alpha- and beta-adrenergic blocking drugs, in Frishman WH, Sonnenblick EH (eds): *Cardiovascular Pharmacotherapeutics*. New York, McGraw-Hill, 1997, pp 59–94.

Frishman WH, Hershman D: β-Adrenergic blocking drugs in cardiac disorders, in Messerli FH (ed): *Cardiovascular Drug Therapy*, 2d ed. Philadelphia, Saunders, 1996, pp 465–474.

Frishman WH, Furberg CD, Friedewald WT: β-Adrenergic blockade for survivors of acute myocardial infarction. *N Engl J Med* 310:830, 1984.

Frishman WH, Skolnick AE: Secondary prevention post infarction: The role of beta-adrenergic blockers, calcium-channel blockers, and aspirin, in Gersh B, Rahimtoola S (eds): *Acute Myocardial Infarction*, 2d ed. New York, Chapman & Hall, 1996, pp 766–796.

Gilbert EM, Abraham WT, Olsen S, et al: Comparative hemodynamic, left ventricular functional, and antiadrenergic effects of chronic treatment with metoprolol versus carvedilol in the failing heart. *Circulation* 94:2817, 1996.

Insel PA: Adrenergic receptors: Evolving concepts and clinical implications. *N Engl J Med* 307:578, 1996.

Lefkowitz RJ, Hoffmann BB, Taylor P: Neurotransmissions: the autonomic and somatic motor nervous system, in Hardman JG, Limbird LE (eds): *Goodman & Gilman's The Pharmacological Basis of Therapeutics*, 9th ed. New York, McGraw-Hill, 1996, p 125.

Luther RR: New perspectives on selective α_1 blockade. *Am J Hypertens* 2:731, 1989.

Opie LH, Sonnenblick EH, Frishman WH, Thadani U: Beta-blocking agents, in Chatterjee K, Frishman W, Gersh BJ, et al (eds): *Drugs for the Heart*, 4th ed. Philadelphia, Saunders, 1997, pp 1–30.

Packer M, Bristow MR, Cohn N, et al: Effect of carvedilol on morbidity and mortality in chronic heart failure. *N Engl J Med* 334:1349, 1996.

Chapter 3 | Parasympathetic Drugs

B. Robert Meyer

The term *parasympathetic nervous system* refers to those portions of the peripheral autonomic nervous system that begin as preganglionic fibers in one of three distinct regions of the central nervous system (CNS), exit the CNS in either the cranial or the sacral regions, and have their postganglionic fibers distributed in a variety of organs throughout the body. One of the three sites of origin for parasympathetic fibers is the midbrain. Fibers originating here join the third cranial nerve and course to the ciliary ganglion. At this ganglion they synapse, and postganglionic fibers innervate the iris and ciliary body. The second site of origin for the parasympathetic system is in the medulla. Fibers originating here join the seventh, ninth, and tenth cranial nerves to exit the CNS. These preganglionic fibers distribute in the pattern of each of these nerves. Fibers in the tenth nerve (the vagus) are distributed to ganglia associated with various visceral organs, including the heart and gastrointestinal (GI) tract. The third and final source of parasympathetic outflow is in the sacral portion of the spinal cord. Preganglionic fibers from this site lead to connections with the bladder, bowel, and pelvic organs.

The anatomic organization of the parasympathetic system differs from that of the sympathetic system. The preganglionic fibers of the parasympathetic system extend from their sites of origin in the CNS to the end organ they are innervating. Ganglia of the parasympathetic system are relatively smaller than those of the sympathetic system, and the postganglionic fibers that emerge from these ganglia are short and localized to a specific organ. The sympathetic system has preganglionic fibers that synapse in large paravertebral ganglia and has an extensive and diffuse postganglionic network that distributes to multiple organs of the body.

Inherent in the structural organization of the parasympathetic system is the ability to act at specific organs to cause very specific responses via localized discharges. In general, where the sympathetic system tends to stimulate activity diffusely through its widespread postganglionic network, the effects of the parasympathetic system are to act at specific organs to accommodate periods of rest and recovery. The system lowers heart rate, increases GI motility, stimulates bladder emptying, increases biliary contraction, and lowers blood pressure.

The parasympathetic nervous system is exclusively cholinergic in character (using acetylcholine as a transmitter), whereas in the sympathetic system the postganglionic fibers are almost exclusively adrenergic. Acetylcholine receptors were first recognized as being of two basic types in 1914, when Dale noted that while acetylcholine could stimulate all types of cholinergic receptors, certain effects could be blocked by the administration of atropine. Effects that are blocked by atropine are termed *muscarinic* effects, named after a substance isolated from the poisonous mushroom *Amanita muscaria* that produces these pharmacologic properties. These effects correspond almost directly to the actions of the parasympathetic system. After atropine blockade, higher doses of acetylcholine can elicit another constellation of effects that appear to be very similar to the properties of nicotine. Dale called these *nicotinic* effects.

Modern investigation into the muscarinic receptors that constitute the parasympathetic system has demonstrated that there are at least five major subtypes of muscarinic receptors (Table 3-1). All muscarinic receptors act via G proteins. Types 1, 3, and 5 activate a G protein that in turn stimulates phospholipase C. Phospholipase C then hydrolyzes phosphatidyl inositol. Ultimately, activation of these receptors leads to increased intracellular calcium concentration. Type 2 and 4 receptors activate a different G protein that inhibits adenylate cyclase, activates K^+ channels, and also may suppress voltage-controlled Ca^{2+} channels.

The most important subgroup of muscarinic receptors for the cardiovascular system are the M_2 or "cardiac" receptors. Activation of these receptors and alteration of potassium transport produce the negative chronotropic and inotropic effects noted in Table 3-1. Most muscarinic receptors are located in the specialized conduction tissue of the heart, and direct innervation of the myocardium itself is sparse. Effects of muscarinic stimulation lead to a decreased rate of spontaneous depolarization of the sinoatrial (SA) node, a consequent delay in the achievement of threshold potential, and a slowing of spontaneous firing. The rate of conduction in the atrioventricular (AV) node is also decreased, and the refractory period to repetitive stimulation is prolonged. The effects of muscarinic receptors on the contractility of the ventricle are substantially less than on the conduction system. Blockade of cholinergic receptors produces positive inotropic effects; negative inotropic effects with cholinergic stimulation can be demonstrated in experimental situations. The clinical relevance of the aforementioned effects remains unknown. All effects of muscarinic stimulation are enhanced in the context of activation of the sympathetic nervous system.

M_3 receptors have vasodilatory properties. Since direct muscarinic innervation of the vasculature has not been demonstrated, and since acetylcholine is a "local" neurotransmitter, the exact role of these receptors as part of the parasympathetic nervous system is debatable. It appears that the pharmacologic effect of M_3 receptors is mediated by receptor-mediated local release of nitric oxide.

Drugs that act at muscarinic receptors can do so by a number of mechanisms to produce their effects. The most common mechanisms of action and the relevant drugs are shown in Table 3-2.

TABLE 3-1 Types of Muscarinic Receptors

Receptor	Location	Effect	Mechanism	Agonists	Antagonist
M_1 (neural)	Cortex, hippocampus	Memory?	Stimulates phospholipase C	Acetylcholine Oxytremorine McNA343	Atropine Pirenzepine
	Gastric parietal cells Enteric ganglia	Gastric acid secretion Gastrointestinal motility	Increased intracellular Ca^{2+}		
M_2 (cardiac)	SA node	Slowed spontaneous depolarization	Inhibition of adenylate cyclase	Acetylcholine	Atropine Gallamine AF-DX 116
	Atrium	Shortened action potential duration, decreased contractile force	Activation of K^+ channels		
	AV node	Decreased speed of conduction			
	Ventricle	Decreased contractile force			
M_3	Smooth muscle Secretory glands	Contraction Vasodilatation secretion	Increased phospholipase C	Acetylcholine	Atropine Hexahydro-siladifenidol
			Vasodilation via nitric oxide		
M_4	CNS	?	Like M_2 via adenylate cyclase	Acetylcholine	?Himbacine
M_5	CNS	?	?Increased phospholipase C	Acetylcholine	?

TABLE 3-2 Mechanisms of Action of Drugs Active at Muscarinic Receptors

Mechanism of Action	Effect	Drug	Comments
Choline esters	Mimic effect of acetylcholine at receptors	Bethanechol Methacholine	Moderate selectivity (see text)
Anticholinesterases	Enhance effect of acetylcholine at receptors	Edrophonium Physostigmine Pyridostigmine Neostigmine	Nicotinic and muscarinic effects both present
Muscarinic receptor antagonists	Compete for binding at postsynaptic receptor	Atropine Scopolamine	Minimal structural selectivity for different muscarinic receptors Selectivity reflects distribution/density of receptors Selectivity may be enhanced by route of administration

DRUGS THAT ENHANCE MUSCARINIC ACTIVITY

Choline Esters

Acetylcholine itself is not a useful drug. Its pharmacologic properties are nonselective and include the stimulation of all muscarinic and nicotinic sites. Therefore, an attempt has been made to develop synthetic analogues of acetylcholine that would have greater selectivity for specific subpopulations of muscarinic receptors. The only clinically useful agents that have thus far emerged from this effort are bethanechol and methacholine. Bethanechol is relatively selective for the urinary bladder and GI tract. It has very little activity at M_2 receptors in the heart. Methacholine is potentially useful in the diagnosis of reactive airway disease and has some activity at cardiac receptors as well. Pilocarpine is a naturally occurring muscarinic agent that has agonist properties principally at muscarinic receptors in the eye and in the GI tract.

Anticholinesterase Agents

The effects of acetylcholine at postsynaptic sites are a function of the concentration of the transmitter at the postsynaptic receptor site. The compound is inactivated by the enzyme acetylcholinesterase, which is readily demonstrable at high concentrations at the postsynaptic sites. Some of the enzyme is bound to the membrane at the synaptic cleft itself, and some floats free in the medium. Acetylcholine effects can be enhanced and prolonged by the inhibition of the action of acetylcholinesterase. Clinically available *anticholinesterases* are listed in Table 3-2. These agents reversibly inhibit cholinesterase activity at all receptor sites. Therefore, their pharmacologic effects reflect not only muscarinic but also nicotinic actions. All these drugs also inhibit the activity of butyrylcholinesterase. This "pseudocholinesterase" is present in many sites of the body, including the liver and plasma. Anticholinesterase drug effects constitute an enhancement of the vagal stimulus on the heart. This leads to a shortening of the effective refractory period, a decrease in SA and AV nodal conduction time, and a diminishment of cardiac output. This is modified somewhat by effects at nicotinic receptors. In addition, with persistent stimulation, a paradoxical decrease in effect will occur. Therefore, with high doses and longer duration of action, a paradoxical decrease in acetylcholine effect can be seen. All these agents have significant potential for noncardiac effects, including GI (increased contraction, acidity, propulsion), skeletal muscle (enhanced activity), and pulmonary effects (enhanced bronchoconstriction).

The anticholinesterase with the shortest duration of action is edrophonium. When given intravenously, it has an onset of effect within 30 to 60 seconds and a duration of effect that is generally less than 10 min, although longer durations of action may be seen in some susceptible individuals. Given this pharmacodynamic profile, edrophonium has been used for the acute diagnosis of myasthenia gravis and for the diagnosis and acute termination of paroxysmal supraventricular tachycardia. Cardiac disease is listed by the manufacturer of edrophonium as a reason for caution in its use, and the drug has not had Food and Drug Administration (FDA)–approved labeling for use in the management of cardiac disease. However, many clinicians have used the drug's capacity to produce acute and intense muscarinic effects as a way of diagnosing atrial arrhythmias after other routine measures have failed. Occasionally edrophonium is used for the acute control of heart rate, for example, slowing heart rate in the context of an evaluation of demand pacemaker functioning. As a single dose, edrophonium should not exceed 10 mg. In older or sicker patients, the maximal dose may need to be reduced to 5 to 7 mg. When the goal of therapy is to gradually decrease heart rate, the drug may be administered in 2-mg boluses up to a total dosage of 10 mg. Significantly higher doses of the drug have been used safely in other clinical contexts.

Recent articles have suggested that the diagnostic use of edrophonium in cardiovascular disease may be extended to include its administration during tilt-table testing as part of the evaluation for possible vasovagal syncope. It is also used in the diagnostic evaluation of patients with atypical chest pain syndromes, where response to acid infusion and edrophonium administration may identify patients with esophageal sources of pain.

Other anticholinesterases include physostigmine, pyridostigmine, neostigmine, and amebonium. These drugs generally have not been found to have any significant role in the management of cardiovascular disease. However, they are used in other areas of medicine, and therefore, it is important to be familiar with the indications for their use and their potential cardiac side effects. Perhaps the most important use for some of these drugs is in the immediate reversal of neuromuscular blockade during general anesthesia. They will reverse the effects of nondepolarizing muscular blocking agents such as tubocurarine, metocurine, gallamine, vecuronium, atracurium, and pancuronium. When titrated appropriately with close monitoring of their effects on neuromuscular blockade, the cardiac effects of these drugs are generally not a problem. On occasion, however, they may produce the syndrome of excessive parasympathetic effect. Since they have no effect on the muscle blockade produced by depolarizing agents such as succinylcholine or decamethonium, these drugs should not be used in that context.

DRUGS THAT DIMINISH MUSCARINIC ACTIVITY

Muscarinic Receptor Antagonists

Atropine is the best known of the muscarinic receptor antagonists. Atropine has a dose-related effect on muscarinic receptors. At its lowest doses, a relatively selective effect on salivary secretion and sweating is demonstrated; at higher doses, it exhibits cardiac effects and more diffuse anticholinergic effects that include nicotinic as well as muscarinic blockade. Atropine's dose-response curve is described in Table 3-3. It has been reported that Chinese individuals show an increased sensitivity to atropine that is independent of resting vagal and sympathetic tone. At low doses (<0.5 mg) it may produce a paradoxical, and usually mild, slowing of heart rate. The mechanism for this mild bradycardia has been debated. It has been attributed by some authors to a central stimulation of vagal afferents. At higher doses, atropine causes a progressive vagolytic effect on the heart, with increased heart rate, decreased refractory period of the AV node, and increased AV conduction velocity. Atropine is indicated for use in the acute treatment of severe symptomatic bradycardias, particularly in the context of acute myocardial infarctions. On rare occasions, where it may be hypothesized that endogenous sympathetic activity is suppressed by parasympathetic effects of vagal stimulation, atropine has been thought to precipitate ventricular arrhythmias. For this reason, it is clear that the drug should not be used casually; its use should be restricted to cases of severe symptomatic bradycardias.

Since atropine will counteract bradycardia or heart block produced by acetylcholine or its analogues, it can be used to counteract the cardiac effects of any syndromes in which vagal nerve stimulation plays an important role. The drug therefore can block the bradycardia and hypotension seen in vasovagal syndromes. Since atropine is only available as a parenteral injection, and since its effects are relatively short lasting, it is useful only for acute reversal of bradyarrhythmias and has no role in chronic management of these conditions.

Atropine also has been investigated recently for its potential utility as an adjunct to dobutamine-stress echocardiography. Atropine has been given as a secondary medication for the enhancement of cardiac response where dobutamine infusion has limited success in producing the desired tachycardia, particularly for patients receiving beta blockers.

TABLE 3-3 Dose-Effect Relationship for Atropine

Dose	Pharmacologic Effect
0.0–0.5 mg	Mild bradycardia, dry mouth, decreased sweating
0.5–1.0 mg	Cardioacceleration, very dry mouth, some pupillary dilation
1.0–2.0 mg	Tachycardia (potentially symptomatic) very dry mouth, pupillary dilation, blurred vision
>3.0 mg	All the preceding, except more marked, and including erythematous, hot skin, increased intestinal tone, urinary retention. At highest doses excitement and agitation leading to delirium or ultimately to coma, accompanied by fevers and scarlet skin.

SUGGESTED READINGS

Bonner TI, Buckley NJ, Young AC, Brann MR: Identification of a family of muscarinic receptor genes. *Science* 237:527–531, 1987.

Caulfield MP: Muscarinic receptors: Characterization, coupling and function. *Pharmacol Ther* 58:319–379, 1993.

Lefkowitz RJ, Hoffman BB, Taylor P: Neurotransmission: The autonomic and somatic motor nervous systems, in Hardman JG, Limbird LE (eds): *Goodman and Gilman's The Pharmacological Basis of Therapeutics*, 9th ed. New York, McGraw-Hill, 1996, pp 105–139.

Levine RR, Birdsall NJM (eds): Symposium: Subtypes of muscarinic receptors V. *Life Sci* 52:405–597, 1993.

Meyer BR: Parasympathetic drugs in cardiovascular disease, in Frishman WH, Sonnenblick EH (eds): *Cardiovascular Pharmacotherapeutics*. New York, McGraw-Hill, 1997, pp 95–100.

Taylor P: Anticholinesterase agents, in Hardman JG, Limbird LE (eds): *Goodman and Gilman's The Pharmacological Basis of Therapeutics*, 9th ed. New York, McGraw-Hill, 1996, pp 161–176.

Chapter 4 | Calcium Channel Blockers

William H. Frishman

The calcium channel blockers are a heterogeneous group of drugs with widely variable effects on heart muscle, sinus node function, atrioventricular (AV) conduction, peripheral blood vessels, and coronary circulation. Eleven of these drugs—nifedipine, nicardipine, nimodipine, nisoldipine, felodipine, isradipine, amlodipine, verapamil, diltiazem, mibefradil, and bepridil—are approved in the United States for clinical use.

PHYSIOLOGIC BACKGROUND

Calcium ions play a fundamental role in the activation of cells. An influx of calcium ions into the cell through specific ion channels is required for myocardial contraction, for determining peripheral vascular resistance through calcium-dependent regulated tone of vascular smooth muscle, and for helping to initiate the pacemaker tissues of the heart, which are activated largely by the slow calcium current.

The concept of calcium channel inhibition originated in 1960 when it was noted that prenylamine, a newly developed coronary vasodilator, depressed cardiac performance in canine heart-lung preparations. Initial studies with verapamil showed that it also exerted negative inotropic effects on the isolated myocardium in addition to having vasodilator properties. These potent negative inotropic effects seemed to differentiate these drugs from the classic coronary vasodilators, such as nitroglycerin and papaverine, which have little, if any, myocardial depressant activity. Unlike β-adrenergic antagonists, many of the calcium antagonists depress cardiac contractility without altering the height or contour of the monophasic action potential and thus interfere with excitation-contraction coupling. Reversible closure of specific calcium ion channels in the membrane of the mammalian myocardial cell was suggested as the explanation of these observed effects.

Subsequently, the effects of verapamil on atrial and ventricular intracellular potentials were studied. Antiarrhythmic compounds were classified into local anesthetics that decreased the maximum rate of depolarization, β blockers, and a third class that prolonged the duration of the cardiac action potential. However, none of these electrophysiologic actions could explain the antiarrhythmic effect of verapamil. Thus a fourth class of antiarrhythmic drug, typified by verapamil, was proposed, with effects separate from those of sodium channel inhibitors and β blockers. It has been shown that the antiarrhythmic actions and negative inotropic effects of verapamil are mediated predominantly through interference with calcium conductance.

CHEMICAL STRUCTURE AND PHARMACODYNAMICS

Structure of the Calcium Channel Blockers

Diltiazem is a benzothiazepine derivative that is structurally unrelated to other vasodilators. Nifedipine is a dihydropyridine derivative unrelated to the nitrates, which is lipophilic and is inactivated by light. Nicardipine, amlodipine, felodipine, isradipine, nisoldipine, and nimodipine are also dihydropyridine derivatives similar in structure to nifedipine. Verapamil ([±] verapamil) has some structural similarity to papaverine. Mibefradil, a drug now approved for use in patients with hypertension and angina pectoris, is from a new structural class of benzomidazolyl-substituted tetraline derivatives. The drug binds competitively at the verapamil binding site and interferes allosterically with the diltiazem site without affecting the dihydropyridine ion binding site.

Bepridil, which is currently available for treatment of angina pectoris, is not related chemically to other cardioactive drugs.

Differential Effects on Slow Channels

The most important characteristic of all calcium channel blockers is their ability to selectively inhibit the inward flow of charge-bearing calcium ions when the calcium ion channels become permeable. Previously, the term *slow channel* was used, but it has recently been recognized that the calcium ion current develops faster than previously thought and that there are at least two types of calcium channels, the L and T. The conventional calcium channel, which has been known to exist for a long time, is called the *L channel.* It is blocked by all the calcium channel antagonists and has its permeability increased by catecholamines. The *T-type channel* appears at more negative potentials than the L-type and probably plays an important role in the initial depolarization of sinus and AV nodal tissue. The function of the L-type channel is to admit the substantial amount of calcium ions required for initiation of contraction via calcium-induced calcium release from the sarcoplasmic reticulum. Mibefradil is the first calcium channel blocker that has selective blocking properties on the T-type channel in addition to its blocking effects on the L-type channel. Specific blockers for the T-type channel are not yet available, but they could be expected to inhibit the sinus and AV nodes profoundly.

Bepridil possesses all the characteristics of the traditional calcium antagonists. In addition, the drug appears to affect the sodium channel (fast channel) and possibly the potassium channel, producing a quinidinelike effect. Bepridil specifically inhibits maximal upstroke velocity (dV/dt max), that is, the influx of sodium in appropriate load dosages. The effect of bepridil on the maximum rate of depolarization has been examined; the action potential height is not changed; however, the action potential duration is extended in a quinidinelike manner.

CARDIOVASCULAR EFFECTS

Effects on Muscular Contraction

Calcium is the primary ionic link between neurologic excitation and mechanical contraction of cardiac, smooth, and skeletal muscle. Actin and myosin are the protein filaments that slide past one another in the adenosine triphosphate (ATP)–dependent contractile process of all muscle cells. In myocardial cells, the regulatory proteins tropomyosin and troponin inhibit this process. When the myocardial cell membrane repolarizes, calcium enters the cell (L channel) and triggers the release of additional calcium from internal stores within the sarcoplasmic reticulum. Calcium released from this large intracellular reservoir then initiates contraction by combining with the inhibitors troponin and tropomyosin. Previously hidden active sites on actin molecules are then available for binding by myosin.

Effects on Coronary and Peripheral Arterial Blood Vessels

The contraction of vascular smooth muscle such as that found in the coronary arteries is slightly different from the contraction of cardiac and skeletal muscles (Table 4-1). Myosin must be phosphorylated, and calmodulin is the regulatory protein to which calcium binds. In addition, vascular smooth-muscle cells have significantly less intracellular calcium stores than do myocardial cells and so rely more heavily on the influx of extracellular calcium.

The observation that calcium channel blockers are significantly more effective in inhibiting contraction in coronary and peripheral arterial smooth muscle than in cardiac and skeletal muscle is of great clinical importance. This differential effect is explained by the observation that arterial smooth muscle is more dependent on external calcium entry for contraction, whereas cardiac and skeletal muscle rely on a recirculating internal pool of calcium. Because calcium-entry blockers are membrane-active drugs, they reduce the entry of calcium into cells and therefore exert a much larger effect on vascular wall contraction. This preferential effect allows calcium-entry blockers to dilate coronary and peripheral arteries in doses that do not severely affect myocardial contractility or that have little, if any, effect on skeletal muscle.

Effects on Veins

The calcium channel blockers seem to be less active in veins than in arteries and are ineffective at therapeutic doses (in contrast to nitrates) for increasing venous capacitance.

Effects on Myocardial Contractility

Force generation during cardiac muscle contraction depends, in part, on calcium influx during membrane depolarization (see Table 4-1). In iso-

TABLE 4-1 Pharmacologic Effects of Calcium Channel Blockers*

	Heart Rate		Conduction						
	Acute	Chronic	SA node	AV node	Myocardial contractility	Peripheral vasodilator	Cardiac output	Coronary blood flow	Myocardial O_2 Demand
Diltiazem	↓	↓	↓	↓	↓	↓	V	↑	↓
Bepridil	↓	↓	↓	↓	V	—	V	↑	↓
Verapamil	↑	↓	↓	↓	↓↓	↓	V	↑	↓
Mibefradil	↓	↓	↓	↓	—	↓	V	↑	↓
Amlodipine	↑	↑—	—	—	↓	↓↓	↑—	↑	↓
Felodipine	↑	↑—	—	—	—	↓↓	↑—	↑	↓
Isradipine	↑	↑—	—	—	—	↓↓	↑—	↑	↓
Nicardipine	↑	↑—	—	—	—	↓↓	↑—	↑	↓
Nifedipine	↑	↑—	—	—	↓	↓↓	↑—	↑	↓
Nimodipine	↑	↑—	—	—	—	V	↑—	↑	↓
Nisoldipine	↑	↑—	—	—	—	↓↓	↑—	↑	↓

*↑= increase; ↓ = decrease; — = no change; V = variable.

Source: From Frishman WH, Stroh JA, Greenberg SM, et al: Calcium-channel blockers in systemic hypertension. *Med Clin North Am* 72:449, 1988, with permission.

lated myocardial preparations, all calcium channel antagonists have been demonstrated to exert potent negative inotropic effects. In guinea pig atria exposed to a drug concentration of 10^{-6} mol/L, the order of potency for depressing the maximal rate of force development during constant pacing was found to be nifedipine > verapamil–diltiazem. In dog papillary muscle, developed tension also was decreased most markedly by nifedipine; the relative potencies (on a weight basis) of verapamil and diltiazem were 1/15 and 1/40, respectively.

The negative inotropic effect of the calcium channel antagonists are dose dependent. The excitation-contraction coupling of vascular smooth muscle is 3 to 10 times more sensitive to the action of calcium channel antagonists than is that of myocardial fibers. Hence the relatively low doses of these drugs used in vivo to produce vasodilatation or beneficial antiarrhythmic effects may not produce significant negative inotropic effects. Furthermore, in intact animals and human beings, the intrinsic negative inotropic properties of these compounds are greatly modified by a baroreceptor-mediated reflex augmentation of β-adrenergic tone consequent to vasodilatation and a decrease in blood pressure. Nifedipine and other dihydropyridines, which exert the greatest vasodilator effects among these agents, accordingly produce the strongest reflex β-adrenergic response and the one most likely to offset the negative inotropic activity of the drugs and lead to enhancement of ventricular performance. Although this mechanism plays an important role in patients with normal or nearly normal left ventricular function, it is unlikely to play a similar role in patients with severe congestive heart failure, in whom the baroreceptor sensitivity is markedly attenuated.

Regarding the newer calcium channel blockers, the hemodynamic profiles of amlodipine and mibefradil were compared with those of verapamil and diltiazem in conscious normotensive rats. Verapamil and diltiazem were negatively inotropic. Amlodipine decreased left ventricular contractility only at the highest dose used. Mibefradil was less negatively inotropic than amlodipine.

Electrophysiologic Effects

While verapamil, nifedipine, diltiazem, and bepridil all depress cardiac contractility with only quantitative differences (see Table 4-1), their effects on the electrophysiology of the heart are different qualitatively. Local anesthetic actions of bepridil, diltiazem, and particularly verapamil may account for some of these differences. Nifedipine and other dihydropyridines have a more selective action at the slow channels, whereas verapamil and diltiazem, at least at higher doses, also inhibit currents in the fast channels in the manner of the local anesthetics. Bepridil has definite class I antiarrhythmic properties.

Verapamil, diltiazem, and mibefradil prolong the conduction and refractoriness in the AV node; the A–H interval is lengthened more than is the H–V interval. In therapeutic concentrations, there are no demonstrable actions on the rate of depolarization or the repolarization phases of the action potentials in atrial, ventricular, and Purkinje fibers. The rate of discharge of the sinus node, which depends on the calcium ion current, is depressed by all calcium channel blockers. In vivo, this effect can be compensated or overcompensated for by activation of baroreceptor reflexes, which increase sympathetic nervous activity.

The antiarrhythmic actions of verapamil and diltiazem relate to their effects on nodal cardiac tissues. In sinoatrial (SA) and AV nodal cells, the drugs modify slow-channel electropotentials in three ways: (1) there is a decrease in the rate of rise and slope of diastolic slow depolarization and an increase in the membrane threshold potential, which reduces the rate of firing in the cell, (2) the action potential upstroke is decreased in amplitude, which slows conduction, and (3) the duration of the action potential is increased. These electrophysiologic effects are dose-related, and above the clinical range electric standstill may occur in SA and AV nodal cells. These observations and others support the concept that slow-channel activity is important in the generation of pacemaker potential in the SA node. Verapamil and diltiazem also exert a depressant effect on the AV node and in low concentrations prolong the effective refractory period. Unlike β-adrenergic blocking drugs and vagomimetic interventions, which depress AV node transmission by altering autonomic impulse traffic, verapamil and diltiazem prolong AV nodal refractoriness directly. However, verapamil may have additional vagomimetic effects.

Bepridil has a modest depressant effect on heart rate and intranodal and infranodal conduction accompanied by a significant increment in the effective and functional refractory periods of the AV node. However, unexpected findings that cannot be explained solely on the basis of slow-channel inhibition of the myocardium include lengthening of the Q–Tc interval and significant prolongation of the atrial and ventricular effective refractory periods.

Mibefradil also has a modest depressant effect on heart rate and intranodal and infranodal conduction.

Effects on Nonvascular Tissues

Calcium ions are required for contraction in all smooth muscles, and these drugs can inhibit contractions in the gastrointestinal tract. Calcium is also important in excitation-secretion coupling. However, there is no evidence that these drugs have significant effects on the endocrine glands in clinical doses. Although antiadrenergic effects of some calcium-entry blockers have been suggested, further studies are needed.

Some calcium-entry blockers may partially inhibit adenosine diphosphate (ADP)–and epinephrine-induced platelet aggregation and thromboxane release from platelets. There are good experimental data that verapamil and diltiazem, and to a lesser extent, nifedipine, can inhibit platelet aggregation in vitro. The drugs appear to be more efficacious in attenuating aggregation when they are present in the reaction mixture before aggregation begins. This can, however, interrupt or slow the rate of aggregation if added after the beginning of the reaction. In addition, the effect of aspirin in attenuating platelet aggregation appears to be potentiated in vitro in the presence of diltiazem. This has led to considerable speculation as to how much this effect may contribute to the efficacy of calcium channel blockers in the treatment of unstable angina. There has been at least one report of patients with unstable angina being treated with verapamil, in which those treated with verapamil demonstrated decreased platelet aggregability and decreased thromboxane A_2 levels. If this is true in vivo, it would substantially support the use of some of these agents as first-line drugs for the treatment of unstable angina.

PHARMACOKINETICS

Although classified together, calcium-entry blockers have differences in their pharmacokinetic properties (Tables 4-2 and 4-3). Differences in completeness of GI absorption, amount of first-pass hepatic metabolism, protein binding, extent of distribution in the body, and the pharmacologic actions of different metabolites may influence the clinical usefulness of these drugs in different patients.

Since many of the calcium channel blockers are relatively short acting, they are now available in various sustained-release delivery systems: diffusion type (diltiazem, verapamil), bioerosion (diltiazem, nifedipine, nicardipine), osmosis (verapamil, nifedipine), and diffusion-erosion (felodipine). Clinical trials are now in progress evaluating isradipine as once-daily therapy with the GI therapeutic system (GITS) formulation (osmosis). Nisoldipine was recently approved as a once-daily therapy in the coat-core formulation and verapamil in a delayed-onset sustained-release osmotic drug delivery system.

After administration of a certain oral dose, the calcium-entry blocking drugs, which are largely metabolized in the liver, show larger interindividual variation in circulating plasma levels. In angina pectoris and hypertension, wide individual differences also exist in the relation between plasma concentrations of calcium-entry blockers and the associated therapeutic effect.

Various dihydropyridine calcium channel blockers (felodipine, nifedipine, nisoldipine) should not be administered with grapefruit juice because it has been shown to interfere with the drug's metabolism, resulting in about a threefold mean increase in C_{max} and an almost twofold mean increase in area under the plasma concentration-time curve (AUC).

TABLE 4-2 Pharmacokinetics of Calcium Channel Blockers and Sustained-Release Preparations*

Agent	Trade name	Absorption, %	Bioavailability, %†	Protein binding, %	VOD, L/kg	$t_{1/2}$ β, h	Clearance, mL/min/kg	Time to peak plasma concentration, h
Diltiazem	Cardizem	>90	35–60	78	5.0	4.1–5.6	15	2–3
Diltiazem SR	Cardizem SR	>90	35–60	78	5.0	5.7	15	6–11
Diltiazem IV	Cardizem		100	78	5.0	3.4	15	
Diltiazem CD	Cardizem CD,	>95	40	70–80	5.0	5–8	15	10–14
Diltiazem XR	Dilacor XR	>95	40	70–80	5.0	5–10	15	4–6
Diltiazem ER	Tiazac	>90	40	70–80	5.0	4–9.5	15	
Verapamil	Calan, Isoptin	>90	10–20	90	4.3	6±4 IV, 8±6 PO	13±7	1–2
Verapamil SR	Calan SR Isoptin SR	>90	10–20	90	4.3	4.5–12	13±7	1–2
	Verelan	>90	20–3	90	162–380 L	12		7–9
Coer verapamil	Covera							
Verapamil IV			100			2–5		
Nifedipine	Procardia, Adalat	>90	65	90	1.32	~5	500–600	0.5
Nifedipine CC	Adalat CC	>90	84–89	92–98	1.32	—	500–600	2–2.5
Nifedipine GITS	Procardia XL	>90	85	>95	1.32	3.8–16.9	500–600	6 to plateau

TABLE 4-2 (*continued*)

Agent	Trade name	Absorption, %	Bioavail-ability, %[†]	Protein binding, %	VOD, L/kg	$t_{1/2}$ β, h	Clearance, mL/min/kg	Time to peak plasma concen-tration, h
Nicardipine	Cardene	>90	~30	>90	0.6	~1 IV	14	0.5–2.0
Nicardipine SR	Cardene SR	>90	35	>95		8.6	0.6	1–4 immediate
Nicardipine IV	Cardene		100	>90	9.3			
Amlodipine	Norvasc	>90	60–65	>95	21	35–45	7	6–12
Isradipine	Dynacirc	90–95	17	97	2.9	8.8	10	1.5
Felodipine ER	Plendil	>95	15–25	>99	10	15.1 ± 2.6	12	2.5–5
Bepridil	Vascor	>90	~60	>95	80	33		5.3
Nimodipine	Nimotop	>90	13	>95	0.94	8–9		0.6
Nisoldipine	Sular	87	5	>99		7–12		6–12
Mibefradil		~90			369	10–15	375	1.2

*VOD = volume of distribution; SR = sustained release; IV = intravenous; CD, XR, CC, XL = extended release; PO = oral; GITS = gastrointestinal therapeutic system.

[†]Extraction ratio.

Source: Adapted from Frishman WH, Sonnenblick EH: Calcium channel blockers, in Schlant RC, Alexander RW (eds): *Hurst's The Heart*, 8th ed. New York, McGraw-Hill, 1994, pp 1291–1308, with permission.

TABLE 4-3 Clinical Characteristics of Calcium Channel Blockers*

	Dosage		Onset of Action, min					
Agent	*Oral*	*IV*	*Oral*	*IV*	*Therapeutic PC, ng/mL*	*Site of metabolism*	*Active metabolites*	*Excretion, %*
Diltiazem	30–90 mg q6–8h	75–150 μg/kg 10–20 mg	<30	<10	50–200	Deacetylation *N* deacetylation *O* demethylation Major hepatic first-pass effect	Yes	60 (fecal) 2–4 (unchanged in urine)
Diltiazem SR	60–120 mg q12h		30–60		50–200		Yes	
Diltiazem IV		0.25 mg/kg (20 mg)						
Diltiazem CD	180–360 mg q24h		30–60		50–200		Yes	
Diltiazem XR	180–540 mg q24h		30–60		40–200		Yes	
Diltiazem ER	120–540 mg q24h				40-200		Yes	
Verapamil	80–120 mg q6–12h	150 μg/kg 10–20 mg	<30	<5	>100	*N* dealkylation *O* demethylation Major hepatic first-pass effect	Yes	15 (fecal) 70 (renal) 3–4 (unchanged in urine)
Verapamil SR	240–480 mg q12 or 24h		<30		>50		Yes	15 (fecal) 70 (renal) 3–4 (unchanged in urine)

TABLE 4-3 (*continued*)

Agent	Dosage		Onset of Action, min		Therapeutic PC, ng/mL	Site of metabolism	Active metabolites	Excretion, %
	Oral	*IV*	*Oral*	*IV*				
Verelan (Verapamil SR)	120–480 mg q24h				>50		Yes	16 (fecal) 70 (renal) 3–4 (unchanged in urine)
Coer verapamil	180–540 mg q24h		4–5h					
Verapamil IV		5–10 mg (0.075–0.15 mg/kg)						
Nifedipine	10–40 mg q6–8h	5–15 μg/kg	<20	3 SL	25–100	A hydroxycarbolic acid and a lactone with no known activity. Major hepatic first-pass effect	No	20–40 (fecal) 50–80 (renal) <0.1 (unchanged in urine)
Nifedipine	30–90 mg/d		<60		25–100		No	
Nifedipine GITS	30–180 mg q24h		2h				No	
Nicardipine	10–20 mg tid	1.15 mg/h	<20	<5	28–50	Major hepatic first-pass effect	No	35 (fecal) 60 (renal) <1 (unchanged in urine)

TABLE 4-3 (*continued*)

Agent	Dosage		Onset of Action, min		Therapeutic PC, ng/mL	Site of metabolism	Active metabolites	Excretion, %
	Oral	*IV*	*Oral*	*IV*				
Nicardipine SR	30–60 mg BID		20		28–50			35 (fecal) 60 (renal) <1 (unchanged in urine)
Nicardipine IV		5-15 mg/h		<2–3	60–800	Hepatic	No	
Nimodipine	60 mg q4h		<30		7	Major hepatic first-pass effect	No	
Nisoldipine ER	20–40 mg q24h					Hepatic hydroxylation	Yes	80 (renal), <1 unchanged in urine
Amlodipine	5–10 mg q24h		90–120 in vitro		6–10	Oxidation Extensive but slow hepatic metabolism	No	20–25 (fecal) 60 (renal) 10 (unchanged in urine)
Isradipine	2.5–10 mg q12h		120		nd	Hepatic deesterification and aromatization	No	30 (fecal) 70 (renal) 0 (unchanged in urine)

TABLE 4-3 (*concluded*)

	Dosage		Onset of Action, min					
Agent	*Oral*	*IV*	*Oral*	*IV*	*Therapeutic PC, ng/mL*	*Site of metabolism*	*Active metabolites*	*Excretion, %*
Felodipine ER	5–20 mg q24h		2–5h		2–20 nmol/L	Hepatic microsomal P450 system oxidation Major hepatic first-pass effect	No	10 (fecal) 60–70 (renal) <0.5 (unchanged in urine & feces)
Bepridil	200–400 mg		30–60		1200–3500			70 (renal) 20 (fecal)
Mibefradil	50–150 mg q24h						No	

*PC = plasma concentrations; BID = twice daily; TID = thrice daily; SL = sublingual; nd = no data.
Source: Adapted from Frishman WH, Sonnenblick EH: Calcium channel blockers, in Schlant RC, Alexander RW (eds): *Hurst's The Heart*, 8th ed. New York, McGraw-Hill, 1994, pp 1291–1308, with permission.

CLINICAL APPLICATIONS

The calcium channel blockers are available in the United States for the treatment of patients with angina pectoris (diltiazem, nifedipine, amlodipine, nicardipine, verapamil, bepridil, mibefradil), for chronic treatment of systemic hypertension (verpamil, isradipine, diltiazem, amlodipine, nicardipine, nisoldipine, felodipine, mibefradil), for the management of hypertensive emergencies and perioperative hypertension (intravenous nicardipine), for treatment and prophylaxis of supraventricular arrhythmias (verapamil, diltiazem), and for reducing morbidity and mortality in patients with subarachnoid hemorrhage (nimodipine). These drugs also have been evaluated and used for a multitude of other cardiovascular and noncardiovascular conditions.

Angina Pectoris

The antianginal mechanisms of calcium-entry blockers are complex (Table 4-4). The drugs exert vasodilator effects on the coronary and peripheral vessels as well as depressant effects on cardiac contractility, heart rate, and conduction; all these actions may be important in mediating the antianginal effects of the drugs. These drugs are not only mild

TABLE 4-4 Hemodynamic Effects of Calcium-Entry Blockers on Myocardial O_2 Supply and Demand*

	Verapamil	Nifedipine	Diltiazem	Bepridil	Mibefradil
Demand					
Wall tension	↑↔	↔ reflex	↔	↔	↑↔
Systolic blood pressure	↓	↓	↓	↔	↓
Ventricular volume	↑	↔	↔	↔	↑
Heart rate	↓†	↑ reflex	↑↔	↑↔	↓
Contractility	↓↓	↓	↓	↓	↔
Supply					
Coronary blood flow	↑	↑↑	↑	↑	↑
Coronary vascular resistance	↓	↓↓	↓	↓	↓
Spasm	↓	↓	↓	↓	↓
Diastolic perfusion time	↑	↓	↑↔	↑↔	↑
Collateral blood flow	↔	↑	↑	↔	↑

*↑ = increase; ↓ = decrease; ↔ = no apparent effect.
†Heart rate may increase sharply but decreases with long-term use.
Source: Adapted from Frishman WH, Sonnenblick EH: Calcium channel blockers, in Schlant RC, Alexander RW (eds): *Hurst's The Heart*, 8th ed. New York, McGraw-Hill, 1994, pp 1291–1308, with permission.

dilators of epicardial vessels not in spasm, but they markedly attenuate sympathetically mediated and ergonovine-induced coronary vasoconstriction; these actions provide a rational basis for effectiveness of the drugs in vasospastic ischemic syndromes. In patients with exertional angina pectoris, the peripheral vasodilator actions of diltiazem, mibefradil, and verapamil and the inhibitory effects on the sinus node serve to attenuate the increases in double product that normally accompany, and serve to limit, exercise.

Stable angina pectoris Multiple double-blind placebo-controlled studies have clearly confirmed the efficacy of diltiazem, nifedipine, amlodipine, nicardipine, verapamil, mibefradil, and bepridil in stable angina pectoris, with patients showing a reduction in chest pain attacks and nitroglycerin consumption and improved exercise tolerance. Calcium-entry blockers, for the most, part appear to be as safe and effective as β blockers and nitrates when used as monotherapies in patients. They also can be used as single-dose therapies in hypertensive patients with angina.

In choosing between a calcium channel antagonist and a β-adrenergic blocking drug in the management of patients with effort-related symptoms, it is apparent that some patients do better with one drug than with the other. Unfortunately, little is known about how to predict with confidence the superior agent in a specific patient without a therapeutic trial. However, verapamil and diltiazem can be used as effective alternatives in patients who remain symptomatic despite therapy with propranolol and other β blockers and as first-time antianginal drugs in patients with contraindications to β blockade; the use of nifedipine as a first-line drug in its original formulation was limited by the reflex tachycardia and potential aggravation of angina that accompanied its use. However, this is probably not a problem with the new nifedipine GITS formulation or with amlodipine. Diltiazem is also approved as a once-daily treatment for angina pectoris in a sustained-delivery formulation. Mibefradil was recently approved in doses of 50 and 100 mg for once-daily treatment of angina pectoris.

Bepridil is available in doses of 200 to 400 mg once daily for use in patients with angina pectoris who are refractory to other antianginal drug therapy. Close monitoring of patients with this drug is necessary at the onset of therapy because a small percentage of patients can have a prolongation of the QT interval on the electrocardiogram. Bepridil can be combined with a β blocker if necessary.

The comparative effects of abrupt withdrawal of verapamil and propranolol in patients with angina pectoris have been studied. Ten percent of patients with stable effort-related symptoms experienced a severe clinical exacerbation of the anginal syndrome on withdrawal of propranolol; no patient experienced rebound symptoms when verapamil was discontinued abruptly. There also appear to be no major withdrawal reactions with nifedipine, mibefradil, or diltiazem.

Angina at rest Patients with angina at rest have a wide spectrum of disorders, ranging from those with variant angina (ST elevation) associated with angiographically normal coronary arteries to those with unstable angina with ST depression or elevation associated with multivessel coronary artery disease. Studies suggest that the coronary vasospasm and/or thrombosis plays a major role in the pathogenesis of ischemia in most patients with angina at rest, regardless of the coronary anatomy. In clinical trials, calcium channel antagonists were effective in this syndrome because of their ability to block spontaneous and drug-induced spasm.

The comparative efficacy of verapamil and propranolol was assessed in a randomized, blind crossover trial in rest angina. Only verapamil reduced symptomatic and asymptomatic episodes of ischemia. These findings are consistent with the concept that coronary vasospasm plays a crucial role in patients with angina at rest; in contrast, rather than providing any benefit, propranolol may exacerbate vasospastic phenomena.

Another study assessed the comparative efficacy of verapamil and nifedipine. Both verapamil and nifedipine proved equally effective, and neither drug depressed ventricular function at rest or during exercise. Accordingly, in the management of patients with variant angina, the choice of a calcium antagonist is likely to be determined not so much by which drug is more effective but by which agent is better tolerated by an individual patient.

The usefulness of calcium channel antagonists in the long-term management of unstable angina was demonstrated in a double-blind, randomized clinical trial showing that the addition of nifedipine to patients receiving nitrates and propranolol can reduce the number of patients with unstable anginal syndromes requiring surgery for relief of pain; the incidence of sudden death and myocardial infarction was similar in the two groups. However, clinical benefits were largely confined to patients whose pain was accompanied by ST-segment elevation.

Combination therapy in angina pectoris Combination therapy with nitrates and/or β blockers may be more efficacious for the treatment of angina pectoris than one drug used alone. The hemodynamic effects of a calcium-blocker/β-blocker combination are shown in Table 4-5. Because adverse effects can occur from this combination (heart block, severe bradycardia, congestive heart failure), patients need careful selection and observation. The hemodynamic effects of combined nitrate/calcium channel blocker therapy are shown in Table 4-6. Hypotension should be avoided. Different calcium blockers also may be combined (nifedipine with verapamil or diltiazem) with added benefit; however, side effects may be prohibitive compared with monotherapy.

TABLE 4-5 Hemodynamic Effects of Calcium-Entry Blockers, β Blockers, and Combination Treatment*

	Calcium blockers	β blockers	Combination
Heart rate	↓↔↑ reflex	↓	↓↔
Contractility	↓↔ reflex	↓	↓↔
Wall tension	↓	↔	↓
SBP	↓	↓	↓
LV volume	↓↔	↑	↑↔
Coronary resistance	↓	↑↔	↓↔

*↑ = increase; ↓ = decrease; ↔ = no change.
Source: From Frishman WH: Beta-adrenergic blockade in the treatment of coronary artery disease, in Hurst JW (ed): *Clinical Essays on the Heart*. New York, McGraw-Hill, 1984, p 48.

Arrhythmias

Atrial fibrillation Except in rare situations, verapamil and diltiazem are ineffective in converting acute and chronic atrial fibrillation to normal sinus rhythm (Table 4-7). However, both diltiazem and verapamil (oral and intravenous) are effective for decreasing and controlling ventricular rate during atrial fibrillation by prolonging AV nodal conduction and refractoriness and thereby increasing AV block both at rest and during exercise. Clinical trials with verapamil in patients with atrial fibrillation have shown that its ability to decrease ventricular rate appears to be unrelated to the chronicity of the arrhythmia, its etiology,

TABLE 4-6 Hemodynamic Rationale for Combining Nitrates and Calcium-Entry Blockers in Angina Pectoris*

	Nitrates	Calcium blockers	Combination
Heart rate	↑ reflex	↓↔↑	↑ reflex
Blood pressure	↓	↓	↓↓?
Heart size	↓/0	↓↔↑	0
Contractility	↑ reflex	↓	0
Venomotor tone	↓	0	↓
Peripheral resistance	↓	↓	↓↓?
Coronary resistance	↓	↓	↓↓?
Coronary blood flow	↑	↑	↑↑?
Collateral blood flow	↑	↑	↑↑?

*↑ = increase; ↓ = decrease; ↓↓? = questionable additive effects; ↔ = no change.
Source: From Frishman WH: Beta-adrenergic blockade in the treatment of coronary artery disease, in Hurst JW (ed): *Clinical Essays on the Heart*. New York, McGraw-Hill, 1984, p 48.

TABLE 4-7 Effects of Diltiazem and Verapamil in Treatment of Common Arrhythmias

Effective	Ineffective
Supraventricular tachycardia AV nodal reentrant PSVT* Accessory pathway reentrant PSVT SA nodal reentrant PSVT Atrial reentrant PSVT	Sinus tachycardia Nonparoxysmal automatic atrial tachycardia Atrial fibrillation and flutter in WPW syndrome† (ventricular rate may not decrease)
Atrial flutter (ventricular rate decreases but arrhythmia will only occasionally convert) Atrial fibrillation (ventricular rate decreases but arrhythmia will only occasionally convert)	Ventricular tachyarrhythmias‡

*PSVT = paroxysmal supraventricular tachycardia.
†Wolff-Parkinson-White syndrome.
‡Only limited experience in this area.
Source: From Frishman WH, LeJemtel T: Electropharmacology of calcium channel antagonists in cardiac arrhythmias. *Pace* 5:402,1982, with permission.

or the patient's age. Verapamil appears to be more effective than digoxin in slowing the rapid ventricular rate in response to physical activity. Either diltiazem and verapamil can be used orally in combination with digoxin in treating acute and chronic atrial fibrillation and flutter.

Paroxysmal supraventricular tachycardia Virtually all cases of supraventricular tachycardia due to intranodal reentry and those related to circus movement type of tachycardia in preexcitation respond promptly and predictably to intravenous verapamil or diltiazem, whereas only about two-thirds of ectopic atrial tachycardias convert to sinus rhythm after adequate doses of the drug (see Table 4-7). Intravenous verapamil and diltiazem are highly efficacious in treating reentry paroxysmal supraventricular tachycardia regardless of etiology or age. The recommended dosage range of verapamil for terminating paroxysmal supraventricular tachycardia in adults is 0.075 to 1.5 mg/kg infused over 1 to 3 min, repeated at 30 min. In patients with myocardial dysfunction, the dose should be reduced. Children have been treated safely with a regimen of 0.075 to 0.15 mg/kg. The recommended dose of diltiazem is 0.25 mg/kg infused over 2 min, repeated at 0.35 mg/kg after 15 min.

There have been few clinical studies comparing intravenous verapamil and diltiazem with other standard regimens in the treatment of paroxysmal supraventricular tachycardia. However, in a number of clinical situations verapamil and diltiazem may offer an advantage over either digitalis preparations or β-adrenergic blockers. For instance, verapamil would be preferable in cases where there is an urgent need to terminate paroxysmal supraventricular tachycardia, since it can produce therapeutic responses within 3 min of infusion, whereas the effects of digoxin are not evident for approximately 30 min. Also, if drug therapy fails to achieve normal sinus rhythm, the short duration of action of verapamil and diltiazem permit earlier cardioversion without some of the dangers that accompany electric cardioversion during digoxin therapy. Verapamil and diltiazem also offer distinct advantages over β-adrenergic blocking drugs in patients whose arrhythmias are associated with chronic obstructive lung disease and/or peripheral vascular disease.

Oral verapamil has been approved for prophylaxis against paroxysmal supraventricular tachycardia in doses of 160 to 480 mg/day, and the treatment experiences have yielded favorable results. Diltiazem is not yet approved in oral form as an antiarrhythmic agent.

Atrial flutter The immediate effect of intravenous verapamil and diltiazem in atrial flutter in most patients is an increase in AV block that slows the ventricular response, rarely followed by a return to sinus rhythm (see Table 4-7). In some, the response occurs through the development of atrial fibrillation with a controlled ventricular response. A single intravenous dose of verapamil or diltiazem has been found to be of diagnostic value in differentiating rapid atrial flutter from paroxysmal supraventricular tachycardia when these two arrhythmias are indistinguishable on the electrocardiogram (ECG). If the rhythm is atrial flutter, the AV block increases immediately, revealing the true nature of the arrhythmia. Oral verapamil also has been used to convert paroxysmal atrial flutter and reduce the rapid ventricular rates associated with this arrhythmia.

Preexcitation Verapamil and diltiazem have been found to induce reversion of most cases of accessory pathway supraventricular tachycardia. Using intracardiac recordings of electric activity during programmed electric stimulation of the heart, data have become available regarding the actions of verapamil on the electrophysiologic properties of the accessory pathway in overt cases of the Wolff-Parkinson-White (WPW) syndrome. The drug has a minimal effect on the antegrade and retrograde conduction times and on the refractory period. Verapamil and diltiazem, therefore, terminate accessory pathway paroxysmal supraventricular tachycardia in the same manner as they do AV nodal reentrant paroxysmal supraventricular tachycardia: by slowing AV nodal conduction and increasing refractoriness. The minimal effect of verapamil and diltiazem on the electrophysiologic properties of the bypass tract is consistent with the observation that the drug is ineffective in atrial fibrillation, complicating WPW syndrome, in which fibrillatory impulses, as with digoxin, conduct predominantly through the anomalous pathway. Under these circumstances, radiofrequency catheter ablation of the accessory pathways appears to be the therapy of choice.

Ventricular arrhythmias Intravenous verapamil and diltiazem have no apparent benefit in ventricular arrhythmias except in acute myocardial infarction. Oral verapamil has no demonstrated role in the management of ventricular tachyarrhythmias. However, bepridil, with its class I antiarrhythmic activity, has been shown to be effective in the short- and long-term control of ventricular arrhythmias. In humans, mibefradil has been shown to protect against malignant ventricular arrhythmias induced by cocaine in an experimental model. However, the drugs are not approved in the United States as ventricular antiarrhythmics.

Precautions in Treating Arrhythmias

A diseased SA node is much more sensitive to slow-channel blockers and may be depressed to the point of atrial standstill. Sinus arrest also can occur without overt evidence of "sick sinus syndrome." Calcium channel blockade also may suppress potential AV nodal escape rhythms that need to arise if atrial standstill occurs. In patients with the brady-tachy form of sick sinus syndrome, either digoxin or β-adrenoceptor blocking drugs probably should not be combined with either verapamil or diltiazem in the prophylaxis of tachyarrhythmias unless a demand ventricular pacemaker is first inserted.

Systemic Hypertension

Calcium channel blockers are effective in the treatment of systemic hypertension and hypertensive emergencies. Calcium channel blocking drugs can be considered potential first-line therapy for initiating treatment in many patients with chronic hypertension. A vast experience in the United States has been collected using verapamil, diltiazem, nifedipine, amlodipine, nicardipine, felodipine, and isradipine in patients with hypertension. Verapamil, nicardipine, nifedipine, felodipine, and diltiazem are available in the United States in both conventional and sustained-release oral formulations, allowing once- and twice-daily dosing. Verapamil is available in a unique delayed-onset sustained-release delivery system to provide a peak blood level at the time of blood pressure elevation during awakening. Whether this will influence morbid and mortal events related to hypertension has not been determined. Innovative combination antihypertensive formulations have been evaluated in clinical trials and are now available: enalapril/extended-release diltiazem, benazepril/amlodipine, trandolapril/extended-release verapamil, and extended-release felodipine/extended-release metoprolol.

Studies are now in progress evaluating various calcium channel blockers in elderly patients with isolated systolic hypertension. Three such projects include a large outcomes study using a new dihydropyridine, lacidipine, in comparison with chlorthalidone [Systolic Hypertension in the Elderly: Lacidipine Long-Term (SHELL) Treatment]; the Study of Mild Isolated Systolic Hypertension (SISH), which is evaluating felodipine and chlorthalidone therapy in elderly patients with systolic blood pressure levels between 140 and 160 mmHg, a clinical situation where, as yet, there are no published treatment outcomes data; and the European Study of Systolic Hypertension (EURO-SYS), which evaluated nitrendipine plus enalapril or hydrochlorothiazide in elderly patients with systolic hypertension. A recent report demonstrated the safety and efficacy of nitrendipine in this population.

The calcium blocker drugs reduce both systolic and diastolic pressures with a minimal amount of side effects, including orthostasis. They can cause left ventricular hypertrophy to regress in patients with hypertension. These drugs also may exhibit antiadrenergic and natriuretic activities and can normalize abnormal coronary vasomotion often observed in hypertensive patients. They can be combined with other antihypertensive drugs if necessary (β blockers, angiotensin converting enzyme inhibitors, and diuretics).

Calcium channel blockers are equally effective in black and white patients and in the young and the old. Women may have greater blood pressure lowering effects than men with comparable doses of drug. They do not lower the pressures of normotensive patients. These drugs may be most useful in patients with low-renin, salt-dependent forms of hypertension. In addition, they have been shown to be useful in treating patients with hypertension following heart transplant.

Despite the widespread clinical use of calcium channel blockers for the treatment of hypertension, there are few long-term studies evaluating cardiovascular and cerebrovascular morbidity and mortality outcomes with these treatments. In 1995, there were two published reports suggesting an increased risk of myocardial infarction and mortality in hypertensive patients receiving the short-acting calcium channel blockers (verapamil, diltiazem, nifedipine) as treatment compared with patients receiving other antihypertensive therapies that included diuretics and β blockers. These reports were case control studies that have built within their experimental design significant methodologic flaws. A great debate appeared in the medical literature regarding the safety of calcium channel blockers as a class for treating hypertension. Based on the available evidence, the FDA has advised physicians not to use the short-acting calcium channel blockers for treating hypertension but has placed no restrictions on the first-line supplementary use of sustained-release calcium channel blocker formulations or longer-acting formulations available for this indication where there appears to be no apparent harm with their use. However, a large number of studies are now in progress comparing calcium channel blockers with other antihypertensive treatments to resolve the safety issue with this treatment modality once and for all. To enlarge the controversy, in a large cohort study of 11,545 patients with chronic coronary artery disease, it was shown recently that calcium channel blockers had no greater risk of causing mortality than other drug treatments.

Hypertensive Emergencies and Perioperative Hypertension

Some of the calcium channel blockers also have been shown to be beneficial and safe in patients with severe hypertension and hypertensive crisis. Single oral, sublingual, and intravenous doses of these drugs have rapidly and smoothly reduced blood pressure in adults and children without causing significant untoward effects. The absolute reduction in blood pressure with treatment appears to be inversely correlated with the height of the pretreatment blood pressure level, and few episodes of hypotension have been reported. Continuous hemodynamic monitoring of patients does not seem necessary in most instances. Intravenous nicardipine is approved for clinical use in the treatment of hypertensive emergencies and perioperative hypertension. Its clinical utility compared with other parenteral treatments still needs to be determined.

"Silent" Myocardial Ischemia

In addition to their favorable effects in relieving painful episodes of myocardial ischemia, the calcium blockers are also effective in relieving transient myocardial ischemic episodes (detected by ECG) that are unrelated to symptoms ("silent" myocardial ischemia). Diltiazem, nifedipine (low-dose), amlodipine, and verapamil alone and in combination with β blockers and nitrates have all been shown to be effective in reducing the number of ischemic episodes and their duration. The prognostic importance of relieving silent myocardial ischemia with calcium blockers and other treatments was evaluated in a study sponsored by the National Heart Lung and Blood Institute, the Asymptomatic Coronary Ischemia Pilot (ACIP).

Myocardial Infarction

Several experimental studies have indicated that nifedipine, verapamil, and diltiazem can reduce the size of myocardial necrosis induced in experimental ischemia. Ischemia can lead to diminished ATP production, which eventually can affect the sodium and calcium ion pumps with the ultimate consequence of calcium ion accumulation in the cytoplasm and calcium overload in the mitochondria. Calcium channel blockers can diminish myocardial oxygen consumption and inhibit the influx of calcium ions to the myofibrils and thus favorably influence the outcome of experimental coronary occlusion. These experimental observations have suggested the use of calcium channel blockers for reducing or containing the extent of myocardial infarction during acute coronary artery occlusions in human beings and as an adjunct to cardioplegia during open heart surgery. However, there have been no adequate studies in human beings to support these approaches.

Compared with the established protective actions of some β-blocking drugs used intravenously or orally in prolonging life and reducing the risk of nonfatal reinfarction in survivors of an acute myocardial infarction, the results with calcium channel blockers (diltiazem, lidoflazine, nifedipine, verapamil) have not been as favorable. The results of a metaanalysis looking at the effects of immediate-release nifedipine in patients surviving myocardial infarction even suggested the potential for harm, which also prompted a debate in the literature regarding the safety of calcium channel blockers as a treatment class for patients surviving myocardial infarction.

The plausibility of these mortality results with calcium blockers is supported by a failure to show a beneficial effect on infarct size, development of myocardial infarctions, or reinfarctions in most trials of patients with myocardial infarctions or unstable angina. A trial using diltiazem in patients with non-Q-wave infarction reported a reduction in recurrent myocardial infarction in the diltiazem-treated patients but no reduction in mortality. In a larger trial with diltiazem in infarction survivors, no favorable effects on mortality were seen. A subgroup of patients with left ventricular dysfunction did worse with diltiazem therapy than with placebo; however, diltiazem therapy appeared effective in patients with relatively normal left ventricular function. Similarly, a more recent study did show benefit of verapamil compared with placebo in infarction survivors, with less benefit observed in patients with left ventricular dysfunction.

A double-blind study is in progress comparing diltiazem and aspirin with aspirin alone [Incomplete Infarction Trial of European Research Collaborators Evaluating Prognosis Post-Thrombolysis (INTERCEPT)] in patients with myocardial infarction who had received thrombolytic therapy. The study is enrolling 920 subjects and will evaluate the effects of treatment on the clinical end points of cardiac death, recurrent nonfatal infarction, and medically refractory ischemia.

Prophylactic use of calcium channel blockers to improve patient survival following myocardial infarction cannot be recommended as a first-line therapy unless there are specific indications for using these drugs. However, in patients with contraindications to β-adrenergic blockade, one can consider using verapamil or diltiazem in survivors of myocardial infarction who have good ventricular function.

Hypertrophic Cardiomyopathy

Propranolol remains the therapeutic agent of choice for symptomatic patients with hypertrophic cardiomyopathy. The beneficial effects produced by propranolol derive from its blocking sympathetic stimulation of the heart.

Clinical studies have shown that the administration of verapamil also can improve exercise capacity and symptoms in many patients with hypertrophic cardiomyopathy. The exact mechanism by which verapamil produces these beneficial effects is not known. Acute and chronic verapamil administration reduces left ventricular outflow obstruction, but examination of indices of left ventricular systolic function during chronic therapy shows that this effect does not result from a reduction in left ventricular hypercontractility. Since patients with hypertrophic cardiomyopathy also exhibit abnormal diastolic function, it is likely that improvement in diastolic filling may be responsible in part for the benefit conferred by verapamil. Enhanced early diastolic filling and improvement in the diastolic pressure-volume relation might be expected to result in an increase in left ventricular end-diastolic volume that would decrease the venturi forces that act to move the anterior mitral valve leaflet across the outflow tract toward the septum. The decrease would cause a diminution of obstruction, reducing left ventricular pressure and myocardial wall stress and thus raising the threshold at which symptoms occur.

In a large study of patients with hypertrophic cardiomyopathy refractory to β blockers, verapamil proved to be effective on a long-term basis, with almost 50% of patients showing either a significant improvement in exercise tolerance, an improvement in symptoms, or a reduction in myocardial ischemia. Approximately 50% of patients who were considered to be candidates for surgery because of moderately severe symptoms unresponsive to propranolol showed significant improvement on verapamil, and surgery was no longer considered necessary.

Other studies have reported that chronic administration of verapamil not only can improve symptoms in patients with hypertrophic cardiomyopathy but also can reduce the left ventricular muscle mass and the ventricular septal thickness measured by echocardiographic and ECG analyses. Verapamil and nifedipine were shown to improve the impaired left ventricular filling characteristics. This beneficial effect on left ventricular diastolic relaxation has not occurred after propranolol.

There may be serious and fatal complications of verapamil treatment in patients with hypertrophic cardiomyopathy. These complications result from the accentuated hemodynamic or electrophysiologic effects of the drug. It is not clear whether the fatal complications occur as a result of verapamil-induced reduction in blood pressure with a resultant increase in left ventricular obstruction or the negative inotropic effects of the drug. Verapamil probably should not be used in patients with clinical congestive heart failure. The loss of sequential atrial ventricular depolarization caused by the electrophysiologic effects of the drug also could compromise cardiac function. The adverse electrophysiologic effects are often transient; however, they could prevent the use of larger drug doses that might provide better relief.

If the calcium-entry blocking effects of verapamil are responsible for its therapeutic actions in hypertrophic cardiomyopathy, other drugs in this class also may be useful. However, the results of a double-blind trial comparing verapamil with nifedipine indicated that verapamil is more effective than nifedipine in improving exercise tolerance and clinical symptoms. Diltiazem was shown recently to improve active diastolic function in patients with hypertrophic cardiomyopathy; however, certain patients had a marked increase in outflow obstruction.

Congestive Heart Failure

The potent systemic vasodilatory actions of nifedipine and other dihydropyridine calcium-entry blockers make them potentially useful as afterload reducing agents in patients with left ventricular failure. Unlike other vasodilatory drugs, however, nifedipine also exerts a direct negative inotropic effect on the myocardium that is consistent with its ability to block transmembrane calcium transport in cardiac muscle cells. The successful use of nifedipine as a vasodilator in patients with left ventricular failure would be dependent on its effect to reduce ventricular afterload exceeding its direct negative inotropic actions, thereby leading to an improvement in hemodynamics and forward flow.

Studies evaluating the effect on hemodynamics of nifedipine used in combination with other vasodilators in patients with heart failure have uniformly demonstrated significant reductions in systemic vascular resistance, usually associated with increases in cardiac output. This group and others have found that resting ejection fractions also rise with nifedipine therapy. Reflex increases in heart rate have been reported, but most investigators have found heart rate to remain the same and, in isolated cases, to fall. Left ventricular filling pressures usually decrease or do not change significantly, but there are instances where pulmonary capillary wedge pressures rise with the use of nifedipine in heart failure. Patients with left ventricular dysfunction and nearly normal levels of left ventricular afterload, that is, disproportionately low wall stress, and those with intrinsic fixed mechanical interference to forward flow, such as aortic stenosis, appear most likely to have unfavorable hemodynamic responses to nifedipine therapy. Most of the published data have dealt only with the acute hemodynamic effects of the agent after single sublingual dosing, with little work done on the use of nifedipine as chronic oral therapy for left ventricular failure.

There is a promising experience in clinical trials with the newer dihydropyridine calcium blockers amlodipine and felodipine in patients with congestive cardiomyopathy. A recent study demonstrated the efficacy and safety of diltiazem in patients with idiopathic cardiomyopathy.

Although evidence is incomplete, there are indications that a cardiac tissue renin-angiotensin system may counteract the actions of calcium channel blockers, especially in patients with heart failure. However, since calcium channel blocking drugs are potent vasodilators, particularly on the arterial circulation, the combination of an angiotensin converting enzyme (ACE) inhibitor and a calcium channel blocker might appear to be useful in further augmenting vasodilation, improving myocardial perfusion and ejection fraction. Hence the V-HeFT III trial was conducted to test the efficacy of the combination of felodipine, enalapril, digoxin, and a diuretic in patients with congestive heart failure. The end points evaluated were exercise tolerance, quality of life, left ventricular function, plasma norepinephrine and atrial natriuretic factor levels, and reduction in occurrence of arrhythmias and mortality. A similar pilot multicenter, placebo-controlled study was carried out using amlodipine in addition to ACE inhibitors, digoxin, and diuretics. This study, known as the Prospective Randomized Amlodipine Survival Evaluation (PRAISE), indicated no clear overall mortality or harm from the use of the drug in patients with severe congestive heart failure. Contrary to the prior experiences of the investigators, there appeared to be little effect in the large subgroup of patients who had coronary artery disease and a barely significant reduction in morbidity and mortality in the minority of patients who did not have coronary artery disease. The investigation is being followed up using amlodipine versus placebo in a study of 1800 patients having cardiomyopathy without coronary artery disease, who are receiving digoxin, diuretics, and ACE inhibitors (PRAISE II). Finally, mibefradil, a new nondihydropyridine calcium blocker with little negative inotropic activity, is being evaluated in a double-blind, placebo-controlled trial of 2000 patients with class II-III heart failure (NYHA) who are already receiving digoxin, ACE inhibitors, and diuretics [Mortality Assessment in Congestive Heart Failure (MACH-1)]. The end points of this study include cardiovascular morbidity and mortality, exercise tolerance, and effects of treatment on neurohormonal activity.

In a recent retrospective analysis of the Studies of Left Ventricular Dysfunction where enalapril was compared with placebo in patients with class I–III heart failure, it was observed that those patients who were receiving concomitant immediate-release calcium channel blocker treatment had a higher mortality than subjects who were receiving concomitant β-blocker therapy.

Use of long-acting dihydropyridine calcium blockers as adjunctive vasodilator therapy in patients with left ventricular failure should be considered only if additional clinical reasons for their administration exist, that is, angina pectoris, systemic hypertension, and aortic regurgitation, particularly if these conditions play important contributory roles in the development or exacerbation of left ventricular dysfunction. Some investigators now suggest that calcium antagonists may provide some benefit to patients with predominant diastolic ventricular dysfunction, but more data are needed to substantiate this claim.

Primary Pulmonary Hypertension

Primary pulmonary hypertension is an entity characterized by excessive pulmonary vasoconstriction and increased pulmonary vascular resistance induced by unknown stimuli. Recently, it was suggested that endothelial cell dysfunction and injury may be responsible for the disease process. Typically, the affected patient is a young to middle-age woman presenting with fatigue, dyspnea, chest discomfort, or syncope. Despite many attempts to develop effective therapy, the results of drug treatment generally have been unsatisfactory, and the syndrome continues to bear a poor prognosis.

Based on the currently available data, it may be concluded that some calcium channel antagonists provide beneficial responses in selected patients with pulmonary hypertension. In general, patients with less severe pulmonary hypertension appear to respond better than do those with more advanced disease. Furthermore, early treatment may serve to attenuate progression of the disease.

In patients with chronic hypoxia-induced pulmonary vasoconstriction, the use of calcium channel blockers may be associated with a worsening of ventilation-perfusion mismatching secondary to inhibition of hypoxic pulmonary vasoconstriction.

Cerebral Arterial Spasm and Stroke

A major complication of subarachnoid hemorrhage is cerebral arterial spasm, which may occur several days after the initial event. Such a spasm may be a focal or diffuse narrowing of one or more of the larger cerebral vessels, which may cause additional ischemic neurologic deficits. Although the exact etiology of this spasm is unknown, a combination of various blood constituents and neurotransmitters has been postulated to produce a milieu that enhances the reactivity of the cerebral vasculature. The final pathway for the vasoconstriction, however, involves an increase in the free intracellular calcium concentration. Accordingly, it is reasonable to postulate that the calcium-channel antagonists may have a beneficial effect in reducing cerebral spasm.

Although verapamil and nifedipine have been shown to prevent cerebral arterial spasm in experimental studies, nimodipine and nicardipine, both nifedipine analogues, have demonstrated a preferential cerebrovascular action in this disorder. The lipid solubility of nimodipine enables it to cross the blood-brain barrier; this may account for its more potent cerebrovascular effects. In a multicenter placebo-controlled study involving 125 patients, it was demonstrated that nimodipine significantly reduced the occurrence of severe neurologic deficits following angiographically demonstrated cerebral arterial spasm. All patients had a documented subarachnoid hemorrhage and a normal neurologic status within 96 h of entry into the study. Although 8 of the 60 placebo-treated patients developed a severe neurologic deficit, only 1 of 55 nimodipine-treated patients suffered such an outcome. Nimodipine is now approved for the improvement of neurologic outcome by reducing the incidence and severity of ischemic deficits in patients with subarachnoid hemorrhage from ruptured congenital aneurysms who are in good neurologic condition after ictus. The recommended dose is 60 mg by mouth every 4 h for 21 consecutive days.

Subsequent investigations have suggested that increased cellular calcium concentration may be implicated in neuronal death after ischemia. Nimodipine administered to laboratory animals after global cerebral ischemia had a more favorable effect on neurologic outcome than did placebo. The results of a prospective double-blind, placebo-controlled trial of oral nimodipine administered to 186 patients within 24 h of an acute ischemic stroke showed a reduction in both mortality and neurologic deficit with active treatment. The benefit was confined predominantly to men. However, subsequent studies where nimodipine therapy was begun up to 48 h after the onset of symptoms revealed no benefit of therapy.

Migraine and Dementia

Classic migraine is characterized by prodromal symptoms with transient neurologic deficits. Cerebral blood flow is reduced during these prodromes and then is increased during the subsequent vasodilatory phase, causing severe headache. Because the entry of calcium ions into the smooth-muscle cells is the final common pathway that controls vasomotor tone, calcium antagonists may prevent or ameliorate the initial focal cerebral vasoconstriction.

Results from controlled studies have demonstrated that 80 to 90% of patients with vascular headaches benefit from nimodipine, confirming the selectivity of this agent for the cerebral blood vessels. Verapamil and nifedipine also have been reported to be effective in the prophylaxis of migraine but are less selective for the cephalic blood vessels and thus cause more systemic side effects. Relief from the migraine prodrome usually began 10 to 14 days after initiation of the drugs but could be delayed 2 to 4 weeks. Cerebral vascular resistance was decreased by all three established calcium antagonists, but only nimodipine reduced the cerebral vasoconstriction induced by inhalation of 100% oxygen. None of the calcium-entry blocking drugs is effective against muscle contraction or tension headaches.

Multiple clinical trials are now being carried out to examine the effects of calcium-entry blockers on the progression of dementing illness, both vascular and Alzheimer types. Preliminary results have shown equivocal benefit from treatment.

Noncardiovascular Uses

Amaurosis fugax Hypoperfusion of the retinal circulation may lead to a brief loss of vision in one eye, a syndrome known as *amaurosis fugax*.

This brief loss of sight has been attributed to embolism from the heart or great vessels or to carotid occlusive disease. In a small group of patients with amaurosis but no signs of emboli or carotid hypoperfusion, administration of aspirin or warfarin did not relieve symptoms. However, oral doses of either verapamil or nifedipine abolished attacks. In several patients, the attacks returned when the calcium blocking agent was discontinued.

High-altitude pulmonary edema Hypoxic pulmonary hypertension appears to play a role in the pathogenesis of high-altitude pulmonary edema. Nifedipine has been used for the emergency treatment of this condition, its benefit coming from its ability to reduce pulmonary artery pressure.

Raynaud's phenomenon Raynaud's phenomenon is characterized by well-demarcated ischemia of the digits with pallor or cyanosis ending abruptly at one level on the digits. Nifedipine has been shown to decrease the frequency, duration, and intensity of vasospastic attacks in approximately two-thirds of patients with primary or secondary Raynaud's phenomenon. Patients with primary Raynaud's phenomenon usually demonstrate the most improvement; digital ulcers have been reported to heal in patients with scleroderma. Doses of 10 to 20 mg of nifedipine thrice daily have been used. Felodipine and isradipine are as effective as nifedipine. Diltiazem, 60 to 360 mg daily, also was useful in patients with primary or secondary Raynaud's phenomenon in multiple placebo-controlled trials.

Atherosclerosis

Atherosclerosis develops through numerous and interrelated processes involving the accumulation of cholesterol, calcium, and matrix materials in the major arteries and at lesion sites. Many of the intracellular and extracellular processes involved in atherosclerotic plaque formation require calcium, and it has been suggested that large deposits of cholesterol may trigger physiologic changes in membranes that favor uptake of calcium into the vascular smooth muscle.

The results of recent controlled studies employing angiography have suggested that some calcium channel blockers may retard the progression of atherosclerosis in humans. In the International Nifedipine Trial on Atherosclerosis Coronary Therapy (INTACT) Study, it was shown that nifedipine reduced the formation of new lesions when compared with placebo. However, nifedipine had no effect on the progression or regression of already existing coronary lesions, and an increased mortality compared with placebo was observed.

The administration of nicardipine for 24 months also had no effect on the progression or retardation of advanced stenoses in patients with coronary atherosclerosis, as confirmed by arteriography. However, the drug did appear to retard the progression of small lesions.

Diltiazem was shown to retard the development of coronary artery disease in heart transplant recipients, an action independent of the drug's blood pressure lowering effect.

In the Multicenter Isradipine Diuretic Atherosclerosis Study (MIDAS), which was a 3-year, double-blind, randomized trial designed to compare the effectiveness of isradipine and hydrochlorothiazide in retarding the progression of atherosclerotic lesions in the carotid arteries, no apparent benefit was seen with either treatment. A similar study to MIDAS is now being carried out with a new dihydropyridine calcium antagonist, lacidipine, in the 4-year European Lacidipine Study on Atherosclerosis (ELSA).

Calcium blockers also have been used to treat patients with intermittent claudication and mesenteric insufficiency.

Other Cardiovascular Uses

Diltiazem has been used as part of an ice-cold cardioplegia solution in patients undergoing coronary surgical procedures. The addition of diltiazem appeared to preserve high-energy phosphate levels with an improvement in hemodynamics in the postoperative period. Concomitant use of nifedipine appears to reduce the incidence of myocardial infarction and transient ischemia in patients undergoing bypass surgery.

Intracoronary diltiazem has been used to reduce the severity and delay the onset of ischemic pain in patients undergoing percutaneous transluminal angioplasty. Calcium blockers also have been used as a long-term treatment to prevent restenosis following balloon angioplasty with questionable benefit.

It has been shown that coronary artery vasospasm may be an important pathophysiologic mechanism in explaining some types of experimental cardiomyopathy. Experimentally, verapamil has been shown to reduce vasospasm in response to myocarditis and by this mechanism to prevent the development of cardiomyopathy.

Calcium blockers (diltiazem and verapamil) also have been found to preserve the functioning of human renal transplants. The drugs dilate the preglomerular afferent arterioles and appear to possess inherent immunosuppressive properties and the ability to ameliorate the nephrotoxic effects of cyclosporine.

ADVERSE EFFECTS

In addition to their widely varying effects on cardiovascular function, these agents also have differing spectra of adverse effects (Table 4-8). Immediate-release nifedipine has a very high incidence of minor adverse effects (approximately 40%), but serious adverse effects are uncommon. The most frequent adverse effects reported with nifedipine and other dihydropyridines include headache, pedal edema, flushing, paresthesias, and dizziness. The most serious adverse effects of this

TABLE 4-8 Adverse Effects of Calcium Channel Blockers*

	Overall	Headache	Dizziness	GI	Flushing	Pares-thesia	Decreased SA &/or AV Conduction	CHF	Hypo-tension	Pedal edema	Worsening of angina
Diltiazem	≈5	+	+	+	+	0	3+	+	+	+	0
Diltiazem SR	≈5	+	+	+	+	0	3+	+	+	+	0
Verapamil	8	+	+	3+	0	0	3+	2+	+	+	0
Verapamil SR	≈8	+	+	3+	0	0	3+	2+	+	+	0
Bepridil	15	0	2+	3+	0	0	+	+	0	0	0
Amlodipine	≈15	2+	+	+	+	+	0	0	+	2+	0
Isradipine	≈15	2+	2+	+	+	+	0	0	+	2+	0
Nifedipine	≈20	3+	3+	+	3+	+	0	+	+	2+	+
Nifedipine GITS	≈10	+	+	+	+	+	0	+	+	+	0
Nicardipine	≈20	3+	3+	+	3+	+	0	0	+	2+	+
Nimodipine	15	+	+	+	+	0	0	+	+	+	0
Nisoldipine	≈15	2+	+	+	+	0	2+	0	+	2+	0
Felodipine	20	2+	2+	+	2+	+	0	0	+	2+	0
Mibefradil	≈10	+	+	+	+	0	3+	0	+	+	0

*GI = gastrointestinal; SA = sinoatrial node; AV = atrioventricular node; CHF = congestive heart failure; 0 = no report; + = rare; 2+ = occasional; 3+ = frequent; SR = sustained release; GITS = gastrointestinal therapeutic system.

Source: Adapted from Frishman WH, Stroh JA, Greenberg SM, et al: Calcium-channel blockers in systemic hypertension. *Med Clin North Am* 72:449, 1988, with permission.

drug include exacerbation of angina, which may occur in up to 10% of patients, and occasional hypotension. These side effects are reduced in number with the new long-acting formulation of nifedipine and also may be fewer in number with some of the new dihydropyridine calcium antagonists.

Diltiazem, verapamil, and mibefradil can exacerbate sinus node dysfunction and impair AV nodal conduction, particularly in patients with underlying conduction system disease. The most frequent adverse effect of verapamil is constipation. The drug also may worsen congestive heart failure, particularly when used in combination with β blockers or disopyramide. There have been recent reports of verapamil-induced parkinsonism. Most of the adverse effects noted with diltiazem and mibefradil have been cardiovascular, with occasional headache and GI complaints. The side effects of calcium blockers may increase considerably when these agents are used in combination.

An increased risk of GI hemorrhage in older patients has been reported with calcium channel blockers, as well as intraoperative bleeding during coronary bypass surgery. An increased risk of developing cancer in older subjects also has been reported.

Bepridil, which has class I antiarrhythmic properties, has the potential to induce malignant ventricular arrhythmias. In addition, because of its ability to prolong the QT interval, bepridil can cause torsades de pointes–type ventricular tachycardia. Because of these properties, bepridil should be reserved for patients in whom other antianginal agents do not offer a satisfactory effect.

Drug Withdrawal

Serious problems that appear to be related to heightened adrenergic activity have been reported with abrupt withdrawal of long-term β-blocker therapy in patients with angina. Clinical experiences with calcium-entry blocker withdrawal suggest that although patients with angina get worse after treatment when a calcium-entry blocker is stopped abruptly, there is no evidence of an "overshoot" in anginal symptoms.

Drug Overdose

Calcium-entry blocker overdosage has been described with increasing frequency. The cardiovascular problems associated with this condition are hypotension, left ventricular conduction, bradycardia, nodal blocks, and asystole. Treatment approaches are described in Table 4-9.

Drug-Drug Interactions

There are few data on the interactions of diltiazem with other drugs. Rifampin severely reduces the bioavailability of oral verapamil by enhancing the first-pass liver metabolism of the drug. Both nifedipine

TABLE 4-9 Cardiovascular Toxicity with Calcium Channel Blockers and Recommendations for Treatment

Effects*	Suggested treatment
Profound hypotension	10% calcium gluconate or calcium chloride; norepinephrine or dopamine
Severe LV† dysfunction	10% calcium gluconate or calcium chloride; isoproterenol or dobutamine; glucagon; norepinephrine or dopamine
Profound bradycardia	Atropine sulfate (not always effective)
Sinus bradycardia	10% calcium gluconate or calcium chloride
SA node and AV node block	Isoproterenol or dobutamine
Asystole	External cardiac massage and cardiac pacing (if above measures fail)

*These effects are seen more frequently in patients who have underlying myocardial dysfunction and/or cardiac conduction abnormalities and who are receiving concomitant β-adrenergic blocker treatment.
†LV = left ventricular.
Source: From Frishman WH, Klein NA, Charlap S, et al: Recognition and management of verapamil poisoning, in Parker M, Frishman WH (eds): *Calcium Channel Antagonists in Cardiovascular Disease*. Norwalk, CT, Appleton-Century-Crofts, 1984, pp 365–370, with permission.

and verapamil increase serum digoxin levels, an observation not made with diltiazem. Verapamil has been reported to increase serum digoxin levels by approximately 70%, apparently by decreasing renal clearance, nonrenal clearance, and the volume of distribution. Studies of the time course of this effect show that it begins with the first dose and reaches steady state within 1 to 4 weeks. Nifedipine also has been reported to increase serum digoxin concentrations in patients but to a lesser extent (about 45%). The mechanism for this interaction is not clear. Verapamil and diltiazem have additive effects on AV conduction in combination with digitalis. They can be used to cause further decreases in heart rate compared with digitalis alone when patients are in atrial fibrillation.

Combinations of propranolol with nifedipine or verapamil have been studied extensively for the therapy of angina pectoris. Several studies have shown improved efficacy for the combination of atenolol and nifedipine compared with any of the drugs used alone. Hemodynamic studies have shown mild negative inotropic effects of verapamil in patients on a β blocker. There are also slight decreases in heart rate, cardiac output, and left ventricular ejection fraction. Combinations of nifedipine and propranolol or metoprolol and of verapamil and propranolol are well tolerated by patients with normal left ventricular function, but there may be a greater potential for hemodynamic compromise in patients with impaired left ventricular function with combined verapamil-propranolol treatment. Combinations of diltiazem, nifedipine, or verapamil with nitrates are well tolerated and clinically useful. When diltiazem is combined with nifedipine, blood levels of nifedipine increase significantly, which may contribute to an increased frequency of adverse reactions with this combination. The combination of verapamil with dihydropyridines has not been well studied.

CONCLUSION

Each of the calcium antagonists exerts its effects through inhibition of slow-channel-mediated calcium ion transport. However, many of the drugs appear to accomplish this by different mechanisms and with differing effects on various target organs. These differences allow the clinician to select the particular drug most suitable for the specific needs of the patient. In addition, the side-effect profiles of these drugs (with little overlap between them) assure that most patients will tolerate at least one of these agents.

SUGGESTED READINGS

Frishman WH: Beta-adrenergic blockade in the treatment of coronary artery disease, in Hurst JW (ed): *Clinical Essays on the Heart*. New York, McGraw-Hill, 1984, p 25.

Frishman WH (ed): *Current Cardiovascular Drugs*, 2d ed. Philadelphia, Current Science, 1995.

Frishman WH: Secondary prevention of myocardial infarction: The role of beta-adrenergic blockers, calcium-channel blockers, angiotensin converting enzyme inhibitors and aspirin, in Willich SN, Muller JE (eds): *Triggering of Acute Coronary Syndromes: Implications for Prevention*. Dordrecht, Kluwer Academic Publishers, 1995, pp 367–394.

Frishman WH: Calcium channel blockers, in Frishman WH, Sonnenblick EH (eds): *Cardiovascular Pharmacotherapeutics*. New York, McGraw-Hill, 1997, pp 101–130.

Frishman WH, LeJemtel T: Electropharmacology of calcium channel antagonists in cardiac arrhythmias, *Pace* 5:402, 1982.

Frishman WH, Sonnenblick EH: Beta-adrenergic blocking drugs and Calcium channel blockers, in R. Wayne Alexander, Schlant RC, Fuster V (eds): *Hurst's The Heart*, 9th ed, New York, McGraw Hill, 1994, pp 1583–1618.

Frishman WH, Sonnenblick EH: Cardiovascular uses of calcium-channel blockers, in Messerli F (ed): *Current Cardiovascular Drug Therapy*, 2d ed, Philadelphia, WB Saunders, 1996, p 891.

Frishman WH, Stroh JA, Greenberg SM, et al: Calcium-channel blockers in systemic hypertension. *Med Clin North Am* 72:449, 1988.

Opie LH, Frishman WH, Thadani U: Calcium channel antagonists, in Opie LH (ed): *Drugs for the Heart*, 4th ed, Philadelphia, Saunders, 1995, pp 50–83.

Packer M, Frishman WH (eds): *Calcium Channel Antagonists in Cardiovascular Disease*. Norwalk, CT, Appleton-Century-Crofts, 1984.

Chapter 5

Drugs That Affect the Renin-Angiotensin System

Michael C. Ruddy, John B. Kostis, and William H. Frishman

PHARMACOLOGIC INHIBITION OF THE RENIN-ANGIOTENSIN SYSTEM

Development of ACE Inhibitors and Angiotensin II Receptor Antagonists

As early as 1956, investigators proposed three separate pharmacologic approaches to interfere with the renin-angiotensin system. These included inhibition of the converting enzyme, antagonism of the effects of angiotensin on the vascular smooth muscle, and inhibition of the action of renin on its substrate. Nine years later, Sergio Ferreira, working in São Paulo, Brazil, reported that venom of the Brazilian pit viper, *Bothrops jararaca*, contains a factor that potentiates the pharmacologic actions of bradykinin. Ferreira teamed up with John Vane's laboratory at the Royal College of Surgeons in London and determined that the venom extract contained a series of small peptides that inhibited angiotensin converting enzyme. From here, the story moved across the North Atlantic to the Squibb Institute for Medical Research in Princeton, New Jersey. Cushman and Ondetti were able to further purify and synthesize the venom-derived peptides with angiotensin converting enzyme inhibitory properties. Of these, a nonapeptide, termed *teprotide*, was found to be the most potent inhibitor of ACE. Teprotide was shown in humans to lower blood pressure, especially in those with high circulating renin activity. The clinical potential of teprotide was limited by its peptide nature, requirement for intravenous administration, and short biologic half-life.

Simultaneously, a different approach directed toward production of a competitive antagonist of the angiotensin II receptor was undertaken in the laboratory of Merril Bumpus in Cleveland. Detailed analyses of the structural requirements of angiotensin and studies of many analogues of angiotensin II eventually led to the development of saralasin, a potent angiotensin II receptor antagonist. Saralasin is an octapeptide that differs in structure from angiotension II at the first (sarcosine) and eighth (alanine) amino acid positions. This compound was shown to lower blood pressure and aldosterone levels in humans in proportion to the circulating levels of angiotensin II. Saralasin was later approved for marketing in the United States as a pharmacologic diagnostic screening agent for renovascular hypertension. However, being a peptide with a short half-life, it had to be administered intravenously. Furthermore, saralasin is both an antagonist and agonist at the receptor sites, which explained the occasional pressor responses to this agent in patients with low plasma renin levels. Because of these limitations, along with the development of the orally active converting enzyme inhibitors, saralasin was eventually withdrawn from the market.

Meanwhile at the Squibb Institute, the search for an orally active converting enzyme inhibitor bore fruit in 1976. Miguel Ondetti, Bernard Rubin, and David Cushman developed a hypothetical model of the active site of angiotensin converting enzyme based on its similarities to carboxypeptidase A, another zinc-containing metalloprotein. They designed an inhibitory molecule containing proline because all the naturally occurring peptidic inhibitors had this amino acid as the carboxyl-terminal residue. At the other end of the compound, placement of a mercapto group to serve as a zinc ion ligand created a remarkably potent and specific inhibitor of angiotensin converting enzyme. This agent, termed *captopril*, was seen to have a high level of oral bioavailability and proved to be an effective blood pressure lowering agent in renin-dependent experimental models of hypertension, such as the two-kidney renal hypertensive rat. Captopril was approved for use by the FDA in 1981. Since then, many additional ACE inhibitors have been developed and marketed by the pharmaceutical industry. These agents differ in bioavailability, pharmacokinetics, affinity for the ACE, effects on enzyme kinetics, tissue solubility, and other properties (see below).

The search for orally active angiotensin II receptor antagonists continued. Timmermans and colleagues at the Dupont Pharmaceutical Company in Delaware investigated an imidazoline derivative originally discovered in Japan. This was structurally modified to losartan, the first orally active angiotensin II receptor antagonist. Unlike saralasin, which blocks both the AT_1 and AT_2 receptor subtypes, losartan blocks only AT_1 receptors. Also, losartan does not have receptor agonist activity. Since the discovery of losartan, there are many other nonpeptide angiotensin receptor antagonists under development with differing pharmacokinetic properties and specificity for the AT_1 and AT_2 receptor subtypes.

Pharmacologic Effects of ACE Inhibitor Therapy

The most important effect of these agents on the renin-angiotensin system is to inhibit the conversion of the inactive decapeptide angiotensin I to the biologically active octapeptide angiotensin II. In this manner they suppress responses to circulating or tissue angiotensin I but not to angiotensin II. All the currently available converting enzyme inhibitors are quite specific in that they do not directly interact with other enzyme systems in the body. However, it is important to keep in mind that converting enzyme itself has many potential substrates. The ACE inhibitors have been shown to slow the metabolic degradation of a number of biologically important peptides, of which bradykinin is the best known. In primary cell cultures, exposure to bradykinin enhances prostaglandin E_2 (PGE_2) generation as a result of stimulation of phospholipase A_2, a cell membrane–bound enzyme responsible for the production of arachidonic acid and its metabolites from phospholipids. ACE inhibitors also have been shown to slow the breakdown of other peptides including humoral mediators such as substance P and LHRH. Thus ACE inhibitors may have an indirect impact on a wide range of physiologically important systems.

Effects of ACE Inhibitors on Blood Pressure of Normotensives

In sodium-replete normotensives, ACE inhibitors have virtually no effect when given acutely. However, with continued chronic administration, there is a small reduction of blood pressure without hypotension. In contrast, a single dose of a rapidly acting ACE inhibitor such as captopril markedly lowers blood pressure in normal subjects who have been sodium depleted by restriction of dietary salt.

Effects of ACE Inhibitors in Hypertensives

Hemodynamic Effects

Blood pressure Primary or essential hypertension is by far the most common form of human hypertension. The view is held that the renin-angiotensin system plays an active or at least permissive role in a large majority of hypertensives. Angiotensin converting enzyme inhibitors have been shown consistently to lower blood pressure when used as monotherapy in more than 50% of patients. Several studies have shown that the initial decline in blood pressure is positively correlated with baseline plasma renin activity and angiotensin II levels. Long-term response to ACE inhibitors is less closely correlated with plasma renin activity at baseline. Nevertheless, white hypertensives generally respond better to this class of agents than do African-American patients, perhaps because of the higher mean plasma renin activity observed in whites. With chronic therapy some individuals may experience an attenuation of the antihypertensive effect. Addition of a thiazide diuretic restored the efficacy in most such patients. It has been suggested that because plasma renin tends to decline with age, the ACE inhibitors might be less efficacious in older patients. However, results of clinical trials indicate that responsiveness to the ACE inhibitors is little if at all affected by age (Table 5-1). ACE inhibitors are effective in reducing pressure in patients with transplantation.

Systemic circulatory effects The fall in systemic blood pressure seen with ACE inhibitor therapy results from a reduction of total peripheral resistance. Heart rate and cardiac output generally remain unchanged during ACE inhibitory therapy. The lack of tachycardic response to the

TABLE 5-1 Antihypertensive Mechanisms of Angiotensin Converting Enzyme Inhibitors

Inhibition of angiotensin II formation
Plasma—endocrine function
Inhibition of vasoconstriction
Inhibition of aldosterone synthesis and release
Tissue—autocrine, paracrine
Potentiation of kallikrein-kinin system
Circulating kinin
Local kinins
Kinin stimulation of phospholipase A leading to production of arachidonic acid
Enhanced production of vasodilatory prostaglandins
Inhibition of sympathetic nervous activity
Peripheral adrenergic terminals
Centrally mediated sympathetic outflow

vasodilating effects of the ACE inhibitors has not been fully explained. It seems likely that attenuation of centrally mediated sympathetic responses, in addition to augmentation of parasympathetic vagal tone, plays a role in maintenance of stable heart rates during ACE inhibitor therapy. With regard to the vasodilatatory effects, there is considerable variability observed in different vascular beds. Pulmonary vascular resistance is not affected by ACE inhibitors, whereas renal resistance is consistently reduced by ACE inhibitors.

Both captopril and enalapril have been shown to attenuate the peak blood pressure increase produced by moderately strenuous physical exercise. The exercise-induced rise in heart rate and cardiac output are not affected by ACE inhibition, although the latter may be reduced by concomitant use of diuretics.

ACE inhibitors also may reduce blood pressure and reverse left ventricular hypertrophy by improving aortic compliance.

Renal circulation Renal vascular tone is generally elevated in the majority of hypertensive patients. Administration of ACE inhibitors augments renal blood flow in proportion to the degree of activation of the renin-angiotensin system. This is thought to be mediated by a preferential vasodilatation of the glomerular efferent arterioles. Thus intraglomerular hydrostatic pressure remains unchanged, and the increase in renal blood flow occurs without an increase in glomerular filtration rate.

Coronary circulation In both hypertensives and normotensives, coronary blood flow depends primarily on autoregulatory mechanisms that adjust blood supply according to myocardial oxygen demand. The coronary vascular bed is less sensitive to the constrictor effects of angiotensin II. Thus, under normal circumstances, the coronary vasodilatory effect of ACE inhibitors is minimal. However, when the renin-angiotensin system is activated, such as with diuretic-induced volume depletion, coronary artery resistance is increased. This effect can be reversed by acute ACE inhibition despite the concurrent fall in systemic blood pressure.

In patients with known coronary artery disease, ACE inhibitors can improve endothelial vasomotor dysfunction perhaps by enhancing endothelial cell release of nitric oxide secondary to diminished breakdown of bradykinin. ACE inhibitors also can protect against nitrate tolerance and nitrate withdrawal–induced vasoconstriction.

Cerebral circulation Cerebral blood flow is normally kept constant over a wide range of systemic blood pressure via autoregulatory mechanisms. Chronic hypertensives tend to exhibit an autoregulation curve that is shifted to the right, that is, toward maintenance of cerebral perfusion at higher pressures. These patients may be especially prone to impairment of cerebral perfusion when blood pressure falls rapidly. It appears that in most circumstances, ACE inhibitor therapy preserves cerebral autoregulation and does not impair cerebral blood flow. Several clinical studies have observed an increase in cerebral blood flow after several days of ACE inhibitor therapy. This effect appeared to be most prominent in those with the greatest initial decline in systemic blood pressure. In spontaneously hypertensive rats, it has been shown that ACE inhibitor administration is associated with a rapid shift in the lower limit of cerebral autoregulation by as much as 20 to 30 mmHg.

Humoral Effects of Neurohumoral Systems

Renin secretion The initial dose of an ACE inhibitor stimulates a rise in plasma renin activity of approximately 25 to 50% in the majority of normotensives and essential hypertensives. With chronic ACE inhibitor monotherapy, plasma renin declines toward baseline but may remain slightly above pretreatment levels. At least two factors are involved in causing the initial rise in renin. First, the initial prompt fall in systemic blood pressure lowers renal perfusion pressure at the level of the preglomerular afferent arteriole. The decline in preglomerular hydraulic pressure promotes local baroreceptor-mediated renin release from the juxtaglomerular apparatus. Second, the juxtaglomerular cells have a high density of AT_1 angiotensin II receptors, which act to mediate negative feedback control of renin release. The ACE inhibitor–induced fall in angiotensin II level disinhibits renin secretion from the juxtaglomerular apparatus, thereby amplifying the baroreceptor-mediated rise in plasma renin activity. The mechanisms responsible for the return toward pretreatment renin secretory rate that has been observed with chronic ACE inhibitor therapy remain poorly understood.

Aldosterone secretion Angiotensin II is the primary secretagogue for aldosterone release by the adrenal zona glomerulosa. Adrenocortical cells of the zona glomerulosa have a very high density of AT_1 receptors. ACE inhibitor–induced fall of angiotensin II predictably and substantially lowers serum and urinary aldosterone levels. With chronic ACE inhibitor treatment, both angiotensin II and aldosterone levels return toward baseline values. Adrenal aldosterone release can be augmented by rises in serum potassium and ACTH, thereby blunting the initial effect of reduced angiotensin II.

Kallikrein-Kinin System

There are important interactions between the renin-angiotensin and kinin system. Angiotensin converting enzyme inactivates the nonapeptide bradykinin by cleavage of the carboxyl-terminal dipeptide. Thus ACE inhibitors can be expected to increase circulating and tissue bradykinin levels. Increased bradykinin levels may have several important implications in the setting of ACE inhibitor therapy. Bradykinin is a vasodilator that may supplement the vasodepressor effect of reducing angiotensin II levels on peripheral resistance and blood pressure. This may explain in part why ACE inhibitors are sometimes quite effective in lowering the blood pressure of patients with low plasma renin activity. Bradykinin also has been found to stimulate the production of vasodilator prostaglandins such as PGE_2 and PGI_2, an action that would tend to further augment the blood pressure lowering actions of the ACE inhibitors. Several of the adverse effects of ACE inhibitor therapy, including cough and angioneurotic edema, have been linked to inhibition of bradykinin metabolism by these agents.

Interactions of ACE Inhibitors with the Sympathetic Nervous System

It has been long known that central administration of angiotensin to experimental animals increases sympathetic efferent nerve activity. The blood-brain barrier is relatively impermeable to components of the renin-angiotensin system. It is still uncertain whether circulating angiotensin can gain access to the brain through some areas such as the subfornical organs or area postrema. Nevertheless, all the components of the renin-angiotensin system can be synthesized within the central nervous system. Furthermore, there is evidence that several of the ACE inhibitors penetrate the blood-brain barrier in sufficient concentration to suppress brain angiotensin II formation. At the periphery, angiotensin II has been shown to facilitate norepinephrine release and inhibit its reuptake by prejunctional sympathetic nerve terminals. It has been proposed that ACE inhibition attenuates peripheral sympathetic activity by reducing systemic and local angiotensin II levels.

Other Metabolic Effects of ACE Inhibitors

In recent decades there has been increasing concern about the possible detrimental effects of several classes of antihypertensive therapy on cardiovascular risk factors. Increases in serum glucose, lipids, and uric acid have all been linked to coronary heart disease risk. Potassium depletion may enhance risk of developing serious cardiac arrhythmia in susceptible individuals.

The weight of evidence indicates that ACE inhibitors have little or no effect on serum levels of total, low-density, and very-low-density cholesterol. Serum triglyceride levels are also generally unchanged. There is some evidence that high-density serum apolipoproteins A-I and A-II are raised somewhat during ACE inhibitor therapy. It appears that carbohydrate disposition may actually be facilitated by captopril treatment. The mechanism for the latter action is not well understood but may be due in part to higher bradykinin levels produced by ACE inhibitor therapy.

There is good evidence that ACE inhibitors have a mild uricosuric action. Moreover, diuretic-induced hyperuricemia is usually lessened somewhat by concomitant use of ACE inhibitors.

Serum potassium levels are usually slightly higher during monotherapy with ACE inhibitors. ACE inhibitors, by blocking angiotensin II formation, suppress adrenal aldosterone secretion. Thus renal excretion of potassium is reduced, resulting in a slight rise in serum levels. This effect of ACE inhibitors may be especially beneficial when diuretics are being used concurrently. Hyperkalemia is a significant risk for patients with renal impairment, diabetes mellitus, or those receiving potassium-sparing or nonsteroidal anti-inflammatory agents (Table 5-2).

ADVERSE EFFECTS OF ACE INHIBITOR THERAPY

In 1981, captopril became the first ACE inhibitor to receive approval for use in the United States. At that time the Food and Drug Administration (FDA)–approved indication for this agent was restricted to treatment of hypertension which had proved resistant to available multidrug antihypertensive therapy. Early concerns about bone marrow suppressive effects of this agent were fortunately allayed with lower dose regimens and appropriate patient selection. Since then, extensive clinical experience with ACE inhibitors has found them to be effective and well tolerated. Since 1981, eight additional ACE inhibitors have been approved for prescription use in the United States. Each has been approved for first-line treatment of all levels of hypertension. Several ACE inhibitors have indications that extend beyond treatment of hypertension. The most recent reports of the Joint National Committee for the Detection, Evaluation and Treatment of Hypertension (JNC-V and JNC-VI) also have included ACE inhibitors among the recommended first-line therapies, especially for patients having concomitant heart failure with systolic dysfunction, and in patients with diabetes mellitus and renal disease.

Nevertheless, ACE inhibitors are not free of the potential for adverse effects, some of which can have serious consequences. Clinicians

TABLE 5-2 Hemodynamic and Hormonal Effects of ACE Inhibition in Patients with Hypertension and Heart Failure*

Hemodynamic parameter	Hypertension	Heart failure
Blood pressure	↓	→↓
Systemic vascular resistance	↓	↓
Heart rate	→	→↓
Stroke volume	→	↑
Cardiac output	→	↑
Ejection fraction	→	↑
Pulmonary capillary wedge pressure	→	↓
Right atrial pressure	→	↓
Renal blood flow	→↑	→↑
Renal vascular resistance	→↓	→↓
Glomerular filtration rate	→	→↑↓
Forearm blood flow	↑	↑
Capacitance of large vessels	↑	↑
Cerebral blood flow	→↑	→↑
Coronary blood flow	→↑	→↑
Exercise capacity	→↑	↑
Angiotensin II	↓	↓
Angiotensin I	↑	↑
Renin	↑	↑
Aldosterone	↑→	↓
Converting enzyme activity	↓	↓
Kinin levels	↑→	↑→
Plasma norepinephrine	→	→↓
Prostaglandins (urinary)	→↑	→↑

* ↑ = increase; ↓ = decrease; → = unchanged.
Source: Modified with permission from Kostis JB, DeFelice EA (eds): *Angiotensin Converting Enzyme Inhibitors*. New York, Alan R Liss, 1987.

should be aware of these problems and be prepared to closely monitor patients at risk.

Hypotension

The initial fall in blood pressure induced by ACE inhibitors is proportional to the pretreatment plasma renin activity. Those patients with a highly activated renin-angiotensin system are most prone to a precipitous decline in blood pressure when starting treatment. There is risk that such a rapid fall in blood pressure can cause impairment of organ function including brain, heart, and kidneys. This may, in susceptible patients, lead to serious ischemic events such as stroke, myocardial ischemia, or acute renal failure. Patients at greatest risk are the elderly but may include anyone with highly renin-dependent blood pressure. Dehydration and diuretic therapy are two of the most common predisposing factors. Patients with severe congestive heart failure, especially if already taking large doses of diuretics, are also at increased risk of acute hypotension. Two other high-risk groups with elevated circulating renin activity include those with occlusive renovascular disease and those with malignant hypertension. When ACE inhibitors are administered in these clinical settings, it's generally prudent to use low initial doses with close patient monitoring. Hypotension, if it does occur, usually can be managed successfully by assumption of the supine position and rapid intravenous infusion of saline solution.

Hyperkalemia

As outlined above, ACE inhibitor–induced decline of aldosterone secretion is associated in most patients with a very small rise in serum potassium level. In patients with normal renal function, clinically significant hyperkalemia is very uncommon. However, patients with even minor degrees of renal impairment, especially those with diabetic nephropathy, are more prone to hyperkalemia. The chronic use of potassium salts, potassium-sparing diuretics, or nonsteroidal anti-inflammatory drugs also may pose an increased hazard. In any of these settings, close monitoring of serum electrolyte levels is warranted, with removal of potentially offending agents as indicated.

Functional Renal Impairment

When ACE inhibitors are given to normal subjects, there is a drop in renal perfusion pressure because the lower angiotensin II levels produce a mild renal vasodilatory effect, predominantly in the postglomerular efferent arterioles. Glomerular filtration rate is generally little affected because there is a concurrent increase in renal blood flow. However, when renal blood flow is impeded by a progressively worsening arterial occlusive process, glomerular filtration rate is preserved at or near normal levels of autoregulation. As renal perfusion pressure declines, baroreceptor-mediated renin release leads to an increase in angiotensin II, which in turn preferentially constricts the postglomerular efferent arterioles. Intraglomerular filtration pressure is thereby preserved until the occlusion becomes advanced. In this setting, administration of ACE inhibitors could be expected to interfere with glomerular autoregulation by attenuating its key element, postglomerular vasoconstriction.

In patients with unilateral renal artery stenosis and a normal contralateral kidney, ACE inhibitors do not produce a clinically evident reduction in renal function. However, when sensitive split renal functional studies are performed, impairment of function in the affected kidney often can be observed. It is not yet known whether this has long-term negative consequences. In patients with bilateral renal artery stenosis or arterial stenosis to a solitary kidney or to a renal allograft,

ACE inhibitors have been shown to cause a deterioration of renal function evidenced by a rise in serum creatinine. It has been suggested that such a rise in serum creatinine after institution of ACE inhibitor therapy may serve as a screening test for one of these forms of renovascular disease. In most but not all cases, renal function returns to pretreatment values following discontinuation of the offending ACE inhibitor.

ACE inhibitor–induced reversible renal impairment also may occur in the setting of underlying renal parenchymal disease of any type if dehydration or concomitant diuretic therapy is present. Another vexing problem is that some patients with severe congestive heart failure experience a rise in serum creatinine following institution of ACE inhibitors. If the rise in creatinine is clinically important, then a reduction or discontinuation of ACE inhibitor therapy or an evaluation for renal vascular disease may be warranted. However, a very slight deterioration of renal function may be acceptable if outweighed by the symptomatic improvement in heart failure.

Before initiating therapy with an ACE inhibitor, all patients should have serum electrolytes, creatinine, and blood urea nitrogen determined. Patients at risk for renal impairment should be monitored especially closely, usually within a few weeks after initiation or adjustment of treatment and following the addition or dose modification of any diuretics. Patients with abnormal renal function noted before treatment with ACE inhibitors should be monitored even more frequently during such therapy.

ACE Inhibitor Cough

It is remarkable that the now well-known association between ACE inhibitors and cough was not generally recognized for more than 5 years after ACE inhibitors were in wide clinical use. This usually nonproductive dry cough, although not a serious problem, can be quite uncomfortable. Patients often describe a "tickle in the throat" that precedes fits of coughing that may be severe enough to cause retching. Estimates of the incidence of dry cough among those receiving ACE inhibitor therapy vary from 5 to 15%. The onset of this symptom is usually within several weeks of starting ACE inhibitor treatment, but it also may begin after several years of uneventful therapy. Typically, the physical examination is unremarkable, with no wheezing or other signs of bronchospasm or pneumonitis evident.

The mechanism of ACE inhibitor cough is thought to be linked to slowed metabolic degradation of the peptides bradykinin and substance P. Bradykinin in turn augments synthesis of arachidonic acid by-products, some of which are protussive in nature. Bradykinin and especially substance P are agonists at peripheral cough receptors found in the lung.

Most controlled studies have failed to demonstrate a beneficial response to changing ACE inhibitors or dose adjustment. However, there are anecdotal reports of benefit derived from the following: reduction of dose, change to a less potent ACE inhibitor, and use of nonsteroidal anti-inflammatory agents or sodium cromoglycate.

Angioneurotic Edema

The risk of angioedema is estimated to be between 0.1 and 0.2% in patients receiving angiotensin converting enzyme inhibitors. Angioedema usually involves the face and oropharyngeal tissues and can result in acute airway obstruction that requires emergency intervention. It has been reported with a first dose as well as after prolonged exposure. Angioedema has been reported to occur when substituting one ACE inhibitor for another. It is generally agreed that ACE inhibitors should not be used at all in an individual who has been so affected. The mechanism for the edema is not certain but is probably linked to inhibition of bradykinin metabolism.

Skin Rash

Early estimates suggested that skin rash developed in 5 to 10% of patients taking captopril. The rash usually manifests as a morbilliform or maculopapular eruption, affecting the upper extremities, torso, and legs. Pruritus is variable but may occur in the absence of a visible rash. There may be associated eosinophilia. The rash invariably disappears on discontinuation of ACE inhibitor therapy and in some milder cases may disappear despite continued treatment. In most recent studies, the incidence of skin rash is much lower than reported earlier. It has been suggested that the reaction is less likely to occur with more recently marketed ACE inhibitors that do not contain a sulfhydryl moiety.

Dysgeusia

Alteration or loss of taste was an interesting side effect seen early on with high doses of captopril. It was variously described as a salty, metallic, or rotten egg taste or simply lack of any taste. In some cases the altered taste sensation resulted in weight loss. Early on it had been suggested that altered taste was the result of chelation with zinc, which is known to play a role in normal gustation. Oral zinc supplementation was recommended but never proved to counteract the high-dose captopril–induced taste disturbances. It has been suggested that more subtle abnormalities of taste may occur with any of the currently available ACE inhibitors, but this has not been well studied.

Hematologic Effects

Neutropenia and agranulocytosis were serious adverse effects seen early in the development of captopril when very high doses, in the range of 150 to 600 mg/day, were utilized. This was most likely to occur in patients with connective tissue disorders such as systemic lupus erythematosus and renal insufficiency. Use of allopurinol or immunosuppressive agents was an additional risk factor. With current dosing regimens for ACE inhibitors including captopril, neutropenia is almost never seen.

A slight reduction of hemoglobin is known to occur commonly with all ACE inhibitors, even when used in recommended doses. This is probably due to a reduction of erythropoietin levels. For many patients this may be a potential benefit in reducing blood viscosity. ACE inhibitors have been employed successfully in patients with erythrocytosis following renal transplantation and may have a therapeutic effect in patients with other forms of polycythemia.

Teratogenic Effects

Studies in experimental animals have suggested that ACE inhibition may pose a significant risk of fetal developmental disorders. In humans, use of ACE inhibitors in the second and third trimesters of pregnancy has been associated with fetal skeletal abnormalities and neonatal renal failure and death. These adverse effects do not seem to have been associated with ACE inhibitor use during the first trimester. However, it is recommended that ACE inhibitor therapy be discontinued when pregnancy is diagnosed and not be employed during pregnancy unless the individual benefits are judged to outweigh the risks.

Idiosyncratic Adverse Experiences

During the first several years of clinical use, there were several well-documented reports of nephrotic syndrome associated with captopril therapy. In most cases, histopathologic studies demonstrated the presence of membranous glomerulopathy. This entity has not been reported in recent years, suggesting that membranous glomerulopathy may be a risk only at high doses of captopril.

Hepatic injury also has been attributed to ACE inhibitor therapy. This takes the form of cholestatic jaundice, hepatocellular injury, or a mixed cholestatic-hepatocellular type. It has been most commonly associated with high-dose captopril or enalapril treatment. Rarely, it has progressed to fulminant hepatic necrosis. In some cases, jaundice has been reported to persist for up to 6 months.

There have been case reports of anaphylactoid reactions in patients undergoing hemodialysis with high-flux dialysis membranes (e.g., AN 69) who were on concomitant ACE inhibitor therapy (Table 5-3).

DRUG INTERACTIONS

Diuretics

Patients on diuretics may experience an excessive reduction of blood pressure after initiation of ACE inhibitor therapy. The possibility of hypotensive effects can be minimized by either discontinuing the

TABLE 5-3 Adverse Effects of ACE Inhibitor Therapy

Hypotension
Renal effects
Hyperkalemia
Functional renal impairment
Acute renal failure
Nephrotic syndrome
Cough
Skin rash
Angioneurotic edema
Taste disturbances
Hemodialysis-associated anaphylaxis
Hematologic
Leukopenia
Anemia
Hepatobiliary
Cholestasis
Hepatocellular dysfunction
Teratogenic effects*
Skeletal malformations
Neonatal renal failure

*Use of ACE inhibitors is contraindicated during pregnancy.

diuretic or increasing salt intake prior to starting ACE inhibitor therapy. If it is necessary to continue the diuretic, use of a small dose of ACE inhibitor along with close medical supervision for the first several hours after the initial dose is indicated.

Use of potassium-sparing diuretics such as triamterene, spironolactone, or amiloride with ACE inhibitors increases the likelihood of developing hyperkalemia. If concomitant use of these agents is indicated because of demonstrated hypokalemia, they should be used with caution and with frequent monitoring of serum electrolytes.

Other Cardiovascular Agents

ACE inhibitors have been used with β blockers, methyldopa, nitrates, calcium antagonists, hydralazine, prazosin, and digoxin without adverse interactions. Aspirin could interfere with the protective effects of ACE inhibitors in patients with heart failure, but this needs to be defined more closely.

Nonsteroidal Anti-Inflammatory Agents

Indomethacin has been shown to impair the blood pressure lowering response to ACE inhibitors, especially in low-renin hypertensives. Hyperkalemia also may be more likely with concomitant use of ACE inhibitors and nonsteroidal anti-inflammatory agents.

Lithium

Lithium toxicity has been reported in patients receiving lithium concomitantly with drugs that cause elimination of sodium, including ACE inhibitors. Thus lithium levels should be monitored more closely when this agent is used in the setting of ACE inhibitor therapy.

CLINICAL USES OF ACE INHIBITORS

Primary (Essential) Hypertension

There is no evidence that the currently available ACE inhibitors have an antihypertensive mechanism of action other than specific inhibition of converting enzyme. The events following inhibition of the enzyme are less well understood.

In experimental animals, ACE inhibitors reduce blood pressure most effectively in models in which the plasma renin level is elevated, such as the 2-kidney-1-clip and sodium-restricted 1-kidney-1-clip hypertensive models. Models in which the plasma renin is low, such as the desoxycorticosterone acetate–salt (Doca/salt) and sodium-replete 1-kidney-1-clip, are less sensitive to the blood pressure lowering effects of ACE inhibitors. In humans with primary hypertension, there is a positive correlation between initial blood pressure response to ACE inhibitors and plasma renin activity. These findings favor a primary role for the reduction of angiotensin II as the mechanism of action. In addition, if low-renin animal models or humans with low plasma renin activity are treated with diuretics, they become more sensitive to the blood pressure lowering effects of ACE inhibitors.

Studies in hypertensive humans have demonstrated that ACE inhibitors given as monotherapy produce an immediate fall in blood pressure in about 70% of patients. The antihypertensive effect is sustained in 50 to 60% of patients. All currently available ACE inhibitors have been approved for use in the treatment of hypertension, and there appears to be little difference among them in antihypertensive efficacy.

Generally, African-American patients, who as a group tend to have lower renin levels, respond less well to ACE inhibitor monotherapy than do whites. Racial differences in blood pressure responses are markedly attenuated by the concurrent use of diuretics. Elderly patients, who also tend to have lower renin levels, seem to respond nearly as well as younger hypertensive subjects. ACE inhibitors are now recognized by the Joint National Committee for the Detection, Evaluation and Treatment of High Blood Pressure as an option for first-line therapy in primary hypertension.

In selecting initial therapy for hypertension, one useful strategy is to take account of concomitant medical disorders. ACE inhibitors have been shown to have a neutral or beneficial effect on levels of serum lipids, glucose, and uric acid. Thus these agents may be especially suitable in patients with dyslipidemia, carbohydrate intolerance, or hyperuricemia. Also, there have been no deleterious effects of ACE inhibitors on pulmonary function tests. ACE inhibitors have been used successfully to treat hypertensives with chronic obstructive pulmonary disease. Furthermore, there appears to be little or no adverse effect of ACE inhibitors on sexual or cognitive function.

Renovascular Hypertension

When hemodynamically significant narrowing of the arterial supply to one kidney is present, plasma renin levels are frequently increased. The hypertension associated with unilateral renovascular occlusive disease is often difficult to treat with agents that do not interfere with action of the renin-angiotensin system. In these patients, ACE inhibitors are usually very effective in reducing blood pressure, often without requiring a multidrug regimen.

In the setting of renal artery stenosis, the diminution of angiotensin II levels following ACE inhibition can have an adverse effect on function of the kidney distal to the stenosis. As renal perfusion pressure declines with progressive arterial narrowing, glomerular filtration pressure becomes more dependent on angiotensin II. Angiotensin II exerts its vasoconstrictive effect predominantly on the postglomerular (efferent) arterioles. This selective action of angiotensin II helps to maintain intraglomerular pressure as preglomerular pressure perfusion is falling. ACE inhibitors, by reducing angiotensin II production, can interfere with glomerular autoregulation and lead to a decline of glomerular filtration rate.

ACE inhibitor–associated azotemia and hypercreatininemia have been observed in patients with bilateral renal artery stenosis and in patients with renal artery stenosis to a solitary kidney. Generally, the impairment of renal function in this setting is reversible after withdrawal of the ACE inhibitor. In many cases of this type, plasma renin levels are low normal and the hypertension is resistant to ACE inhibitor monotherapy. Addition of diuretics is often helpful in lowering the blood pressure but may significantly amplify the risk of renal impairment.

Reduction of glomerular function has been shown to occur in the affected kidney in cases of unilateral renal artery stenosis where the contralateral renal circulation is intact. However, renal failure does not develop because the intact kidney compensates for the decrease in the affected side. Major determinants of the response of a stenotic kidney to ACE inhibition include the degree of fall in systemic blood pressure, the severity of occlusion, and the level of plasma renin.

The presence of renal artery stenosis does not completely preclude the use of ACE inhibitors. However, there are certain precautions that should be followed in this setting. Serum creatinine level should be assessed at baseline and, depending on the pretreatment value, within a few days to weeks of initiating or altering ACE inhibitor therapy. Renal function also should be rechecked following the addition or modification of supplemental antihypertensive agents, especially diuretics. If renal function is seen to decline, then a dose reduction or discontinuation of the ACE inhibitor or diuretic may be indicated.

Hypertensive Emergencies

Idiopathic malignant hypertension and accelerated hypertension in the setting of renovascular disease are two conditions in which the renin-angiotensin system is likely to be highly activated. Most oral ACE inhibitors have an onset of action within a few hours of dosing. Of these, captopril has the shortest onset of action, within 30 to 60 min, a special advantage in the emergent setting. Orally administered captopril also has the shortest duration of action, a property that allows more frequent dose adjustment. Enalaprilat, the hydrolyzed, active form of enalapril, has an onset of action within a few minutes of bolus intravenous administration. For patients unable to receive oral medication because of neurologic or GI impairment, parenteral enalaprilat may be lifesaving.

Scleroderma renal crisis is another hypertensive emergency in which angiotensin II levels are often quite elevated. In patients with scleroderma this complication can be recognized by an acute or subacute rise in blood pressure and serum creatinine, the presence of proteinuria, decreased platelet count, and marked retinal arterial vasospasm. Hypertensive scleroderma renal crisis tends to occur most frequently during the winter months, presumably due to Raynaud-like effects of the environmental temperatures on the renal vasculature. ACE inhibitor therapy with oral captopril or intravenous enalaprilat are considered first-line treatments.

It is important to be aware that the depressor effect from ACE inhibitors is often not predictable in the acute hypertensive setting. In some severely hypertensive patients, renin levels are not elevated, and the initial blood pressure response may be minimal, leading to important therapeutic delays. In contrast, caution is necessary in patients suspected of having a markedly activated renin-angiotensin system, since sudden hypotension may develop and result in renal, cerebral, or cardiac injury.

Primary Hyperaldosteronism

Hypersecretion of aldosterone from one or both adrenal glands in the absence of known physiologic stimuli is responsible for approximately 1% of hypertension in the United States. Renal renin secretion is typically suppressed under these conditions, partly because of sodium retention and consequent plasma volume expansion. As expected, the blood pressure response to acute administration of ACE inhibitors in patients with primary hyperaldosteronism is usually minimal. However, more prolonged use of ACE inhibitors is sometimes associated with significant blood pressure reduction. Long-term blood pressure response to ACE inhibitors is enhanced by the concomitant use of diuretics. In patients with bilateral adrenal hyperplasia of the adrenal zona glomerulosa, aldosterone secretory rate is usually hypersensitive to angiotensin II. The finding that aldosterone release is hyperresponsive to angiotensin II in the hyperplastic form of primary hyperaldosteronism has been exploited to differentiate this disorder from the adenomatous type, using captopril in the diagnostic setting (Table 5-4).

Cardiac Disorders

Congestive heart failure Left ventricular dysfunction results in neurohormonal activation (e.g., sympathetic nervous system, renin-angiotensin system, lysine vasopressin) that initially compensates adequately for decreased perfusion while exacting its toll in harmful effects over the long term. These mechanisms result is an increase in systemic vascular resistance and salt and water retention, which in turn depresses cardiac performance further to complete the vicious circle. Conventional treatment of congestive heart failure (CHF) with diuretics and digitalis does not interrupt this vicious cycle and may actually aggravate it through vasoconstrictive effects of these agents. ACE inhibitors help to interrupt this cycle and improve symptoms and exercise tolerance without unacceptable side effects. In addition, they lower mortality, hospitalization rates, and the occurrence of myocardial infarction.

In congestive heart failure, ACE inhibitors cause significant hemodynamic improvement, including lowering of the right atrial, pulmonary arterial, and pulmonary capillary pressures, and systemic

TABLE 5-4 ACE Inhibitors, Classification

I. Natural
  a. Peptides
    1. Snake (e.g., teprotide, BPP_{5a})
    2. Human (e.g., [des-pro^3] bradykinin, enkephalins, substance P)
    3. Microbial (e.g., uracein [nocardia], ancovenin [strep], talopectin [actinomadura])
  b. Nonpeptides (e.g., bicyclic lactams, phenacein)
II. Synthetic
  a. Peptides (e.g., val-trp, phe-ala-pro)
  b. Peptide analogues (di- or tripeptide, etc.)
    1. Sulfur as zinc ligand (e.g., captopril, alacepril, phentiapril,* pivalopril,* zofenopril)
    2. Carboxyl as zinc ligand (e.g., enalapril, perindopril, ramipril, quinapril, delapril, pentopril, lisinopril, cilazapril*)
    3. Phosphinyl as zinc ligand (e.g., fosinopril)

*Conformationally restricted.

Source: Modified with permission from Kostis JB, DeFelice EA (eds): *Angiotensin Converting Enzyme Inhibitors*. New York, Alan R Liss, 1987.

vascular resistance associated with an increase in cardiac output and improvement of left ventricular function. These effects have been attributed primarily to inhibition of plasma and tissue ACE and decreased production of angiotensin II. However, other mechanisms such as sympathetic withdrawal and decreased inactivation of bradykinin may play a role. Moreover, ACE inhibitors improve functional capacity. During long-term administration, improvements in duration of treadmill exercise, cardiothoracic ratio, left ventricular ejection fraction, congestive symptoms, and New York Heart Association functional class were observed in controlled studies.

In addition to the improved exercise tolerance, controlled studies have shown lower mortality in patients with heart failure who are treated with ACE inhibitors. Large prospective studies of these agents in patients with left ventricular dysfunction with and without congestive heart failure have shown decreased mortality as well as myocardial infarction and hospitalization for congestive heart failure. Vasodilator therapy with nitrates and hydralazine also was found to reduce mortality of patients with chronic CHF in the Vasodilator Heart Failure Trial (VHeFT). However, in VHeFT-2, enalapril was superior to the combination of vasodilators from the mortality point of view. On the other hand, hypotension and dysregulation of intrarenal hemodynamics may worsen the clinical picture. Thus the effects of these agents will vary from patient to patient.

An antiarrhythmic effect, that is, a decrease in ventricular ectopic activity, when studied by ambulatory electrocardiography at rest and exercise, has been observed in some but not all studies. Also, the lack of a reduction in sudden death mortality in some studies, for example, Cooperative North Scandinavian Enalapril Survival Study (CONSENSUS) and Studies on Left Ventricular Dysfunction (SOLVD), may reflect the ambiguity of classification of death in severely ill patients with high-density complex ventricular ectopy.

Side effects of ACE inhibition in CHF are primarily related to hypotension. Patients with severe congestive heart failure on diuretics and borderline blood pressure, hyponatremia, and high plasma renin activity may develop profound hypotension with the first dose of an ACE inhibitor. This may lead to renal failure. In addition, hyperkalemia due to decreased glomerular filtration as well as decreased aldosterone secretion may occur. Because of concern about hypotension and deterioration of renal function, it is prudent to initiate therapy with a low dose of ACE inhibitor. In patients with low blood pressure, the diuretic dose may be omitted temporarily or decreased before initiation of ACE therapy. Therapy of the hypotensive episodes may include atropine for the bradycardia that sometimes accompanies these episodes and the cautious use of volume expansion or pressors.

ACE inhibitors and congestive heart failure—perspective It is clear that the use of ACE inhibitors is now accepted in a broad group of patients with left ventricular dysfunction, including those with acute pulmonary edema. In patients with chronic congestive heart failure who remain symptomatic despite treatment with digitalis and diuretics, it favorably affects symptoms, function, and prognosis. In asymptomatic left ventricular dysfunction without clinical CHF, it prevents the development of CHF. In patients with mild CHF, addition of diuretics to ACE inhibitors may be needed. In patients with mild congestive symptoms and sodium and water retention, diuretics have been shown to be more effective than ACE inhibitors in reducing excess water load. In patients who are completely asymptomatic but have left ventricular dysfunction, therapy with ACE inhibitors rather than with inotropic or diuretic agents is indicated. ACE inhibitors may potentiate a diuretic effect by lowering aldosterone and ADH levels and also probably through an effect on renal prostaglandins. On the other hand, lowering of blood pressure and glomerular filtration rate may tend to cause water retention. The combination of other vasodilators such as isosorbide dinitrate with ACE inhibitors may enhance their individual beneficial hemodynamic effects. Digoxin has not yet been shown to alter risk of mortality.

Myocardial infarction Recent clinical trials have shown the benefit of using ACE inhibitors in acute myocardial infarction. The Survival and Ventricular Enlargement Trial (SAVE) enrolled patients within 3 to 16 days following myocardial infarction with an ejection fraction of 40% or less but without overt heart failure or symptoms of myocardial ischemia, with an average follow-up of 42 months. Captopril improved survival and reduced morbidity and mortality due to major cardiovascular events including recurrent myocardial infarction.

The majority of patients enrolled in SOLVD had history of earlier myocardial infarction as well as chronic left ventricular dysfunction. The incidence of symptomatic heart failure and related hospitalizations was significantly reduced by ACE inhibition with enalapril in asymptomatic patients (SOLVD prevention trial). In symptomatic CHF patients, a statistically significant reduction in mortality was also seen.

Patients with clinical evidence of heart failure after acute myocardial infarction were enrolled in Acute Infarction Ramipril Efficacy (AIRE). Treatment with ramipril was associated with lower (27% reduction) mortality from all causes. In the second Cooperative North Scandinavian Enalapril Survival Study (CONSENSUS II), enalapril (enalaprilat IV) was given within 24 h of acute myocardial infarction. There was no survival benefit with this early ACE inhibitor intervention during follow-up ranging from 41 to 180 days.

On the other hand, in the third Gruppo Italiano per lo Studio della Sopravivenza nell'Infarcto Miocardico (GISSI-3), lisinopril started within 24 h of acute infarction produced a small but statistically significant reduction in overall mortality. Similar benefits were observed with oral captopril within the first 24 h of acute myocardial infarction in the Fourth International Study of Infarct Survival (ISIS-4).

ACE inhibition in acute myocardial infarction can cause hypotension. The Chinese Cardiac Study (CCS-1) examined the safety and efficacy of acute interventional use of captopril in patients experiencing their first anterior myocardial infarction. Captopril (or placebo) was started immediately and titrated to 25 mg tid. Captopril was well tolerated, but first-dose hypotension was more common than with placebo. In the acute phase of the infarction, catecholamine levels and repetitive ventricular arrhythmias were reduced. Enzymatic infarct size was smaller. In the chronic phase, the incidence of heart failure was reduced.

Thus there is general agreement that acute infarction patients with left ventricular dysfunction (LVD) or with clinical evidence of heart failure benefit from ACE inhibition as well as patients with LVD and healed infarction. Some of the ACE inhibitors are FDA approved for this indication. The benefit of ACE inhibition when given to all patients with acute myocardial infarction in the acute phase appears smaller. Clinical guidelines for the use of ACE inhibitors in acute coronary syndromes are being formulated.

Studies are now in progress evaluating the effects of long-term ACE inhibition in survivors of acute myocardial infarction who have minimal impairment of ventricular function.

Left ventricular hypertrophy ACE inhibitors can reduce left ventricular hypertrophy in patients with hypertension, but the prognostic implications of this finding are not known. Studies are in progress in hypertensive patients with left ventricular hypertrophy to determine whether ventricular mass regression can be associated with an improved cardiovascular prognosis.

Mitral and aortic regurgitation The short-term administration of ACE inhibitors can produce favorable hemodynamic effects in patients with mitral and aortic valvular regurgitation. In patients with aortic regurgitation, ventricular ejection fraction increases and forward stroke volume remains unchanged. In patients with mitral regurgitation, ejection fraction remains unchanged and stroke volume increases. In patients with chronic aortic regurgitation, a reduction in left ventricular volume and regurgitant fraction has been observed with ACE inhibitors and other vasodilators. In symptomatic patients with mitral valve regurgitation, excluding patients with hypertrophic cardiomyopathy and mitral valve prolapse, ACE inhibitors are considered the drug of choice.

Renal Disease

Renal parenchymal disease For patients with hypertension and normal renal function, the reason for therapeutic reduction of blood pressure is to prevent strokes, coronary heart disease, and premature vascular disease. For patients with renal dysfunction, the situation is more complex. Most renal diseases, especially those affecting the glomeruli, lead to or worsen preexisting high blood pressure. Although it is clear that renal dysfunction may be a cause of systemic hypertension, the kidney is also a victim of hypertension. Early clinical observations suggested that the systemic hypertension that accompanies renal insufficiency is associated with a more rapid progression to end-stage renal failure. In several animal models with experimentally induced renal insufficiency, progressive renal failure can be slowed or halted by adequate blood pressure control.

The mechanisms involved whereby systemic hypertension accelerates the decline of renal function are not yet fully established. Experimental studies in rats have demonstrated that the sustained increase in intraglomerular capillary pressure in response to the initial loss of functioning nephrons provokes a destructive sclerosing injury in the remaining and previously intact renal tissue. Thus, according to one hypothesis, glomerular hypertension plays a key pathogenic role in the inevitable progression of kidney disease to advanced renal insufficiency. Because angiotensin II has a preferential vasoconstrictor effect on the glomerular efferent arteriole, it had been hypothesized that reduction of angiotensin II by ACE inhibitors might lower intraglomerular pressure and thereby slow or prevent progression of renal impairment.

In one experimental model by which rats were subjected to subtotal nephrectomy, treatment with ACE inhibitors decreased systemic and glomerular pressure and was associated with a marked reduction of the glomerular sclerosis that normally develops in this model. In the same remnant kidney model, an equivalent reduction of systemic blood pressure with reserpine, hydralazine, and hydrochlorothiazide failed to attenuate glomerular hypertension and failed to affect the sclerotic process in the remnant kidney tissue.

In humans, the rate of decline of renal function is affected by the nature and degree of underlying renal pathology, the magnitude of proteinuria, dyslipidemia, glycemic control, protein intake, and degree of blood pressure elevation. Wee and Epstein performed an extensive review of clinical studies of the effects of ACE inhibitor therapy on renal function of patients with a diverse group of nondiabetic renal diseases. In approximately 29 of 35 short-term studies of the effects of ACE inhibitor therapy on renal function (durations 2 weeks to 6 months), measures of glomerular filtration remained stable, whereas in 4 studies there was deterioration and in 2 there was improvement. Effective renal blood flow remained stable in 13 studies and increased in 4. Of the 23 studies in which proteinuria was assessed, treatment with an ACE inhibitor was associated with a significant decline in 20 studies and no change in 3. In long-term observations, measures of glomerular filtration rate remained stable in 12 of 16 studies. Proteinuria seemed to benefit less in that there was a decrease reported in only 6 of

15 studies in which this had been determined. Recently, the degree of proteinuria has been questioned as a surrogate end point for the surveillance of patients with nondiabetic chronic renal disease.

In a recently completed 3-year placebo-controlled trial, the ACE inhibitor benazepril was shown to protect against the progression of renal insufficiency in patients with various renal diseases except for those having polycystic kidney.

Diabetic nephropathy Progressive renal failure is a significant cause of morbidity and death in both insulin- and non-insulin-dependent diabetics. The triad of hypertension, proteinuria, and decreased glomerular filtration rate appears in approximately 40% of all type I insulin-dependent diabetics and is nearly as prevalent in non-insulin-dependent diabetes. Diabetic nephropathy represents the summation of metabolic and hemodynamic effects of this disorder on kidney structure and function. Hyperglycemia-induced glycosylation of structural proteins of the glomerular mesangium and basement membrane may contribute to protein leakage across the glomerulus. Elevated growth hormone or other growth factors may be responsible for glomerular hypertrophy. In experimental models of diabetes, intraglomerular pressure and flow are increased owing to an imbalance between efferent and afferent resistance, with a relative deficiency at the preglomerular end. This causes the diabetic kidney to become exquisitely sensitive to the detrimental effects of hypertension.

In human diabetics, treatment of hypertension has long been known to slow the rate of loss of renal function. More recently it has been suggested that ACE inhibitors, by preferentially reducing postglomerular resistance, might have a special role in protecting the kidney function of diabetics with and without hypertension. The use of ACE inhibitors in experimental models of diabetes has revealed that these agents reduce intraglomerular pressure and slow progression of disease to a greater extent than conventional antihypertensive drugs. Early short-term studies of hypertensive and nonhypertensive patients with diabetic nephropathy showed a slower rate of decline of renal function when treated with captopril than no therapy. Bjork and colleagues reported an investigation of 40 patients with type I diabetes mellitus and nephropathy who were randomized to either enalapril or metoprolol. It was found that the ACE inhibitor group had a greatly reduced rate of decline of renal function in comparison with the metoprolol-treated patients. More recently, Lewis and the Collaborative Study Group published their findings from a randomized study of insulin-dependent diabetics in which 409 patients with diabetic nephropathy received either captopril or placebo for a median follow-up of 3 years. Captopril treatment was associated with a highly significant reduction in the rate of rise of serum creatinine and a 50% reduction in the risk of end-stage renal failure or death. It has been proposed and widely accepted that captopril or other ACE inhibitor therapy be used in normotensive and hypertensive patients with type I insulin-dependent diabetes. Whether ACE inhibitor therapy will have a similar protective effect on the renal function of non-insulin-dependent diabetics is under investigation.

Practical aspects of ACE inhibitor therapy in renal insufficiency In clinical practice, blood pressure control of many patients with hypertension and renal insufficiency is quite difficult. Single-drug therapy is often not sufficient. Sodium retention appears to participate in the etiology of elevated blood pressure in the setting of renal impairment. Therefore, to achieve blood pressure control, such patients may end up on a combination of drugs that includes diuretics. Diuretics increase renin dependency of blood pressure, thereby amplifying the potential depressor action of ACE inhibitors. It also has been postulated that volume depletion can increase the dependency of glomerular autoregulation on angiotensin II levels. From the known effects of angiotensin II on the postglomerular efferent arteriole, there is risk that diuretics also may augment the likelihood of an ACE inhibitor–induced decline in glomerular filtration rate, even in the absence of renal artery stenosis. This phenomenon has been documented with a variety of renal parenchymal disorders.

It is prudent to determine the serum creatinine in all patients before initiating ACE inhibitor therapy. Those with renal insufficiency of any cause should have renal function monitored closely, especially so with any increment of ACE inhibitor or diuretic dose. It is also important to be aware that most ACE inhibitors are excreted primarily through a renal mechanism. Reports of idiosyncratic adverse experiences such as skin rash and bone marrow suppression may be more likely in patients receiving high doses of these agents in the setting of renal impairment. Thus it is important to follow specific guidelines for dose adjustment of the ACE inhibitor for each agent.

Cerebrovascular Disease

In humans, administration of ACE inhibitors is associated with either no change or an increase in cerebral blood flow despite decreased systemic blood pressure. In patients with congestive heart failure, studies utilizing positron emission tomography (PET) scanning and xenon clearance have demonstrated that administration of captopril preserved cerebral blood flow while decreasing systemic blood pressure by 5 to 40%. ACE inhibitors dilate large vessels such as the aorta and carotid arteries, as well as smaller arterioles downstream. Thus both the lower and upper limits of cerebral autoregulation tend to shift to the lower levels of blood pressure by ACE inhibitor therapy.

ACE inhibitors have been shown to reduce the consequences of experimental carotid occlusion on cerebral lactate and ATP production in spontaneously hypertensive rats. In this study, cerebral blood flow monitoring by H_2 clearance indicated that changes in cerebral hemodynamics were not a prerequisite for the anti-ischemic effect of ACE inhibitors. It is possible that reduction of angiotensin levels or increase in bradykinin levels or other peptide hormones might help to protect neuronal metabolism against ischemic insult.

The case for ACE inhibitors in prevention and treatment of stroke is not yet resolved. There are no clinical trials on the effect of ACE inhibitors in stroke reduction in hypertensives. It is generally accepted that all currently available antihypertensive agents may provide protection from stroke by virtue of their blood pressure lowering action. ACE inhibitors reset cerebral autoregulation to lower blood pressure, thereby protecting the brain against sudden hypotensive events. On the other hand, lowering of the upper limit of autoregulation by ACE inhibitors could prove to be detrimental by limiting protection against sudden surges in blood pressure. A full-scale clinical investigation of the effects of ACE inhibition on primary and secondary prevention of ischemic strokes is warranted.

ACE Inhibitors and Quality of Life

Quality of life is a notion that refers to a subjective perception of physical and psychological sense of well-being. Hypertension, in the absence of target-organ damage, has long been considered to be asymptomatic. Recent studies have shown that self-awareness of the diagnosis is associated with increased absenteeism from work and decreased sense of well-being. Hypertensives may suffer from or be more aware of a number of symptoms often observed in the general population. In 1986, Croog and colleagues reported that captopril therapy, in comparison with propranolol and methyldopa, was associated with improved measures in quality of life. These questionnaire-based assessments included vitality, cognitive function, work performance, and sexual function. Animal studies also have pointed to improved learning in several models during ACE inhibitor administration, such as food-reinforced alteration of T-maze task in rats and objective discrimination task in primates. Since then, a number of clinical studies have attempted to compare the effects of ACE inhibitors with each other and with other types of antihypertensive drugs on quality of life and cognitive function.

The mechanisms for differential effects on quality-of-life measures are poorly understood. The clinical studies are often confounded by varying levels of blood pressure control and by different types and rates of drug-related adverse effects. The CNS is known to contain all the principal elements of the renin-angiotensin system, including renin, angiotensinogen, and angiotensin converting enzyme. Stimulation of angiotensin receptors in the brain has been demonstrated to affect multiple biochemical, behavioral, and functional responses. Conceivably,

ACE inhibitor–induced altered release or degradation of neurotransmitter peptides may contribute to the putative changes in sense of well-being.

ACE INHIBITORS IN COMBINATION THERAPY

Diuretics and ACE Inhibitors

Early observations suggested that the antihypertensive effect of ACE inhibitors is amplified when the renin system is activated. Correspondingly, the blood pressure lowering ability of ACE inhibitors was shown early on to be enhanced by volume depletion. Several multicenter trials have unequivocally demonstrated the synergistic interaction of ACE inhibitors and diuretic therapy in hypertension. Of importance, the antihypertensive action of this form of combination therapy was similar in blacks and whites. Also, several of the adverse metabolic effects of diuretics, including hypokalemia, hyperglycemia, hyperuricemia, and hypercholesterolemia, were attenuated in combination with ACE inhibitors.

When diuretic–ACE inhibitor combination therapy is selected for a patient, an important consideration is the sequence in which the ACE inhibitor and diuretic are initiated. Diuretic-induced volume depletion may predispose patients to a precipitous decline of blood pressure following administration of an ACE inhibitor. Thus it is prudent to begin therapy with the ACE inhibitor with addition of the diuretic 1 to 2 weeks later as needed. For patients already taking a diuretic, it is sometimes not medically practical to withhold this agent prior to initiation of ACE inhibition, such as for the patient with congestive heart failure. In this setting, the patient may need to be observed closely for several hours following a low first dose of the ACE inhibitor.

A number of ACE inhibitors are currently available in fixed-dose combinations with hydrochlorothiazide. These are generally best utilized in patients who have or are expected to have a suboptimal response to ACE inhibitor monotherapy. Careful attention should be directed to choosing the particular fixed-dose combination that is most suitable for the individual patient.

β Blockers and ACE Inhibitors

Clinical experience with β-blocker–ACE inhibitor combination therapy is less extensive than with diuretic–ACE inhibitor combinations. One of the important mechanisms by which β blockers lower blood pressure is via antagonism of the β-adrenergic receptor–mediated renin release by the renal juxtaglomerular apparatus. Thus it can be expected that combination therapy with ACE inhibitors might be of little value. Most of the published data have derived from studies of short duration. In general, these results indicate a modest additive effect of ACE inhibitors with β blockers. It has been suggested that the additive effects of β blockade on ACE inhibitor therapy may be greater in patients with high renin forms of hypertension. Because the additive effect of combining β blockade with ACE inhibition on blood pressure appears to be modest, there has been little interest in the development of fixed-dose combinations of these two classes of antihypertensive agents.

Calcium Entry Antagonists and ACE Inhibitors

Calcium antagonists affect blood pressure via mechanisms independent of the renin-angiotensin system. In turn, the calcium antagonists have a modest stimulatory effect on renin release. Systemic vasodilatation induced by the calcium antagonists, especially the dihydropyridines, signals a reflex increase in centrally mediated outflow of sympathetic nervous activity, which thereby enhances renal renin secretion. Based on the differing actions of calcium antagonists and ACE inhibitors on the circulation, it is reasonable to expect that the combination of these two classes would have an additive or synergistic effect. A number of controlled clinical trials have confirmed that there is a consistent and significant additive effect on blood pressure reduction when ACE inhibitors are used in combination with calcium antagonists. Neither ACE inhibitors nor calcium antagonists have been shown to adversely affect levels of such metabolic parameters as blood glucose, lipids, and uric acid. Thus these agents may be especially advantageous to use in combination for patients with resistant hypertension who have derangement of carbohydrate, lipid, or uric acid metabolism. Currently, four fixed-dose formulations are available in the United States, which comprises benazepril and amlodipine, enalapril and diltiazem, enalapril and felodipine, and trandolapril and verapamil. Besides an additive antihypertensive effect of the two agents, it was found that edema associated with calcium antagonist therapy was significantly reduced during combination therapy with the two agents. Other fixed-dose combinations are currently under development.

DIAGNOSTIC USE OF ACE INHIBITORS

Renal Artery Stenosis

The screening and diagnosis of renovascular disease has received increasing attention in light of recent advances in surgical and percutaneous angioplasty techniques. The first use of renin-angiotensin inhibition in the diagnosis of renal artery stenosis was that of the angiotensin receptor antagonist saralasin, approved for this purpose in 1979. Patients with unilateral disease were found to have a greater decline in blood pressure during the infusion of this peptide analogue of angiotensin II. Because saralasin is a peptide, it requires administration by the parenteral route. Furthermore, the antihypertensive effect, although sensitive, has a low specificity for renovascular disease. The use of saralasin fell out of favor with the development of the orally active converting enzyme inhibitors and was eventually taken off the market in the United States. Captopril, the first available orally active ACE inhibitor, was found to have a similar but equally nonspecific effect on the blood pressure of patients with unilateral renal artery stenosis. In 1986, Muller and colleagues at Cornell reported that the captopril test could be vastly improved by the determination of plasma renin activity before and 60 to 90 min after an initial dose of the drug. The diagnostic accuracy of this form of the captopril–plasma renin challenge test has been in the range of 85 to 95%, depending on the diagnostic criteria employed and the pretest probability based on clinical screening.

Considerable experience has accrued with the use of [^{123}I]hippuran (a marker for renal blood flow) and ^{99m}Tc-DTPA (a marker for glomerular filtration) renography for diagnostic screening. Sensitivity of these nuclear imaging techniques for hemodynamically significant renovascular disease is 60 to 80%, depending on the criteria used to define a diagnostically positive study. Autoregulation of renal blood flow and glomerular filtration rate by the stenotic kidney may have limited the diagnostic sensitivity of nuclear renography. Angiotensin II plays a critically important role in renal hemodynamic autoregulation by maintaining vascular tone in the efferent postglomerular arteriole. Reduction of angiotensin II formation by ACE inhibition may thereby result in a fall in glomerular filtration pressure. The effect of ACE inhibitors on glomerular autoregulatory function has led to the development of captopril-stimulated renography.

Specific protocols vary somewhat among centers. Generally, patients suspected of having renovascular occlusive disease by clinical criteria are administered a dose of a rapidly acting oral ACE inhibitor such as captopril or intravenous enalaprilat 1 to 2 h prior to injection with the nuclear imaging tracer. Subtle differences of intraglomerular pressure between the two kidneys are amplified by the sudden decline in local and circulating angiotensin II levels that result from administration of the ACE inhibitor. Published results indicate that the diagnostic sensitivity of captopril-stimulated nuclear renography is 90 to 100%.

The diagnostic value of captopril–plasma renin challenge test followed by renal ^{99m}Tc-DTPA renography is also currently under assessment.

Primary Hyperaldosteronism

The syndrome of primary hyperaldosteronism results from the hypersecretion of the mineralocorticoid aldosterone by the adrenal cortex in the absence of known stimuli. In the earlier literature, most reported cases of primary hyperaldosteronism were due to a solitary benign adenoma with autonomous secretion and release of the hormone, so-called Conn's syndrome. In more recent years, a greater number of patients with primary hyperaldosteronism are found to have bilateral hyperplasia of the adrenal zona glomerulosa. These patients tend to have milder biochemical and hormonal abnormalities. Differentiation of the adenomatous from the hyperplastic form of hyperaldosteronism is important since the former is usually best managed with surgical removal of the offending gland. In patients with unprovoked hypokalemia, the diagnosis of primary hyperaldosteronism can usually be made based on finding elevated serum and urinary aldosterone with suppressed plasma renin activity. There is evidence that the hyperplastic type derives from cells of the zona glomerulosa that become hypersensitive to the stimulatory effects of angiotensin II on aldosterone production. Thus aldosterone levels remain elevated even in the setting of reduced plasma renin-angiotensin levels. By determining the suppressive effect of captopril on plasma aldosterone it is possible to differentiate the adenomatous from the hyperplastic form of this disorder. Failure of serum aldosterone levels to decline even partially following an initial dose of the ACE inhibitor is more consistent with an adenoma, whereas aldosterone levels usually decline by approximately 50% in the hyperplastic type.

STRUCTURE-ACTIVITY RELATIONSHIP OF ACE INHIBITORS

It has been known that angiotensin converting enzyme is a peptidase similar to carboxypeptidase A and that both enzymes are zinc-containing metalloproteins. Based on the hypothesis of a structural similarity between ACE and carboxypeptidase, Cushman et al. synthesized captopril, a drug that resembles the carboxyl-terminal dipeptide residue to teprotide, a naturally occurring ACE inhibitor. The sulfhydryl group of captopril enhanced its potency, since the sulfur moiety binds tightly with the zinc ion of ACE. However, highly potent ACE inhibitors, with a carboxyl group as a zinc ligand and additional binding sites, were later synthesized. Newer ACE inhibitors may have other chemical functions as zinc ligands, such as the phosphinic acid residue in fosinopril (Table 5-5).

DIFFERENCES AMONG ACE INHIBITORS

Although there are differences among ACE inhibitors, they are not as pronounced as those seen among calcium antagonists or beta blockers. ACE inhibitors may differ in the ways shown in the following paragraphs (Tables 5-5, 5-6).

Chemical Class

The presence or absence of the sulfhydryl group, a strong zinc ligand, may enhance the potency of ACE inhibitors but has been implicated in

TABLE 5-5 ACE Inhibitors, Differences*

1. Chemical class
   Zinc ligand, etc.
2. Potency
   K_i
   IC_{50} (ACE, conversion of angiotensin I to angiotensin II, bradykinin degradation)
3. Prodrugs
   Site and time course of bioactivation, etc.
4. Pharmacokinetics
   Absorption (e.g., %, C_{max}, T_{max})
   Bioavailability (e.g., %, AUC)
   Volume of distribution
   Metabolism (e.g., $t_{1/2}$, total clearance, renal clearance)
   Excretion (e.g., urine %, feces %)
   Protein binding
5. Tissue effects
   Tissue penetration, time course, dissociation constants
6. Side effects
7. Additional pharmacologic properties, e.g., neutral endopeptidase activity, diuretic activity
8. Drug interactions

*AUC, area under the plasma concentration time curve; IC_{50}, inhibitory concentration 50%.

Source: Modified with permission from Kostis JB, DeFelice EA (eds): *Angiotensin Converting Enzyme Inhibitors*. New York, Alan R Liss, 1987.

taste disturbances and skin rashes. It also may confer a shorter duration of action, since it is easily oxidized. On the other hand, a direct effect of the sulfhydryl functionality of captopril on phospholipase A_2 may lead to an increase in vasodilatory prostaglandins, thereby potentially augmenting the blood pressure lowering effects of this agent.

Potency

Potency of ACE inhibitors is related to the dissociation constant of the inhibitor-enzyme complex (K_i value). However, for potent ACE inhibitors a steady-state kinetic approach may not be ideal. The potency of an ACE inhibitor also may be described by the concentration able to inhibit 50% of the activity of the enzyme.

Prodrugs

Most ACE inhibitors are administered orally as pro-drugs to improve absorption. The prodrugs are hydrolyzed after absorption into the active compounds. The speed of biotransformation affects the time of onset of action. Cirrhosis or CHF may delay the onset and prolong the duration of action of prodrugs, and variation of biotransformation may increase the variability of clinical effects.

TABLE 5-6 FDA-Approved Indications for ACE Inhibitors

ACE inhibitor	Proprietary name(s)	Hypertension	CHF	Post-MI CHF	Diabetic nephropathy	Asymptomatic LV dysfunction
Benazepril	Lotensin	+				
Captopril	Capoten	+	+	+	+	+[a]
Enalapril	Vasotec	+	+			+[b]
Enalaprilat	Vasotec IV	+				
Fosinopril	Monopril	+	+			
Lisinopril	Prinivil, Zestril	+	+	+[c]		
Moexipril	Univasc	+				
Quinapril	Accupril	+	+			
Ramipril	Altace	+	+[d]			
Trandolapril	Mavik	+		+		

[a]Captopril is indicated in clinically stable patients with left ventricular dysfunction (EF ≤ 40%) following myocardial infarction to improve survival and to reduce the incidence of overt heart failure.
[b]Enalapril is indicated in clinically stable asymptomatic patients with left ventricular dysfunction (EF ≤ 35%) to decrease the rate of development of overt heart failure and to decrease the incidence of hospitalization due to CHF.
[c]Lisinopril is indicated for hemodynamically stable patients within 24 h of acute MI to improve survival.
[d]Ramipril is indicated in stable patients who have demonstrated clinical signs of CHF within the first few days after sustaining acute myocardial infarction to decrease mortality and progression to severe heart failure.

Pharmacokinetic Properties

Long duration of action associated with long elimination half-lives, as seen, for example, in ramipril, cilazapril, lisinopril, and quinapril, allows once-a-day dosing especially in hypertension. Most marketed ACE inhibitors are excreted by the kidney and may require dosage adjustment in severe renal insufficiency and CHF. Some ACE inhibitors, for example, spirapril and fosinopril, are also metabolized by the liver and may not need dosage adjustment.

Protein binding may have clinical significance when ACE inhibitors are administered together with highly protein-bound drugs, such as nonsteroidal anti-inflammatory agents. The drugs are widely distributed in most tissues. Captopril is partially oxidized at the sulfhydryl group, and both captopril and its metabolites are excreted primarily in the urine, with minor elimination in the feces. Enalapril and lisinopril are excreted unchanged. Excretion is usually by tubular secretion. Elimination half-life of unchanged captopril is approximately 2 to 3 h. The elimination half-life increases progressively with the degree of renal impairment, so that the dose should be reduced or the intervals between dosing should be increased in patients with moderate to severe renal dysfunction. Enalapril is metabolized to the active (diacid) compound enalaprilat, mostly in the liver. Peak action of enalapril is usually around 4 h and of lisinopril around 6 h after oral administration, and the long duration of action is a reflection of the long half-life. The serum concentration versus the time curve of enalaprilat and lisinopril has been shown to be polyphasic, with a prolonged terminal phase with an elimination half-life of approximately 35 h. Patients with severe heart failure may accumulate captopril and its disulfide metabolite and may have slower clearance of enalapril, enalaprilat, and lisinopril.

Inhibition of Tissue ACE

Inhibition of plasma ACE does not fully explain the spectrum of clinical effects of ACE inhibitors such as their effect in low renin and the lack of a relationship between plasma ACE inhibition and clinical effect. The duration of the antihypertensive effect exceeds the duration of ACE inhibition in plasma.

ACE is expressed and probably has functional significance in blood vessels, heart, kidney, adrenals, etc. The effects on bradykinin, prostaglandins, and other substrates and the inhibition of ACE in different tissues such as the aorta, other arteries, lung, kidney, testes, and plasma may have different time courses or different intensities and may characterize pharmacodynamic properties. They may be due to differences in tissue penetration, binding, and dissociation characteristics and kinetics in content of ACE in different tissues.

Additional Pharmacologic Properties

The synthesis of ACE inhibitors with added pharmacologic properties may in the future add to the diversity of these agents. Molecules with ACE inhibitory and diuretic properties that were synthesized did not reach clinical practice. Combined neutral endopeptidase and ACE inhibitor agents are now in clinical development.

ANGIOTENSIN II RECEPTOR ANTAGONISTS

Angiotensin II Receptors

Angiotensin II receptor antagonists, a new class of pharmacologic blockers of the renin-angiotensin system (RAS), have been shown recently to be safe and effective antihypertensive agents in both animal and human studies. This section reviews the biology of A-II receptors, the pharmacology of the prototype A-II receptor antagonist losartan, and the clinical experiences with A-II receptor antagonism as an antihypertensive treatment, while exploring other potential clinical uses for this new class of drugs.

As described earlier, angiotensin exerts its effects by binding to specific receptors in the plasma membrane of various tissues. Using the photoaffinity ligand binding method, a single protein has been isolated with a molecular weight of 65,000 to 67,000 that showed angiotensin receptor binding activity. However, structure-activity relationship studies and competitive binding experiments showed a variable antagonist and/or agonist response to angiotensin analogues. The same analogue could elicit different responses depending on the target tissue. For example, an agent considered to be a pure antagonist in a given tissue may be a pure agonist in other tissue. These studies suggest that there are multiple angiotensin receptor subtypes among various tissues. In fact, the mechanism of action of angiotensin II in various effector tissues seems to be quite different. Multiple signal transduction pathways have been proposed, including inhibition of adenylate cyclase, stimulation of the phosphatidylinositol conversion by coupling to phospholipase C, activation of ligand-gated calcium channels, and modulation of voltage-dependent calcium channels. These findings support angiotensin receptor heterogeneity and led to the discovery of distinct angiotensin receptor subtypes.

Angiotensin receptors may be differentiated into two distinct subtypes by radioligand receptor binding studies using the specific, nonpeptide antagonists losartan (DuP 753) and PD123177, as well as by their sensitivity to reducing agents (Fig. 5-1). The type 1 angiotensin receptor is inactivated by pretreatment with the reducing agent dithiothreitol (DTT) and is a losartan-sensitive site because of its high affinity for losartan but low affinity to PD123177. AT_1 mediates its physiologic functions by coupling to a transmembrane G protein and can be inhib-

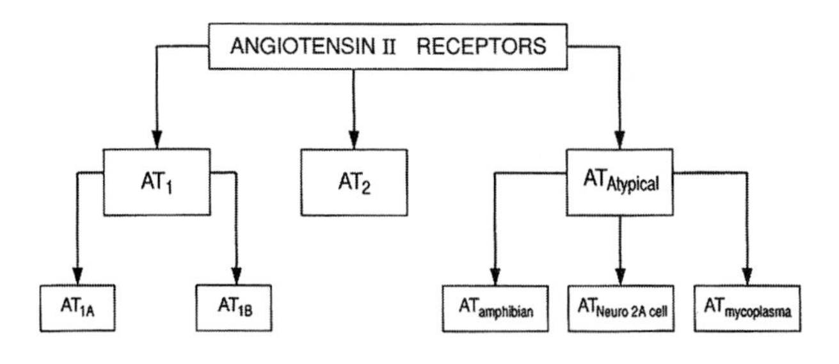

FIG. 5-1 The classification and characteristics of angiotensin II receptors. DTT = dithiothreitol. *(From Kang PM, Landau AJ, Eberhardt RT, Frishman WH: Angiotensin II receptor antagonists: A new approach to blockade of the renin-angiotensin system. Am Heart J 127:1388, 1994, with permission.)*

ited by guanine nucleotides. The type 2 angiotensin receptor is resistant to DTT inactivation and is PD123177 sensitive. Both receptor subtypes appear to be found in different tissues in varying proportions. The AT_1 receptor predominates in virtually all vascular tissue and is the only type present in the liver and in rat spleen. In other tissues the A-II receptor subtypes exhibit different distributions. For example, in rat brain, the AT_1 receptor is present in pituitary and periventricular organs, but AT_2 receptors are found in the thalamus, locus coeruleus, and cerebellum. AT_1 predominates in the kidney glomeruli, but the AT_2 receptor predominates in the renal capsule. Recent data show that AT receptors extend beyond the current definition of AT_1 and AT_2. "Atypical" angiotensin receptors have been described in amphibians, mouse neuroblastoma cells, and *Mycoplasma*. Furthermore, isoforms of AT_1 have been cloned and sequenced in mice and subsequently named AT_{1A} and AT_{1B} (see Fig. 5-1). They are structurally, if not functionally, different and appear to be involved in various mechanical pathways of the A-II receptors.

LOSARTAN AND OTHER ANGIOTENSIN II RECEPTOR BLOCKERS

Losartan {2-*n*-butyl-4-chloro-5-hydroxymethyl-1-[2′-(1*H*-tetrazole-5-yl) biphenyl-4-yl] imidazole, potassium salt} is the most potent, orally active, specific, competitive A-II receptor antagonist of this drug group.

Losartan was shown to inhibit the specific binding of labeled A-II to its receptor sites in various experimental models. In rabbit aorta, losartan also was shown to antagonize the A-II-induced contraction response. At different concentrations, losartan did not show any response to KCl or norepinephrine, nor did it influence ACE or renin activities. Losartan, at effective A-II inhibitory doses, did not enhance the bradykinin vasodepressor response, whereas captopril potentiated it.

Losartan, given either orally or intravenously, lowered blood pressure in furosemide-treated animals with high plasma renin activity (PRA) but did not lower blood pressure in conscious normotensive or deoxycorticosterone acetate hypertensive rats with low PRA. Using a high-renin hypertensive rat model, losartan was shown to decrease blood pressure when given orally or intravenously, with similar efficacy to the ACE inhibitors. The hypotensive effect lasted more than 24 h for oral losartan administration without affecting the heart rate. In conscious, spontaneously hypertensive rats (SHRs) with normal PRA, losartan given orally decreased mean arterial pressure. This same effect was not observed with saralasin, due to its agonistic activity. Bilateral nephrectomy abolished the antihypertensive effects of losartan, suggesting that losartan is dependent on an active RAS. An infusion of losartan abolished the A-II-induced pressor response and aldosterone release in SHRs, whereas PD123177 had no effect on these parameters. Finally, oral administration of losartan for 2 weeks caused a marked decrease in blood pressure in SHRs. PRA, A-I, and A-II levels were increased, whereas aldosterone levels were decreased.

In the rat kidney, losartan, in a dose-related manner, was shown to displace A-II from its specific binding sites and antagonize the vasoconstrictive effects of A-II. Losartan reversed A-II-mediated renal afferent and efferent arteriolar constriction in hydronephrotic rat kidneys and markedly decreased fluid and electrolyte absorption in the proximal convoluted tubule. In rats with high PRA, losartan increased renal blood flow, urine flow, and sodium excretion without changing arterial pressure and glomerular filtration rate (GFR). However, in normal-renin or low-renin models, losartan produced minor or no changes in sodium and water excretion. Losartan showed similar effects on renal hemodynamics in a canine model of essential hypertension. In anesthetized dogs, losartan caused renal vasodilatation and natriuresis similar to captopril. The renal hemodynamic effects were more pronounced in the sodium-depleted state with both losartan and captopril treatment.

Preliminary studies with losartan suggested the existence of an active metabolite. Intravenous (IV) injection of losartan exhibits a biphasic response. Blood pressure initially falls rapidly after the injection, followed by slower reduction, with maximal blood pressure reduction being observed after 3 h. The ED_{30} of orally administered losartan is comparable with IV injection, even though the observed oral bioavailability of losartan is only 33%. These findings prompted further investigation, which led to the discovery of EXP3174, a major active metabolite of losartan that has high potency and a long duration of action without agonistic activity. EXP3174 has an IC_{50} of 3.7×10^{-8} mol/L in rat adrenal cortical membranes and shows noncompetitive inhibition of A-II-induced contraction with a pA2 value of 10.09 (slope = 1.32) in the isolated rabbit aorta. IV injection of EXP3174 revealed a 20-fold more potent antihypertensive effect than losartan, with an ED_{30} of 0.04 mg/kg. However, the oral ED_{30} of EXP3174 is 0.66 mg/kg, which is comparable to oral ED_{30} of losartan. In furosemide-treated conscious dogs with high PRA, losartan and EXP3714, but not PD123177, were as effective as captopril in lowering blood pressure.

A number of new oral, nonpeptide, A-II receptor antagonists similar to losartan have been tested. These include valsartan, irbesartan, eprosartan, candesartan, tasosartan, telmisartan, forasartan, and ripisartan. Valsartan and irbesartan, were recently approved and marketed for use in hypertension.

Losartan Pharmacokinetics

Losartan has an oral bioavailability of about 33%, indicating a considerable first-pass effect with no effect from food. The drug is metabolized by hepatic carboxylation to form the active metabolite E 3174; a small percentage of patients lack the enzymes for this reaction. The time to achieve peak plasma concentration (C_{max}) is 1 h for losartan and 3 to 4 h for E 3174. The antihypertensive effect correlates closest with the plasma levels of the active metabolite. The pharmacokinetics of the drug are not influenced by renal disease, whereas in patients with hepatic dysfunction, the blood levels of both losartan and E 3174 increase, necessitating a reduced dose. Drugs that induce the P450 CYP_{max} systems may increase the rate of losartan metabolism. There are no known drug interactions with warfarin or digoxin.

Clinical Studies with Losartan in Hypertension

Oral administration of losartan to normal male volunteers was shown, in a dose-dependent manner, to reduce the peak systolic blood pressure response resulting from an injection of A-II. Three, six, and thirteen hours after administering a 40-mg dose of losartan, blood pressure decreased by 31 ± 5%, 37 ± 6%, and 45 ± 3%, respectively, when compared with controls. Losartan (5, 10, 20, or 40 mg) given orally once a day for 8 days also reduced the systolic blood pressure response to A-II injections in a dose-dependent manner, on the 1st, 4th, and 8th days. There was a persistent antihypertensive effect present 24 h after the 40-mg dose. In healthy volunteers, losartan had no significant side effects and did not affect the basal heart rate or the arterial pressure; however, losartan did induce a dose-dependent compensatory rise in

PRA and the A-II level. A study designed to measure the plasma concentration of losartan and its active metabolite EXP3174 in six healthy volunteers showed that at 40, 80, or 120 mg, the peak plasma levels of the parent compound were attained less than an hour after the oral administrations of 40, 80, and 120 mg, and the levels rapidly disappeared within 6 h after drug administrations. On the other hand, the active metabolite EXP3174 accumulated and was eliminated more slowly. With 80- and 120-mg doses, the peak levels of EXP3174 were observed about 3 h after the administrations, with plasma levels detectable past 24 h. Also, significant dose-dependent inhibition of the systolic blood pressure response to exogenous A-II was observed for up to 24 h with these doses of losartan compared with the placebo.

Inpatient and outpatient studies also have demonstrated the antihypertensive efficacy of losartan. In eight hospitalized patients with essential hypertension, oral losartan was administered for 2 to 4 weeks, and doses were increased until diastolic blood pressure (bp) fell below 90 mmHg. With an average losartan dose of 59.4 $\pm$ 43.7 mg/day, supine bp decreased significantly without any changes in pulse rate or in renal function. In another study, losartan given at 50 to 150 mg once a day to hospitalized patients caused significant decreases in systolic and diastolic bp when compared with placebo. Preliminary findings from the first large dose-finding outpatient study with losartan given in doses of 10, 25, 50, 100, or 150 mg once a day have shown a statistically significant peak (6 h after the dosing) and trough (24 h after the dosing) effect on bp with doses of 50 mg or higher compared with the placebo. Doses above 50 mg did not show a greater reduction in bp. At doses lower than 50 mg, there was a statistically significant peak reduction but no significant trough reduction, suggesting that giving the lower doses more frequently may produce antihypertensive effects that are comparable to giving 50 mg once daily.

In clinical trials in patients with essential hypertension, losartan at a daily dose of 50 to 100 mg has been found to be as efficacious as ACE inhibitors, felodipine, and atenolol in reducing bp. Blood pressure lowering with losartan used once and in two divided doses is evident within 1 week and is maximal at 6 weeks. This bp lowering effect of losartan is enhanced by the simultaneous administration of a diuretic agent.

Potential Advantages of Losartan Compared with ACE Inhibitors

ACE inhibitors have proved to be safe and effective drugs in the treatment of hypertension and congestive heart failure. However, there are relatively frequent side effects with these drugs which are observed more commonly in certain groups of patients (e.g., underlying renal abnormality). This has stimulated a search for inhibitors of the RAS without ACE-related side effects. During the early ACE inhibitor era when higher doses were used, the incidence of adverse skin reactions approached 50%. Today, a maximal dose of captopril rarely exceeds 150 mg/day, producing a pruritic maculopapular rash in 4 to 7% of cases. In addition, ACE inhibition–induced angioneurotic edema is rare, as it is with losartan.

Neutropenia (<1000 WBC/mm^3) is a serious but uncommon side effect that is mainly associated with captopril and is almost always reversible on discontinuation. In patients with uncomplicated hypertension, the incidence is 0.01% with captopril. However, among a subset of patients with both underlying renal impairment and collagen vascular disease, the incidence is as high as 3.7%. It is hypothesized that the sulfhydryl group present in captopril, similar to the sulfhydryl group of penicillamine, may contribute to this side effect. Enalapril, which has no sulfhydryl group, has resulted in a lower incidence of neutropenia.

GI toxicity with ACE inhibitors includes dysgeusia (1.4 to 2.1%), nausea, vomiting, and diarrhea (2%). These effects are usually self-limiting and do not require discontinuation of the drug. In fact, disappearance of dysgeusia has been observed after 3 months despite continual treatment with ACE inhibitors. Thus, adverse skin reactions, angioedema, neutropenia, and GI disturbances are class-specific side effects of ACE inhibition that may be avoided by using losartan.

Another common side effect of ACE inhibitors is a dry cough. ACE, also known as *kinase II*, is responsible for the degradation of bradykinin, substance P, and other biologically active peptides in the kallikrein-kinin-prostaglandin system. The mechanism of ACE inhibitor–induced cough is thought to be related to increased bronchial reactivity secondary to reduced degradation of proinflammatory mediators such as bradykinin and substance P. A direct histamine-releasing effect of mast cells and basophils by ACE inhibitors, resulting in an airway inflammation, is also thought to be involved. The prevalence of ACE inhibitor–induced cough in patients is approximately 5%, with about 2% of them requiring discontinuation of the medication. However, some studies reported the incidence to be as high as 34%. Because of high substrate specificity, losartan has no effect on the kallikrein-kinin-prostaglandin system and does not increase the concentration of bradykinin and other peptides, bypassing this undesirable side effect of ACE inhibition.

Drug-induced renal failure is a serious side effect of ACE inhibitors. Normally, the reduction of intrarenal A-II will increase renal blood flow and GFR. However, patients with underlying compromised renal perfusion (secondary to bilateral renal artery stenosis or severe congestive heart failure with markedly reduced cardiac output) may develop a paradoxical decrease in GFR resulting in azotemia. The accepted mechanism for this is a reduction in intrarenal A-II-mediated efferent arterial tone, with a resultant fall in glomerular filtration. This renal abnormality is reversible on discontinuation of ACE inhibitors. Also, induction of hypoaldosteronism by ACE inhibition results in approximately 0.1 to

0.2 mEq/L increase in potassium. Clinically significant hyperkalemia is rare in patients with normal renal function, but it may occur in patients with underlying renal impairment, or those receiving potassium supplements or potassium-sparing diuretics. About 0.3% of patients require discontinuation of ACE inhibition secondary to hyperkalemia. The effects of losartan on renal function and hyperkalemia are not yet fully known.

One of the mechanisms by which ACE inhibition causes hypotension involves the vasodilating effect of increased levels of bradykinin. In animals the renal vasodilator effect of ACE inhibition is partly related to inhibition of bradykinin degradation. Since the antihypertensive effect of losartan is dependent on an active RAS, it was thought that losartan would be a less effective antihypertensive agent compared with ACE inhibitors. However, studies have shown that antihypertensive efficacy of losartan is similar to ACE inhibition. A comparison of the antihypertensive effect of furosemide, losartan, and enalapril in spontaneously hypertensive rats showed that furosemide produced a marked diuresis and tachycardia without changes in blood pressure, but losartan and enalapril decreased mean blood pressure by 41.89 ± 7.17 and 47.13 ± 8.67 mmHg, respectively. In fact, in SHRs the acute, maximal, antihypertensive effect of losartan was greater than that of captopril. For captopril to reduce blood pressure to a similar extent, it would need to be supplemented with a diuretic.

Other Cardiac Applications

Cardiac hypertrophy Angiotensin II promotes a growth response in vascular smooth muscle by stimulating mRNA synthesis, protein synthesis, growth factor expression, and cellular hypertrophy. These responses play a critical role in the pathogenesis of cardiac hypertrophy. Therefore, by blocking the RAS, cardiac hypertrophy can be attenuated. In rats, losartan prevents and decreases cardiac hypertrophy independent of mechanical stimulation. Chronic losartan administration increased PRA and A-II levels, but left ventricular A-II concentration was lowered, suggesting that local RAS, rather than circulating A-II, is involved in the development of cardiac hypertrophy. Furthermore, only losartan was effective in blocking the hypertrophic response of A-II, but not PD123177, suggesting that AT_1 receptors are the main receptors responsible for the hypertrophic response.

An ongoing study, the Losartan Intervention for Endpoint Reduction in Hypertension (LIFE), is designed to assess whether there are clinical benefits associated with regression of LVH with either atenolol or losartan. The study will enroll 8300 patients and will continue for 4 years or until 1040 patients have sustained an acute myocardial infarction, stroke, or cardiovascular death.

Myocardial infarction The local intracardiac RAS may play an important role both in the development of myocardial infarction (MI) and its complications. In patients with high-renin essential hypertension, there is a sevenfold increase in the risk of developing MI compared with patients with low renin levels. In dogs whose coronary arteries were ligated, both the size of the infarct-related area and the area at risk were reduced by pretreatment with an ACE inhibitor. A-II blockade during myocardial ischemia in rat hearts has been shown to significantly lower lactate dehydrogenase activity, creatinine kinase activity, and the incidence and duration of ventricular arrhythmias during the reperfusion period. Similarly, studies using the isolated perfused rat heart have shown that the duration of ventricular arrhythmia is reduced by losartan, captopril, and a renin inhibitor if given before and during the reperfusion. However, if given during reperfusion, only losartan had significantly reduced the duration of ventricular arrhythmias.

The safety of losartan and other A-II receptor blockers needs to be determined in patients with ischemic heart disease. A recent case report described the new onset of angina pectoris in a patient just starting losartan therapy.

Congestive heart failure In early stages of heart failure, compensatory mechanisms are evoked to maintain cardiac output and tissue perfusion. The RAS is stimulated to increase preload and afterload to help maintain cardiac output. These compensatory mechanisms actually worsen heart failure by causing progressive ventricular dilatation. By blocking the RAS, ACE inhibitors decrease systemic vascular resistance and increase venous compliance, thereby decreasing left ventricular end-diastolic pressure. These favorable hemodynamic parameters in turn reduce the development of heart failure and may improve mortality related to CHF. ACE inhibitors have been shown to improve hemodynamics, exercise tolerance, symptoms, and mortality in heart failure. Directly blocking the effect of A-II with losartan may show a similar hemodynamic response and theoretically provide favorable clinical results. Experimental hemodynamic studies in ischemic heart failure have shown that losartan and captopril cause similar acute hemodynamic, hormonal, and renal effects without changing the left ventricular weight/body weight ratio, mean aortic pressures, or heart rates when compared with placebo. These findings demonstrate that inhibition of the RAS creates favorable hemodynamic changes in heart failure. Furthermore, it suggests that losartan may be as effective in the treatment of heart failure as ACE inhibitors.

Losartan has been evaluated as a treatment for CHF. Favorable hemodynamic effects from direct angiotensin II receptor blockade and reductions in left ventricular volumes, left ventricular mass, and collagen content have been demonstrated. In 66 patients with NYHA classes II–III CHF and mean ejection fraction $<40\%$, Gottlieb et al. demonstrated reductions in systemic vascular resistance and mean arterial pressure but were not able to demonstrate more than a trend in the reduction of pulmonary capillary wedge pressure or increases in cardiac index. Crozier et al., in 134 patients with NYHA classes II–III CHF and mean ejection fraction $\leq$ 24%, demonstrated significant improvement in hemodynamics associated with angiotensin receptor antagonism characterized by reduced pulmonary capillary wedge pressure, reduced heart rate, reduced systemic vascular resistance, reduced norepinephrine levels, and an increase in cardiac index. Additional evidence for the effect of angiotensin blockade on hemodynamics in heart failure comes from studies using direct renin antagonists as a means toward decreasing angiotensin II activity. Patients who received either of the direct renin antagonists remikiren or enkiren alone experienced increased cardiac index, reduced left ventricular filling pressures, and reduced systemic vascular resistance. Remikiren and enalaprilat, when given individually, result in nearly identical hemodynamic changes. The addition of enalaprilat to remikiren did not result in additional hemodynamic changes. Selective inhibition of the effects of angiotensin II on the cardiovascular system can result in favorable hemodynamic changes in heart failure that parallel those seen with ACE inhibition. These results also imply that elevated levels of bradykinin, which result from ACE inhibition, do not produce clinically significant hemodynamic changes. Whether angiotensin blockade will produce the same reduction in filling pressures as ACE inhibitors has yet to be widely demonstrated.

In a rat model of heart failure induced by myocardial infarction, Raya et al. demonstrated comparable effects of captopril and losartan on left ventricular volume, left ventricular end-diastolic pressure, and venous compliance. When given for 2 weeks in the period following ligation of the left anterior descending coronary artery, both captopril and losartan reduced left ventricular volume, left ventricular end-diastolic pressure, and central venous pressure when compared with controls. There were no significant differences in infarct size, and left ventricular mass was not significantly different among the three groups. Smits et al. ligated the left anterior descending coronary artery of laboratory rats. Treatment with losartan compared with untreated and sham-operated animals resulted in a decrease in collagen content of the noninfarcted myocardium. Hemodynamic parameters, with the exception of blood pressure, were not significantly changed. Taken together, limited data support the beneficial effects of angiotensin II receptor antagonism in the treatment of severe heart failure following myocardial infarction. Comparisons of angiotensin II receptor blockade with ACE inhibitors are limited.

Lastly, the autocrine-paracrine RAS has been defined at the myocyte level, and a non-ACE tissue, chymase, that can generate angiotensin II has been localized within the myocardium. Although controversial, this chymase may be responsible for 80% of the angiotensin II produced in the human heart. Thus this tissue-based RAS might be a more specific target for therapy than ACE inhibition. Angiotensin II receptor blockade, which should be effective regardless of the pathway through which the angiotensin II is generated, may be an effective therapy. Angiotensin II receptor blockade combined with ACE inhibition might produce more complete angiotensin II blockade while maintaining the favorable effects of ACE on bradykinin and prostaglandin. Preliminary studies do suggest an additive beneficial hemodynamic action when ACE inhibitors are combined with A-II receptor blockers. The importance of this issue remains to be defined.

The extent to which bradykinin and prostaglandins mediate the effects of ACE inhibition is uncertain. Sources of ambiguity arise from species-specific effects of ACE inhibitors on the endothelium or vascular reactivity of laboratory animals and the small number of studies in humans. The evidence supports an important role for prostaglandins and bradykinin, and possibly an increasingly important understanding of the role that intact endothelial function has in patients with left ventricular dysfunction and ischemic heart disease. However, the role of angiotensin in the pathogenesis of ACE inhibition and left ventricular remodeling should not be diminished. The available evidence demonstrates hemodynamic and potential effects of angiotensin inhibition on myocardial growth and left ventricular dilation after myocardial infarction in the absence of changes in bradykinin metabolism. A large-scale trial comparing traditional ACE inhibition with angiotensin receptor inhibition appears both warranted and safe. Multiple studies evaluating mortality outcomes, including the Evaluation of Losartan in the Elderly Trial (ELITE) with angiotensin II receptor blockers in patients with CHF have been completed. A favorable mortality benefit was seen with losartan compared with captopril in elderly patients with CHF.

Postangioplasty vascular restenosis The RAS may modulate the response of the blood vessel wall to an injury, and hence RAS blockade may have inhibitory activity against intimal lesion formation following vessel injury. Inhibition of bovine aortic endothelial cells with lisinopril and losartan leads to an increased expression of the protooncogene c-*src* by increasing endothelial cell migration and urokinaselike plasminogen activator (u-PA) activity. In fact, interruption of the RAS was shown to result in an improvement of vessel patency in animal models of hypertension, hyperlipidemia, and angioplasty. Another cellular response in injured vessels involves smooth-muscle cell (SMC) migration into the intima, followed by SMC proliferation, resulting in intimal lesion formation. The AT_1 receptor seems to be involved in neointimal formation and myointimal proliferative responses after balloon-catheter injury.

There are two different phenotypes of SMCs that have been identified. The contractile or quiescent phenotypes contain contractile proteins α-actin, smooth-muscle myosin, and thick filaments and contract in response to appropriate stimuli, but cannot undergo cytokinesis. On the other hand, the synthetic or activated phenotypes have fewer contractile proteins but have greatly increased synthetic and proliferative capacity. In restenotic lesions after angioplasty, activated phenotypes seem to predominate. Also, A-II stimulates cell proliferation in activated cells, and this effect is blocked by losartan but not PD123177. In situ hybridization studies of 20 coronary-atherectomy specimens demonstrated that restenosis developed in 8 of 10 patients with positive baseline hybridization results (increased expression of activated phenotypes before angioplasty) but in only 1 of 10 patients with negative baseline hybridization results ($p = 0.007$).

In the SHR, after balloon injury of an artery, inhibition of the RAS by ACE inhibitor (benazeprilat or cilazapril) and losartan resulted in a significant reduction in intimal lesion formation. SMC migration was reduced by both benazeprilat and losartan, but SMC proliferation was reduced only by losartan. In the recent MERCATOR restenosis trial, the ACE inhibitor cilazapril did not prevent restenosis or improve clinical outcomes after angioplasty.

Similarly, losartan also was unsuccessful in preventing postangioplasty restenosis.

Renal Disease

The RAS may be involved in renal hemodynamic and glomerular actions that may cause a deterioration in renal function in specific patients. A renal protective effect of A-II blockade by ACE inhibitors has been shown in hypertensive, normotensive, and/or hypertensive patients with diabetic nephropathy and nondiabetic patients with proteinuria. The mechanism by which this occurs is thought to be an ACE inhibitor–induced decrease in efferent arteriolar resistance with reduction of intraglomerular, capillary hydraulic pressure, resulting in a gradual decrease of glomerular membrane permeability to proteins. Losartan inhibits A-II-induced vasoconstriction of the renal and mesenteric vasculature in cats. Losartan causes increased GFR and renal blood flow and decreased renal vascular resistance without changing mean arterial pressure, cardiac output, or systemic vascular resistance. In rats with reduced renal mass, losartan can attenuate the development of proteinuria and segmental glomerular sclerosis. However, in patients with compromised renal perfusion, changes in renal hemodynamics with losartan may paradoxically worsen renal impairment. Losartan has been shown to have similar effects on renal hemodynamic as ACE inhibitors. Therefore, losartan also may be clinically useful in slowing the progression of renal insufficiency secondary to hypertension or diabetes. AT_1 receptors, located in the glomerulus, tubules, and medulla, have been implicated in physiologically important renal functions. However, PD123177 also shows a diuretic effect on renal tubules without affecting renal hemodynamics and vasopressin levels.

Cerebrovascular and Other Neurologic Diseases

There are several major effects of the RAS on the CNS. The RAS participates in the autoregulation of cerebral blood flow, which is a process that maintains relatively constant cerebral blood flow despite wide changes in arterial blood pressure. In fact, locally produced A-II may be involved in cerebral autoregulation. In experimental and clinical studies, overstimulation of RAS has been implicated in the development of end-organ damage such as stroke. A favorable shift in cerebral autoregulation occurs with blockers of the RAS so that systemic lowering of blood pressure by A-II blockade does not result in decreased cerebral blood flow. A-II blockade with losartan has shown a decreased mortality from strokes in stroke-prone SHRs fed a high sodium diet.

Central blood pressure control involves central AT_1 receptors located mainly in the anterior hypothalamic area. In SHRs, microinjection of losartan into the anterior hypothalamic area causes a significant dose-related decrease in mean arterial pressure without change in heart rate. Infusion of intracerebroventricular (ICV) losartan in salt-sensitive rats also produces inhibition of an A-II-induced pressor effect. The AT_1 receptor seems to be involved with both central pressor and dipsogenic effects, because AT_2 antagonists do not inhibit these effects. Also, A-II is a dipsogen that raises blood pressure. In rats, ICV or IV administration of losartan inhibited the dipsogenic effect of ICV- or IV-administered A-II. However, losartan does not readily cross the blood-brain barrier in rats, since oral losartan did not antagonize the ICV-administered A-II nor did ICV losartan block the IV A-II-induced pressor response.

In the peripheral nervous system, losartan abolishes A-II-induced pre- and postsynaptic potentiation of noradrenergic neurotransmission in animals. Another CNS function of A-II is in the synapse and specifically involves interactions with neurotransmitters such as acetylcholine, catecholamines, serotonin, and other neuropeptides. These interactions may lead to alterations in motivation (e.g., thirst, pain), memory, and motor control. Performance deficit measured in a passive avoidance task in rats by ICV administration of renin was attenuated by concomitant ICV administration of losartan and ACE inhibitor, but not PD123177, suggesting that only the AT_1 receptor is involved in these responses. The significance of the interactions is not yet known.

Oncogenesis

There is speculation regarding an association between the RAS and tumorigenesis. In smooth and cardiac muscle cells, a growth-promoting effect of A-II is suspected, since A-II has been shown to stimulate cellular proliferation and mRNA and protein synthesis, as well as enhancing the expression of protooncogene and growth factors such as PDGF (platelet-derived growth factor) and TGF-β (transforming growth factor β). Jackson et al. reported that the *mas* oncogene product may be a "neuronal-type" angiotensin receptor and induction of the *mas* oncogene may require stimulation by A-II. Since the *mas* oncogene has been shown to be oncogenic in nude mice and has transforming activity on NIH 3T3 cells, there is concern that by interfering with the RAS one may induce tumorigenesis. In large clinical trials, the incidence of cancer was not statistically significant between ACE inhibitor–treated groups versus placebo groups. Currently, information on oncogenic properties of losartan is not available. Therefore, any conclusions regarding possible tumorigenesis from ACE inhibition and losartan are premature, and further studies, including long-term follow-ups of patients who are being treated with ACE inhibition and losartan, need to be conducted.

UNRESOLVED ISSUES

A-II receptor blockers appear to be efficacious and safe drugs for the treatment of systemic hypertension. However, losartan and other A-II receptor blockers are specific blockers of the AT_1 receptor and do not block the AT_2 receptors. AT_1 blockade with losartan leads to an increase in all angiotensin peptides, and the consequences of heightened AT_2 receptor stimulation have not been defined.

It is also not known what effects the A-II receptor blockers have on overall mortality, morbidity, and quality of life, issues being evaluated in clinical trials such as the Trial for Usual Care of Hypertension.

SUGGESTED READINGS

The CONSENSUS Trial Study Group: Effects of enalapril on mortality in severe congestive heart failure: Results of the Cooperative North Scandinavian Enalapril Survival Study (CONSENSUS). *N Engl J Med* 316:1429, 1987.

Frishman WH (ed): Angiotensin converting enzyme inhibitors, in *Current Cardiovascular Drugs*. Philadelphia, Current Medicine, 1995, pp 11–25.

Kang PM, Landau AJ, Eberhardt RT, Frishman WH: Angiotensin II receptor antagonists: A new approach to blockade of the renin-angiotensin system. *Am Heart J* 127:1388, 1994.

Kostis JB, DeFlice EA (eds): *Angiotensin Converting Enzyme Inhibitors*. New York, Alan R Liss, 1987.

Landzberg BR, Frishman WH, Lerrick K: Pathophysiology and pharmacological approaches for prevention of coronary artery restenosis following coronary artery balloon angioplasty and related procedures. *Prog Cardiovasc Dis* 34:361, 1997.

Loeb HS, Johnson G, Henrick A, et al: Effect of enalapril, hydralazine plus isosorbide dinitrate, and prazosin on hospitalization in patients with chronic congestive heart failure: The V-HeFT VA Cooperative Studies Group. *Circulation* 87(6 Suppl):V178, 1993.

Markham A, Goa KL: Valsartan: A review of its pharmacology and therapeutic use in essential hypertension. *Drugs* 54:299, 1997.

Pfeffer MA, Braunwald E, Moye LA, et al, on behalf of the SAVE Investigators: Effect of captopril on mortality and morbidity in patients with left ventricular dysfunction after myocardial infarction: Results of the Survival and Ventricular Enlargement Trial. *N Engl J Med* 327:669, 1992.

Pitt B, Segal R, Martinez FA, et al, on behalf of ELITE Study Investigators: Randomised trial of losartan versus captopril in patients over 65 with heart failure (Evaluation of Losartan in the Elderly Study: ELITE). *Lancet* 349:747, 1997.

Ruddy MC, Kostis JB, Frishman WH: Drugs that affect the renin-angiotensin system, in Frishman WH, Sonnenblick EH (eds): *Cardiovascular Pharmacother*apeutics. New York, McGraw-Hill, 1997, pp 131–192.

The SOLVD Investigators: Effect of enalapril on survival in patients with reduced left ventricular ejection fractions and congestive heart failure. *N Engl J Med* 325:293, 1991.

The SOLVD Investigators: Effect of enalapril on mortality and the development of heart failure in asymptomatic patients with reduced left ventricular ejection fractions. *N Engl J Med* 327:685, 1992.

Chapter 6 Diuretic Therapy in Cardiovascular Disease

Michele H. Mokrzycki, Praveen Tamirisa, and William Frishman

Diuretics have been employed widely for more than 30 years and have been the mainstay of treatment for congestive heart failure (CHF) and systemic hypertension during that period. Despite the advent of newer agents for treating both conditions, diuretics continue to be utilized and are among the most commonly prescribed drugs in the world.

Diuretics are classified into three main categories determined by their structure, their site of action, and their effects on electrolyte excretion. The three main types of diuretics are the thiazides (and related drugs), the loop diuretics, and the potassium-sparing agents. Different pharmacologic approaches to diuresis are also available or are under development.

In this chapter, the diuretic drugs are discussed, focusing on their use in the treatment of CHF, systemic hypertension, and angina pectoris.

DIURETIC CLASSES

Loop Diuretics

The most potent diuretics are those whose action is in the medullary thick ascending limb of Henle (mTAL) because of the percentage of filtrate reabsorption that occurs at this segment of the nephron. In the euvolemic state, ~20% of filtered sodium load is reabsorbed in the mTAL, compared with only 7% in the distal tubule and 5% in the collecting duct. Drugs in this diuretic class include furosemide, bumetanide, torsemide, and ethacrynic acid. The loop diuretics (Table 6-1) are > 98% protein-bound and therefore are not freely filtered by the glomerulus. They access the tubular lumen by secretion via an organic anion transporter. Secretion of loop diuretic may be impaired by the presence of elevated levels of endogenous organic acids, such as in renal failure, and by probenecid, salicylates, and nonsteroidal anti-inflammatory agents. Once in the lumen of the tubule, the loop diuretics compete with chloride for binding to the $Na^+/K^+/2Cl^-$ cotransporter situated on the apical membrane of the mTAL, thereby inhibiting the reabsorption of sodium and chloride. The urinary diuretic concentration best represents the fraction of drug delivered to the mTAL and significantly correlates with the natriuretic response following diuretic administration.

Furosemide is the most widely used diuretic in this class. In normal patients, the oral bioavailability of furosemide is 50%. Following an oral dose, the onset of action is within 30 to 60 min, peaks at 1 to 2 h, and has a duration of action of 6 h. The normal half-life of furosemide

TABLE 6-1 Diuretic Drugs

	Half-life, h	Route of elimination
Thiazide and thiazide-like drugs		
Bendroflumethiazide	8.5	30% R, 70% M
Benthiazide	NA	NA
Chlorthiazide	15 (normal)	R
Chlorthalidone	35–50	
Cyclothiazide	NA	R
Hydrochlorothiazide	13 (normal)	R
Hydroflumethiazide	17	50% R, 50% M
Indapamide	14	M
Methyclothiazide	NA	R
Metolazone	14	80% R, 20% B
Polythiazide	26	25% R, 75% M
Quinethalone	NA	R
Trichlormethiazide	6	R
Loop diuretic drugs		
Bumetanide	1.5	60% R, 40% M
Ethacrynic acid	1	65% R, 35% M
Furosemide	0.5–1 (normal)	60% R, 40% M
Torsemide	2–4	20% R, 80% M
Potassium-sparing drugs		
Amiloride	6–9	50% R, 50% B
Triamterene*	3	M
Spironolactone	13–24	M
Osmotic agents		
Glycerin	0.5	M
Mannitol	1 (normal)	R
Urea	NA	R
Carbonic anhydrase inhibitors		
Acetazolamide		

Note: R = renal excretion of intact drug; M = metabolized to inactive compounds; B = biliary.
* = Metabolized to active metabolite canrenone that is excreted in urine; NA = not available.

is 50 min. Furosemide may be given intravenously (IV) over 1 to 2 min. Following IV administration, diuresis begins within 15 min and peaks at between 30 and 60 min. The duration of action is up to 2 h when given intravenously.

Sixty percent of a furosemide dose is excreted unchanged in the urine; the rest is conjugated with glucoronic acid in the kidney. In renal insufficiency (GFR < 30 mL/min), the elimination half-life of furosemide is prolonged and the diuretic response is impaired, largely owing to reduced drug delivery to its site of action within the tubule. In CHF, the pharmacokinetics of oral furosemide are altered: delayed furosemide absorption leads to a delay in the time at which peak concentration occurs. Altered furosemide pharmacodynamic properties also characterize the state of heart failure. This occurs independently of the route of administration (oral versus IV) and is caused by adaptations within the glomerular microcirculation and renal tubule (which are present) during chronic diuretic administration. The pharmacokinetic and pharmacodynamic properties of ethacrynic acid are similar to furosemide.

Bumetanide is 40 times more potent than furosemide and is available in both oral and IV preparations. In normal patients, the bioavailability of bumetanide is 80% following an oral dose, and the onset of diuretic effect occurs within 30 min and peaks within 1 h. The duration of action of oral bumetanide is between 3 and 6 h, and its half-life is between 1 and 3.5 h. In healthy subjects, 60% of a bumetanide dose is excreted unchanged in the urine. The remaining dose is metabolized in the liver, via the cytochrome P450 system, a pathway that is unaltered in renal insufficiency. In renal failure, the hepatic clearance of bumetanide sufficiently compensates for the impaired renal clearance such that the elimination half-life of bumetanide is not prolonged. Similar to furosemide, the delayed absorption of oral bumetanide results in lower peak concentrations, as well as in delayed time to peak concentration.

Torsemide is a new loop diuretic that differs from others in its class in that 80% of a dose undergoes hepatic metabolism. Because only 20% of the drug is excreted unchanged in the urine, its half-life is minimally altered in renal failure. Torsemide is absorbed rapidly and is 80 to 90% bioavailable. In patients with chronic renal insufficiency or cirrhosis, the natriuretic response following torsemide is unaffected by route of administration (oral versus IV). Maximal sodium excretion occurs within the first 2 h after either route. In healthy subjects, the half-life of torsemide is 3.3 h, but it is prolonged to 8 h in cirrhosis. When selecting an oral agent in patients with heart failure, torsemide may be particularly advantageous in that its absorption is unimpaired and is less variable than with oral furosemide. In fact, torsemide pharmacokinetics in patients with heart failure are comparable with those in healthy subjects. However, as is the case with all loop diuretics, dose-response curves for torsemide in patients with CHF are shifted downward and to the right, suggesting altered drug pharmacodynamics and a diminished diuretic response.

In addition to their natriuretic properties, loop diuretics modulate renal prostaglandin synthesis, particularly prostaglandin E_2 (PGE_2). Following furosemide or ethacrynic acid administration, urinary PGE_2 excretion is enhanced and accompanied by a significant improvement in renal plasma flow. This effect has not been demonstrated with the thiazide class of diuretics. Clearance studies support the fact that renal prostaglandins, particularly PGE_2, possess important diuretic properties. PGE_2 inhibits sodium reabsorption in both the mTAL and the collecting duct and increases free water clearance in the collecting duct by antagonizing vasopressin.

Thiazides

The thiazide diuretics (see Table 6-1) may be reasonable first-line natriuretic agents in early left ventricular (LV) dysfunction, during which renal perfusion is not yet significantly compromised. In overt ventricular failure, however, thiazides are usually ineffective. Thiazides are 50% protein-bound, and more than 95% of a dose is excreted unchanged in the urine. They gain access into the tubular lumen by both glomerular filtration and tubular secretion. In the kidney, they inhibit sodium chloride reabsorption in the early distal tubule where they compete for the chloride site on the apically located Na^+/Cl^- cotransporter.

Hydrochlorothiazide (HCTZ) is the most widely prescribed drug in this class of diuretics. Seventy-one percent of an oral dose of HCTZ is absorbed. The onset of diuresis is within 2 h, peaks between 3 and 6 h, and continues for up to 12 h. HCTZ's pharmacokinetics follow a two-compartment model of elimination (α phase 5 h, β phase 6 to 15 h), and the half-life of HCTZ is prolonged in decompensated heart failure and with renal insufficiency.

Metolazone is a quinazoline diuretic and is similar to the thiazides in structure and mechanism of action. Although its major effect is in the cortical diluting segment, metolazone has a minor inhibitory effect on proximal tubular sodium reabsorption. Metolazone is lipid-soluble and easily accesses the tubular lumen during states of renal insufficiency, unlike the thiazides. Another advantage of metolazone is its longer duration of action of 12 to 24 h.

With chronic thiazide diuretic use, a *ceiling effect* is observed. This term refers to the limited period of time (~3 days) during which thiazides produce a net sodium loss while on a constant sodium diet. After this relatively brief period of negative sodium balance, a new steady state is established in which sodium intake and output are matched. This phenomenon is caused by renal tubular adaptation to volume contraction associated with diuretic use. In hypovolemia, a larger fraction of filtered sodium load is reabsorbed proximally compared with baseline when euvolemic (80% versus 67%, respectively). In addition, high aldosterone levels increase sodium retention in more distal nephron segments; often referred to as the *braking phenomenon*.

Potassium-Sparing Diuretics

Spironolactone is a lipid-soluble potassium-sparing diuretic and competes with aldosterone for binding to its receptor in the principal cell of the collecting duct. Spironolactone is particularly advantageous during states of reduced renal perfusion because the drug's delivery to its site of action is not dependent on glomerular filtration rate (GFR). Amiloride and triamterene are similar to spironolactone in that they are potassium-sparing and act on the principal cell; however, they must be delivered intralumenally to be effective (see Table 6-1). More specifically, they reduce Na^+ flux into principal cells by blocking the apically located sodium channel. When used alone, the potassium-sparing diuretics are relatively weak diuretics. In heart failure they are useful when combined with a loop diuretic to overcome diuretic resistance and reduce potassium wasting.

Carbonic Anhydrase Inhibitors

Acetazolamide, a nonbacteriostatic sulfonamide, inhibits carbonic anhydrase, an enzyme that plays an important role in bicarbonate reabsorption in the proximal tubule (see Table 6-1). Bicarbonate (HCO_3) reabsorption in the nephron is dependent on proton (H^+) secretion into the lumen, where the two combine to form carbonic acid. Carbonic acid is rapidly metabolized in the presence of carbonic anhydrase. When this enzyme is absent, intraluminal H^+ concentration rises, thereby inhibiting additional H^+ secretion and impairing HCO_3 absorption by as much as 80%. Acetazolamide is an effective diuretic when the filtered load of bicarbonate is high, as when the serum bicarbonate is > 28 mEq/L. In the absence of a metabolic alkalosis, acetazolamide is a relatively weak diuretic because sodium absorption is enhanced at more distal sites: the mTAL, distal tubule, and collecting duct. Although not a first-line agent, acetazolamide is useful in the setting of heart failure when a significant primary metabolic alkalosis occurs, such as is seen with contraction alkalosis, vomiting, nasogastric aspiration, or transfusion of citrate-containing blood products. Significant urinary potassium losses occur with acetazolamide use.

Osmotic Diuretics

Mannitol is a nonreabsorbable polysaccharide and is freely filtered by the glomerulus (see Table 6-1). It exerts an osmotic effect by trapping water in the lumen resulting in obligatory water and solute losses. This class of diuretics is contraindicated in the setting of CHF for obvious reasons. Mannitol mediates the movement of extravascular fluid into the intravascular compartment, which in the setting of CHF may precipitate acute pulmonary edema and worsen heart failure. Other drugs in this class include urea and glycerin, which, along with mannitol, are used to treat cerebral edema in patients with normal renal function.

FACTORS INFLUENCING DIURETIC EFFICACY IN HEART FAILURE

Altered Pharmacokinetics

The efficacy of furosemide and other loop diuretics is often significantly reduced in decompensated heart failure. Impaired drug absorption has been implicated as one of the causes of the drug's variable efficacy when administered orally. Reduced gastric and intestinal motility, edematous bowel wall, and decreased splanchnic blood flow have been demonstrated in heart failure and may be responsible for delayed furosemide absorption; however, the total amount of furosemide absorbed in 24 h is similar to that found in normal patients.

In patients with stable, compensated heart failure given oral furosemide, the time to peak urinary excretion is prolonged to ~190 min (normal = 90 min) and peak urinary excretion rate is reduced by 50%. Furosemide and bumetanide, when given in doses of equivalent potency, induce a similar natriuretic response in patients with heart failure. The pharmacokinetic properties of IV furosemide are unaltered in heart failure compared with healthy patients with similar creatinine clearances. In decompensated heart failure, the IV route of administration is preferable when possible, since the onset of diuresis is shorter and more predictable.

The potency of a loop diuretic is determined by the amount that enters the tubular lumen of the mTAL. Delivery of furosemide to its intralumenal site of action is dependent on renal plasma flow and proximal tubular secretion. As renal plasma flow and peritubular capillary flow decline, so will the delivery of furosemide to the basolateral membrane of the proximal tubular cell. The secretion of furosemide is altered when the GFR is severely reduced (< 30 mL/min) because of the accumulation of endogenous organic acids. These end products of protein metabolism compete with furosemide for secretion by the organic anion exchanger. With this degree of renal insufficiency, the loop diuretics must be administered in higher doses to ensure adequate delivery to their site of action.

In the setting of normal renal function, the duration of the natriuretic effect of furosemide and bumetanide with IV administration is between 1 and 2 h and, when given by oral route, is 6 h. This relatively brief period of natriuresis is followed by a state of sodium avidity, referred to as *postdiuretic sodium retention.* The degree of salt retention is enhanced when a high salt diet is ingested. Ways in which this can be averted are by restricting sodium intake and by increasing the frequency of diuretic dosing to a twice or thrice daily schedule.

High-Dose Loop Diuretic Administration

In patients with CHF refractory to standard furosemide doses, high-dose furosemide may be efficacious. Marangoni and colleagues administered high-dose IV furosemide (500 to 2000 mg daily) for a mean of 10 days to 20 patients with severe CHF previously resistant to lower doses of IV furosemide. An improvement in diuresis and reduction in body weight were observed. Sixteen of 20 patients were upgraded from New York Heart Association (NYHA) class IV to III and one patient from NYHA class IV to II. Similar studies have reported improved furosemide efficacy in refractory heart failure using high-dose oral furosemide. Kuchar and O'Rourke found a clinical improvement, as assessed by NYHA classification criteria, in 17 of 21 patients using high-dose oral furosemide (> 500 mg daily) for 1 month.

When moderate to severe renal impairment is present in decompensated heart failure, a brief trial of high-dose furosemide is reasonable. Gerlag and Van Meijel treated patients with renal insufficiency (mean GFR = 32 mL/min) and refractory CHF with high-dose oral (960 ± 688 mg daily) and IV (up to 1-g boluses or 4-g continuous infusion) furosemide. Over a 4-week period, the mean weight reduction was 11.1 ± 5.2 kg, and an improvement in NYHA classification was observed in all patients. Hypokalemia was the most common side effect observed, and dehydration, gout, tinnitus, and reversible renal impairment also were reported. In general, when treating decompensated heart failure in the setting of severe renal impairment, if urine output does not improve within 2 to 4 h following repeated administration of high-dose furosemide, the initiation of dialysis or hemofiltration for volume removal should be considered.

Continuous IV Loop Diuretic Infusion

Continuous IV administration of loop diuretic is an effective method of overcoming diuretic resistance in heart failure and is preferable to intermittent IV administration. In a randomized crossover study comparing continuous infusion versus bolus bumetanide injection in chronic renal failure (mean GFR = 17 mL/min), Rudy and colleagues observed a greater net sodium excretion during continuous infusion despite comparable total 14-h drug excretion. The rate of urinary bumetanide excretion remained constant when infused. With intermittent administration, peak bumetanide excretion was observed within the first 2 h and tapered thereafter. Furthermore, the maximum serum bumetanide concentration was lower during continuous infusion when compared with intermittent dosing (155 versus 1118 μg/L).

In CHF, continuous infusion of furosemide produces a similar natriuresis at serum concentrations 20 times lower than after a comparably effective bolus dose (0.5 mg/L versus 10 mg/L). Only one prospective, randomized crossover study is available that compares continuous IV infusion of furosemide (loading dose of 30 to 40 mg followed by infusion at a rate of 2.5 to 3.3 mg/h for 48 h) versus intermittent IV bolus administration (30 to 40 mg every 8 h for 48 h) in NYHA class III and IV heart failure. Although a small study, Lahav and colleagues observed a significantly greater diuresis and natriuresis using continuous furosemide infusion compared with intermittent administration; this was accomplished at a lower peak furosemide concentration. When continuously infused, the pattern of furosemide delivery produced more effective drug utilization, that is, sodium excretion relative to total furosemide excretion, whereas with intermittent bolus furosemide, wide fluctuations in urine output and sodium excretion were observed. Theoretically, infusion of furosemide at a constant rate may be safer than intermittent IV dosing, although a larger study is needed to confirm this.

Altered Pharmacodynamics

Dose-response curves relating the urinary furosemide excretion rate to the sodium excretion rate in both compensated and decompensated heart failure reveal an impaired response to diuretics when compared with normal patients. This occurs independently of the mode of administration and is caused by tubular adaptation to chronic diuretic use. Extracellular volume contraction is accompanied by reduced GFR and filtered sodium load, as well as increased reabsorption of sodium in the proximal nephron. The end result is impaired delivery of sodium to the mTAL. Following the prolonged administration of a loop diuretic, a compensatory increase in sodium reabsorption in nephron segments distal to the mTAL occurs in response to increased sodium delivery to these segments. Stanton and Kaissling observed alterations in the cellular ultrastructure on electron microscopy in the early distal tubule and collecting duct during chronic diuretic therapy. These changes included an increase in cell volume and proliferation of the basolateral membrane of distal convoluted tubule cells and principal cells, and were independent of changes in aldosterone concentration or extracellular volume. Other investigators have reported a marked increase in Na^+/K^+-ATPase activity and cellular hypertrophy in the distal convoluted tubule, connecting segment, and collecting tubule in rats after furosemide therapy.

Combination Diuretic Use

A reasonable approach to overcome distal sodium retention is the addition of distal-acting diuretics to loop diuretic therapy. Numerous reports have demonstrated a rapid profound diuresis (1 to 2 L daily within 24 to 48 h), accompanied by clinical improvement, following the addition of metolazone to furosemide in CHF patients previously resistant to furosemide alone. Metolazone, a thiazide-like diuretic, is particularly advantageous because duration of action is prolonged, it is lipophilic, and it remains effective in states of renal impairment. However, in a study comparing metolazone with a thiazide, when either was used in combination with a loop diuretic, no significant difference in sodium excretion or urine output was observed between the two drugs. Spironolactone, when used in combination with a loop diuretic, also has been associated with an improvement in diuretic response in CHF patients previously resistant to loop diuretics.

OTHER PHARMACOLOGIC APPROACHES TO DIURESIS

Dopamine in Heart Failure

Since the 1960s, dopamine has been used as a natriuretic agent in the setting of heart failure. Goldberg and colleagues, in 1963, were the first to report a natriuresis using low-dose dopamine in four patients with

CHF when used alone, without conventional diuretic agents. Uncontrolled studies show a modest improvement in GFR and renal plasma flow in patients with CHF when low-dose dopamine was used in the absence of other diuretics; however, these findings have not been duplicated in all reported series. In fact, several investigators were unable to demonstrate a diuretic effect at low doses but did so at higher doses of dopamine infusion. Only recently have properly controlled clinical trials become available that critically evaluate the renal-enhancing effects of low-dose dopamine as an adjunct to standard diuretic therapy in the setting of heart failure.

Dopamine's actions are dose-dependent. At low doses (0.5 to 2 mg/kg per minute), dopamine stimulates D1 receptors located in the renal, mesenteric, coronary, and cerebral arterioles, mediating vasodilation. In the kidney, both the afferent and efferent arterioles dilate in response to dopamine, actions that result in an increase in renal plasma flow, but with little to no increase in GFR. At this dose, dopamine exerts a direct effect in the proximal tubule, where it interferes with sodium reabsorption. This may be enhanced by dopamine's inhibitory effect on aldosterone secretion and by its vasodilatory effect on the peritubular capillary, which impairs reabsorption of filtrate. With higher doses (2 to 5 mg/kg per minute), the β_1-receptor effect predominates, which is characterized by enhanced cardiac contractility, cardiac output, and stroke volume. At doses of 5 to 10 mg/kg per minute, α-receptor-mediated vasoconstriction and elevated systemic vascular resistance are present.

Even when administered in the low-dose range, it is difficult to separate the D1-receptor effect of dopamine from the β-adrenergic effect, since there is much overlap. Substantial adverse effects may occur at this dose of dopamine, including elevated LV end-diastolic pressure, pulmonary capillary wedge pressure, and increased frequency of ventricular ectopy. It should be pointed out that when dopamine is infused for longer than 24 h, D1-receptor-mediated hemodynamic changes are attenuated. This may be due to upregulation of the receptor on chronic stimulation.

More recently, several prospectively randomized, controlled studies became available that evaluated dopamine's efficacy in heart failure. Swan and colleagues were unable to demonstrate an improvement in GFR when dopamine was infused at low doses (1 to 3 mg/kg per minute) in patients with compensated heart failure (NYHA class II or III). Furthermore, when low-dose dopamine was infused with furosemide, no additional improvement in natriuresis was observed. In a similar study, Good and colleagues evaluated the effect of dopamine on a furosemide-induced diuresis in patients with stable chronic heart failure. They reported no increase in urine volume or sodium excretion with either low (1 mg/kg per minute) or high (10 mg/kg per minute) doses of adjunctive dopamine. The efficacy of low-dose dopamine also has been evaluated in elderly patients with CHF who were resistant to diuretics and angiotensin converting enzyme inhibitors. Dopamine did not significantly alter the GFR, renal plasma flow, urine volume, or sodium excretion. The use of low-dose dopamine in heart failure is not supported by recent controlled trials, particularly when used as an adjunct to conventional diuretics.

The risks of dopamine, even at low doses, are not without consequence. Serious adverse effects have been reported while using low doses, although they were reported in studies of small sample size and that lacked placebo controls. These include reports of myocardial infarction, ventricular arrhythmia, digital necrosis, and reduced ventilatory drive in response to hypoxemia. Mucosal ischemia and translocation of bacteria and bacterial toxins have been demonstrated in animal models of shock in which low doses of dopamine were utilized.

Diuretics, Angiotensin Converting Enzyme Inhibition, and Renal Function

In the past decade, the angiotensin converting enzyme inhibitors (ACEI) have revolutionized the treatment of LV dysfunction and overt heart failure. However, functional renal insufficiency occurs in about 30% of patients with severe CHF during ACEI and diuretic therapy. This is most common in the acute setting, during which abrupt changes in mean arterial pressure (MAP) cause a deterioration in renal function and impair the diuretic effect of furosemide. At times of reduced renal perfusion pressure, angiotensin II's (AT_2's) vasoconstrictive effect on the efferent arteriole increases intraglomerular pressure, thereby maintaining GFR. During volume depletion, if the MAP falls below the range of glomerular autoregulation, the addition of an ACEI will result in a decline in GFR. This is due to ACEI-induced efferent arteriolar relaxation. When AT_2 is inhibited to a lesser degree such that GFR remains stable, as with low dose of ACEI (captopril 1 mg), an enhanced natriuretic response to furosemide is observed.

Risk factors for developing functional renal insufficiency when using an ACEI in heart failure are hyponatremia < 135 mEq/L, diabetes, and the use of long-acting forms of ACEI. Packer found enalapril to be more frequently associated with prolonged hypotension, lack of natriuretic response, and a fall in creatinine clearance by ~20% in severe chronic heart failure when compared with captopril. Sodium balance plays an important role in modulating the renal response to ACEI in heart failure. Patients with hemodynamic findings of salt and volume depletion before ACEI and who receive large diuretic doses are also at risk for developing functional renal insufficiency [higher PRA (plasma renin activity), mean RAP (right atrial pressure) < 5 mm, MAP < 60 mm, and LVFP (left ventricular filling pressure) < 15 mm].

In heart failure, the concomitant use of diuretics, ACEIs, and prostaglandin inhibitors [nonsteroidal anti-inflammatory agents (NSAIDs), aspirin] may result in acute renal insufficiency. Locally produced prostacyclin plays an important role in opposing afferent arteriole vasoconstriction and augmenting or maintaining renal blood flow (RBF) in states of reduced renal perfusion. In this setting, NSAID use is most commonly associated with reversible, hemodynamically mediated renal insufficiency but may progress to acute tubular necrosis. Mild functional renal insufficiency is usually well tolerated during combination diuretic and ACEI therapy and does not necessarily require withdrawal of ACEI therapy. However, when clinically significant worsening of GFR occurs, reasonable initial therapeutic measures include a reduction in the diuretic dose and liberalization of dietary sodium intake. ACEI dose should be adjusted when the severity of heart failure worsens. Discontinuation of ACEIs should be considered when modest to severe renal insufficiency or severe hyperkalemia (> 5 mEq/L) occurs.

DIURETICS IN SYSTEMIC HYPERTENSION

Hypertension is one of the most common indications for prescribing medications in the United States. Current estimates report that as many as 50 million people in the United States are hypertensives, as defined by a systolic blood pressure (SBP) > 140 mmHg and/or diastolic blood pressure (DBP) > 90 mmHg. Both cardiovascular and cerebrovascular events, renal disease, and mortality from all causes increase in a continuous and etiologically significant manner with higher levels of both SBP and DBP. In its most recent reports, the Joint National Committee on the Detection, Evaluation, and Treatment of High Blood Pressure (JNC V and JNC VI) advocated the use of diuretics and β blockers as optimal first-line antihypertensive agents. This is based on outcome studies utilizing diuretics and β blockers that reported a reduction in strokes and other cardiovascular end points. However, the prognosis and appropriate treatment for individual patients should be based on considerations that go beyond the absolute blood pressure reading.

Salt-Sensitive Hypertension

Essential hypertension is a heterogeneous disease, and patients vary in their response to different therapies and cardiovascular risk. Renin-sodium profiling has been proposed by Alderman, Laragh and others as a way of categorizing hypertensive patients and of identifying the relative contribution of salt-volume sensitivity and renin-mediated vasoconstriction to the pathophysiology of hypertension. Renin-sodium profiling is determined by plotting the PRA with the concurrent 24-h urine Na^+ excretion. Alderman and colleagues determined the renin-sodium profile in more than 1700 subjects with mild to moderate hypertension. Low renin-sodium profiling, indicative of sodium-volume mediated hypertension, was found in 30% of patients and was more prevalent among blacks, women, and those older than 55 years of age. High renin profiles were found in 10 to 20% of patients; the remaining

50% of the population studied exhibited renin values within the normal range. The fact that hypertensives had any renin presence is abnormal, since data in normotensive subjects report suppressed renin values associated with a rise in blood pressure.

To better interpret the renin-sodium relationship in hypertension, an analytical model entitled the *vasoconstriction-volume analysis* has been proposed by Laragh. According to this model, a high renin-Na^+ product represents one end of the spectrum of hypertension. This group includes malignant and renovascular hypertension, in which excessive renin secretion creates a "dry," intensely vasoconstricted, and volume-contracted state. At the other end of the spectrum are the patients with low-renin hypertension, largely owing to salt retention and extracellular volume expansion. Most hypertensive patients fall somewhere between these extreme groups and have inappropriate amounts of renin relative to total body Na^+. According to these data, one may conclude that sodium retention is a contributing factor to the development of essential hypertension in ~80% of patients. Theoretically, the renin-sodium profiling data provide strong support for the first-line use of diuretics with or without the addition of β blockers in most patients. Renin-sodium profiling also has prognostic importance and is of value in predicting cardiovascular risk. In Alderman's study, patients with high renin-sodium profiles (young patients, whites, and men) were found to have a higher risk of myocardial infarction despite similar blood pressure control when compared with those with medium and low renin-sodium profiles (incidence per 1000 person years 14.7 versus 5.6 and 2.8). This relation did not apply to cerebrovascular accidents, noncardiovascular disease, or overall mortality.

Mechanisms by Which Diuretics Lower Blood Pressure

The exact mechanisms by which diuretics reduce blood pressure are not known. Initially the drugs reduce intracellular volume and cardiac output. However, with long-term diuretic use, blood pressure remains reduced because of reduced peripheral vascular resistance, with cardiac output returning to pretreatment levels. Diuretics do not have a direct effect on vascular smooth muscle, and the mechanism for the effect on vascular resistance may relate to a persistent reduction in body sodium. A reduced concentration of sodium in vascular smooth muscle may reduce intracellular calcium concentrations, making the smooth muscle cells more resistant to contractile stimuli and vasoconstrictor hormones.

Diuretics in Clinical Trials

Diuretics and β blockers have been associated with a reduction in the risk of stroke, cardiovascular events, and overall mortality in long-term controlled clinical trials. No other class of antihypertensive agents has been shown to affect outcome in terms of cardiovascular end points or mortality. Fourteen major trials in which diuretics and/or β blockers were used as first-line agents were recently reviewed. Active treatment of hypertension in these trials was associated with a significant reduction in the incidence of strokes and a small reduction in cardiovascular events, including mortality.

Five studies were specifically aimed at the elderly hypertensive (age > 60): the Systolic Hypertension in Elderly Program (SHEP), the Swedish Trial in Old Patients (STOP), the Medical Research Council Trial in the treatment of older adults (MRC 2), the European Working Party on High Blood Pressure in the Elderly (EWPHE), and the trial of Coope and Warrender. The impact of antihypertensive treatment on mortality was greater in elderly subjects than in those < 60 years of age. Stroke reduction was similar and consistent in all the trials regardless of age group; however, active treatment was associated with a greater protective effect against myocardial infarction and CHF in older patients than in younger patients. In addition to their beneficial effects on mortality and cardiovascular end points, diuretics have been shown to improve the quality of life as assessed by exercise capacity.

Four clinical trials are available in which diuretics were compared with β blockers: the International Prospective Primary Prevention Study in Hypertension (IPPPSH), Heart Attack Primary Prevention in Hypertension Research Group (HAPPHY), Medical Research Council (MRC), and MRC 2. In combination, these trials consisted of 34,676 patients who were treated and followed for 5 years. The two drug classes were comparable with regard to the incidence of stroke. With regard to myocardial infarction, two studies suggested that β blockers were superior and two studies supported greater benefit with diuretics. In fact, the MRC 2 was the only trial to show a statistical difference in incidence of myocardial infarction between the groups and found diuretics to be superior to β blockers. It has been argued, however, that these results may be skewed because many patients on β blockers were withdrawn from therapy for bradycardia. Since the greatest benefits in postinfarction studies were in those patients who had maximum β blockade, many potential responders may have been inappropriately taken off therapy.

Special Groups of Hypertensives

Elderly

There are approximately 25 million people over the age of 65 and as many as 50% are hypertensive, as defined by blood pressure (BP) > 160/90 mmHg. In patients older than 64 years, there is a disproportionate amount of isolated systolic hypertension (ISH) as defined by SBP > 160, DBP < 90. Data from the Framingham Heart Study in men and women age 65 to 89 report the prevalence of ISH to be 14.4% in men and 22.8% in women. In comparison, for this age group the prevalence of systolic-diastolic hypertension was 7.6% in men and 9.7% in women. The major determinants of ISH from this study were age, female sex, obesity in women, and prior SBP readings in middle age (i.e., 140 to 149 mmHg $\gg$ risk than 120 to 129 mmHg). The significance of SBP as a predictor of cardiovascular morbidity and mortality increases in the elderly and may exceed that associated with systolic-diastolic hypertension.

In this population, an important factor in the development of ISH is reduced distensibility of arteries and arterioles leading to decreased compliance. Age-related arterial wall thickening occurs at the expense of cross-sectional diameter and is associated with a rise in systemic peripheral resistance, as well as in SBP, DBP, and MAP. ISH is characterized by an increased pulse pressure and by an increased LV mass. Data using renin-sodium profiling categorized hypertension in the elderly to be predominately of the low- and medium-profile classifications.

The most recent data in elderly patients are from three major multicentered prospective trials: the SHEP, STOP, and MRC 2 trials. The SHEP study was a large, double-blind, placebo-controlled trial that comprised 4736 men and women of age > 60 years with ISH. In the treatment arm, patients were randomized to receive low-dose diuretics as initial therapy; β blockers were added as a second step. At the end of the 5-year follow-up period, 46% of subjects had adequate blood pressure control using only a low dose of chlorthalidone. Another 23% of patients were controlled when a β blocker was added to the diuretic. Outcome included a 36% reduction in strokes ($p < 0.05$). Myocardial infarction risk was reduced by 27%, and overall mortality was reduced by 13%; however, these results did not reach statistical significance.

Both the MRC 2 and STOP trials studied the effect of antihypertensive treatment in elderly patients with both systolic-diastolic hypertension (SBP > 180 mmHg and DBP > 90 mmHg, or DBP $>$ 105 mmHg). In the STOP trial, 1627 patients aged > 70 years were randomized to placebo versus diuretic (HCTZ plus amiloride) versus β blocker. In the diuretic group, β blockers were used as a second-line antihypertensive agent. At the end of the study, about two-thirds of patients were on combination therapy. After 25 months of follow up, there were significant reductions in fatal and nonfatal strokes by 47% and in overall mortality by 43% in the treated groups (diuretics and β blockers). In addition, cardiac mortality was reduced by 13%, although not of statistical significance. In the MRC 2 trial, 4396 patients were randomized to one of three arms—placebo versus HCTZ plus amiloride versus atenolol—and were followed for > 6 years. Outcome was similar to those found in the SHEP and STOP trials with regard to stroke reduction and reduction in myocardial infarction. From the preceding data it may be concluded that, in elderly patients, antihypertensive therapy using low-dose diuretics or β blockers alone or in combination have a proven benefit in terms of stroke reduction, as well as a reduction in cardiovascular and overall mortality.

Blacks

In black patients, hypertension is more prevalent at a younger age and is usually more severe than in white patients. Hypertension in blacks is associated with a three- to fivefold greater incidence of target-organ damage compared with that in white hypertensives, including cardiomegaly, strokes, CHF, hypertensive retinopathy, and renal insufficiency. The majority of black hypertensives fall into the low-renin category. Alderman and colleagues found that black women had the highest proportion of low-renin profiles of all subjects (63%). Black men were twice as likely as white men to have low-renin profiles (40% versus 18%); only 9% had high-renin profiles. This low-renin state cannot be explained by volume expansion alone, since no consistent relationship between these two factors has been found in this population. The INTERSALT study, a multicenter, cross-sectional study that evaluated the relationship between electrolytes and blood pressure, was unable to correlate excessive salt intake as a contributing factor to the development of hypertension in black people. However, both normotensive and hypertensive blacks have been shown to have a salt-sensitive blood pressure response as compared with the white population. This has been attributed to reduced renal handling of large sodium loads.

Although the pathogenesis of hypertension in the black population has not been well elucidated, as a group, black patients respond very well to diuretic therapy. Black patients made up appoximately half the study participants in the Veterans Administration Cooperative Study and the Hypertension Detection and Follow-Up Program (HDFP) Study, both of which were diuretic-based. In the VA "moderately severe" hypertension trial, diuretic treatment was associated with a reduction in morbid events from 26 to 10% in black patients. In the HDFP study, the reduction in mortality in the group in which diuretics were administered as first-line therapy was 18.5% for black men and 27.8% for black women, whereas mortality was reduced by only 14.7% in white men and −2.1% for white women.

It has been reported that between 40 and 67% of younger black patients and 58 and 80% of elder blacks respond favorably to diuretics when administered alone. As a rule, diuretics are more efficacious than β blockers and ACEIs in blacks. However, when thiazide diuretics are added to other classes of antihypertensives in black patients, their efficacy is improved. Although shown to be efficacious for blood pressure control and for reducing morbidity and mortality in black hypertensives, the ability of diuretics to reduce the risk of target-organ damage is unclear. The Multiple Risk Factor Intervention Trial (MRFIT) study reported that treatment in hypertensive blacks did not delay or prevent loss of kidney function.

Women

Because women outnumber men in the general population, there are more hypertensive females than males. The attributable risk percentage for cardiovascular complications caused by hypertension is higher for females than it is for males. At present, there is a paucity of data on the treatment of hypertension in women, since most of the major trials did not include a sufficient number of female participants. The earliest available data on the treatment of hypertension in women was from the HDFP. Forty-six percent of 10,940 subjects were women. As mentioned previously, the HDFP study demonstrated a clear benefit in treating hypertensive black women, reporting a 27.8% reduction in mortality. However, in white women, a small but not statistically significant increase in mortality was found in the treated group (−2.5%). The MRC included 17,354 subjects, 48% of whom were white women. When analyzed by gender, the overall mortality significantly increased in women by 26% but declined in men by 15%. The data from MRC and HDFP are worrisome and have generated much controversy regarding antihypertensive treatment in women. These data, however, are difficult to interpret owing to inadequate sample size and lower incidence of end points in women.

The Australian Therapeutic Trial of Mild Hypertension comprised 3427 patients, of whom 37% were white women. In contrast to the results of MRC and HDFP, in this study women demonstrated a 36% reduction in total end points (death and cardiovascular/cerebrovascular events); however, this did not reach statistical significance because of the small number of women in the study and low event rates. More recent data on antihypertensive treatment in women come from the EWPHE and the SHEP trials. In the EWPHE study, 70% of 840 subjects were women, and although treatment in women was associated with an 18% reduction in cardiovascular mortality, men benefited to a greater extent (47% reduction). The SHEP study recruited 4736 participants, of whom 48% were white women, and demonstrated a favorable effect of active treatment in women. Overall, a 36% reduction of stroke incidence and a 32% reduction in all cardiovascular events were demonstrated. When analyzing women as a separate group, the findings included a reduction in stroke incidence in the women receiving treatment (white women, 48 versus 66 events, and black women, 7 versus 21 events). Unfortunately, only 9% of participants in this study were black women.

In summary, the current JNC V and JNC VI guidelines for the treatment of hypertension in women are not entirely supported by the few clinical trials available. Future studies evaluating the treatment of hypertension in women, with particular regard to adverse effects, are needed to establish firm treatment guidelines and to dispel current controversy.

Regression of Cardiac Hypertrophy and Diuretic Therapy

In the setting of hypertension, left ventricular hypertrophy (LVH) is an important adaptive mechanism that occurs in response to increased afterload. Electrocardiographically and echocardiographically determined LV mass has been recognized as a powerful independent risk indicator for cardiovascular-associated morbidity and mortality. Although controversial, theoretically, it is reasonable to consider regression of LVH a desirable therapeutic goal when prescribing an antihypertensive medication.

Despite similar levels of blood pressure control, clinical studies have demonstrated that some classes of antihypertensive agents are more efficacious than others in their ability to reverse LVH. In 1991, Moser and Setaro compiled an overview of all studies evaluating LVH regression in diuretic-treated hypertensive patients. Six studies were cited that supported the efficacy of diuretics on reduction of LV mass. Five studies were found in which no significant reduction in LV mass was observed. Criticism of the negative studies included the relative short duration of follow-up, small patient number, and lack of a control group in these trials.

In 1992, Dahlöf performed a metaanalysis of 109 studies comprising 2537 patients to determine the differences of antihypertensive classes on regression of LVH. He included only studies with echocardiographically determined LVH and analyzed data regarding changes in left ventricular wall thickness, diameter, and mass. Diuretics were associated with an 11% reduction in LV mass; however, this was primarily due to a reduction in LV internal diameter. On the other hand, the reduction of LV mass associated with ACEIs (15%), β blockers (8%), and calcium antagonists (8.5%) was largely due to a reversal of posterior and intraventricular septal thickness. Well-designed, prospective, controlled, randomized trials are needed to determine the effect of different antihypertensive agents on LV mass reduction and whether qualitative differences in LV mass reduction correlate with cardiovascular end points.

Diuretics in Combination with Other Antihypertensives

Diuretics are commonly used with other classes of antihypertensive drugs to control systemic hypertension. There are many fixed combination formulations having various thiazide diuretics combined with reserpine, hydralazine, ACEIs, AT_2 receptor blockers, β-adrenergic blockers, clonidine, and α-methyldopa. Recently, very-low-dose diuretic–β-blocker combinations have become available, combining HCTZ with bisoprolol and chlorthalidone with betaxolol; these formulations have received first-line approval by the FDA.

Combination antihypertensive therapy is reviewed in Chapter 16. The potential of combination therapy is to provide additive blood pressure actions from agents having different modes of action. At the same time, the adverse effects from one antihypertensive component can be counteracted by that of the other component.

DIURETICS FOR ANGINA PECTORIS

There is growing evidence that diuretic therapy may provide a useful adjunctive therapy in patients with chronic stable angina. Diuretics were first suggested as a treatment for angina decubitus because of their ability to reduce intravascular volume and ventricular wall tension when patients were recumbent. They also were suggested as a treatment for nitrate tolerance by preventing the volume expansion seen with vasodilator treatment. However, in a recent study it was observed that the addition of a diuretic to nitroglycerin patch treatment in patients with angina without CHF did not prevent nitrate tolerance. However, diuretic treatment alone did improve exercise tolerance on a treadmill, suggesting an antianginal benefit of diuretics. Diuretic therapy also increased the rate-pressure product achieved by patients at the angina threshold.

The mechanism of benefit was a reduction in LV preload during exercise, thereby reducing myocardial oxygen demand. However, with other antianginal therapies available, diuretics are not being recommended as a routine part of antianginal treatment because of their adverse metabolic effects with chronic use. Diuretics can be considered for patients having refractory anginal symptoms despite other treatment or for those who are intolerant to other medications.

ADVERSE EFFECTS OF DIURETICS

Hypokalemia

Hypokalemia is common finding in patients treated with diuretics; however, the relationship between diuretic-induced hypokalemia and the development of clinically significant arrhythmias remains controversial. Hypokalemia has been associated with an increased frequency of ventricular premature contractions (VPCS) in several studies of hypertensive patients treated with diuretics. The largest of these is the MRFIT, which found a significant inverse relationship between the serum potassium concentration and VPC frequency. In contrast, however, some studies have failed to show a relationship between the two.

One explanation for these conflicting results may stem from the fact that many were small studies and because those which lacked a correlation between serum potassium concentration and VPC frequency were of brief duration (4 weeks) compared with those in which a positive association was shown (24 to 40 weeks). This observation is supported by the findings of the Medical Research Council study involving

324 patients with mild hypertension, of whom 287 underwent ambulatory electrocardiographic monitoring. Although after 8 weeks of diuretic therapy there was no difference in frequency of VPCs from baseline, after 24 months there was a significant difference in VPCs in those patients receiving diuretics compared with those receiving placebo (20 versus 9%). The presence of VPCs was significantly related to the serum potassium concentration, ($p = 0.04$). Patients with LVH, CHF, or myocardial ischemia are at particularly high risk of developing lethal ventricular arrhythmias in the setting of potassium depletion.

Despite the association of increased VPC frequency with diuretic-induced hypokalemia, in recent clinical trials (SHEP, STOP, MRC) the treatment of hypertensive patients with low-dose thiazides was associated with a 20 to 25% reduction in cardiovascular events. In these studies, the use of lower doses of thiazides or thiazides in combination with potassium-sparing diuretics may explain why the more favorable results compared with those of earlier trials, such as MRFIT, in which higher doses of diuretics where utilized and were associated with increased risk of sudden cardiac death.

In 1994, Siscovick and colleagues examined the association between thiazide treatment and the risk of primary sudden cardiac death in a retrospective, case-controlled study. The risk of cardiac arrest among patients receiving combined thiazide and potassium-sparing diuretic therapy was lower than that among patients treated with a thiazides alone (odds ratio 0.3:1). Compared with low-dose diuretic therapy (25 mg), intermediate-dose therapy (50 mg) was associated with a moderate increase in the risk of cardiac arrest (odds ratio 1.7:1), and high-dose therapy (100 mg) was associated with an even greater increase in risk (odds ratio 3.6:1). In contrast with potassium-sparing diuretics, the addition of potassium supplements to thiazide therapy had little effect on the risk of sudden cardiac death (odds ratio 0.9:1). Furthermore, among patients receiving only one antihypertensive drug, risk of cardiac arrest was no higher with diuretic treatment than with β blockers (odds ratio 1:1). Combined therapy with thiazide (25 mg) and a potassium-sparing agent was associated with an estimated relative risk of 0.3 when compared with β blockers. Severely reduced serum potassium levels (< 3 mEq/L) are infrequently associated with thiazide diuretic use and are more likely to occur with loop diuretics and carbonic anhydrase inhibitors, particularly when oral intake is reduced. Severe hypokalemia (< 2.5 mEq/L) may cause profound muscle weakness, rhabdomyolysis, and acute tubular necrosis.

Hypomagnesemia

Few controlled trials are available that evaluate the role of diuretics in promoting magnesium deficiency. In an extensive review of the literature, Davies and Frasier found both positive and negative fluctuations in both serum and plasma magnesium levels associated with diuretic use (−10 to +5.9% from baseline). However, this review consisted primarily of thiazide-based trials. Potassium-sparing diuretics were consistently found to be associated with an increase in serum and intracellular magnesium concentration.

Theoretically, the chronic administration of large doses of loop diuretics could induce negative magnesium balance. The site of action of loop diuretics is the medullary thick ascending limb, where ~60% of the filtered load of magnesium is reabsorbed. Magnesium is an important enzymatic cofactor for NA^+/K^+-ATPase and for renal potassium reabsorption in the medullary thick ascending limb. In the presence of magnesium deficiency, significant amounts of urinary potassium wasting occur and often lead to hypokalemia. In one study, 41% of patients with hypokalemia were found to have low serum magnesium levels. Two studies report hypomagnesemia in 19 to 37% of CHF patients treated with loop diuretics. The data regarding the association of hypomagnesemia with increased prevalence of VPCs, sudden death, and overall survival are conflicting, and a definite causal relationship is lacking.

Hyponatremia

Almost all cases of diuretic-induced hyponatremia have been reported with thiazide diuretics. This can be explained by the differential effects of thiazides and loop diuretics on renal concentrating ability. Free water excretion is more severely impaired with thiazide diuretics because of their cortical site of action. With thiazide use, renal medullary tonicity is unaltered and is therefore "primed" for maximal water reabsorption in the presence of ADH. On the other hand, loop diuretics inhibit sodium chloride transport into the renal medulla and prevent the generation of a maximal osmotic gradient. In addition, a combination of factors, which include increased free water ingestion, reduced GFR, and elevated ADH concentration, commonly accompanies thiazide use and contributes to the generation of hyponatremia. Severe hyponatremia is most prevalent in elderly women and occurs within the first 2 weeks of therapy.

Glucose Intolerance

Thiazide diuretics have been associated with elevated fasting glucose levels and impaired glucose tolerance in nondiabetic patients in long-term studies. On average, fasting plasma glucose increases by 0.3 to 0.5 mmol/L during thiazide use. Equally well established is the fact that thiazide diuretics worsen glucose control in established diabetic patients. Evidence relating glucose intolerance with diuretic-induced hypokalemia is inconclusive. Hypokalemia may impair insulin release from β-islet cells and mediate peripheral insulin resistance. Potassium-sparing diuretics do not alter glucose homeostasis. However, the use of potassium supplementation with thiazide diuretics has not been shown to prevent the development of impaired glucose tolerance.

Diuretic-associated glucose intolerance appears to be dose-related and is reversible on withdrawal of the agent, although data regarding the association of improved glucose tolerance using low-dose HCTZ are conflicting. Ramsay and colleagues recently reviewed this issue and found several studies that support unaltered glucose homeostasis using low-dose HCTZ (25 to 50 mg daily). However, they also cite three long-term trials that reported elevated fasting blood glucose levels and impaired glucose tolerance using between 12.5 and 50 mg of HCTZ.

During low-dose HCTZ therapy, elevated fasting plasma insulin levels and reduced glucose disposal are important contributing factors in generating a state of glucose impairment. The frequency of treatment initiation for hyperglycemia during various antihypertensive therapies was evaluated by Gurwitz and colleagues. Patients receiving thiazides alone did not require treatment for hyperglycemia in any greater frequency than those receiving other agents.

It is not known whether the metabolic changes in previously glucose-tolerant patients lead to the development of microvascular complications or cause clinical diabetes. Evidence from several trails suggests that thiazide diuretic–induced glucose intolerance and insulin resistance do not adversely affect coronary artery disease risk in hypertensive patients. In patients with established diabetes mellitus, thiazide diuretic use should be avoided when possible, since there is an association, although rare, of diuretic use and the hyperosmolar nonketotic syndrome. Glucose intolerance occurs less commonly with loop diuretics.

Lipid Metabolism

Short-term studies (< 1 year) report a 5 to 7% increase in cholesterol levels with diuretic use. However, data from long-term clinical trials (VA Cooperative Study, MRC trial, HDFP Study, HAPPHY trial, SHEP, and others) have reported unchanged cholesterol levels after 1 year of diuretic therapy. In fact, data from the HDFP Study indicate that hypertensives with baseline marked hypercholesterolemia (> 250) who were treated with diuretics experience a decline in cholesterol levels from the second to fifth years of therapy. Those with less severe hypercholesterolemia at baseline (< 250) had no significant alteration in serum cholesterol levels in the 2- to 5-year follow-up period.

Postural Hypotension

Net negative sodium balance occurs during the first 3 days of thiazide therapy. The elderly are particularly prone to postural hypotension because of an age-related decrease in baroreceptor activity. They may be particularly sensitive to sudden reductions in blood pressure, especially with underlying cerebrovascular or coronary disease. In the SHEP trial, the prevalence of postural hypotension was 12.8% in the treated group versus 10.6% in the placebo group, and the incidence of syncope was 2.2% in the treated patients, compared with 1.3% in the placebo group. Reports of fatigue and unsteadiness or imbalance also were slightly more frequent in the treated patients.

Ototoxicity

The association of otoxicity and loop diuretics is well documented in both experimental and clinical studies. The exact mechanism by which loop diuretics cause hearing loss in unknown. Loop diuretic–induced ototoxicity usually occurs within 20 min of infusion and ususally is reversible, although permanent deafness has been reported. Ototoxicity has been associated with ethacrynic acid, furosemide, and bumetidine with both IV and oral routes of administration. Patients with renal failure and those receiving concomitant aminoglycoside therapy are at greatest risk of developing loop diuretic–associated ototoxicity.

Ototoxicity is clearly related to the rate of infusion and to peak serum concentrations. Heidland and Wigand conducted audiometric studies during the infusion of furosemide at a constant rate of 25 mg/min and reported reversible hearing loss in two-thirds of patients. Fries and colleagues found no hearing loss in renal failure patients receiving between 500 and 1000 mg over 6 h. High plasma levels of furosemide (50 μg/mL) are associated with a greater incidence of auditory disturbances, and Brown and colleagues found patients with levels greater than 100 μg/mL to be at risk for permanent deafness. In general, the rate of furosemide infusion should be no faster than 4 mg/min, and serum concentrations should be kept below 40 μg/mL.

Gout

Diuretics have been shown to precipitate secondary hyperuricemia and gout. In the MRC trial, compared with placebo, patients receiving thiazide diuretics had significantly more withdrawals for gout (4.4 versus 0.1 per 1000 patient years). Serum urate levels are elevated during diuretic use due to reduced intravascular volume, increased proximal tubular reabsorption, reduced proximal tubular secretion, and impaired GFR. Hyperuricemia is dose-related and reversible on discontinuation of diuretic therapy.

Allergic Interstitial Nephritis

Renal insufficiency due to diuretic-induced interstitial nephritis is a relatively rare occurrence and has been reported using loop diuretics, thiazides, and potassium-sparing diuretics. The classic clinical presentation is acute renal failure and sterile pyuria, accompanied by the triad of rash, fever, and eosinophilia. Renal biopsy shows intense interstitial inflammation with lymphocytes, eosinophils, noncaseating granulomas, and normal glomeruli. In most cases, renal function rapidly improves with cessation of diuretics.

Cutaneous Reactions

Cutaneous skin reactions are not uncommon with diuretics.

DRUG-DRUG INTERACTIONS

There are many drug-drug interactions that involve diuretics. Some of these interactions are summarized in Chapter 22.

SUGGESTED READINGS

LeJemtel TH, Sonnenblick EH, Frishman WH: Diagnosis and management of heart failure, in Alexander RW, Schlant RC, Fuster V (eds): *Hurst's The Heart*, 9th ed. New York, McGraw-Hill, 1998, pp 745–781.

Mokrzycki MH, Tamirisa P: Diuretic therapy in cardiovascular disease, in Frishman WH, Sonnenblick EH (eds): *Cardiovascular Pharmacotherapeutics*. New York, McGraw-Hill, 1997, pp 193–222.

Schuller D, Lynch JP, Fine D: Protocol-guided diuretic management: comparison of furosemide by continuous infusion and intermittent bolus. *Crit Care Med* 1997; 25:1969–1975.

The Sixth Report of the Joint National Committee on Prevention, Detection, Evaluation, and Treatment of High Blood Pressure. *Arch Intern Med* 1997; 157: 2413–2446.

Chapter 7 Magnesium, Potassium, and Calcium as Potential Cardiovascular Disease Therapies

William H. Frishman, Erdal Cavusoglu, and Joel Zonszein

Both deficiency states and abnormalities in the metabolism of the electrolytes magnesium, potassium, and calcium have been associated as etiologic factors in systemic hypertension, ischemic heart disease, congestive heart failure, atherosclerosis, diabetes mellitus, and arrhythmia. Replacement and supplementation of these substances in experimental animals have been shown to both prevent and treat these cardiovascular conditions. In this chapter, magnesium, potassium, and calcium are discussed as potential cardiovascular disease therapies.

MAGNESIUM

Magnesium is the second most common intracellular cation in the human body, second only to potassium. Overall, it is the fourth most abundant cation. Magnesium is involved in well over 300 different enzymatic reactions in the body, particularly those which are concerned with the utilization of energy. It is important in many cell membrane functions, including the gating of calcium ion channels, serving to mimic many effects of calcium channel blockade. Magnesium is a necessary cofactor for any biochemical reaction involving adenosine triphosphate (ATP) and is essential for the proper functioning of the Na^+/K^+- and calcium-ATPase pumps, which are helpful in maintaining the normal resting membrane potential. Magnesium deficiency can lead to abnormalities in myocardial membrane potential that can result in cardiac arrhythmias. Deficiency states or abnormalities in magnesium metabolism also play important roles in ischemic heart disease, congestive heart failure, sudden cardiac death, diabetes mellitus, preeclampsia-eclampsia, and hypertension.

Cardiovascular Effects of Magnesium

There are numerous properties and actions of the magnesium ion that could theoretically have beneficial effects on the cardiovascular system. At vascular membranes, magnesium lowers systemic vascular resistance, dilates coronary and cerebral arteries, relieves vasopasm, and lowers arterial blood pressure. At cardiac membranes, magnesium slows heart rate, protects mitochondrial function and high-energy phosphate levels, and acts as an antiarrhythmic. In addition, magnesium possesses antiplatelet, anticoagulant, and antiatherosclerotic properties and can protect against the formation of oxygen free radicals.

Magnesium deficiencies or metabolic abnormalities can cause abnormalities in cardiovascular function.

Role of Magnesium in Ischemic Heart Disease and Myocardial Infarction

For many years, magnesium deficiency has been linked to ischemic heart disease and myocardial infarction. Although innumerable animal and human studies have attempted to define the relevance of magnesium and its deficiency to both the incidence and management of ischemic heart disease, much confusion still remains in this regard. Epidemiologic studies comparing death rates from ischemic heart disease from different regions of many countries have attempted to link low magnesium concentrations in soil and water with higher cardiovascular mortality. Several autopsy series also have suggested that patients dying of acute myocardial infarction tend to have reduced myocardial magnesium concentrations compared with those dying of other causes. In addition, magnesium deficiency has been implicated as an etiologic factor for many of the risk factors for coronary artery disease, such as diabetes mellitus, hypertension, and hyperlipidemia.

Autopsy studies dating back to the 1970s have consistently demonstrated that fatal acute myocardial infarctions were associated with depressed myocardial magnesium concentrations. Such studies have shown that patients dying of cardiac causes, compared with those dying of noncardiac causes, had lower myocardial concentrations of magnesium. A number of basic science studies subsequently have demonstrated that acute ischemia is in fact associated with a dramatic increase in the efflux of magnesium from the cell. Furthermore, the ischemically injured myocyte appears to be rich in both calcium and sodium. Finally, low myocardial magnesium concentrations also have been demonstrated in chronic ischemic heart disease as well.

Studies in animals have suggested a beneficial role of magnesium in ischemia and infarction. It has been theorized that by preventing calcium overload, magnesium may protect against reperfusion injury. Reports of the use of magnesium in acute myocardial infarction in humans date back as early as the 1950s. Magnesium administration was found to have beneficial effects in patients with myocardial infarction in several small studies, and a metaanalytic review reported on a lower morbidity and mortality rate with this treatment.

The advantageous effects of intravenous (IV) magnesium sulfate given immediately to patients with suspected acute myocardial infarction was initially documented in a large prospective, double-blind trial (LIMIT-2) with a lower mortality of 7.8 versus 10.3% in the placebo group. The side effects of magnesium treatment in this study were minimal, with transient flushing and an increased incidence of sinus bradycardia. However, the routine administration of magnesium during acute myocardial infarction has been discontinued after the outcome of a larger study, ISIS-4, which included 58,050 patients and found no beneficial effects of magnesium administration when compared with control. The timing of the loading of magnesium dose in relation to thrombolytic therapy or spontaneous reperfusion has been offered as an explanation for the different results in LIMIT-2 and ISIS-4. Early treatment is essential, since serum magnesium concentrations must be raised by the time of reperfusion because injury is immediate. Other studies using an earlier magnesium loading dose also have not demonstrated a significant difference in cardiac arrhythmias.

Magnesium administration may have a greater therapeutic role in those patients experiencing acute myocardial infarction who are unable to receive thrombolytic therapy, a population with a high in-hospital mortality rate. Magnesium therapy in this group of patients has been found to have a reduced incidence of arrhythmias and therefore less mortality and decreased incidence of congestive heart failure by preserving left ventricular ejection fraction. Similarly, a beneficial effect of magnesium therapy has been reported in patients with unstable angina undergoing bypass grafting, but other studies have not been able to confirm these cardioprotective effects.

The discrepancy in the results of these studies has dampened the enthusiasm for routine magnesium use in the management of patients with acute myocardial infarction. The disparate results between these two large clinical trials (LIMIT-2 and ISIS-4) are puzzling. However, the ISIS-4 trial was not specifically designed to test the hypothesis that magnesium may limit reperfusion injury, and the time factor in which magnesium is given needs to be further clarified. It is also important to determine if those patients with magnesium deficiency are the ones who benefit or whether magnesium should be used as a true cardioplexic agent in the non-magnesium-deficient individual. At this time, magnesium therapy cannot be recommended as routine treatment in the management of acute myocardial infarction. Ongoing studies, such as the Magnesium in Coronaries (MAGIC) and Pressure Controlled Intermittent Coronary Sinus Occlusion (PICSO) projects may help define a future role for magnesium in ischemic heart syndromes.

Magnesium in Diabetes and Congestive Heart Failure

Magnesium scarcity is associated with various medical disorders but is particularly common in diabetes mellitus, congestive heart failure, and diuretic use. Whereas recognition of potassium deficiency and replacement are common in these conditions, this is not the case with magnesium. Further, adequate potassium repletion can be impaired in some unless magnesium deficiency is corrected. The incidence of both hypokalemia and hypomagnesemia can be lessened by using potassium-sparing diuretics or angiotensin converting enzyme inhibitors and angiotensin II receptor blockers for the treatment of patients with heart failure and hypertension.

Excessive glycosuria is the main cause of magnesium deficiency in diabetes mellitus, and its severity is inversely correlated with glycemic control. Increased fat and protein mobilization during acute metabolic decompensation, as well as other factors, also play a role. The prevalence and severity of magnesium deficiency can be aggravated by other conditions, particularly congestive heart failure and diuretic use. In these cases, many electrolyte imbalances can develop that adversely affect patient survival. Hyponatremia is closely associated with a poor prognosis, hypokalemia with increased ventricular dysrhythmias, and hypomagnesemia with arrhythmias and refractory hypokalemia. However, magnesium deficiency has yet to be identified as an independent risk factor for mortality in such conditions.

Magnesium in Arrhythmias

There is an inverse correlation between myocardial irritability and serum magnesium concentrations that can be effectively reversed by IV administration of either magnesium SO_4 or magnesium Cl_2. Oral magnesium replacement also can reduce the frequency of ventricular irritability during the chronic therapy of congestive heart failure. The risk of hypomagnesemia-induced cardiac arrhythmias is particularly important in individuals treated with digitalis, since this association has a synergistic adverse effect on the Na^+/K^+-ATPase pump.

As stated, magnesium is an essential cofactor for the Na^+/K^+-ATPase enzyme. Magnesium deficiency leads to impaired functioning of this enzyme, resulting in lowered intracellular potassium concentrations. The resting membrane potential thus becomes less negative or more positive, which, in turn, makes the cell more susceptible to depolarization. This makes the cell theoretically more prone to premature excitation, thereby lowering its threshold for the development of arrhythmias. In addition to its effect on the Na^+/K^+-ATPase pump, magnesium has been shown to have profound effects on the several different types of potassium channels that are known to exist within cardiac cells. Studies in animals appear to support the theory that magnesium makes the cell more resistant to the development of arrhythmias. For example, magnesium infusion has been shown to raise the threshold for both ventricular premature contractions (VPCs) and ventricular fibrillation induction in dog heart models. Furthermore, much evidence exists linking magnesium deficiency with an increased incidence of both supraventricular and ventricular arrhythmias.

Evidence of the salutary effects of IV magnesium in treating both supraventricular and ventricular tachyarrhythmias has been known for many years. In addition, numerous anecdotal reports have been published attesting to the utility of magnesium in cases of refractory ventricular arrhythmias, although most of these cases were probably associated with magnesium deficiency. Despite these observations and the theoretical benefits of magnesium with regard to the development of arrhythmias, there has actually been no controlled study looking at the efficacy of magnesium as an antiarrhythmic agent in the treatment of ventricular arrhythmias. Furthermore, it is unclear whether the potential effectiveness of magnesium in these situations represents a pharmacologic effect of magnesium or whether it merely reflects repletion of a deficiency state. Whatever its potential role in the management of "run-of-the-mill" ventricular arrhythmias, magnesium clearly does have a time-honored and proven place in the treatment of ventricular arrhythmias due to digoxin toxicity.

Magnesium in Hypertension

Multiple studies have shown a relative hypomagnesemia in patients with essential hypertension. This reduction in serum magnesium might be enough to induce peripheral vasoconstriction and raise blood pressure.

Epidemiologic studies have shown an inverse relationship between magnesium in the diet and the level of blood pressure. In addition, successful drug therapy of hypotension appears to be associated with elevations in the levels of intracellular free magnesium in erythrocytes. However, the results of studies where magnesium was used to treat hypertension demonstrated conflicting results regarding blood pressure reduction. Methodologic issues in study designs were raised to explain the different findings in these various trials. Nevertheless, magnesium supplementation may be of benefit in hypertensive patients receiving thiazide diuretics. Magnesium supplementation was found not to affect blood pressure in a primary hypertension prevention study.

Clinical Use of Magnesium

There is a high incidence of magnesium deficiency in hospitalized patients, particularly in those with other precipitating conditions that may aggravate magnesium deficiency, such as poor nutrition and multisystemic disorders. This is particularly important in patients treated with a myriad of medications, such as diuretics and aminoglycoside antibiotics.

Difficulty in establishing the diagnosis of magnesium deficiency is due to the minimal or often absent clinical manifestations as well as a lack of reliable laboratory tests. Clinical manifestations, when present, are nonspecific and confined to mental changes or neuromuscular irritability. Tetany, one of the most striking and better-known manifestations, is found only rarely; instead, less specific signs such as tremor, muscle twitching, bizarre movements, focal seizures, generalized convulsions, delirium, and coma are more common. Magnesium deficiency occurs more frequently and should be suspected when other electrolyte abnormalities coexist. Electrocardiographic changes such as prolongation of the QT and PR intervals, widening of the QRS complex, ST-segment depression, and low T waves, as well as supraventricular and ventricular tachyarrhythmias, may further lead to diagnosis and treatment. Once suspected, serum magnesium concentration continues to be the routine screening test, and although a low level may be indicative of low intracellular stores, there is a poor correlation, and therefore, serum magnesium determination is unreliable. Intracellular magnesium measurements, as well as other technologies, are available but so far clinically impractical. A more practical probe is the "magnesium loading test," which is both therapeutic and diagnostic. It consists of the parenteral administration of $MgSO_4$ and assessment of urinary magnesium retention. Individuals with normal magnesium balance eliminate at least 75% of the amount given. This approach is recommended in all patients with a high index of suspicion, particularly those with ischemic heart disease or cardiac arrhythmias. Magnesium administration is contraindicated in anuric individuals and those with significant renal impairment. In mild deficiency cases, magnesium restoration is often achieved after eliminating the causative factors and restarting a normal diet. Parenteral magnesium administration, however, is more effective and should be the route used when replacement is necessary during medical emergencies. A recommended regimen is 2 g of $MgSO_4$ (16.3 mEq) given IV over 30 min, followed by a constant infusion rate of 1 mEq/kg for the first day and 0.5 mEq/kg per day for 3 to 5 more days. Ampules of 10, 25, and 50% solutions are available, containing 8.1 mEq/g. Oral magnesium is not recommended for acute situations, since high doses are needed and may result in diarrhea. The intramuscular route is useful but painful and should be avoided when an IV infusion is possible. The available formulations of magnesium are listed in Table 7-1.

POTASSIUM

A relationship between a high dietary intake of potassium and a reduced risk of cardiovascular disease has been suggested by animal experiments and clinical investigations. Drugs affecting membrane potassium channels also have been shown to have a favorable impact on various cardiovascular conditions.

Cardiovascular Effects of Potassium

Potassium in Systemic Hypertension

In experimental animals, high dietary potassium appears to protect against the development of stroke, cardiac hypertrophy, and systemic

TABLE 7-1 Magnesium Formulations

Magnesium chloride	64-mg tablets
Magnesium citrate	IV solutions
Magnesium gluconate	30-, 500-, and 550-mg tablets
Magnesium hydroxide	Milk of magnesia
Magnesium oxide	140-mg capsules, 420-mg tablets
Magnesium sulfate	IV solutions

hypertension. From human epidemiologic studies, arterial blood pressure levels seem to correlate with dietary and urinary sodium-potassium ratios and inversely with urinary potassium levels. Many black hypertensives have been shown to ingest less than the optimal 90 mEq of potassium recommended in the adult diet.

Potassium has multiple effects in humans, which suggests its use as a blood pressure lowering agent (Table 7-2). Potassium supplementation in humans has a natriuretic action, even in the presence of elevated aldosterone, and can decrease cardiac output. Potassium can increase kallikrein and increase nitric oxide production from the endothelium, factors that could lower blood pressure. Potassium supplementation has been shown to attenuate sympathetic activity and to decrease the amount and effect of vasoactive hormones. Finally, potassium may have a direct systemic vasodilatory action by enhancing Na^+/K^+-ATPase activity and the compliance of large arteries.

In clinical trials, oral potassium supplementation (as opposed to dietary potassium) has been shown to lower blood pressure in hypertensive patients on normal or on high-sodium diets. Similar observations also have been made in elderly hypertensive subjects. In patients receiving salt-restricted diets, potassium supplementation is less effective in reducing elevated blood pressure, suggesting that this form of treatment is most effective in the management of salt-sensitive hypertensives.

Dietary potassium (60 mEq/day) also has been examined as a blood pressure lowering supplement in patients already receiving antihypertensive drugs such as diuretics and β blockers, providing additional effectiveness in reducing pressure.

In summary, there is good evidence to suggest that dietary potassium supplementation can cause a mild reduction in blood pressure, especially in hypertensive patients on high-salt diets. It is still not known for how long the blood pressure lowering effect of potassium is maintained. In patients receiving diuretics who become hypokalemic, potassium supplementation can correct the deficiency while providing additional blood pressure lowering effects. Rather than recommending potassium supplements for the entire population of hypertensive

TABLE 7-2 Proposed Mechanisms of Blood Pressure Reduction with Potassium

Increased natriuresis—direct effect on renal tubule
Increased renal kallikrein and prostacyclin
Increased nitric oxide (increased vasodilatory response to acetylcholine)
Attenuation of sympathetic activity
Decreased amount and effect of vasoactive hormones (renin)
Direct arterial effect—enhanced activity of Na^+/K^+-ATPase
Enhanced vascular compliance

patients or patients at risk for developing hypertension, biologic markers need to be obtained that can easily identify subgroups of patients who would best respond to this type of therapeutic regimen.

Electrophysiologic Effects

Hypokalemia

Hypokalemia leads to a decrease in the rate of repolarization of the cardiac cell, leading to a prolongation of the recovery time. Hypokalemia results in the slope of phase 3 of the transmembrane action potential becoming less steep. As a result, there is an increase in the interval during which the difference between the transmembrane potential and the threshold potential is small. Consequently, the period of increased excitability is prolonged and the appearance of ectopic complexes is facilitated. A decrease in the extracellular potassium concentration increases the difference in potassium concentrations across the cell membrane and tends to hyperpolarize the cell during diastole.

Electrocardiographically, hypokalemia produces a flattening or inversion of the T wave with concomitant prominence of the U wave. This occurs without any significant change in the QT duration. When hypokalemia is severe, the QRS complex may widen slightly in a diffuse manner. The ECG pattern of hypokalemia is not specific and may follow administration of digitalis, antiarrhythmic agents, or phenothiazines and can occur with ventricular hypertrophy or bradycardia.

Potassium Supplementation

General Considerations

Potassium may be administered for the purpose of replacing a total-body deficit or treating decreased serum levels. Additionally, subjects with salt-sensitive hypertension may be responsive to the beneficial effect of potassium supplementation. Furthermore, dietary potassium may be as effective as supplementation, although the data in this regard are not as abundant. Finally, some investigators have proposed that small elevations of potassium concentration related to high levels of dietary potassium intake may be sufficient to inhibit free radical formation, smooth-muscle proliferation, and thrombus formation. In this way, the rate of progression to atherosclerotic lesion formation may be slowed and thrombosis in atherosclerotic vessels diminished.

Oral Therapy

If a patient consumes a diet deficient in potassium-rich foods (e.g., fruit, vegetables), dietary alterations may be sufficient. Such dietary modifications can provide 40 to 60 mEq/day of potassium. Salt substitutes provide another economical alternative to prescription potassium supplements; they contain 7 to 14 mEq potassium per gram (5 g equals approximately 1 tsp). Potassium supplements are usually given as

TABLE 7-3 Oral Potassium Formulations

Liquid potassium chloride products	10–40 mEq/15 mL
Potassium chloride products for reconstitution	20–50 mEq: Powders, effervescent powders, and tablets
Prolonged-release potassium chloride products	1.3–10 mEq: Wax-matrix tablets, enteric coated tablets, and microencapsulated capsules
Other potassium formulations	Potassium gluconate, potassium citrate, potassium acetate, potassium carbonate: for use in hyperchloremia and hypokalemia

potassium chloride, although other forms are available (Table 7-3). Potassium chloride elixir and slow-release KCl tablets or capsules are common preparations. The most common side effect of such KCl oral supplements is gastric irritation. The non-chloride-containing potassium supplements provide an alternative for those unable to tolerate the KCl preparations or for use in hyperchloremic acidosis. Since severe hyperkalemia can occur as a consequence of oral supplementation, serum potassium levels always should be monitored during therapy.

IV Therapy

Potassium can be administered intravenously in patients with severe hypokalemia and in those unable to tolerate oral preparations. A detailed discussion of the approximation of potassium deficit is beyond the scope of this chapter. However, in the absence of ECG changes and a potassium level greater than 2.5 mEq/L, potassium can be administered at a rate of up to 10 mEq/h in concentrations as high as 30 mEq/L. Maximum daily administration should not exceed 100 to 200 mEq. If the serum potassium level is under 2 mEq/L and is associated with either ECG changes and/or neuromuscular symptoms, potassium can be administered intravenously at a rate of 40 mEq/h and at concentrations as high as 60 mEq/L. This should be accompanied by continuous ECG monitoring as well as measurement of serum potassium levels every several hours. In cases of life-threatening hypokalemia, potassium should be given initially in glucose-free solutions, since glucose may cause further lowering of potassium.

Summary

Potassium traditionally has been used as a replacement in hypokalemia related to systemic illness and drug use (diuretics). Magnesium often must be used with potassium to correct hypokalemia successfully. Recent evidence is mounting that potassium could be useful to prevent and treat cardiovascular diseases such as hypertension and atherosclerosis with favorable effects on morbidity and mortality outcomes.

CALCIUM

Similar to magnesium and potassium, abnormalities in calcium homeostasis appear to play an important role in the pathogenesis of cardiovascular disease.

Cardiovascular Effects of Calcium

Calcium in Systemic Hypertension

Calcium metabolism is linked closely to the regulation of systemic blood pressure, and calcium supplementation has been proposed as a treatment for systemic hypertension. Increased concentrations of free calcium found within the cytosol of vascular smooth-muscle cells are thought to be responsible for the increased contractility of vessels in hypertension. In animal models, acute intracellular calcium overload of vascular smooth-muscle cells can produce hypercontractility. Hypertension can develop if a general increase in systemic arteriolar tone leads to a rise in peripheral flow resistance. Furthermore, with progressive elevation of calcium, the structural integrity of the arterial and arteriolar walls is destroyed. Thus, in various animal models, calcium overload initiates lesions of an arteriosclerotic character. The increased concentrations of free calcium within the vascular smooth-muscle cells could be secondary to alterations in calcium entry, binding, or extrusion from the cells. Studies on human cells have shown changes related to all three of these mechanisms.

Beyond the probability that an increased intracellular calcium is involved in the pathogenesis of hypertension, there are other observed relationships between calcium and hypertension. These include the relationship between serum calcium levels and blood pressure, the effect of dietary and supplemental calcium on blood pressure, and the renal excretion of calcium and serum parathyroid hormone (PTH) levels in patients with hypertension.

Serum Calcium and Hypertension

Hypertension is more common in the presence of hypercalcemia, and in many but not all studies, there appears to be a direct relationship between the total serum calcium level and blood pressure. However, the relationship between serum ionized calcium and blood pressure does not appear to be as strong. Nevertheless, there are enough data to suggest a vasoconstrictive effect of increasing extracellular calcium levels, presumably by a stimulation of catecholamine release.

Increased Renal Excretion of Calcium

Compared with normotensive subjects, hypertensive individuals excrete more calcium both under basal circumstances and during a calcium infusion. This may be due to the increase in calcium excretion known to occur following intravascular volume expansion with the resulting rise in sodium excretion. Alternatively, it may be secondary to a decreased binding of calcium to kidney cells. Whatever the precise mechanism, it is known that patients with volume-expansion forms of hypertension excrete calcium in excess.

Observational Studies and Clinical Trials with Calcium Supplements

There have been more than 30 reports on observational studies of calcium and hypertension, with the majority demonstrating an inverse relationship between calcium intake in the diet and level of blood pressure.

However, clinical trials of calcium supplementation (1 to 2 g/day for up to 4 years) have been less consistent in this regard, with only approximately two-thirds of such studies demonstrating a beneficial effect of supplemental calcium on blood pressure. The rationale for supplemental calcium therapy is based on the assumption that PTH levels are elevated in response to low levels of ionized calcium, resulting from the hypercalciuria seen in some forms of volume-expanded hypertension. Additional calcium, by raising plasma calcium, would shut off PTH and thereby lower blood pressure. Indeed, in selected populations of hypertensive patients characterized by either increased urinary calcium excretion, low ionized calcium, or increased PTH levels, calcium supplements often cause a significant fall in blood pressure. In addition, increased calcium intake acts to increase sodium excretion in the urine and may lower blood pressure by this mechanism. However, in unselected populations of hypertensive patients, most clinical studies have shown little or no effect of calcium supplementation on blood pressure. Furthermore, even those patients with lower serum calcium and higher PTH levels who may benefit from calcium supplementation may do so with the potential risk of developing kidney stones.

In contrast, studies in pregnant women have shown that calcium supplementation can provide important reductions in both systolic and diastolic blood pressures and can reduce the risk of preeclampsia.

In summary, based on the available data, calcium supplementation or an increased intake of calcium by enriched foods cannot be recommended as a treatment for the general hypertensive population or for the prevention of hypertension. Individual patients may benefit from this approach, such as pregnant women, but there are no screening methods for identifying those patients in the general population who would benefit by it.

Calcium Use in Cardiac Arrest

Calcium plays an essential role in excitation-contraction coupling, and for many years calcium chloride administered intravenously was used in cardiac resuscitation efforts in patients with bradyasystolic arrest. It is no longer used for this indication, since no survival benefit has been observed and there is evidence that calcium may induce cerebral vasospasm and increase the extent of reperfusion injury in the heart and brain.

Calcium Use in Arrhythmia

IV calcium can slow the heart rate and has been used to treat tachycardias. The drug must be used cautiously, however, in patients receiving digoxin because it can precipitate digitalis toxicity and ventricular arrhythmias related to afterdepolarization. Afterdepolarizations are membrane potential voltage oscillations that are dependent on a preceding action potential. There are two types of afterdepolarizations. Early afterdepolarizations (EADs) occur during phase 2 or 3 of the action potential, whereas delayed afterdepolarizations (DADs) occur after reestablishment of resting membrane potential (phase 4). DADs have been shown in vitro to occur in the setting of digitalis toxicity or catecholamine excess as well as in hypertrophied myocardium and in Purkinje cells after myocardial infarction. DADs appear to result from the oscillatory release of calcium ions from sarcoplasmic reticulum during conditions of calcium overload. The clinical significance of DADs and triggered activity is not completely clear, but this mechanism has been invoked to explain at least an etiology for some ventricular arrhythmias. Although much remains to be learned, it seems likely that triggered activity will emerge as an important mechanism of human arrhythmia.

Decreases in extracellular calcium concentration can result in an increased action potential duration, resulting from an increase in duration and a decrease in amplitude of phase 2 of the cardiac action potential. Hypocalcemia may cause a clinically insignificant decrease in the QRS duration; cardiac arrhythmias are uncommon.

IV calcium has been used to treat intoxications from calcium channel blockers complicated by bradyarrhythmia and hypertension.

Clinical Use of Calcium

Calcium is available as an oral calcium carbonite formulation providing 170 to 600 mg of elemental calcium in tablet form. Calcium citrate tablets (200 to 500 mg of elemental calcium), calcium gluconate syrup, and calcium lactate tablets are also available. In cases where hypocalcemia may persist despite adequate calcium supplementation, a vitamin D supplement may be required to enhance calcium absorption.

IV calcium is available as calcium chloride (27.2 mg/mL), calcium gluceptate (18 mg/mL), and calcium gluconate (9 mg/mL). Calcium chloride is the preferred formulation because it produces more predictable levels of ionized calcium in plasma.

Summary

Except for specific situations, such as calcium entry blocker overdose, pregnancy, and hypocalcemia, treatment with calcium is not recommended for prevention and treatment of cardiovascular disease. Calcium, however, should be maintained in the diet for general health maintenance.

SUGGESTED READINGS

Altura BM, Altura BT: Role of magnesium in the pathogenesis of hypertension updated: Relationship to its actions on cardiac, vascular smooth muscle, and endothelial cells, in Laragh JN, Brenner BM (eds): *Hypertension: Pathophysiology, Diagnosis and Management.* New York, Raven Press, 1995, pp 1213–1242.

Eichhorn EJ, Tandon PK, DiBianco R, et al: Clinical and prognostic significance of serum magnesium concentration in patients with severe chronic congestive heart failure: The PROMISE Study. *J Am Coll Cardiol* 21(3):634, 1993.

Frishman WH, Cavusoglu E, Zonszein J: Magnesium, potassium, and calcium as potential cardiovascular disease therapies, in Frishman WH, Sonnenblick EH (eds): *Cardiovascular Pharmacotherapeutics.* New York, McGraw-Hill, 1997, pp 223–236.

Harlan WR, Harlan LC: Blood pressure and calcium and magnesium intake, in Laragh JH, Brenner BM (eds): *Hypertension: Pathophysiology, Diagnosis and Management.* New York, Raven Press, 1995, pp 1143–1154.

Hatton DC, Young EW, Bukoski RD, McCarron DA: Calcium metabolism in experimental genetic hypertension, in Laragh JH, Brenner BM (eds): *Hypertension: Pathophysiology, Diagnosis and Management.* New York, Raven Press, 1995, pp 1193–1211.

Siani A, Strazzullo P: Relevance of dietary potassium intake to antihypertensive drug treatment, in Laragh JH, Brenner BM (eds): *Hypertension: Pathophysiology, Diagnosis and Management.* New York, Raven Press, 1995, pp 2727–2737.

Svetkey LP, Klotman PE: Blood pressure and potassium intake, in Laragh JH, Brenner BM (eds): *Hypertension: Pathophysiology, Diagnosis and Management.* New York, Raven Press, 1990, pp 217–227.

Tobian L: The protective effects of high-potassium diets in hypertension, and the mechanisms by which high-NaCl diets produce hypertension—A personal view, in Laragh JH, Brenner BM (eds): *Hypertension: Pathophysiology, Diagnosis and Management.* New York, Raven Press, 1995, pp 299–312.

Woods KL, Fletcher S: Long-term outcome after intravenous magnesium sulphate in suspected acute myocardial infarction: The second Leicester Intravenous Magnesium Intervention Trial (LIMIT-2). *Lancet* 343:816, 1994.

Woods KL, Fletcher S, Raffe C, Haider Y: Intravenous magnesium sulphate in suspected acute myocardial infarction: Results of the second Leicester Intravenous Magnesium Intervention Trial (LIMIT-2). *Lancet* 339:1553, 1992.

Chapter 8 Digitalis Preparations and Other Inotropic Agents

Edmund H. Sonnenblick, Thierry H. LeJemtel, and William H. Frishman

DIGITALIS GLYCOSIDES

Digitalis glycosides have had a long and venerable history in the treatment of congestive heart failure. In 1785, William Withering reported on his use of the digitalis leaf as a purported diuretic agent to treat anasarca, presumably caused by congestive heart failure. Indeed, the major effects of digitalis were thought to be on the kidneys, although important effects on heart rate were noted. Only in the latter part of the nineteenth century did it become apparent that there was a direct action of digitalis glycosides to increase cardiac contractility, whereas in the earlier part of the twentieth century its effects on the peripheral circulation and the autonomic nervous system were noted.

Pharmacologic Action

Digitalis glycosides have important effects on multiple systems in addition to augmenting the contractility of the myocardium. Electrophysiologically, digitalis glycosides speed conduction in the atrium while inhibiting conduction at the atrioventricular node. In the normal circulation, digitalis glycosides also produce generalized arteriolar vasoconstriction while affecting the central nervous system to enhance parasympathetic and reduce sympathetic nervous system activation. Digitalis sensitizes baroreflexes to decrease efferent sympathetic activity, which acts to reduce sinus node activity and thus reduce heart rate. The increase in baroreflex sensitization also increases parasympathetic tone, while central vagal nuclei are also stimulated. The broad enhancement of parasympathetic activity with digitalis glycosides helps to explain the sinus heart rate slowing observed with the drugs, as well as their therapeutic efficacy in control of supraventricular arrhythmias. As discussed later, in the failing state, the effects of sympathetic withdrawal may be dominant so as to reduce arterial vascular resistance, while in the normal circulation arterial vasoconstriction may be dominant. Integration of these various actions adds to the inotropic activity of and therapeutic usefulness of digitalis glycosides.

The action of digitalis glycosides to increase contractility and alter electrophysiology of heart muscle occurs through inhibition of the enzyme Na^+/K^+-ATPase on the surface membrane of myocardial cells, which results in an increase in the amount of Ca^{2+} to activate contraction. The Na^+/K^+-ATPase is an energy-requiring "sodium pump" that extrudes three Na^+ ions that enter the cell during depolarization in exchange for two potassium ions, thus creating an electric current and a negative resting potential. Contraction is brought about by an action potential that depolarizes the surface membrane of the cell. This action potential is created by a rapid inward current of Na^+ into the cell that opens Ca^{2+} channels and permits Ca^{2+} to enter the cell. This releases substantially more Ca^{2+} from stores in the sarcoplasmic reticulum within the cell, which in turn activates the contractile mechanism by binding to a component of the troponin-tropomyosin system that had been maintaining the resting state. With Ca^{2+} bound to troponin, actin and myosin can interact to produce force and shortening. The greater the amount of activating Ca^{2+}, the greater the force and shortening. When Ca^{2+} is released from troponin and taken up by the sarcoplasmic reticulum, relaxation occurs. The relatively small amount of Ca^{2+} that enters the cell with activation is ultimately removed by an electrogenic Na^+/Ca^{2+} exchange that extrudes one Ca^{2+} for three Na^+ ions. When intracellular Na^+ is increased, less exchange occurs and the net amount of intracellular Ca^{2+} is increased. Thus, by inhibiting the Na^+/K^+-ATPase, digitalis glycosides produce a decrease in intracellular K^+ and an increase in intracellular Na^+ that increases intracellular Ca^{2+}.

In general, the main way in which all inotropic agents, including digitalis glycosides, increase contractility is by increasing the amount of Ca^{2+} available for activation. This is the case in both normal and failing myocardium. In the failing heart, there appears to be a decrease in the Ca^{2+} released into the cytosol with activation. The inotropic effects of digitalis glycosides are apparently due to an increase in intracellular Ca^{2+} that augments Ca^{2+} stores in the sarcoplasmic reticulum, resulting in a subsequent increase in the extent of myocyte activation.

The electrophysiologic actions of digitalis glycosides are complex, since they are intimately related to autonomic actions as well as K^+ effects and also the type of cardiac tissue affected. In pacemaker cells in the atria there is little effect except for increased automaticity at toxic levels. In the sinoatrial node and atrioventricular conduction system, the refractory period is prolonged. At toxic levels, conduction block can be produced through decreasing resting potential, which results in slowed conduction. At toxic levels of glycoside, the Purkinje system may become autonomous because of decreased resting potentials. All these effects are magnified by decreased extracellular K^+ so that toxicity is enhanced by a low serum K^+ and reduced by an increased K^+.

At therapeutic levels, the effects of digitalis glycosides reflect the direct electrophysiologic actions of the drug and the indirect actions of neurohormonal stimuli. In the atria, increased parasympathetic tone decreases refractory period that overrides the direct digitalis effect to prolong refractory period. Increased parasympathetic stimulation may reduce automatically through hyperpolarization of pacemaker cells, whereas sinus node activity, which is not affected directly by digitalis, is reduced through both increased parasympathetic and increased sympathetic tone.

Toxic levels of digitalis glycosides tend to exaggerate the parasympathetic augmentation, which may actually lead to atrial arrhythmias. Sympathetic activity may be increased with toxic levels, which, added to the direct actions of digitalis glycosides, can potentially result in life-threatening ventricular tachyarrhythmias.

In addition to effects on heart muscle to increase contractility and on vascular smooth muscle to increase contraction, digitalis glycosides exert significant actions on the autonomic nervous system, and these effects may provide a major part of purported beneficial actions. These effects include both stimulation and inhibition and may vary with dose of drug and underlying state of disease. In addition, short- and long-term effects may differ and alter ultimate efficacy. Relatively low doses of digitalis glycosides increase parasympathetic tone through apparent increased sensitivity of the efferent limb of both ventricular and arterial baroreceptors. Increased sensitivity of arterial baroreceptors enhances efferent parasympathetic activity while leading to withdrawal of reflex sympathetic tone, resulting in sinus bradycardia as well as arterial and venous dilatation. This indirect effect is opposite to the direct effect of glycosides to produce smooth-muscle vasoconstriction. Added effects of this sympathetic withdrawal include increased renal blood flow, renin release inhibition, and decreased antidiuretic hormone (ADH) release. Release of acetylcholine by vagal fibers is also thought to inhibit norepinephrine release from nerve endings as well as reduce β-receptor responses.

The overall effects of digitalis glycoside in the healthy individual are the result of the sum of its actions on the heart, the circulation, and the central nervous system, so it is difficult to establish direct from indirect effects of glycosides in many instances. Digitalis glycosides increase myocardial contractility directly in both the normal and failing heart, although the effects are relatively greater in the latter situation. However, hemodynamic results differ. In the absence of congestive heart failure, where both sympathetic and parasympathetic tone are minimal, digitalis glycosides increase peripheral arterial resistance directly, with a concomitant modest increase in arterial pressure, accompanied by a shift in blood volume to the splanchnic bed with decline in venous return and cardiac output. In contrast, with congestive heart failure, with withdrawal of elevated sympathetic nerve activity and increased parasympathetic tone, a fall in peripheral arterial resistance occurs with an increase in cardiac output. In terms of the heart, a decrease in ventricular filling pressure also occurs while stroke volume increases. These effects are increased by enhancing parasympathetic tone in the failing circulation, which may mimic some of the beneficial effects of β blockers and unloading agents, as noted elsewhere.

Whether the effects of digitalis glycosides are always beneficial and, if so, at what dose remain controversial. Studies in the elderly and in patients with myocardial infarction have demonstrated an increased threat of digitalis toxicity without careful monitoring. However, in the presence of severe failure [New York Heart Association (NYHA) class III], withdrawal of digoxin has resulted in substantial and rapid clinical deterioration despite concomitant therapy, including angiotensin converting enzyme (ACE) inhibitors and diuretics. When used in mild congestive heart failure, glycosides have increased ejection fraction, while ACE inhibitors were largely effective only in increasing exercise performance. These beneficial effects are observed whether the patients were in atrial fibrillation or in sinus rhythm. Recently, the placebo-controlled multicenter Digitalis Investigation Group (DIG) study, in more than 7000 patients with congestive heart failure, showed that digoxin did not affect mortality when compared with control. Digoxin therapy also was shown to improve both ventricular function and patient symptoms.

Digitalis Preparations: Structure, Pharmacokinetics, and Metabolism

All cardiac glycosides contain a ring structure termed an *aglycone* to which are attached up to four sugar molecules at the C-3 position. The aglycone itself is formed by a steroid nucleus to which a β-unsaturated lactone ring is attached at the C-17 position. Hydroxyl groups are generally found at C-3 and C-14, whereas a glucose moiety is generally attached through the C-3 hydroxyl group. At present, digoxin and digitoxin are the glycosides that are used clinically; they differ structurally only by the presence in digoxin of a hydroxyl group in the C-12 position. Cardiac activity, which correlates with the binding of drug to Na^+/K^+-ATPase on the cell surface sarcolemma, depends on the unsaturated lactone ring, the hydroxyl at C-14, and a cis configuration in carbons 8 to 17 in the aglycone ring. As the number of sugars on C-3 is reduced, water solubility increases and hepatic metabolism rather than renal excretion is favored. Thus digoxin is excreted primarily by the kidneys, whereas digitoxin is metabolized in the liver. Digitoxin is 90% bioavailable as compared with 60% for digoxin. A major difference between these agents is that digoxin is 25% protein-bound while digitoxin is 93% bound, such that the half-life of digoxin is 1.7 days and that of digitoxin is quite long at 7.0 days.

At present, digoxin and digitoxin are the only glycosides readily available in the United States, and digoxin is used in most instances. Digoxin has an onset of action from 30 min to 2 h when given orally and 5 to 30 min when given intravenously. Peak action occurs in 6 to 8 h when given orally and in 1 to 4 h when given intravenously. The plasma half-life of digoxin is 32 to 48 h, and it is excreted by the kidneys in a 50 to 70% unchanged state. Renal impairment may delay excretion of digoxin, which may lead to accumulation and development of toxicity. Digitoxin has a much larger half-life of several days and is metabolized largely by the liver.

Clinical Use

A loading dose for both digoxin and digitoxin is necessary to reach stable state rapidly, although with digoxin this is attained in 5 to 7 days with only a maintenance dose. Although intravenous digoxin is available, the oral dosage is generally adequate, except in urgent settings. The average loading dose of digoxin is 1.0 to 1.5 mg, given in divided doses over 24 h, with a maintenance dose of 0.125 to 0.25 mg/day. These doses are commonly halved in the elderly or in patients with renal insufficiency. The maintenance dose commonly needs adjustment to regulate resting heart rate in atrial fibrillation (between 55 and 70 beats per minute). In sinus rhythm, the dose is more uncertain, and a desired serum level of approximately 1.0 mg/kg should be sought.

As noted previously, the beneficial effects of augmented parasympathetic tone and sympathetic withdrawal may be obtained with relatively small doses of digitalis while not encountering potentials of toxicity. Thus the issue of dosage of digoxin remains unsettled relative to benefit sought.

Digitoxin requires a loading dose, since steady state on maintenance is attained only after several weeks. The loading dose is about 1.0 mg in divided doses, with maintenance of 0.1 to 0.15 mg/day. The advantage of digitoxin is its hepatic excretion in the presence of renal insufficiency and the lessened impact of poor patient compliance because of its much longer duration of action. Its disadvantage is the long time required for washout should toxicity occur or be suspected.

The serum level of digoxin can be affected by several other drugs. Cholestyramine, kaolin-pectin, neomycin, and bran can decrease digoxin absorption. Erythromycin, omeprazole, and tetracycline can increase digoxin absorption. Thyroxine can increase the volume of distribution of digoxin and enhance renal clearance. Quinidine increases serum digoxin levels, doubling levels in most patients over 1 to 2 days. The mechanism remains unclear, but if digoxin intake is not reduced, toxicity can occur. Verapamil reduces renal excretion and can increase serum digoxin levels by as much as 50% over a period of time. Amiodarone and propafenone appear to have a similar effect. With concurrent verapamil, amiodarone, and propafenone use, digoxin doses should be halved. Other antiarrhythmic agents do not exhibit interactions with digoxin.

Both thiazides and loop diuretics may lead to K^+ depletion, which augments myocardial sensitivity to digitalis glycosides with resulting arrhythmias, often requiring oral K^+ substitutes or the use of K^+-sparing diuretics such as amiloride. This may lead to arrhythmias of digoxin toxicity at even relatively low serum digoxin levels. Spironolactone, which inhibits the effects of aldosterone and thus serves to save K^+, also may have an opposing effect to reduce renal clearance of digoxin, thus raising its serum level.

In general, digoxin is used most commonly and thus will be the focus of the remaining discussion.

Digoxin in the Treatment of Congestive Heart Failure

As noted above, digoxin has its most beneficial hemodynamic actions when substantial ventricular depression is evident along with congestive heart failure. In this circumstance, it augments myocardial performance while reflexly reducing peripheral resistance. Slowing of the heart rate, whether via enhanced parasympathetic tone and reduced sympathetic activity to reduce sinus rate or via control of heart rate in atrial fibrillation (as discussed later) will greatly benefit ventricular filling and reduce pulmonary congestion. Thus the actions of digitalis glycosides not only affect the performance of the depressed myocardium but also have a central action to favorably alter the neurohumoral milieu that may impact adversely on the heart and circulation. In the treatment of congestive heart failure, digoxin is generally employed along with diuretics and vasodilator agents. By reducing peripheral resistance, digoxin and peripheral vasodilators act in a complimentary manner.

In acute heart failure, characterized by acute pulmonary edema, severe limitations of cardiac output, and perhaps hypotension, more rapidly acting inotropic agents such as intravenous dobutamine or milrinone may be required along with loop diuretics and vasodilators. This situation may occur in the setting of rapid deterioration of the patient with more chronic heart failure or following a large myocardial infarction. In this circumstance, the main aim is to increase cardiac output and reduce filling pressures as a setting for longer-term stabilization.

While rapidly acting inotropic agents are being used, digitalization may be started cautiously for its longer-term effects. In the setting of myocardial infarction, the situation is more complex. Because of fear that arrhythmias may be induced or oxygen consumption increased, which may be detrimental, digoxin is generally avoided in the first few days following the infarction, although in the longer term, digitalization, especially if dosing is carefully controlled, may be of value along with other agents, especially ACE inhibitors. In the absence of clear congestive heart failure with only lower ejection fraction (NYHA classes I and II), digitalis has had an apparent adverse effect on long-term mortality and should be avoided. For chronic congestive failure, digoxin is of use over the long term when administered in association with loop diuretics and ACE inhibitors. Benefits are most evident in patients with NYHA class III or IV congestive heart failure. In this circumstance, the response of the circulation is characterized by a decrease in venous pressures and ventricular filling pressures and an increase in cardiac output. Heart rate is slowed, and ejection fraction tends to rise, while peripheral resistance falls with little or no change in arterial pressure. These salutary effects are attributed to a combination of augmented myocardial contractility and restoration of baroreceptor sensitivity, which results in enhanced parasympathetic and decreased sympathetic tone. Myocardial oxygen consumption tends to be reduced in heart failure owing to a decrease in heart size, and thus ventricular wall tension, and a slowing of heart rate. Earlier concepts supported the view that digoxin was of greatest benefit when atrial fibrillation was present and controlled. It is now clear that efficacy is present also when the patient with heart failure is in sinus rhythm. Withdrawal of digoxin from such patients has lead to rapid deterioration, even when both diuretics and ACE inhibitors were used. Although digoxin has been associated with an increase in ejection fraction, vasodilators have shown more significant increments in exercise performance. These considerations would justify the combined use of these agents. However, whereas the use of ACE inhibitors may well be indicated when the ejection is reduced but symptoms are limited (classes I and II), digoxin probably should be reserved for use with more overt symptoms (classes III and IV).

Although digoxin can be given once a day without tolerance or tachyphylaxis, the dose is a matter of issue. In general, a serum level of 0.5 to 1.5 mg/L is believed to be therapeutic. This level may vary from patient to patient, and a clear dose-response relation has not been established. Indeed, some of the greatest benefits may be gained from lower doses (e.g., 0.125 mg/day), which may induce the neurohumoral benefits of lower sympathetic and higher parasympathetic tone while reducing the incidence of possible toxic side effects, as discussed later. There appear to be no adverse effects from digoxin usage in terms of mortality in patients with congestive heart failure, and substantially increased morbidity is noted when the drug is withdrawn. Effects on mortality with digoxin are complicated by the fact that the nature and progression of the underlying process that has led to failure in the first place may well be the ultimate determinant of mortality. If morbidity is reduced substantially with digoxin, as has been demonstrated, a neutral effect on ultimate mortality, as has been demonstrated, would be acceptable. This was demonstrated recently in the National Institutes of Health–sponsored DIG study, a controlled trial in patients with congestive heart failure (CHF), which showed no effect on survival compared with placebo, a reduction in hospitalizations, and a low incidence of digoxin toxicity.

Digoxin has been of limited value in treatment of right-sided heart failure, as may occur in cor pulmonale or left-to-right shunts. Digoxin also has limited value in the face of acute left ventricular failure due to acute myocardial infarction. After the first few days of an infarction have passed, longer-term digoxin use has been employed as it would be in any form of chronic failure, but its effects on mortality have remained controversial. Nevertheless, since mortality may be increased by digoxin after infarction, especially when clear evidence of heart failure is absent, its use is best reserved for those with overt congestive heart failure.

Digitalis Toxicity

Digoxin levels can be measured readily in the serum by immunologic techniques, and the therapeutic level is thought to be 1.0 to 2.0 mg/mL. Administration of other drugs may alter the serum level by altering either absorption or elimination and may contribute to toxicity, as noted previously. For example, verapamil and quinidine may increase plasma levels.

The signs and symptoms of digitalis toxicity have been amply described, although some may be very subtle. These include nausea and anorexia that may lead to weight loss, fatigue, and visual disturbances. Psychiatric disturbances may occur less commonly, including delirium, hallucinations, or even seizures. Electrocardiographic alterations occur with variable degrees of AV block and ventricular ectopy. Sinus bradycardia, junctional rhythm, paroxysmal tachycardia with variable AV block, Wenckebach AV block, and ventricular tachycardia leading to ventricular fibrillation may be seen. Such arrhythmias are potentiated by hypokalemia as well as digitalis-mediated enhanced parasympathetic tone. Such arrhythmias may be life-threatening in the presence of severe heart failure and should be avoided or controlled as possible.

The diagnosis of digitalis toxicity is suggested by signs and symptoms, as well as electrocardiographic alterations, and supported by an elevated serum digoxin level. A certain diagnosis may be made only with drug withdrawal accompanied by subsidence of these findings. With the therapeutic level of digoxin between 1.0 and 2.0 mg/mL, digitalis toxicity levels would be unlikely but not excluded; levels beyond 3.0 mg/mL would suggest toxicity, while levels below 1.5 mg/mL, when not complicated by hypokalemia, would suggest other problems. It is important to note that only steady-state serum drug concentrations show any relationship with cardiac glycoside toxicity. Thus, for example, when monitoring serum digoxin concentration, the samples should be collected at least 6 to 8 h after drug administration. Nevertheless, there is great crossover between patients reflecting variable sensitivity such that withdrawal of digoxin on suspicion is always advisable for treatment as well as diagnosis. This is especially true because some patients elicit profound vagal responses with relatively small amounts of digoxin.

While withdrawal of digoxin and correction of hypokalemia may be adequate treatment of digitalis toxicity in most instances, a temporary pacemaker may be required for severe bradycardia or complete heart block. Lidocaine is useful to treat ventricular ectopy or ventricular tachycardia. Dilantin also has been used, while quinidine, which may displace digoxin from binding sites and thus raise serum digoxin levels further, should be avoided. Amiodarone and intravenous magnesium also have been utilized successfully for this purpose.

In the presence of massive digoxin overdosage, most commonly associated with suicide attempts, digitalis-specific antibodies (digoxin-specific Fab fragments) have been remarkably effective. In general, such an approach in the usual therapeutic setting is unnecessary but provides a backup to more conservative approaches such as normalizing serum K^+ and withholding digoxin if they are not proceeding well.

Digoxin reduction should be considered and individualized in the elderly patient with renal insufficiency. Since electrical conversion is accompanied by ventricular arrhythmias, reduction of dosage 1 to 2 days before is advisable.

CATECHOLAMINES AND SIMILAR INOTROPIC AGENTS

In general, positive inotropism is based on enhancing the delivery of Ca^{2+} to the contractile system so as to increase force and shortening. Increasing Ca^{2+} in the serum will effect this transiently, while, as noted previously, digitalis glycosides increase Ca^{2+} for activation by inhibiting sarcolemmal Na^+/K^+-ATPase. Catecholamines increase activating Ca^{2+} via β-adrenergic receptors and the adenylcyclase system.

β Receptors are located in the sarcolemma and make up a complex structure that spans the membrane. The β receptor is connected with G proteins that either activate (G_s) or inhibit (G_i) a secondary system, adenylate cyclase, which, when activated by G_s, induces the formation of 3′,5′-cyclic adenosine monophosphate (cyclic AMP). Cyclic AMP in turn activates certain protein kinases that lead to intracellular phosphorylation of proteins that enhance both the entry and removal of intracellular Ca^{2+}. By providing more Ca^{2+} to the troponin-tropomyosin system, a greater interaction between actin and myosin occurs, increasing force and shortening. Increasing the rate of Ca^{2+} removal from the cytoplasm speeds the rate of relaxation.

In the normal heart, norepinephrine is synthesized and stored in sympathetic nerve endings that invest the entire heart, atria, conduction system, and ventricle. When activated, these nerve endings are depolarized, and norepinephrine is released from granules in nerve endings into myocardial clefts containing β-adrenergic receptors, which, when activated, turn on the sequence of events noted earlier. Not only does this enhance Ca^{2+} entry into the myocyte to augment contraction, but it also phosphorylates phospholambam, which enhances relaxation. Subsequently, most of the released norepinephrine is taken back and restored in the sympathetic nerve endings. Released norepinephrine is also inactivated by two enzymes, catechol-*O*-methyltransferase (COMT) and monoamine oxidase (MAO), and the products are excreted largely by the kidneys.

In very severe heart failure, stores of norepinephrine in the ventricle are largely depleted, and the sympathetic nerve endings fail to take up norepinephrine normally. At the same time, circulating norepinephrine released from peripheral sympathetic nerve endings may be increased, especially in severe failure. In less severe heart failure, the decreased norepinephrine levels may reflect enhanced release due to increased sympathetic nerve activity.

In both the normal and failing myocardium, activation of the adenylcyclase system can augment contractility. Agents that do this may be divided into two categories. The first comprises the catecholamines (e.g., norepinephrine, epinephrine) and their synthetic derivatives (e.g., dobutamine, isoproterenol), which act via cell-surface adrenergic receptors. The second includes agents that inhibit the breakdown of cyclic AMP by inhibition of phosphodiesterase type III (e.g., amrinone, milrinone, and pimobenden). Some of these agents, such a pimobenden, also may increase myofibrillar sensitivity to calcium and then further augment contraction.

Catecholamines constitute an endogenous hormonal system exerting reflex control of the heart and circulation. Their effects depend on localized controlled neural release and receptor specificity in terms of action.

Dopamine is the naturally occurring precursor of both norepinephrine and epinephrine. Although epinephrine is released from the adrenal medulla, norepinephrine is the primary mediator in the heart and peripheral circulation.

The actions of both endogenous and exogenous catecholamines depend on their activation of specific α- and β-adrenergic receptors (Table 8-1). α Receptors include α_1 receptors, which are postsynaptic and are located in vascular smooth muscle and in the myocardium. In smooth muscle, they mediate vasoconstriction; in the heart, weak positive inotropic and negative chronotropic effects. α_2 Receptors are presynaptic and, when stimulated, decrease norepinephrine release from peripheral nerve endings as well as sympathetic outflow from the central nervous system. α_2 Receptors also may mediate vasoconstriction in specific peripheral vascular beds.

β-Adrenergic receptors can be divided into β_1 and β_2. β_1 Receptors are located in the myocardium where they mediate positive inotropic, chronotropic, and dromotropic effects. Their activation occurs primarily by norepinephrine released from neurons in the heart. β_2 Receptors are located in vascular smooth muscle, where they mediate vasodilata-

TABLE 8-1 Adrenergic Receptor Activity of Sympathomimetic Amines

	α_1	β_1	β_2	Dopaminergic	Dose
Dopamine	+++	++	+	++++	<2 μg/kg/min—vasodilation effects on peripheral dopaminergic receptors; 2–10 μg/kg/min—inotropic effects, β_1-receptor activation; 5–20 μg/kg/min—peripheral vasoconstriction, α effects
Norepinephrine	++++	++++	0	0	Initiate with 8–12 μg/min; maintain 2–4 μg/min
Epinephrine	+++	++++	++	0	
Isoproterenol	0	++++	++++	0	0.5–5 μg/min
Dobutamine	+++	++++	++	0	Start at 2–3 μg/kg/min and titrate upward

tion, and in the sinoatrial node, where they are chronotropic. In general, β_2 receptors are activated by circulating catecholamines released from peripheral sites such as the adrenal medulla.

Another type of receptor has been termed the *dopaminergic receptor*, which is localized to the mesenteric and renal circulations and mediates arterial vasodilatation. The physiologic and pharmacologic actions of various catecholamines depend on which receptor they activate in both the heart and the periphery (Table 8-2).

Norepinephrine has potent α_1 and β_1 activity. When norepinephrine is released from cardiac nerve endings, as occurs in normal exercise, myocardial contractility and heart rate are augmented. When norepinephrine is administered exogenously, its major action is to stimulate α_1 receptors, leading to marked peripheral arterial vasoconstriction. Thus norepinephrine has been used for severe hypotension to increase arterial blood pressure so as to maintain blood flow to vital organs. Long-term renal vasoconstriction from continued norepinephrine administration may produce ischemic renal damage, including acute tubular necrosis, so prolonged use, that is, more than 24 to 48 h, is usually untenable. For the failing heart, this peripheral vasoconstriction also provides an undesirable added pressure load (afterload), which tends to vitiate the potential benefits of β_1 stimulation.

Dopamine has both α_1 and β_1 activity but also stimulates dopaminergic receptors in the renal vasculature to produce arterial dilation and increased renal blood flow. Its β_1 effects in the heart occur largely through the release of endogenous norepinephrine, which may be largely depleted in the failing heart. As doses of dopamine are increased, conversion to norepinephrine also occurs, which tends to produce relatively more pressor effects than myocardial inotropic stimulation. As such, the benefits of dopamine administration, if any,

TABLE 8-2 Physiologic and Pharmacologic Actions of Catecholamine Receptors

Receptor	Receptor activity	Primary location
β_1	Positive inotropic and chronotropic action; increased AV conduction	Heart (atria, ventricle, AV node)
β_2	Peripheral vasodilation	Arterioles, arteries, veins, bronchioles
α_1	Arteriolar vasoconstriction	Arterioles
α_2	Presynaptic inhibition of norepinephrine release	Sympathetic nerve endings, CNS
Dopaminergic	Renal and mesenteric vasodilation, natriuresis, diuresis	Kidneys

are at low doses (e.g., 0.02 mg/kg per minute), where they may induce renal arterial vasodilatation in association with administration of other more potent inotropic agents (e.g., dobutamine).

Dobutamine is a synthetic variant of the catecholamines whose structure has been altered to optimize hemodynamic response in the dog characterized by an increase in cardiac output and a decrease in ventricular filling pressure with little change in heart rate. Since arterial pressure also rises modestly, peripheral vascular resistance must of necessity fall. The positive inotropic activity of dobutamine is mediated by direct stimulation of β_1-adrenergic receptors in the myocardium (see Tables 8-1 and 8-2). It is unclear why a concomitant increase in heart rate does not always occur. One possibility is that an increase in cardiac output that increases arterial pressure serves to reflexly buffer any heart rate increase. Given the capacity of dobutamine to increase cardiac output and reduce filling pressures without substantial heart rate change, dobutamine has been used widely to treat severe acute left ventricular failure in the absence of profound hypotension, which is poorly responsive to diuretics and vasodilators, as may be seen following a very large myocardial infarction or in acute decompensation in the course of chronic congestive heart failure. In the presence of severe hypotension, the β_2 stimulation of dobutamine may be harmful, and administration of an α_1-stimulating vasoconstrictor such as norepinephrine or higher-dose dopamine also may be necessary to increase arterial peripheral resistance.

Dobutamine infusion is generally begun at 2 μg/kg per minute and titrated to optimize cardiac output while reducing left ventricular filling pressure. Tachycardia is carefully avoided so as not to increase ischemia. The effects on myocardial oxygen consumption (MVO_2) are complex. Whereas the increase in contractility will increase MVO_2, a decrease in heart size will tend to reduce it. The end result is generally a modest increase in MVO_2 induced by dobutamine. With a better maintained arterial pressure and reduced left ventricular diastolic pressure in the absence of tachycardia, coronary perfusion pressure also may be increased. The major side effects of dobutamine are an excessive increase in heart rate with high doses and ventricular arrhythmias, both of which may mandate dose reduction and even drug discontinuation. Tachyphylaxis also may occur to a variable degree. In general, once hemodynamic benefits are attained, dobutamine is slowly withdrawn. (In some cases this has not been possible, and sustained administration becomes necessary, which may require portable pumps for administration. The outcome in this circumstance is generally dire.)

In chronic congestive heart failure, the patient is commonly maintained on vasodilators such as angiotensin converting enzyme inhibitors, loop diuretics, and digoxin. Nevertheless, episodes of acute decompensation characterized by increased pulmonary congestion and edema and reduced renal function with increasing fluid accumulation may intervene. The addition of dobutamine with or without milrinone provides an increase in cardiac output with a decrease in filling pressures, which with added diuretics may help to restore a steady state for a variable period of time. Dopamine, at a low dose, is commonly used concomitantly to augment renal blood. This generally requires a short hospitalization and temporary hemodynamic monitoring.

PDE INHIBITORS AND OTHER AGENTS

The adenylcyclase–cyclic AMP system also can be activated beyond the β receptor. Hormones such as glucagon activate the system and can increase myocardial contractility acutely despite β_1 blockade. Although useful in overcoming β-adrenergic blockade if necessary, glucagon may induce gastric atony and nausea, which has limited its more generalized use.

Amrinone and milrinone are prototypes of a new class of cardiotonic agents that activate the adenylcyclase system through inhibition of the enzyme that breaks down cyclic AMP, phosphodiesterase III (PDE III). Type III PDE inhibitors decrease the breakdown of cyclic AMP in the myocardium and increase cyclic guanidine monophosphate (cyclic GMP) in vascular smooth muscle, resulting in an increase in myocardial contractility as well as arterial and venous vasodilatation. Other members of this class of drugs include enoximone and pimobendan, although only amrinone and milrinone have been approved by the Food and Drug Administration (FDA) for treatment of acute heart failure. The mechanism by which vasodilatation occurs is not completely understood. Increased cyclic GMP induces phosphorylation of myosin light-chain kinase, which decreases sensitivity to calcium and calmodulin. In the heart, inotropism may relate not only to increased cyclic AMP–mediated calcium availability for contraction and increased rates of its removal for relaxation but also to increased sensitivity of the contractile system for calcium. Both amrinone and milrinone, which are available as intravenous agents, have substantial ability to augment cardiac output while reducing both right and left ventricular filling pressures. The lowering of filling pressures is greater than that seen with dobutamine. Dilatation of the pulmonary vasculature is also a very useful therapeutic effect. Arterial pressure tends to be reduced, whereas an increase in heart rate may occur. Since dobutamine increases cyclic AMP and milrinone reduces its breakdown, the combination of these agents is substantially more potent than either agent alone. When either dobutamine or milrinone is utilized, ectopic activity may be increased, which requires careful supervision in their use.

PDE III inhibitors are also orally active and produce the same hemodynamic improvement as seen with intravenous use. However, in longer-term oral use, increased mortality was seen with the use of milrinone, especially in the presence of class IV heart failure. This increased mortality may have been due to the relatively short action of this agent (1.5-h half-life), which leads to large peaks and valleys in dosing and concomitant arrhythmias. For the time being, this has vitiated clinical study of these agents, but more stringent control of the use of this class of agents as adjuncts to other agents ultimately may increase their value.

Clinical Use of Noncatecholamine Inotropes

Amrinone and milrinone are administered intravenously, starting with a loading dose followed by a continuous infusion. For amrinone, a 0.5 μg/kg bolus is followed by a 5 to 10 μg/kg per minute infusion. Milrinone, which is 10 times more potent, is administered as a 50 μg/kg bolus followed by a 0.25 to 1.0 μg/kg per minute infusion. Because of its higher selectivity for phosphodiesterase and ease of use, milrinone has become the agent of choice compared with amrinone. Milrinone's half-life is 30 to 60 min and amrinone's is 2 to 3 h, and the half-lives of both drugs are prolonged in severe heart failure. Thrombocytopenia has been reported with amrinone in 3% of patients and is rare with milrinone. Ventricular ectopy leading to more severe ventricular arrhythmias is reported with both drugs and is not dose-related. Supraventricular arrhythmias are seen less commonly, hypotension is seen in 3%, and chest pain is seen in 1% of patients receiving the drugs.

REFERENCES

The Digitalis Investigation Group: The effect of digoxin on mortality and morbidity in patients with heart failure. *N Engl J Med* 336:525, 1997.

Frishman WH (ed): *Current Cardiovascular Drugs*, 2d ed. Philadelphia, Current Medicine, 1995, p 194.

LeJemtel TH, Sonnenblick EH, Frishman WH: Diagnosis and management of heart failure, in Alexander RW, Schlant RC, Fuster V (eds): *Hurst's The Heart*, 9th ed. New York, McGraw-Hill, pp 745–781, 1998.

Nielsen-Kudsk JE, Aldershvile J: Will calcium sensitizers play a role in the treatment of heart failure? *J Cardiovasc Pharmacol* 26(Suppl 1):S77, 1995.

Packer M, Gheorghiade M, Young JB, et al: Withdrawal of digoxin from patients with chronic heart failure treated with angiotensin-converting-enzyme inhibitors. RADIANCE Study. *N Engl J Med* 329:1, 1993.

Sonnenblick EH, LeJemtel TH, Frishman WH: Digitalis preparations and other inotropic agents, in Frishman WH, Sonnenblick EH (eds): *Cardiovascular Pharmacotherapeutics*. New York, McGraw-Hill, pp 237–251, 1997.

Tauke J, Goldstein S, Gheorghiade M: Digoxin for chronic heart failure: A review of the randomized controlled trials with special attention to the PROVED and RADIANCE Trials. *Prog Cardiovasc Dis* 37:49, 1994.

Uretsky BF, Young JB, Shahidi FE, et al: Randomized study assessing the effect of digoxin withdrawal in patients with mild to moderate chronic congestive heart failure: Results of the PROVED Trial. *J Am Coll Cardiol* 22:955, 1995.

Chapter 9 | The Organic Nitrates and Nitroprusside

Jonathan Abrams

The organic nitrates and sodium nitroprusside make up a class of drugs known as the *nitrovasodilators*. The common denominator of these agents is the production of nitric oxide (NO) within vascular smooth-muscle cells or platelets (Fig. 9-1). Nitric oxide activates the enzyme guanylate cyclase, which in turn results in an accumulation of intracellular cyclic guanosine 3′5′-monophosphate, or cGMP. Smooth-muscle cell relaxation is induced by cGMP through fluxes in intracellular calcium. In the platelet, increases in cGMP exert an antiaggregatory action, and thus decreased platelet activation, resulting in less thrombosis.

The predominant actions of the nitrovasodilators are the hemodynamic perturbations resulting from vascular dilatation. In contrast to the majority of vasodilating agents available to the clinician, the nitrates and nitroprusside (NP) relax the venous capacitance bed as well as arteries and arterioles. The role of the antiplatelet and antithrombotic actions of these compounds remains somewhat controversial, although much recent evidence supports a true benefit for nitrate-induced decreases in platelet-thrombus activation.

Nitroglycerin (NTG) has been utilized in medicine for well over 100 years. This drug, initially employed for anginal chest pain, became a mainstay of the homeopathic tradition in the early part of the 20th century. For the past three decades or more, NTG and the organic nitrates have been used widely for the acute and chronic therapy of ischemic chest pain. More recently, these compounds have been employed in acute and post-myocardial infarction and, importantly, as adjunctive therapy of congestive heart failure. Nitroprusside, available only as an intravenous agent, is effective in the treatment of severe or acute hypertension, acute or chronic congestive heart failure, and pulmonary edema. As a general rule, NP is not used to alleviate myocardial ischemia.

Attenuation of nitrate effects, or *nitrate tolerance*, is the major obstacle to successful utilization of these drugs in clinical practice. There does not appear to be a significant degree of tolerance to the actions of NP, however. In recent years, a wide variety of nitrate formulations and compounds has become available, whereas some older nitrate compounds (e.g., pentaerythritol tetranitrate) are no longer in use (Table 9-1).

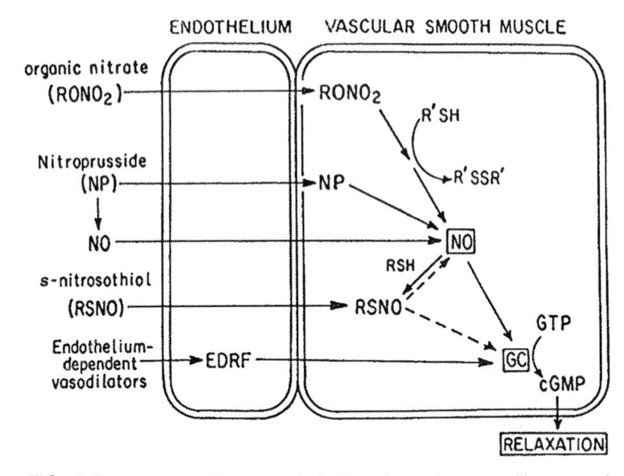

FIG. 9-1 Nitrovasodilators, endothelium-dependent vasodilators, and vascular smooth-muscle relaxation. Abbreviations: NO = nitric oxide; EDRF 5 endothelium-derived relaxing factor; R′SH and RSH = two distinct pools of intracellular sulfhydryl groups; R′SSR′ = disulfide groups; GC = guanylate cyclase. *(From Kowaluk E, Fung H-L: Pharmacology and pharmacokinetics of nitrates, in Abrams J, Pepine C, Thadani U (eds): Medical Therapy of Ischemic Heart Disease: Nitrates, Beta Blockers, and Calcium Antagonists. Boston, Little, Brown, 1992, p 152, with permission.)*

THE ORGANIC NITRATES

Mechanisms of Action

Cellular

Nitroglycerin, isosorbide dinitrate (ISDN), and 5-isosorbide mononitrate (ISMN) are metabolized by vascular tissue near the plasma membrane of smooth muscle cells of veins and arteries (see Fig. 9-1). It was previously believed that nitrates underwent a stepwise dinitration process that resulted in NO via the production of nitrite ion (NO_2^-). However, it now appears that these compounds may form NO directly through an enzymatic process that does not necessarily involve nitrite production as an intermediary. Furthermore, the obligatory role of *s*-nitrosothiols (SNO) remains controversial (see Fig. 9-1) Nitrates can be converted to SNO but are dominantly a direct precursor of NO. Both NO and SNO can activate guanylate cyclase, leading to the production of cGMP, a second messenger that leads to vascular smooth-muscle cell relaxation.

TABLE 9-1 Nitrate Formulations: Dosing Recommendations and Pharmacokinetics

	Usual dose, mg	Onset of action, min	Effective duration of action
Sublingual NTG	0.3–0.6	2–5	20–30 min
Sublingual ISDN	2.5–10.0	5–20	45–120 min
Buccal NTG	1–3 bid-tid	2–5	30–300 min*
Oral ISDN	10–60 bid–tid	15–45	2–6 h
Oral ISDN-SR	80–120 once daily	60–90	10–14 h
Oral ISMN	20 bid†	30–60	3–6 h
Oral ISMN-SR	60–120 qd	60–90	10–14 h
NTG ointment	0.5–2.0 tid	15–60	3–8 h
NTG patch	0.4–0.8 mg/h‡	30–60	8–12 h

*Effect persists only while tablet intact in buccal cavity.
†Two daily doses 7 h apart (e.g., 8 am, 2 pm).
‡Patch should be removed daily for 10–12 h.
Abbreviations: NTG = glyceryltrinitrate (nitroglycerin); ISDN = isosorbide dinitrate; ISMN = isosorbide mononitrate; SR = sustained release.
Note: Higher doses are often required in heart failure.

The enzymatic conversion of the nitrovasodilators is not homogeneous; NP and SNO appear to require different enzymes or "receptors," which presumably accounts for some of the differences in the hemodynamic spectrum among these agents and also could relate to the different susceptibility to tolerance between organic nitrates and NP or SNO. Intracellular chemical processes also result in NO formation in a nonenzymatic manner; this is much less important for the organic nitrates than for NP.

In the platelet, increases in cGMP have been correlated with the degree of vasodilation in the coronary arteries. Presumably, platelet activation is modulated by nitrates via cGMP-induced actions.

Nitrate Tolerance

Whereas the precise mechanisms of tolerance remain the subject of intense investigation, it is known that NO production and cGMP responses become attenuated in the setting of nitrate tolerance. Furthermore, the obligatory role of thiols during nitrate activation remains controversial as regards tolerance phenomena. Although it now seems clear that intracellular glutathione or cysteine stores are adequate, and thiol deficiency per se is not a factor in tolerance development, thiol or —SH groups are critical to SNO formation. Furthermore, a thiol moiety is a component of the enzyme that converts nitrates to NO. Thus tolerance development may in part be related to thiols within the vascular smooth-muscle cell in relationship to the production of SNO or the nitrate enzyme(s) responsible for NO formation.

Nitrate Effects on Regional Circulations

Administration of NTG or other nitrates in sufficient dosage results in dilatation of veins and large- to moderate-sized arteries, with a fall in vascular impedance. At high concentrations, nitrates dilate the smaller arteries, and at very high doses, nitrates can relax arterioles and the microcirculation. Venodilatation is seen at low nitrate concentrations and is near maximal at moderate dosage (Fig. 9-2). Interesting studies by Harrison's group have suggested that the enzymes responsible for nitrate conversion to NO apparently are not present in the coronary microvessels, thus limiting the degree of increase in coronary blood flow and decrease in coronary vascular resistance that can be achieved with NTG through dilatation of these small coronary vessels. Nitroprusside, on the other hand, directly forms NO in the microcirculation and readily relaxes the resistance vessels; this can cause a fall in distal coronary bed pressure and also may allow for a coronary steal phenomenon in vessels beyond a coronary atherosclerotic obstruction (See below).

FIG. 9-2 Vasodilatory actions of organic nitrates in the major vascular beds. Note that the venous or capacitance system dilates maximally with low doses of organic nitrates. Increasing the amount of drug does not cause appreciable additional venodilatation. Arterial dilatation and enhanced arterial conductance begin with low doses of nitrate. With further vasodilatation, appearing with increasing dosage at high plasma concentrations, the arteriolar or resistance vessels dilate, resulting in a decrease in systemic and regional vascular resistance. *(From Abrams J: Hemodynamic effects of nitroglycerin and long acting nitrates. Am Heart J 110:216–224, 1985, with permission.)*

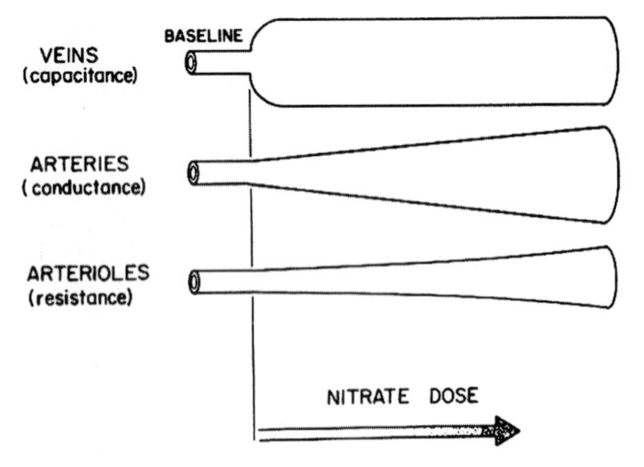

Nitrates dilate the epicardial coronary arteries and, to a lesser degree, the smaller or distal coronary vessels. Coronary blood flow transiently increases and then declines below baseline as myocardial energy needs decrease. Systemic venous relaxation in the extremities and splanchnic circulation results in sequestration of the circulating blood volume away from the heart and lungs, with a fall in cardiac output.

Nitrates also relax the splanchnic and mesenteric arterial beds, possibly contributing to the decrease in blood flow return to the heart. Renal blood flow is marginally affected by NTG; it may decrease to a modest degree. The cerebral vascular bed dilates with nitrates, and blood volume to the brain may increase. Thus these agents are contraindicated when intracranial pressure is elevated.

An important clinical action of nitrates relates to the pulmonary circulation. These drugs consistently lower pulmonary venous and pulmonary capillary pressures, which contributes significantly to their efficacy in heart failure as well as myocardial ischemia. Pulmonary arterial bed relaxation is beneficial to subjects with secondary pulmonary hypertension; nitrates do not generally have a useful role in primary pulmonary hypertension.

Hemodynamic Correlates of Clinical Nitrate Efficacy

Table 9-2 indicates the presumed mechanisms of action for the various clinical conditions for which these agents are prescribed. In general, the traditional view has been that nitrate-induced reversal and/or prevention of myocardial ischemia is due to reductions in myocardial oxygen consumption related to reduced cardiac chamber size and decreased systolic and diastolic pressures within the heart. These alterations are predominantly related to the venous and arterial vasodilating actions discussed above. The presumed paradigm is a major nitrate-induced decrease in cardiac work to match available coronary blood supply. However, in recent years much evidence has contributed to the view that the organic nitrates have important actions in increasing regional or nutrient coronary blood flow, particularly to areas of myocardial ischemia. In addition to epicardial coronary artery dilatation, prevention or reversal of coronary artery vasoconstriction or spasm, increased coronary collateral size and flow, enhanced distal vessel and collateral caliber when constrictor forces predominate, coronary atherosclerotic stenosis enlargement, and improved coronary endothelial function are all mechanisms that may interact in a favorable fashion to alleviate or prevent ischemia by directly enhancing coronary blood supply to myocardium downstream from a fixed or dynamic coronary obstruction (see Table 9-2).

In congestive heart failure, the beneficial effects and rationale for the nitrates are more obvious and are related to a predictable lowering of left and right ventricular filling pressures, as well as the "unloading"

TABLE 9-2 Mechanism of Action of Nitrates: Relationship to Clinical Indications

Acute attacks and prophylaxis of stable angina pectoris	Decreased myocardial oxygen consumption • Decreased LV dimension • Decreased LV filling pressure • Decreased LV systolic pressure • Decreased vascular impedance Increased coronary blood supply • Epicardial coronary artery dilation • Coronary stenosis enlargement • Improved coronary endothelial function • Dilation of coronary collaterals or small distal coronary vessels
Unstable angina	Same as above, plus antiplatelet, antithrombotic action
Acute myocardial infarction	Same as above, plus anti-platelet, antithrombotic action
Congestive heart failure Systolic dysfunction	Decreased LV and RV dimensions (little data in CHF) Decreased LV and RV filling pressure Decreased systemic vascular resistance Decreased arterial pressure Decreased PA and RA pressure Improved endothelial function CAD patients: increased coronary blood flow Decreased mitral regurgitation
Diastolic dysfunction	Decreased LV filling pressure
Hypertension	Decreased systolic blood pressure Decreased systemic vascular resistance Decreased LV preload - uncertain importance

Abbreviations: LV = left ventricular; RV = right ventricular; PA = pulmonary artery; RA = right atrial; CAD = coronary artery disease; CHF = congestive heart failure.

actions that arise from decreased arterial pressure and impedance to left ventricular ejection. These afterload-reducing actions contribute to a modest increase in stroke volume and cardiac output in subjects with impaired left ventricular systolic function, in contradistinction to the typical fall in forward cardiac output in the normal heart. In addition, NTG appears to improve impaired vascular endothelial function common to heart failure.

Nitroglycerin: The Exogenous Endothelium-Derived Relaxing Factor

Normal endothelial function vasodilatory and counters platelet activity. In the presence of coronary atherosclerosis, even mild, the dilating actions of the endothelium are impaired in both the coronary and systemic circulations. Thus diminished vasodilation to physiologic stimuli (e.g., shear stress, platelet release products) and impaired platelet anti-adhesion and aggregation responses are present in many to most individuals with clinical coronary artery disease. Vasoconstrictor responses to exercise, mental stress, cold pressor testing, and with the administration of endothelium-dependent dilator stimuli (e.g., acetylcholine, bradykinin) have been well documented in coronary artery disease (CAD) subjects. Diminished availability of NO and prostacycline, as well as increased endothelin expression, is common in these patients; increased superoxide anions may play a major role in inducing the endothelial dysfunction common to CAD. Stenosis constriction or collapse is an advanced manifestation of impaired endothelial function and may substantially contribute to the precipitation of myocardial ischemia in patients with angina or silent ischemia. NTG prevents or reverses this phenomenon, which has been documented with acetylcholine administration as well as exercise.

In congestive heart failure, disordered endothelial vasodilator activity is also common, importantly contributing to the vasoconstrictor state common to heart failure. Enhanced sensitivity to catecholamines is part of the abnormal vascular physiology in association with endothelial dysfunction; this phenomenon should be deleterious in heart failure as well as CAD.

Nitrates, as donors of NO, have been called *exogenous endothelium-derived relaxing factor* (ERDF) agents; these drugs improve responses to a variety of stimuli in the presence of endothelial dysfunction. Thus, in the patient with CAD, administration of organic nitrates can partially or completely normalize impaired endothelial-related vasodilation and presumably, but as yet unproved, restore endothelium-modulated antiplatelet activity toward normal. In fact, NTG vascular responses appear to be more robust in the setting of endothelial dysfunction than in the normal state. Nitrates also may improve endothelial function in heart failure.

CLINICAL INDICATIONS FOR NITRATES

The major cardiovascular conditions for which nitrates are effective are listed in Table 9-2. The roles of NTG and the other organic nitrates in CAD are well established. Treatment and prophylaxis of anginal attacks as well as prevention of chest pain in chronic angina pectoris are the most important uses of these drugs. More problematic is the usefulness of nitrates in acute myocardial infarction (MI). Although sublingual or intravenous NTG is excellent for recurrent ischemic chest pain, hypertension, or heart failure in the setting of an acute infarct, there is considerable uncertainty as to the benefits of *routine* 24- or 48-h infusions of NTG or the use of any nitrate when obvious clinical indications are absent in the setting of infarction. Despite promising but limited older animal and human data, the recently completed European megatrials

GISSI-3 (Gruppo Italiano per lo Studio della Supravivenza nell'Infarcto Miocardico) and ISIS-4 (Fourth International Study of Infarct Survival) have failed to show an important role for early administration of nitrates continued for 5 to 6 weeks after an acute MI.

Nitrates are underutilized in congestive heart failure. These drugs are effective in improving symptoms and exercise tolerance and, in conjunction with the angiotensin converting enzyme inhibitors, are useful for the treatment of symptomatic heart failure. Large doses are often required in these patients. Nitrate resistance, as well as the necessity to use huge amounts of these drugs, has been described in advanced heart failure. In the first Veterans Administration cooperative heart failure mortality study, the combination of ISDN 40 mg four times daily and hydralazine 300 mg/day reduced mortality. However, the combination of hydralazine and oral ISDN proved less effective in improving survival in heart failure patients than the angiotensin converting enzyme (ACE) inhibitor enalapril.

Intravenous NTG is an effective formulation for lowering blood pressure in the setting of acute hypertension or for the control of mean arterial pressure during a variety of delicate surgical procedures. This agent has been successfully employed for post-coronary bypass patients with elevated blood pressure. Oral nitrates, while utilized extensively in the early part of this century for hypertension, are not part of contemporary conventional therapy of essential hypertension, in part because of the appearance of tolerance to the systolic pressure lowering effects of these drugs. One report from France indicates a potential benefit for oral ISDN in systolic hypertension of the elderly.

NITRATE FORMULATIONS AND NITRATE PHARMACOKINETICS

Three organic nitrate compounds—NTG, ISDN, and ISMN—are currently used throughout the world and have been shown to provide benefits in angina pectoris and congestive heart failure. There does not appear to be any difference in clinical efficacy among these compounds. Choice of formulation, dosage, use of a tolerance-avoidance regimen, and physician experience and bias are major factors influencing which nitrate is prescribed for which patient. Tolerance is a problem for all nitrate formulations except for sublingual NTG and ISDN or transmucosal NTG; appropriately designed dosing regimens can prevent the appearance of significant nitrate tolerance (See Tables 9-1 and 9-3).

Nitroglycerin

The classic prototype nitrate is NTG, which is available in many formulations (see Table 9-1). This molecule has a very short half-life of several minutes; cessation of an intravenous NTG infusion or removal

TABLE 9-3 Factors That Influence Nitrate Tolerance

Induce tolerance	Prevent tolerance
Continuous or prolonged nitrate exposure (e.g., transdermal patches, intravenous)	Intermittent dosing
Large doses	Small doses
Frequent dosing	Infrequent dosing
Sustained-action formulations	Short-acting formulations
No or brief nitrate-free interval	Provision of adequate nitrate-free interval

of a transdermal patch results in a rapid fall in NTG plasma levels within 20 to 40 min. The metabolism of NTG occurs within the vascular wall (see Fig. 9-1). Veins take up NTG more avidly than arteries. It is not useful or practical to measure NTG plasma levels in clinical practice; this assay is technically difficult. Early studies with sublingual NTG suggest that the therapeutic NTG level is at least 1 ng/mL; plasma concentrations with the NTG patch are substantially lower. The minimum recommended dose of the patch is 0.4 mg/h, with larger amounts often being more effective. Several recent studies confirm a true anti-ischemic action of these agents, which should be administered in an on-off fashion. The patch should be applied for only 12 to 14 h each day. Rebound angina and vasoconstriction are possible effects of intermittent therapy.

Several dosing systems for NTG have been available to physicians but are not widely used and may not be available in pharmacies. These include the buccal or transmucosal formulation, NTG ointment, and oral sustained-release NTG capsules. Ointment and buccal NTG are effective but difficult for patients to use. NTG ointment is recommended for hospitalized or housebound patients with nocturnal angina or symptomatic congestive heart failure. Oral NTG has virtually no reliable data supporting its effectiveness.

Isosorbide Dinitrate

Isosorbide dinitrate (ISDN) is perhaps the most widely used long-acting nitrate in the world. It is available in short-acting and sustained-release formulation; the majority of clinical studies in the literature have used short-acting oral ISDN. Table 9-4 outlines the relevant pharmacokinetic features of ISDN and ISMN. Sustained-release ISDN should be used only once daily. In Europe, intravenous ISDN is commercially available. Sublingual or chewable ISDN has long been available for acute attacks of chest pain or angina prophylaxis, but these compounds are infrequently utilized in the United States.

When ISDN is administered, the parent compound is converted to two active metabolites, 2- and 5-isosorbide mononitrate. The latter is a

TABLE 9-4 Pharmacokinetics of Isosorbide Dinitrate and 5-Mononitrate

	ISDN	5-ISMN
Bioavailability	20–25%*	100%
Half-life	30–60 min	4–5 h
Metabolites	2-ISMN, 5-ISMN	None
Plasma levels	Low	High
Formulations†	IV, SL, oral, oral sustained-release, ointment, spray	Oral, oral sustained release

*Extensive hepatic first-pass effect.
†Only oral and sublingual compounds available in the United States.

pharmacologically active molecule that is commercially synthesized and available in short-acting and sustained-release formulations. A dose of the parent compound ISDN results in plasma concentrations of all three molecules. Note that ISDN itself has a short half-life of 50 to 60 min and rapidly disappears from the circulation. ISMN has a much longer half-life of 4 to 6 h and accounts for the protracted nitrate effects following administration of ISDN. Approximately 50 to 60% of ISDN is converted to 5-ISMN. Thus, although only 20 to 25% of ISDN itself is bioavailable when taken orally, a substantial component of the administered dose becomes pharmacologically active as 5-ISMN (see Table 9-4).

Isosorbide 5-Mononitrate

The 5-mononitrate formulation is the newest nitrate formulation released in the United States. It was initially available only in the short-acting form; to avoid tolerance, short-acting 5-ISMN is recommended to be taken in a twice-daily regimen, with 7 to 8 h between doses (see Table 9-1). Scandinavian and European experience indicated that a q12h regimen was satisfactory to avoid tolerance, but American trials with this compound indicated that a longer overnight interval was necessary to avoid attenuation of clinical effectiveness. Sustained-release 5-ISMN is effective on a once-daily basis. A minimum of 60 mg/day is recommended; a large American multicenter trial suggested that higher doses, such as 120 or 240 mg daily, may be necessary for sustained antianginal efficacy without tolerance.

SUGGESTIONS FOR NITRATE DOSING

It is important to start nitrate therapy with small doses and to build up to a predetermined end point or maximally tolerated amount over time. Headache and dizziness are the limiting symptoms with nitrate administration. Some individuals are extremely sensitive to organic nitrates; others experience little to no side effects. Many if not most patients are underdosed with long-acting nitrates, at least with respect to clinical trial data. For instance, 10 mg of oral ISDN, 30 or 60 mg of ISMN-SR, and 0.2 to 0.4 mg/h of the NTG patch are less likely to be clinically effective doses. If the patient's angina is well controlled with these amounts, it is satisfactory to continue such therapy. However, the physician should be satisfied that a more desirable clinical response is not indicated; if so, higher amounts of the nitrate should be tried. In congestive heart failure, the dosage of nitrates to achieve a significant hemodynamic effect is usually considerably higher than in patients with normal left ventricular function.

Often patients who are troubled with nitrate headaches with initial nitrate dosing can be treated effectively with analgesics (aspirin, acetaminophen) to control the headache symptoms, which usually decrease or disappear over time. Nitrate hypotension is best handled by reducing the dose; concomitant therapy with calcium channel antagonists or angiotensin converting enzyme inhibitors or hypovolemia increases the likelihood of dizziness and even syncope owing to low blood pressure following nitrate administration.

ADVERSE EFFECTS

In addition to headache and hypotension-related dizziness, nitrates occasionally can cause nausea. Patients with congestive heart failure tolerate large doses of nitrates surprisingly well. Rare cases of nitrate syncope have been reported, as have marked vasovagal responses and even AV block. Nitrates should be given with great care in the setting of right ventricular infarction complicating inferior myocardial infarction, since these drugs lower right ventricular filling pressure and can further depress cardiac output.

Intravenous NTG has been suggested to interfere with the actions of heparin, resulting in increased heparin requirements to achieve the desired prolongation of the activated clotting time. This interaction remains controversial. One report suggests the NTG may impair tissue plasminogen activator activity during thrombolysis.

In general, the organic nitrates are well-tolerated drugs with little serious adverse sequelae. Headache, the most problematic symptom related to nitrate therapy, can be controlled in many to most patients. However, upward of 20 to 30% of individuals cannot tolerate long-acting nitrate therapy.

NITRATE TOLERANCE

Clearly, the most vexing issue regarding nitrate therapy is the attenuation of nitrate efficacy with repeated dosing. This subject has an enormous literature and continues to engender considerable controversy. However, almost all experts agree that tolerance will predictably appear when protolerant dosing regimens are utilized. Dozens of high-quality clinical and basic research studies underscore the magnitude of this problem. The rapid onset of tolerance can be substantiated after several repeated doses of oral nitrate given with too short an interdose interval. Major attenuation of nitrate action in angina has been repeatedly demonstrated with continuous 24-h application of transdermal NTG; in fact, an antianginal effect can no longer be demonstrated by the second day of continuous patch therapy, even when very large doses are used. Similar findings have been demonstrated for intravenous NTG, as well as the oral agents ISDN and ISMN, when these drugs are not administered in a tolerance-avoidance regimen. Table 9-3 lists the cardinal principles for avoiding nitrate tolerance. Table 9-1 outlines the recommended dosing schedules for the available nitrates. Intravenous NTG administered for the acute ischemic syndromes of unstable angina pectoris or acute myocardial infarction should not be terminated abruptly so as to avoid tolerance; rebound phenomena are well known, and sudden withdrawal of intravenous NTG may be dangerous in this setting, even if some degree of hemodynamic tolerance is present.

The mechanisms of nitrate tolerance are not discussed here. Table 9-5 lists some current theories about tolerance mechanisms. Recent but preliminary studies suggest that ACE inhibitor therapy, angiotensin II receptor blockade, diuretics, or hydralazine may limit the appearance of nitrate tolerance.

NITROPRUSSIDE

Sodium nitroprusside is an inorganic nitrovasodilator that results in abundant NO availability in vascular smooth-muscle cells. It is likely that NP has antiplatelet activity, but there are limited data in this regard. Nitroprusside is a ferrocyanide compound with a nitroso moiety. Cyanide molecules are released as the molecule undergoes metabolism to NO, but in general, plasma cyanide and thiocyanate concentrations in

TABLE 9-5 Recently Proposed Mechanisms of Nitrate Tolerance

Sulfhydryl depletion: Inadequate generation of reduced —SH or cysteine groups required for organic nitrate biotransformation to NO
Desensitization of soluble guanylate cyclase; impaired activity of the enzyme guanylate cyclase
Counterregulatory neurohormonal activation: nitrate-induced increases in catecholamines, arginine vasopressin (AVP), plasma renin, aldosterone, and angiotensin II activity, with resultant vasoconstriction and fluid retention
Plasma volume shifts: increased intravascular blood volume related to decreased capillary pressure
Oxygen free radical destruction of nitric oxide with production of peroxynitrates resulting in enhanced sensitivity to vasoconstrictors (especially angiotensin II)

clinically utilized dosages are too low to cause toxicity in subjects with normal renal function. NP provides NO throughout the vasculature; metabolic conversion to NO does not depend on enzymatic conversion to NO to any significant degree. Thus NO is abundantly available in the microcirculation following NP infusion; these distal small vessels have a decreased capacity to metabolize the NTG molecule. This is an important dissimilarity between the two compounds, since their spectrum of vasodilatation differs significantly. Because NP has a potent effect on the small resistance vessels of the heart, there is a greater possibility for a coronary steal phenomenon than with NTG. NP induces relaxation of the microcirculation throughout the myocardium, potentially allowing for diversion of nutrient coronary blood flow away from regions of ischemia distal to a coronary obstruction. NP appears to dilate collateral vessels to a lesser degree than NTG, which could exacerbate a potentially deleterious diversion of blood from ischemic zones. (See below.)

Nitroprusside is a potent venodilator. On the arterial side, it is more hemodynamically active than NTG, particularly regarding the smaller arterioles and resistance vessels. In general, there is a more equivalent degree of venous and arterial vasodilatation with NP than NTG, which has more dominant venodilator action than arterial, particularly at lower doses.

Indications for Nitroprusside

Sodium NP is a drug used exclusively in critical-care units and the operating suite. It is a highly effective vasodilator of great potency. NP was investigated extensively in the early days of vasodilator therapy of acute myocardial infarction and congestive heart failure. Its balanced venous and arterial actions make it an ideal drug for the immediate therapy of acute and/or severe heart failure associated with high ventricular filling pressure and low stroke volume. The drug is also a first-line choice for treatment of severe hypertension and is probably preferable to intravenous NTG in this capacity because of its greater arterial dilator potency at lower dosage. At very high concentrations, the hemodynamic activity of intravenous NTG is quite similar to NP.

A series of older animal and human investigations has suggested a potential hazard for the use of NP in nonhypertensive ischemic states, such as acute myocardial infarction and unstable angina pectoris. Decreases in regional myocardial blood flow and collateral flow, associated with increased ischemia, have been demonstrated in human and dog studies when NP was compared with intravenous NTG. One early animal investigation suggested a more potent vasodilating action on the smaller coronary vessels than NTG, which was more active in the larger coronary arteries. Another trial successfully treated patients with immediate post-coronary bypass grafting hypertension with NP or

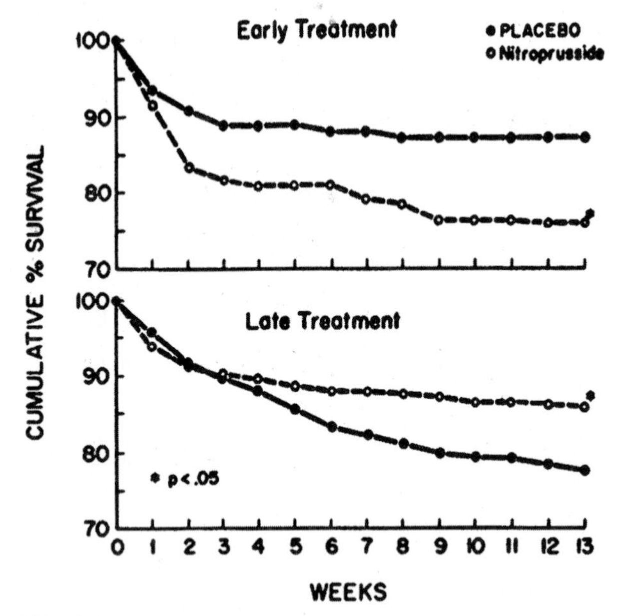

FIG. 9-3 Intravenous nitroprusside in acute myocardial infarction. There were approximately 400 patients in each group, NP versus placebo. Cumulative percentage of patients surviving after early treatment (within 9 h of onset of acute myocardial infarction) and late treatment (later than 9 h). *(From Cohn JN, Franciosa JA, Francis GS, et al: Effect of short-term infusion of sodium nitroprusside on mortality rate in acute myocardial infarction complicated by left ventricular failure. N Engl J Med 306:1129–1135, 1982, with permission.)*

intravenous NTG. Two conflicting trials of NP in the setting of acute myocardial infarction were published in 1982 (Fig. 9-3). In the VA cooperative study, NP offered no advantage to patients given a 48-h infusion of NP versus placebo when the infusion was instituted a mean of 17 h after onset of chest pain. However, a retrospective analysis suggested that patients treated early (within 9 h of onset of symptoms) fared less well with NP than with placebo, whereas later-treated subjects had a decreased mortality rate (see Fig. 9-3). It was speculated that the former group may have had lower left ventricular filling pressures within the first day or two and thus may have been exposed to an NP-induced risk of hypoperfusion of the coronary bed or a coronary steal;

TABLE 9-6 Indications for Nitroprusside

Severe hypertension
Acute pulmonary edema
Severe congestive heart failure
Acute and/or severe mitral or aortic regurgitation
Acute myocardial infarction complications:
Heart failure or uncontrolled hypertension
Use extreme caution:
• Hypotension or borderline systolic blood pressure
• Acute myocardial ischemia in the absence of heart failure
• Renal insufficiency

the late-treated cohort presumably had more patients with left ventricular dysfunction and an elevated filling pressure, and in these subjects NP would have been of benefit when compared with placebo. However, another study from the Netherlands demonstrated a decrease in mortality in acute MI patients randomized to NP. The reasons for the different results are unknown, although it has been speculated that the second study included a number of hypertensive subjects who may have derived additional benefits from NP that may have affected the final outcome. In any case, this dilemma has not been resolved by subsequent studies. Warnings about the use of NP in acute MI are not new, and current guidelines for the therapy of myocardial infarction include intravenous NTG but not NP.

Tables 9-6 and 9-7 list the indications and precautions for the use of sodium nitroprusside.

Dosage

The infusion of NP should begin with 0.5 to 1 μg/kg per minute, increasing to no more than 10 μg/kg per minute. Most experts recommend reducing the mean or systolic arterial pressure by 10%, avoiding central aortic hypotension. Meticulous care must be given to the patient with actual or potential myocardial ischemia so as to prevent an excessive central aortic pressure decrease.

Sodium nitroprusside must be given with appropriate precautions, including protection from ambient light to prevent an accelerated re-

TABLE 9-7 Precautions in the Use of Nitroprusside

Exposure of NP solution to light
Prolonged infusion (more than 48 h)
Renal insufficiency
Infusion rates greater than 10 μg/kg per minute
Measure thiocyanate levels in high-risk subjects (prolonged infusion, azotemia)

lease of NO and cyanide. The infusion should be limited in duration to 48 h, since NP toxicity can occur over time as the cumulative dose increases. Renal and hepatic insufficiency are risk factors for adverse reactions to NP, with excessive concentrations of cyanide and thiocyanate, the metabolic by-product of NP metabolism. Thiocyanate toxicity should be suspected in patients receiving NP who develop abdominal pain, mental status changes, or convulsions. Cyanide toxicity can be manifest by a reduction in cardiac output and metabolic or lactic acidosis. Methemoglobinemia can be observed as a relatively pure manifestation of NP toxicity.

CONCLUSION

The available nitrovasodilators remain important cardiovascular drugs for management of patients with ischemic heart disease, emergent hypertension, and congestive heart failure. Their actions appear to simulate many of the normal vascular physiologic processes involved in vasodilation and have provided tremendous insights into the pathophysiology of vascular disease. Informed and judicious use of the nitrates and NP should provide benefit for many individuals with cardiovascular disease.

SUGGESTED READINGS

Abrams J: Hemodynamic effects of nitroglycerin and long acting nitrates. *Am Heart J* 110:216, 1985.

Abrams J: Mechanisms of action of the organic nitrates in the treatment of myocardial ischemia. *Am J Cardiol* 70:30B–42B, 1992.

Abrams J: The role of nitrates in coronary heart disease. *Arch Intern Med* 155:357–364, 1995.

Abrams J: Beneficial actions of nitrates in cardiovascular disease. *Am J Cardiol* 77:31C–37C, 1996.

Abrams J: The organic nitrates and nitroprusside, in Frishman WH, Sonnenblick EH (eds): *Cardiovascular Pharmacotherapeutics*. New York, McGraw-Hill 1997, pp 253–265.

Abrams J: Role of endothelial dysfunction in coronary artery disease: A symposium—Myocardial ischemia: New perspectives on prevention and stabilization of coronary syndromes. *Am J Cardiol* 79 (Suppl 12B):2, 1997.

ACC/AHA guidelines for the management of patients with acute myocardial infarction: A report of the American College of Cardiology/American Heart Association Task Force on Practice Guidelines (Committee on Management of Acute Myocardial Infarction). *J Am Coll Cardiol* 28:1328, 1996.

Cohn JN, Franciosa JA, Francis GS, et al: Effect of short-term infusion of sodium nitroprusside on mortality rate in acute myocardial infarction complicated by left ventricular failure. *N Engl J Med* 306:1129, 1982.

Diodati J, Theroux P, Latour J-G, et al: Effects of nitroglycerin at therapeutic doses on platelet aggregation in unstable angina pectoris and acute myocardial infarction. *Am J Cardiol* 66:683–688, 1996.

Flaherty JT: Role of nitrates in acute myocardial infarction, in Abrams J, Pepine C, Thadani U (eds): *Medical Therapy of Ischemic Heart Disease*. Boston, Little, Brown, 1992, pp 309–328.

Fung H-L, Chung S-J, Bauer JA, et al: Biochemical mechanism of organic nitrate action. *Am J Cardiol* 70:4B–10B, 1992.

Gruppo Italiano per lo Studio della Supravivenza nell'Infarcto Miocardico: GISSI-3: Effects of lisinopril and transdermal glyceryl trinitrate singly and together on 6-week mortality and ventricular function after acute myocardial infarction. *Lancet* 343:1115–1122, 1994.

Harrison DG, Bates JN: The nitrovasodilators: New ideas about old drugs. *Circulation* 87:1461–1467, 1993.

ISIS-4 (Fourth International Study of Infarct Survival) Collaborative Group: ISIS-4: A randomized factorial trial assessing early oral captopril, oral mononitrate, and intravenous magnesium sulphate in 58,050 patients with suspected acute myocardial infarction. *Lancet* 345:669–685, 1995.

Kowaluk E, Fung H-L: Pharmacology and pharmacokinetics of nitrates, in Abrams J, Pepine C, Thadani U (eds): *Medical Therapy of Ischemic Heart Disease: Nitrates, Beta Blockers, and Calcium Antagonists*. Boston, Little, Brown, 1992, p 152.

Lewin HC, Berman DS: Achieving sustained improvement in myocardial perfusion: Role of isosorbide mononitrate: A symposium—Myocardial ischemia: New perspectives on prevention and stabilization of coronary syndromes. *Am J Cardiol* 79 (Suppl 12B):31, 1997.

Münzel T, Bassenge E: Long-term angiotensin-converting enzyme inhibition with high-dose enalapril retards nitrate tolerance in large epicardial arteries and prevents rebound coronary vasoconstriction in vivo. *Circulation* 93:2052–2058, 1996.

Schwarz M, Katz SD, Demopoulos L, et al: Enhancement of endothelium-dependent vasodilation by low-dose nitroglycerin in patients with congestive heart failure. *Circulation* 89:1609–1614, 1994.

Thadani U: Management of patients with chronic stable angina at low risk for serious cardiac events: A symposium—Myocardial ischemia: New perspectives on prevention and stabilization of coronary syndromes. *Am J Cardiol* 79 (Suppl 12B):24, 1997.

Chapter 10 Antiadrenergic Drugs with Central Action, Ganglionic Blockers, and Neuron Depletors

Lawrence R. Krakoff

Drugs that reduce arterial pressure by interruption of the sympathetic nervous system are among the oldest used to treat hypertension. Indeed, antihypertensive therapy became feasible with the discovery of such agents as reserpine and the autonomic ganglion blockers before 1965. However, many of the older preparations are now of historic interest, having been superseded by more specifically targeted drugs that inhibit action of the sympathetic nervous system with greater selectivity and also reduce pressure with fewer of the adverse effects that severely limited use of their predecessors. Nonetheless, some of those antiadrenergic drugs, which became useful before the appearance of α- and β-adrenergic receptor blockers, remain valuable for specific situations and thus have become "niche" drugs rather than widely used therapeutics. There is, however, a new class of centrally acting agents, those whose major effect is agonism at imidazole I_1 receptors, and these agents have promise for broader application. This class was discovered through the detection of clonidine-like substances in brain tissue having characteristics distinct from catecholamines (e.g., classic adrenergic agonists) and binding with high affinity to imidazole receptors found in central regulatory sites of the baroreflex arc and sympathetic outflow. Definition of the imidazole I_1 receptor led to evaluation of drugs for their binding activity to these sites. Two agents have thus been characterized and developed for clinical trial as antihypertensive drugs. This chapter focuses primarily on three groups of antihypertensive drugs: (1) those whose action lies primarily within the central nervous system, (2) the ganglionic blockers, and (3) peripheral adrenergic neuron depletors. Emphasis is placed on the specific clinical circumstances where some of these agents may play a helpful role.

CLASSIFICATION AND PHARMACOLOGY

Centrally Active Agents

Several antihypertensive drugs seem to have their predominant effect by an action within the brain at sites that regulate sympathetic tone, as listed in Table 10-1. For other agents, central action represents a minor fraction of their overall effect, for example, the β-receptor blockers and possibly the angiotensin converting enzyme (ACE) inhibitors; the latter reduce pressure with minimal or no activation of sympathetic reflexes.

TABLE 10-1 Centrally Active Antihypertensive Drugs

α_2-receptor agonists Clonidine Guanabenz Guanfacine	These agents reduce peripheral sympathetic tone by central stimulation of α_2 receptors, mostly within brain stem centers. They also act on recently described imidazole receptors.
Methyldopa	This drug has mixed action: α_2-receptor agonist, false transmitter, and dopadecarboxylase inhibitor.
Reserpine	Depletes central and peripheral aminergic (noradrenergic and serotoninergic) neurons.

Classic α_2-Receptor Agonists

The classic α_2-receptor agonists are perhaps the best characterized of the centrally acting drugs. They reduce sympathetic tone within the brain stem by stimulating α_2 receptors on neurons of vasomotor centers that inhibit outflow of impulses to spinal preganglionic neurons. In addition, they also may achieve their effect by stimulation of recently described imidazole receptors. In peripheral postganglionic noradrenergic neurons, stimulation of α_2 receptors diminishes release of transmitter, a feedback system for control of intrasynaptic norepinephrine concentration. α_2-Receptor agonists such as clonidine then have a peripheral action by adding to inhibition of norepinephrine release. However, α_2 receptors at post- or nonsynaptic sites on cardiac or smooth-muscle cells may be stimulated by α_2 agonists, causing an increase in pressure. Thus a transient rise in pressure may occur within the first hour after giving a single dose of clonidine. Thereafter, blood pressure falls to well below pretreatment levels in parallel with a demonstrable decrement in sympathetic neural function reflected by a fall in plasma norepinephrine concentration or decreased sympathetic neural impulse rate. The suppression of sympathetic tone by the α_2-receptor agonists has been used to treat essential hypertension. In congestive heart failure, increased sympathetic activation (reflected by elevated plasma norepinephrine levels) conveys a poor prognosis. A preliminary study has shown that clonidine can reduce plasma norepinephrine in this syndrome. However, no outcome studies have yet established that α_2 agonists are beneficial in the heart failure syndrome.

The usual decrease in plasma norepinephrine concentration after clonidine administration is about 45 to 50% in normal subjects and those with essential hypertension. Patients with the catecholamine-secreting tumor pheochromocytoma have little change in plasma norepinephrine concentration after clonidine is given, providing the rationale for the clonidine suppression test as a diagnostic assessment for these tumors.

Clonidine is the prototype α_2 agonist. Guanabenz and guanfacine are similar to clonidine except for having a longer duration of action. All the α_2 agonists are effective antihypertensive drugs, and all have a similar pattern of adverse effects: sedation, dry mouth, and a tendency to overshoot or rebound hypertension on withdrawal. In sleep studies, clonidine has been found to reduce rapid eye movement (REM) sleep when compared with the β blocker atenolol. Clonidine also has been studied in sleep apnea with inconsistent effects.

All α_2 agonists are active as oral preparations. Clonidine, in addition, is available for administration as a trandermal delivery system (TTS), which releases medication at a relatively constant rate over 7 days. Clonidine TTS is an effective antihypertensive; some but not all studies suggest that its use is associated with fewer adverse effects compared with tablets. It has been suggested that clonidine TTS is useful for selected noncompliant patients who do not like to take pills. For patients already taking clonidine tablets and who must have surgery with general anesthesia, the TTS formulation can be used to maintain control of blood pressure and avoid rebound hypertension during the perioperative period when medications cannot be given by mouth. Prolonged use of the TTS patch can cause a skin reaction severe enough that a change to alternative therapy is necessary.

α-Methyldopa

α-Methyldopa is also a centrally active antihypertensive agent. Its mechanism of action is complex. Originally developed as an antagonist of dopa-decarboxylase, α-methyldopa was conceived as a drug that would inhibit catecholamine synthesis (preventing the conversion of dihydroxyphenylalanine, dopa, to dopamine by dopa-decarboxylase). However, this effect was far too small to account for methyldopa's antihypertensive effect, since dopa-decarboxylase is not a rate-limiting enzyme but usually present in excess in a variety of tissues. Later studies led to recognition that α-methyldopa could be converted to α-methyldopamine, a false neurotransmitter, but also an α_2 agonist, with the central and peripheral actions of the other members of this group. More recently, it has been proposed that conversion of α-methyldopa to α-methyl-epinephrine (by *N*-methylation) also may participate in this drug's hypotensive action.

α-Methyldopa is an effective antihypertensive agent, given by mouth or intravenously. The intravenous formulation (an ester of the parent drug) has been used for hypertensive emergencies including toxemia of pregnancy. Prolonged treatment with α-methyldopa is often associated with salt and water retention, reversing the antihypertensive effect (pseudotolerance) and requiring addition of a diuretic agent.

Adverse effects related to α-methyldopa are fatigue, somnolence, possible memory impairment, and diminished sexual function (reduced libido and impotence). Several of these are common to other centrally active agents. Unique to α-methyldopa, however, are (1) a positive Coombs' test (owing to appearance of an antibody directed against red cell Rh determinants), which occasionally causes significant hemolysis, and (2) a drug-induced hepatitis with fever, eosinophilia, and increased serum levels of hepatic enzymes. The acute drug-induced hepatitis is self-limited once α-methyldopa is discontinued. There have been several case reports and small series of patients with chronic hepatitis and even cirrhosis found after many years of exposure to α-methyldopa. Whether these were truly drug-induced or the consequence of undetected viral hepatitis (e.g., prior to the discovery of hepatitis C virus) is not certain.

Reserpine

Reserpine is a distinct antihypertensive drug whose action is not related to either α_2 agonism or any effect on imidazole receptors. Originally derived from an Indian vine, *Rauwolfia serpentina*, reserpine is absorbed by the gastrointestinal tract and enters central and peripheral adrenergic and serotoninergic neurons where it specifically eliminates amine storage granules. This action leads to irreversible depletion of neurotransmitter through intraneuronal metabolism by monoamine oxidase and a resulting fall in arterial pressure due to a functional and long-lasting catecholine deficit. Reserpine itself is rapidly eliminated from the circulation, its metabolism still remaining unknown. However, because of the time necessary for regeneration of new intraneural amine storage granules, the pharmacologic action of reserpine is quite long. It may take days to weeks for full adrenergic neuronal functional recovery after cessation of reserpine administration. Although an effective antihypertensive agent, reserpine adminstration is accompanied by many adverse effects. Fatigue, depression, nasal congestion, and gastric hyperacidity often have been observed. The depression may occur insidiously only weeks to months after initiation of treatment and may be severe, even leading to suicide. Like α-methyldopa, reserpine use may cause salt/water retention and pseudotolerance, making diuretic treatment necessary to keep pressure controlled.

Ganglionic Blocking Agents

Transmission from preganglionic neurons of the autonomic nervous system to postganglionic neurons is achieved by acetylcholine acting on receptors defined as *nicotinic* in classic pharmacology. Nicotinic receptors are blocked by quaternery ammonium compounds, interrupting ganglionic transmission and sympathetic tone. This action lowers blood pressure, particularly during standing, that is, orthostatic hypotension. Ganglionic blockers also impair neurotransmission of the parasympathetic nervous system, accounting for several adverse effects: adynamic intestinal ileus, acute urinary retention, and pupillary dysfunction. Patients taking ganglionic blockers are quite "volume sensitive" in that their pressure may fall substantially if even slightly hypovolumic yet remain hypertensive if minimally in volume excess. Judicious use of fluid replacement and diuretic administration is required if ganglionic blockers are to be used effectively.

Before the 1960s, several ganglionic blockers, namely, hexamethonium, pentolinium, and mecamylamine, were used successfully to treat malignant hypertension. At present, only two drugs in this class are available in the United States; these are mecamylamine and trimethaphan camsylate. Mecamylamine is given by mouth as 10-mg tablets twice daily. Trimethaphan is available only for intravenous infusion, and its use is limited to hypertensive emergencies, such as dissecting hematoma of the aorta or for controlled hypotension during surgery. For all practical purposes, the oral ganglionic blockers are obsolete, given the development of antihypertensive drugs over the past 30 years.

Peripheral Neuron Depletors

Guanethidine and guanadrel enter peripheral noradrenergic nerve terminals via amine uptake channels, where these drugs bind to norepinephrine storage vesicles, inhibiting transsynaptic release or transmitter. In addition, norepinephrine stores are depleted by displacement from vesicles and intraneuronal metabolism by monoamine oxidase. Both cardiac and vascular postganglionic sympathetic neurons are depleted by these drugs. Unlike reserpine, the peripheral neuron depletors do not damage or eliminate storage vesicles. Consequently, sympathetic neurotransmission returns to normal as drug concentration falls, with dissociation of the drug-vesicle complex. Duration of action is longest for guanethidine, ~24 h, and shorter for guanadrel, 6 to 10 h. Reduction of sympathetic transmitter release during treatment with the neuron depletors affects basal or resting blood pressure but is much more prominent during standing or exercise, when sympathetic activity is normally increased. Orthostatic hypotension and/or exercise weakness, even syncope, often have been observed during treatment. It is therefore necessary to monitor both supine and standing blood pressures when these agents are used as antihypertensive therapy. Bradycardia and possibly heart block may occur as a result of diminished cardiac adrenergic transmission. Other effects of reduced peripheral sympathetic function that may be observed during treatment with these agents are (1) retrograde ejaculation, (2) diarrhea-like change in bowel function, and (3) loss of normal adrenergic pupillary responses.

Because the peripheral neuron depletors enter the nerve terminal via norepinephrine uptake, their action is prevented by drugs such as cocaine or tricyclic antidepressants (e.g., imipramine). This unique drug interaction accounts for the reversal of blood pressure control in patients receiving the peripheral neuron depletors, when tricyclics are given concurrently.

EFFECTIVENESS OF THE CENTRAL ACTING DRUGS, GANGLIONIC BLOCKERS, AND PERIPHERAL NEURON DEPLETORS

Assessment of antihypertensive drugs includes, as a primary measure, whether they have been found to prevent cardiovascular mortality and morbidity in randomized clinical trials. In this context, reserpine and α-methyldopa deserve attention. Reserpine, in combination with a thiazide diuretic and hydralazine, reduced major trial end points compared with placebo in the Veterans Administration trial for severe and moderate hypertension and in combination with a diuretic for treatment of isolated systolic hypertension in the elderly. α-Methyldopa was used for active therapy in combination with a thiazide diuretic in several clinical trials of mild to moderate hypertension that are now considered pivotal in establishing the benefit of antihypertensive drug treatment. However, there is insufficient evidence for concluding that either of these two drugs is beneficial as *monotherapy*. The other available centrally acting agents, the α_2 agonists, have been employed infrequently in the large, randomized clinical therapeutic trials. Both the ganglionic blockers and guanethidine were evaluated for treatment of severe or malignant hypertension. Observational studies suggested that reduction of pressure in such patients was beneficial in comparison with historical controls or untreated patients by altering the rapidly fatal course of those with the highest blood pressure levels and evidence of extensive target-organ damage.

SUMMARY OF CURRENT AND RECOMMENDED USE

Most of the approved antihypertensive drugs reviewed in this chapter (Table 10-2) will have little or no role to play in the management of a large number of patients with essential hypertension, having been largely replaced by more recently developed classes. However, the long-term safety record for these drugs cannot be discounted. If hypertensive patients are well controlled on these older agents and have no related adverse effects, there is no compelling rationale for changing medication. As a last consideration, the goal of reducing sympathetic tone for treatment of hypertension remains theoretically desirable, if it could be achieved without the adverse reaction characteristic of reserpine, the α_2-agonists, and α-methyldopa. The imidazole I_1 receptor agonists have promise for central reduction of sympathetic function with fewer side effects and deserve further exploration as a potentially valuable class.

TABLE 10-2 Dose Range, Special Indications, and Adverse Effects of the Centrally Acting Agents, Ganglionic Blockers, and Peripheral Neuron Depletors

Name	Indications for use	Dose range	Adverse effects
Reserpine	Essential hypertension in addition to a diuretic; parenteral form can be used for hypertensive emergencies	0.1–0.5 mg PO daily; same dose for parenteral use	Sedation, depression, hyperacidity, nasal congestion
α-Methyldopa	Essential hypertension, in addition to a diuretic	250–1000 mg twice daily	Sedation, positive Coombs' test, hepatitis
α-Methyldopa ester	IV form for hypertensive emergencies, toxemia of pregnancy	125–1000 mg as IV slow bolus	Sedation, drowziness
Clonidine	Essential hypertension, usually with diuretic	0.1–0.3 mg twice daily; TTS patch once weekly	Sedation, dry mouth, constipation
Guanabenz	Essential hypertension, usually with diuretic	4–16 mg once or twice daily	Same as clonidine
Guanfacine	Essential hypertension, usually with diuretic	1–3 mg daily	Same as clonidine
Mecamylamine	Rare, severe refractory hypertension	1.5–10 mg daily	Orthostatic hypotension, ileus, urinary retention, blurred vision
Trimethaphan	Hypertensive emergencies only	0.5–3 mg/min intravenously	Same as mecamylamine; tachyphylaxis may be due to hypervolemia
Guanethidine	Severe refractory hypertension	10–50 mg daily	Orthostatic hypotension, diarrhea, bradycardia
Guanadrel	Severe refractory hypertension	20–25 mg daily	Orthostatic hypotension, bradycardia

SUGGESTED READINGS

Hoffman BB, Lefkowitz RJ, Taylor P: Neurotransmission: The autonomic and somatic nervous systems, in Hardman JG, Limbird LE, Gilman AG (eds): *Goodman and Gilman's The Pharmacological Basis of Therapeutics*. New York, McGraw-Hill, 1996, pp 105–139.

Krakoff LR: Clinical trials, in *Management of the Hypertensive Patient*. New York, Churchill-Livingstone, 1995, pp 33–48.

Krakoff LR: Antiadrenergic drugs with central action, ganglionic blockers and neuron depletors, in Frishman WH, Sonnenblick EH (eds): *Cardiovascular Pharmacotherapeutics*. New York, McGraw-Hill, 1997, pp 267–273.

Taylor P: Agents acting at the neuromuscular junction and autonomic ganglia, in Hardman JG, Gilman AG, Limbird LE (eds): *Goodman and Gilman's The Pharmacological Basis of Therapeutics*. New York, McGraw-Hill, 1996, pp 177–197.

Chapter 11 Nonspecific Antihypertensive Vasodilators

Lawrence R. Krakoff

Increased systemic vascular resistance is the hemodynamic characteristic of arterial hypertension. In established essential hypertension and various forms of secondary hypertension, raised systemic vascular resistance is invariably found, irrespective of the underlying cause of high arterial pressure. It is not then surprising that vasodilators were among the first to be developed for treatment of hypertension, specifically hydralazine. Yet it became evident during the initial assessment of vasodilators that their antihypertensive effect led to activation of sympathetic baroreflexes with tachycardia and increased cardiac output in compensation for the reduction in peripheral (systemic) vascular resistance. Furthermore, fluid-volume retention and activation of the renin-angiotensin system also were a consequence of unopposed systemic arteriolar vasodilation. Thus, by the 1970s, the orally active nonselective vasodilators became classified as third-line antihypertensive drugs, to be used only in combination with diuretics and antiadrenergic agents, usually β-receptor blockers, as the triple-drug regimen for severe hypertension. There are, however, a few specific places where these vasodilators may play more specific or important therapeutic roles, as is described in this chapter.

PHARMACOLOGY AND CLASSIFICATION OF THE NON-SPECIFIC VASODILATORS

Hydralazine

1-Hydrazinophthalazine (hydralazine) was one of the first available orally active antihypertensive drugs. The hydrazine (HN—NH2) in position 1 of the double-ringed phthalazine confers activity as a vasodilator. Hydralazine is a direct arteriolar vasodilator, independent of any receptor antagonism. Its mechanism of action remains somewhat unclear but seems to be dependent on endothelial cells and may be related to formation of nitric oxide and/or hyperpolarization of vascular smooth-muscle cells and interruption of intracellular calcium action. The hemodynamic effect of hydralazine is reduction of systemic vascular resistance with activation of sympathetic reflexes and increased heart rate and cardiac output on a neurogenic basis. The reflex-mediated changes in cardiac function after hydralazine treatment can be prevented by β-receptor antagonists. Chronic administration of hydralazine stimulates renin release, raising plasma renin activity; salt and water retention with gain in weight is also observed. While the half-life of hydralazine, reflected by plasma concentrations, is 1 to 2 h, the antihypertensive effect may last 6 to 12 h. Effective dosing schedules are provided by having the drug taken two to three times daily.

After absorption from the gastrointestinal tract, hydralazine may be acetylated in the liver to a varying degree depending on the genetics of the patient. Slow and fast acetylators are represented almost equally in the population of the United States. Hydralazine is relatively less bioavailable for slow acetylators, who require higher oral doses for equal antihypertensive effect. Extrahepatic metabolism also occurs and accounts for the drug's elimination, once reaching the circulation.

Adverse effects of hydralazine may be divided into two categories: (1) those related to the hemodynamic effect of the drug and (2) those specifically linked to its unique biochemical characteristics. Headaches, flushing, tachycardia, palpitations, angina-like chest discomfort or true angina of myocardial ischemia, dizziness, and orthostatic hypotension are the consequences of the vasodilating action of hydralazine and the significant sympathetic reflex activation as a physiologic response. In contrast, the hydralazine lupus syndrome, serum-sickness-like reaction, hemolytic anemia, and glomerulonephritis syndromes seem best related to hydralazine itself and are more likely to occur in slow acetylators, often white women. Many patients treated with hydralazine who develop positive antinuclear antibodies do not proceed to symptomatic lupus. However, with so many alternative drugs, there is little basis for continuing antinuclear antibody (ANA)–positive patients on hydralazine in most situations. Vitamin B_6 (pyridoxal-responsive)–dependent polyneuropathy is a rare adverse effect of sustained hydralazine administration explainable by a direct chemical combination of the drug with pyridoxine, reducing supply of the cofactor for many enzymes. Both hydralazine lupus syndromes and polyneuropathy usually occur during treatment with high doses, more than 50 mg daily.

Hydralazine has been used for cardiovascular therapy of four specific disorders: essential hypertension, pregnancy-induced hypertension, congestive heart failure, and aortic valvular insufficiency. Treatment of essential hypertension is usually limited to those patients with very high pretreatment pressures, typically $>$ 110 mmHg diastolic pressure, who do not respond adequately to other agents or combinations. Hydralazine is then added as the third or fourth drug to prior use of a diuretic and β-receptor blocker. While effective, recent comparative studies suggest that the dihydropyridine calcium channel blockers, such as felodipine, or the angiotensin converting enzyme (ACE) inhibitors reduce blood pressure just as well as hydralazine and tend to have fewer adverse effects in some studies. Hydralazine remains useful for treatment of pregnancy-induced hypertension, including toxemia. It and α-methyldopa have been employed for this purpose over several decades with acceptable efficacy and safety. Nonetheless, in a comparison study, the calcium channel blocker nifedipine was found to be superior to hydralazine for treatment of severe preeclamptic pregnancies. Treatment of congestive heart failure not responding to diuretic agents, digoxin, and ACE inhibitor therapy may benefit from addition of hydralazine in doses of 300 to 600 mg daily in selected patients. The drug does not appear to stimulate the sympathetic nervous system in chronic congestive heart failure unless symptomatic hypotension occurs. It may have a direct inotropic action and appears to have more favorable effects on renal blood flow than ACE inhibitors in patients with heart failure and renal dysfunction. Studies need to be done to determine whether there is *additional benefit* from giving hydralazine to patients with heart failure already receiving diuretics, digoxin, and ACE inhibitors.

In combination with isosorbide dinitrate, orally administered hydralazine (300 mg daily) has been shown to reduce mortality in patients with advanced congestive heart failure already receiving digoxin and diuretics when compared with placebo and prazosin. In a subsequent study, however, enalapril was shown to be more effective than hydralazine-isosorbide dinitrate on clinical outcomes (Fig. 11-1).

Patients with asymptomatic nonrheumatic aortic regurgitation theoretically might benefit from vasodilatory therapy. Hydralazine has been studied in such patients and indeed does reduce systolic pressure. However, activation of the renin-angiotensin system may offset any benefit. In a randomized comparison trial of hydralazine and enalapril in patients with aortic regurgitation, over 1 year both drugs reduced systolic pressure, but only enalapril reduced left ventricular mass index and left ventricular diastolic volume index. Thus more recently developed antihypertensive agents have reduced the need for hydralazine in several cardiovascular diseases.

Nitroprusside (See also Chapter 9)

Sodium nitroprusside has been known as a blood pressure lowering inorganic salt for more than 50 years, but its utility as an intravenous agent for fast and controlled reduction of arterial pressure in hypertensive emergencies was recognized in the 1950s. The action of nitroprusside has been compared with that of intravenous nitroglycerin but has been found to be the result of an interaction between the ferricyanide salt and red blood cell enzymes that causes decomposition of the parent compound to nitric oxide, now recognized as the endogenous endothelial cell–derived relaxing factor (EDRF).

ATP-K^+ Channel Openers: Minoxidil and Diazoxide

The powerful arteriolar vasodilators minoxidil and diazoxide were developed in the 1970s for use in the treatment of severe and refractory hypertension and hypertensive emergencies. Minoxidil became a part of the triple drug regimen for treatment of severe hypertension, especially for patients who were unresponsive or had significant adverse

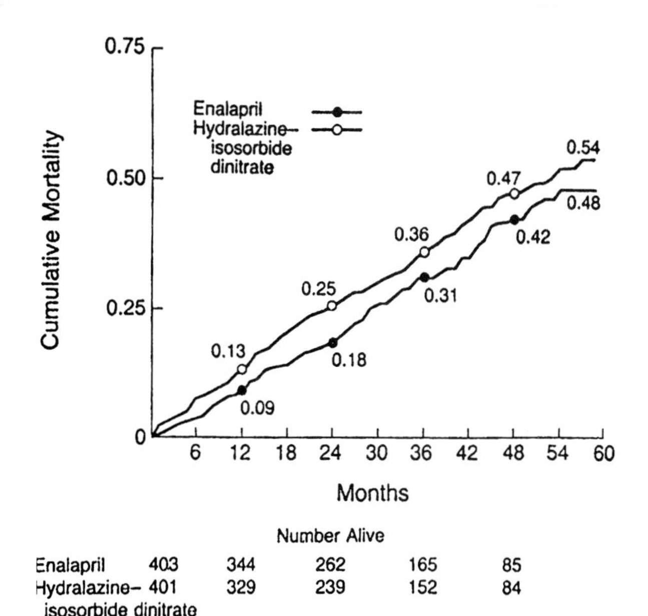

FIG. 11-1 Cumulative mortality in the enalapril and hydralazine-isosorbide dinitrate treatment arms over the entire follow-up period. Cumulative mortality rates are shown after each 12-month period. For the comparison of the treatment arms after 2 years and overall, P = 0.016 and *P* = 0.08, respectively (log-rank test). The number of patients alive after each year is shown below the graph. *(From Cohn JN, Johnson G, Ziesdne S, et al: A comparison of enalapril with hydralazine-isosorbide dinitrate in the treatment of congestive heart failure. N Engl J Med 325:303, 1991, with permission.)*

reactions to hydralazine. Diazoxide, given as an intravenous bolus, was used for hypertensive emergencies as an alternate to sodium nitroprusside.

Minoxidil is a prodrug that becomes active with sulfation of an N—O site by a hepatic sulfotransferase. Minoxidil's mechanism of action is mostly due to activation of the ATP-K^+ channel, causing hyperpolarization of smooth-muscle cell membranes with relaxation (vasodilation), an action shared by diazoxide and pinacidil. Other ATP-K^+ channel activators, such as nicorandil, cromokalim, aprikalim, bimakalim, and emakalim, are being assessed for either systemic or coronary artery vasodilatation. Some of the ATP-K^+ channel activators inhibit release of insulin from pancreatic islet β cells (long recognized as an effect of diazoxide), antagonizing the effect of the sulfonylureas at the K^+ channel. Experimental studies suggest that diazoxide is the most potent agent for inhibition of hypoglycemia due to a sulfonylrea with pinacidil having a detectable but lesser effect.

The hemodynamic action of the ATP-K^+ channel openers is a profound reduction in systemic vascular resistance with activation of sympathetic reflexes causing tachycardia, increased cardiac output, and plasma norepinephrine. β-receptor blockade diminishes both the degree of tachycardia and the increase in cardiac output. These drugs cause fluid retention in part by activation of the renin-angiotensin-aldosterone system and by intrarenal proximal and distal tubular mechanisms. Sustained use of minoxidil may lead to increased pulmonary artery pressures, that is, pulmonary hypertension, perhaps the result of the prolonged hyperdynamic state resulting from reduced precapillary vascular resistance and an arteriovenous shunt-like state. Other side effects of minoxidil include effects on myocardial repolarization.

The currently available ATP-K^+ channel openers minoxidil and diazoxide are used only for severe hypertension when other agents are ineffective. At a dose of 5 to 20 mg twice daily, minoxidil in combination with a β-receptor blocker and potent diuretic (most often a loop-active agent such as furosemide) is almost always effective in reducing blood pressure. Weight gain, despite diuretic use, often occurs. Hair growth is inevitable and may become disfiguring. Diazoxide is used only as an intravenous injection for hypertensive emergencies at doses of 150 to 300 mg by bolus injection or rapid intravenous infusion. Hypotension can occur, since the response to a given dose is unpredictable. Prolonged use of diazoxide often causes hyperglycemia, due to inhibition of insulin release, another action explained by activation of ATP-K^+ channels.

SUMMARY: EFFECTIVENESS AND CURRENT USE OF THE VASODILATORS

The historical importance of hydralazine, the first orally active vasodilator to be used for treatment of hypertension, is apparent because it was a component of the active drugs (with reserpine and chlorothiazide) first used to demonstrate the value of antihypertensive drug treatment for prevention of cardiovascular mortality and morbidity in the Veterans Administration trials. In addition, hydralazine was shown to be effective in a randomized trial for retarding the progression of symptomatic congestive heart failure and is still considered useful for treatment of hypertension in pregnancy. These are good reasons to maintain hydralazine in current formularies; perhaps this drug has been underused in recent years. In contrast, newer agents like the dihydropyridine calcium channel entry blockers have largely replaced the need for minoxidil in refractory severe hypertension when hydralazine is ineffective or unacceptable. Last, both intravenous nitroprusside and intravenous nicardipine are effective and safe titratable drugs much better suited for treatment of the hypertensive emergencies compared with diazoxide.

SUGGESTED READINGS

Andersson, KE: Clinical pharmacology of potassium channel openers. *Pharmacol Toxicol* 70:244, 1992.

Cohn JN, Archibald DG, Ziesche S, et al: Effect of vasodilator therapy on mortality in chronic congestive heart failure. *N Engl J Med* 314:1547, 1986.

Cohn JN, Johnson G, Ziesche S, et al: A comparison of enalapril with hydralazine-isosorbide dinitrate in the treatment of chronic congestive heart failure. *N Engl J Med* 325:303, 1991.

Krakoff LR: Nonspecific antihypertensive vasodilators, in Frishman WH, Sonnenblick EH (eds): *Cardiovascular Pharmacotherapeutics*. New York, McGraw-Hill, 1997, pp 275–279.

Oates, JA: Antihypertensive agents and the drug therapy of hypertension, in *Goodman and Gilman's The Pharmacological Basis of Therapeutics*. New York, McGraw-Hill, 1996, pp 780–808.

Chapter 12 Antiarrhythmic Drugs

Scott E. Hessen, Eric L. Michelson,
William H. Frishman

Cardiac arrhythmias form a spectrum from clinically insignificant rhythms to life-threatening and lethal arrhythmias. Effective pharmacologic treatment of arrhythmias requires an understanding of the underlying mechanism of arrhythmia as well as the pharmacokinetics, pharmacodynamics, and electropharmacology of available antiarrhythmic medications. Whereas mechanisms have been established with some certainty for a number of arrhythmias, for many the mechanisms remain to be elucidated. Interrelationships between cardiac anatomy, nature and extent of structural heart disease, severity of functional impairment, cellular electrophysiology, metabolic fluxes, and factors such as ischemia and autonomic state are only beginning to be understood. With these diverse factors acting within each patient, it should come as no surprise that antiarrhythmic drug action is often unpredictable and must be applied empirically to individual patients.

CLASSIFICATION

Several different classifications of antiarrhythmic drugs have been proposed in the past. A useful classification scheme should relate drug class, cellular electrophysiologic effects, and utility of various antiarrhythmic agents in specific clinical situations. Today, the most widely used classification system is a modification of the one proposed by Vaughn Williams (Table 12-1). This classification classifies drugs according to their effects on action potentials in individual cells. In this scheme, class I drugs block sodium channels responsible for the fast response in atrial, ventricular, and Purkinje tissues, depressing conduction velocity. Class I drugs are further divided into three subclasses based on (1) the kinetics of association and dissociation of the drug with the sodium channel, (2) the strength of channel blockade, and (3) the effects on repolarization. Class II drugs are β-adrenergic receptor antagonists. Class III agents prolong cardiac repolarization, predominantly by blocking potassium channels during phases 2 and 3 of the action potential, thereby increasing tissue refractoriness. Class IV drugs block calcium channels, depressing the slow response in sinus nodal, atrioventricular (AV) nodal, and perhaps other cells. Admittedly, such a classification is a considerable oversimplification and does not account for autonomic nervous system effects or the action of agents such as digoxin or adenosine, for example, all of which need to be considered in discussing antiarrhythmic drugs.

In addition, it has become clear that a single antiarrhythmic drug may have multiple effects on cardiac cells. For example, sotalol has β-blocking activity (class II) and also significantly prolongs the action

TABLE 12-1 Modified Vaughn Williams Classification of Antiarrhythmic Drugs

Class	Main electrophysiologic properties	Examples
Ia	Sodium channel blockade Intermediate channel kinetics Repolarization lengthened	Quinidine Procainamide Disopyramide
Ib	Sodium channel blockade Rapid channel kinetics	Lidocaine Mexiletine Tocainide Phenytoin
Ic	Sodium channel blockade Slow channel kinetics	Flecainide Propafenone
II	β-Adrenergic blockade	Propranolol Esmolol Acebutolol
III	Potassium channel blockade Sodium channel activation	Sotalol Amiodarone Ibutilide
IV	Calcium channel blockade	Verapamil Diltiazem

potential duration (class III). Amiodarone has been shown to have class I, II, III, and IV effects and perhaps other effects as well. Similarly, individual stereoisomers of drugs may have diverse effects. For example, the dextro isomer of sotalol possesses class III activity with only minimal β-blocking activity, while the levo isomer possesses both β-blocking and class III activity. Finally, many drugs undergo metabolism to electrophysiologically active metabolites that may have different electrophysiologic effects than the parent compound. Procainamide, a class Ia drug, is metabolized in the liver to *N*-acetylprocainamide (NAPA), a drug with significant class III effects.

A more recent classification scheme, called the *Sicilian gambit*, attempts to relate the various clinical effects of antiarrhythmic drugs to specific anatomic or physiologic "weak points" of target arrhythmias. Although clinically based and therefore more appealing, it is not clear that this new classification will be more useful than the Vaughn Williams classification.

Successful clinical application of antiarrhythmic agents requires not only an understanding of the cellular electrophysiology of the drugs and a thorough understanding of their pharmacology but also knowledge of drug-drug interactions, hemodynamic effects, and the ancillary properties of these agents. Failure to consider these factors often results in drug inefficacy or toxicity. This chapter presents most antiarrhythmic drugs currently available in the United States. The pharmacology, electrophysiology, pharmacokinetics, antiarrhythmic effects, drug interactions, hemodynamic properties, side effects, indications, and dosing are presented. A complete discussion of these agents is beyond the scope of this chapter, and data for recently released drugs are often incomplete and based to a large measure on animal data and preliminary data from clinical studies. Adverse effects reported for new agents represent those effects seen in highly selected patient populations and are subject to investigator interpretation; they may not be representative of those seen in clinical practice. It also should be noted that virtually all antiarrhythmic drugs have the potential to depress automaticity, conduction, and contractility; all have potential proarrhythmic effects. In addition, in many cases there is relatively little information available on the effects of various drugs on abnormal myocardium or in patients with more advanced cardiac pathologic conditions.

Antiarrhythmic drugs also must be considered potential cardiac toxins. A physician treating a patient with an arrhythmia hopes the drug is "more toxic" to tissue involved with the arrhythmia than to the rest of the heart or patient. Often this is not the case, since the therapeutic index of these drugs can be quite low. In addition, noncardiac side effects are frequent. Achievement of "therapeutic" drug levels does not guarantee efficacy or eliminate the risk of toxicity. Furthermore, agents effective for the acute management of arrhythmias may not be effective for chronic prophylaxis. The failure to reduce or paradoxically increase mortality also exists with antiarrhythmic drugs, as demonstrated by the Cardiac Arrhythmia Suppression Trial (CAST). Thus antiarrhythmic therapy should be used cautiously and ideally should be reserved for those situations which significantly impact on a patient's duration or quality of life.

OPTIMAL ANTIARRHYTHMIC MANAGEMENT OVERVIEW

Although a complete discussion of the clinical use of antiarrhythmic drugs is beyond the scope of this chapter, the following generalizations for commonly occurring arrhythmias may be made.

Atrial Fibrillation

Atrial fibrillation is the most common sustained tachyarrhythmia encountered in clinical practice. Management goals include (1) prevention of thromboembolism and stroke, (2) control of ventricular rate, and (3) restoration and maintenance of sinus rhythm. Almost all patients with atrial fibrillation, paroxysmal or sustained, should be anticoagulated with warfarin to reduce the risk of thromboembolism. Exceptions include those patients with a contraindication to warfarin and those younger than 65 years of age with no structural heart disease ("lone atrial fibrillation"). Aspirin therapy may be useful for patients with a contraindication to warfarin.

Control of ventricular rate by slowing impulse conduction through the AV node has been achieved for more than a century with digitalis preparations. Although effective at rest, digitalis is unable to control ventricular rate adequately during exercise or other clinical states with elevated levels of catecholamines. In many patients, better control may be achieved by utilizing β-blocking agents or calcium channel blockers such as verapamil or diltiazem. Intravenous agents such as esmolol or diltiazem can be used to rapidly achieve rate control; longer-acting drugs can then be used for chronic therapy. Other antiarrhythmics, such as class Ic drugs and amiodarone, also slow the ventricular rate. Patients with excessive tachycardia due to inadequate rate control (heart rate chronically greater than 130 beats per minute) may develop cardiomyopathy with progression to congestive heart failure. Patients whose heart rate is uncontrollable using combinations of agents (i.e., digoxin and verapamil or propranolol) should be considered for catheter ablative techniques and permanent pacemaker implantation.

Antiarrhythmic drugs are useful to restore sinus rhythm and lessen the duration between episodes of atrial fibrillation. Agents used for these purposes include class Ia drugs quinidine, procainamide, or disopyramide; class Ic drugs propafenone and flecainide; class II agents; and class III agents sotalol and amiodarone. In general, antiarrhythmic drugs do not eliminate recurrent episodes of atrial fibrillation but can increase the duration of sinus rhythm between recurrences. β-Blocking drugs are especially useful for this purpose in patients after cardiac surgery. Class III agents amiodarone and sotalol are being used more frequently for control of atrial fibrillation, even though they are not approved for this indication in the United States. A unique class III agent, ibutilide, is used in bolus fashion to chemically cardiovert patients to sinus rhythm. It has been effective in approximately 40 to 70% of patients.

A large multicenter study is now in progress that is comparing whether optimized antiarrthythmic drug therapy administered to maintain sinus rhythm in patients having episodes of atrial fibrillation/flutter has an impact on total mortality and disabling stroke when compared with optimized therapy that merely controls heart rate in atrial fibrillation/flutter patients [atrial fibrillation follow-up investigation of rhythm management (AFFIRM)].

Nonpharmacologic techniques for control of atrial fibrillation include the MAZE surgical operation and catheter ablative procedures.

Atrial Flutter

In many ways, management of atrial flutter is similar to that of atrial fibrillation. Acute control of ventricular rate is usually achieved using intravenous therapy, either using a β-blocking agent such as esmolol or propranolol or a calcium channel blocking drug such as verapamil or diltiazem. Infusions of esmolol or diltiazem may be preferred due to their short half-life, which permits finer control of ventricular rate with a faster offset in case hypotension or excessive bradycardia develops. Chronic control of ventricular rate with atrial flutter is difficult, but similar types of agents, given orally, are commonly used. Digoxin, used alone, is rarely sufficient.

Direct current cardioversion or atrial overdrive pacing are the most rapid methods used to restore sinus rhythm, although pharmacologic conversion may become more frequent in the future. Ibutilide appears uniquely able to rapidly terminate established atrial flutter in a majority of patients. The risk of embolization and stroke after conversion from atrial flutter appears to be less than with atrial fibrillation, although many clinicians also anticoagulate patients with atrial flutter. Oral antiarrhythmic drugs, such as quinidine, procainamide, disopyramide, sotalol, amiodarone, flecainide, moricizine, and propafenone, may be used to restore and maintain sinus rhythm.

Particular care must be used when administering class Ia or Ic agents to patients with atrial flutter. These drugs may slow the atrial rate, whereas the anticholinergic effects of some of these agents may facilitate AV nodal conduction, resulting in an acceleration of ventricular rate. Occasionally, 1:1 conduction of the flutter impulse may occur, resulting in a ventricular rate between 220 and 250 beats per minute, which invariably causes hemodynamic compromise. This complication may be averted by ensuring adequate AV nodal blockade prior to instituting therapy with these agents. Amiodarone slows AV conduction and may be used as a single agent. Administration of adenosine to patients with atrial flutter will increase AV block, allowing visualization of flutter waves. Atrioventricular conduction may paradoxically improve after adenosine administration and also has caused 1:1 AV conduction.

Nonpharmacologic therapy for atrial flutter is increasingly being used. Radiofrequency catheter ablation of the isthmus of atrial tissue between the tricuspid valve and inferior vena cava annulae appears effective at preventing recurrences of atrial flutter. Alternatively, for intractable cases, ablation of the AV junction to create complete heart block with insertion of a permanent pacemaker may be performed.

AV Nodal Reentrant Tachycardia

After atrial fibrillation and atrial flutter, AV nodal reentrant tachycardia is the most common form of supraventricular tachycardia. This arrhythmia is caused by a reentrant circuit within the AV node and perinodal tissues. Therefore, pharmacologic therapies are directed toward the AV node. Acute management includes vagal maneuvers such as carotid sinus massage or Valsalva. Administration of adenosine or verapamil intravenously will universally terminate this arrhythmia. Similarly, intravenous β blockers, diltiazem, or verapamil can be effective. Agents useful for long-term pharmacologic management include digoxin, β-adrenergic receptor antagonists, and calcium channel antagonists such as verapamil or diltiazem. In unusual cases, propafenone, flecainide, or amiodarone may be useful. Patients with this arrhythmia are increasingly being treated with radiofrequency catheter ablation of the AV nodal "slow pathway."

AV Reentrant Tachycardia (Wolff-Parkinson-White Syndrome)

Patients with Wolff-Parkinson-White (WPW) syndrome have an anatomic fiber of myocardium that directly connects the atria and ventricles. This fiber may conduct cardiac impulses unidirectionally from atria to ventricles or from the ventricles to atria; bidirectional impulse conduction is also common. Because of the presence of dual pathways (the normal AV conduction system is the other one) for impulse conduction from atria to ventricles, reentrant arrhythmias are possible.

The most common tachycardia, orthodromic reciprocating tachycardia, utilizes the bypass tract in a retrograde (ventriculoatrial) direction and generally results in a narrow QRS tachycardia. Atrial fibrillation or flutter commonly occurs in conjunction with the WPW syndrome, and if the accessory pathway is capable of antegrade (atrioventricular) conduction, an irregular rhythm with both wide and narrow QRS complexes, often at rapid rates, will occur. Rarely, such patients will develop ventricular fibrillation from exceedingly rapid ventricular rates. The least common arrhythmia, antidromic reciprocating tachycardia, utilizes the bypass tract in an antegrade direction and results in a regular wide complex arrhythmia resembling ventricular tachycardia (VT).

Any of the preceding arrhythmias should be terminated using synchronized direct current cardioversion if hemodynamic collapse is present. Patients with a narrow QRS tachycardia are best treated with vagal maneuvers, followed, if necessary, by intravenous adenosine or verapamil. Caution should be used with adenosine in patients with known WPW syndrome because adenosine may produce atrial fibrillation. If rapid antegrade conduction over the bypass tract is possible, hemodynamic collapse may occur. A direct current (dc) defibrillator should always be immediately available whenever adenosine is used. Other acute therapies include intravenous esmolol or diltiazem. Patients with wide complex tachycardias and WPW syndrome should be treated as if they had VT. Intravenous procainamide is the therapy of choice if cardioversion is not required. Digoxin should not be used to treat patients with a bypass tract capable of antegrade conduction because it may accelerate impulse conduction over the tract.

The need for chronic pharmacologic therapy for patients with WPW syndrome has almost been completely eliminated by the success of radiofrequency catheter ablation. When necessary, patients without antegrade bypass tract conduction often may be treated with either a β blocker or calcium channel blocking drug. Patients with antegrade bypass tract conduction or patients with arrhythmia recurrences during therapy with β blockers or calcium channel blocking drugs should be treated with a class Ia, Ic, or III drug. Flecainide, propafenone, procainamide, disopyramide, or moricizine may be used, often in conjunction with a β-blocking agent. Sotalol, with β-blocking and class III activity, also may used. Amiodarone, while effective, is rarely necessary.

Atrial Tachycardia

Atrial tachycardia is an uncommon supraventricular tachycardia caused by abnormal automaticity or reentry within the atria. Patients with structural heart disease, especially after surgical correction of congenital heart disease, have reentrant atrial tachycardias due to atrial suture lines. Automatic atrial tachycardias are often self-limited and may disappear after several months to years. Patients with atrial tachycardias are often symptomatic, and pharmacologic treatment is justified. Long-standing tachycardias, with heart rates in excess of 130 beats per minute, may produce a dilated cardiomyopathy and congestive heart failure.

Automatic tachycardias are often amenable to treatment with β-blocking or calcium channel blocking drugs such as propranolol or verapamil. In more resistant cases, class Ic drugs such as flecainide or propafenone may be helpful. Some cases of atrial tachycardia are refractory to pharmacologic therapy and require catheter ablation for control.

Reentrant atrial tachycardias often require therapy with class Ia, Ic, or III antiarrhythmic drugs. Sotalol, flecainide, and amiodarone are often used. Unlike automatic arrhythmias, reentrant arrhythmias rarely are self-limited, requiring therapy for life. Patients with these arrhythmias often undergo catheter ablation to avoid lifelong antiarrhythmic drug therapy.

Multifocal atrial tachycardia appears to result from a diffuse increase in atrial automaticity. It is commonly seen in patients with severe lung disease and may be facilitated by theophylline, inhaled or oral β-adrenergic stimulants, and possibly digoxin. Therapy with either verapamil or metoprolol has been shown to be helpful, although any long-term therapy should include improving underlying lung function.

Ventricular Tachycardia

Ventricular tachycardia is a heterogeneous collection of ventricular tachyarrhythmias caused by several different arrhythmia mechanisms that occur in patients with varying degrees of structural heart disease. Most commonly, VT is a reentrant arrhythmia occurring in a patient with coronary artery disease, prior myocardial infarction, and frequently left ventricular dysfunction. Hemodynamic collapse is a common result of VT that is not self-terminating; sudden cardiac death is often the final result.

Occasionally, VT may be hemodynamically tolerated. In these individuals, intravenous infusion of either lidocaine or procainamide may result in arrhythmia slowing and often termination. Ventricular overdrive pacing is also effective, but synchronized dc cardioversion (with appropriate sedation and anesthesia) is the quickest method to restore a normal rhythm. Most episodes of VT terminate spontaneously and produce no symptoms, however. Optimal management of these patients is currently unknown.

Intravenous lidocaine, procainamide, bretylium, and amiodarone are useful acutely for prevention of VT recurrences. Class III agents sotalol and amiodarone are increasingly being used as chronic therapy for symptomatic VT. Other useful agents include mexiletine, quinidine, procainamide, disopyramide, propafenone, flecainide, and moricizine. All these agents have appreciable cardiac and noncardiac side effects, and depending on the method used to judge efficacy, each may be effective in only 10 to 30% of patients. It does appear certain that whatever pharmacologic agent is employed must be proved effective, either by suppression of ambient ectopy by Holter monitoring or by means of electrophysiologic testing. Empirical therapy is rarely effective, although amiodarone is currently being evaluated for such use.

Ventricular tachycardia with a continuously changing QRS morphology occurring in the setting of a prolonged QT interval (torsades de pointes) is a unique form of VT. This arrhythmia is often due to effects of antiarrhythmic drugs that prolong the action potential (classes Ia and III). Although this form of VT often terminates spontaneously, ventricular fibrillation and sudden death may occur. Acute therapy consists of normalization of potassium and magnesium levels, along with acceleration of the heart rate to 110 to 120 beats per minute by pacing or infusion of isoproterenol. Chronic therapy consists of elimination of all agents that prolong action potential duration. If necessary to treat other arrhythmias, amiodarone appears safe for use in patients with torsades de pointes despite its ability to markedly prolong the QT interval. Torsades de pointes also can occur as a familial form of arrhythmia as a result of mutations to DNA encoding either the cardiac sodium or potassium channel proteins.

Unusual forms of VT may occur in apparently structurally normal hearts. Ventricular tachycardia with a left bundle branch morphology and an inferior frontal plane axis often originates from the right ventricular outflow tract. This arrhythmia is often catecholamine-sensitive; it is frequently induced by exercise. β-Blocker drugs or catheter ablation usually is effective. Another unique type of VT, idiopathic left ventricular VT, has a right bundle branch QRS morphology with a superior frontal plane axis. This VT is often responsive to verapamil; catheter ablation is also effective. However, most patients with right bundle superior axis VT will not have the verapamil-sensitive type. It is also worth noting that verapamil should not be administered to patients during VT, except when the VT is known by prior electrophysiologic testing to be verapamil-sensitive. Administration of verapamil to patients with VT and coronary artery disease has resulted in hypotension and several deaths.

Implantable cardioverter defibrillators are increasingly being used for patients with recurrent hemodynamically destabilizing VT. It is not yet clear that use of this technology results in an improvement of overall mortality, however. Other therapies, such as endocardial resection and catheter ablative techniques, may be useful in selected patients.

Ventricular Fibrillation

Immediate dc countershock is the appropriate response to ventricular fibrillation. After a hemodynamically stable rhythm has been restored, antiarrhythmic therapy may be useful to prevent recurrences of this lethal arrhythmia. Acceptable intravenous medications include lidocaine, procainamide, bretylium, or amiodarone. Adjunctive therapies, such as relief of myocardial ischemia and correction of electrolyte imbalance are often helpful. Small doses of an intravenous β-blocking agent, such as propranolol, metoprolol, or esmolol, can have a surprisingly beneficial effect as well. Patients with frequent recurrences of ventricular fibrillation and whose intrinsic rhythm is relatively bradycardic may be helped by temporary atrial or ventricular pacing at heart rates of approximately 100 to 120 beats per minute.

Chronic antiarrhythmic drug therapy for prevention of recurrences of ventricular fibrillation should ideally be guided by either serial electrophysiologic testing or serial Holter monitoring to ensure drug efficacy. Common choices include sotalol or amiodarone. Empirical therapy with amiodarone is also commonly employed and is currently being evaluated as one therapy arm in the multicenter antiarrhythmic drug versus implantable defibrillator (AVID) study. Implantable cardioverter defibrillators are being used increasingly in high-risk patients; these devices have been proved effective in reducing sudden cardiac death, although their effects on overall mortality are less certain. Of course, implantable cardioverter defibrillators do not prevent recurrences of ventricular tachyarrhythmias, but immediately resuscitate patients when these arrhythmias are detected. Often combined therapy with an implantable cardioverter defibrillator with antiarrhythmic drug therapy is necessary in patients with frequent episodes of ventricular tachyarrhythmias.

CLASS IA AGENTS

Class Ia drugs block the sodium channel and fast response, predominantly in atrial, ventricular, and Purkinje tissue. The maximum rate of rise of phase 0 of the action potential is depressed, slowing conduction velocity. The potency of channel blockade is moderate, and repolarization (action potential duration) is prolonged. In addition, the drugs' kinetics of channel association and dissociation are on the order of several seconds, and consequently, drug effects are typically more profound at more rapid heart rates. Class Ia antiarrhythmic drugs are effective for many atrial and ventricular tachyarrhythmias.

Quinidine

Pharmacologic Description

Quinidine, an optical isomer of quinine, is an alkaloid derived from cinchona bark. First described by van Heynigen in 1848, quinidine was given its present name by Pasteur in 1853. Use of cinchona in patients with atrial fibrillation was described by Jean-Baptiste de Senac of Paris in 1749.

Electrophysiologic Action

Quinidine is a prototypic class Ia antiarrhythmic agent. It decreases the slope of phase 0 of the action potential, decreases the amplitude of the action potential, and slows conduction velocity in atrial, ventricular, and Purkinje tissue. In addition, quinidine delays repolarization, thereby increasing action potential duration. Electrocardiographic effects include prolongation of the QT, corrected QT (QTc), and QRS intervals. QRS prolongation greater than 35 to 50% of baseline is usually associated with toxicity.

Pharmacokinetics and Metabolism

Quinidine is currently available as quinidine sulfate, quinidine gluconate, and quinidine polygalacturonate. The bioavailability of quinidine ranges from 47 to 96%, averaging 75%. The milligrams of quinidine base in different preparations varies and thus should be considered in dosing, particularly when switching formulations. The bioavailability of the gluconate preparation is 10% less than that of the quinidine sulfate. After oral ingestion of quinidine sulfate, peak plasma concentrations occur within 60 to 90 min. The gluconate preparation is more slowly absorbed, with peak levels occurring 4 h after dosing. The elimination half-life ranges between 6 and 8 h. The clearance of quinidine is decreased in patients with significant hepatic insufficiency and with advancing age. Smaller maintenance doses are required in these patients. Advanced renal disease has only minimal effects on quinidine clearance. Approximately 90% of quinidine is bound to plasma proteins. Several cardioactive metabolites have been identified, including (3*S*)3-hydroxyquinidine (3OH-Q) and quinidine-*N*-oxide (QNO). Although these metabolites are less active than the parent compound (approximately 25% and 4% for 3OH-Q and QNO, respectively), in approximately one-fourth of patients their concentrations may approach or even exceed that of quinidine and contribute significantly to the overall electrophysiologic effects of the drug. Since these metabolites are not measured in all assays, quinidine levels may underestimate the potential activity of the drug under steady-state conditions.

Hemodynamic Effects

Quinidine is an α-adrenergic receptor antagonist that lowers peripheral vascular resistance. Whereas large oral doses can produce hypotension through this mechanism, the problem is most common with intravenous dosing. Although quinidine directly depresses myocardial contractility, clinically significant myocardial depression usually does not occur except with large intravenous doses.

Antiarrhythmic Effects

Quinidine can suppress a wide variety of supraventricular and ventricular arrhythmias. In life-threatening ventricular tachyarrhythmias, quinidine has shown long-term efficacy in 15 to 30% of patients with ventricular tachycardia or cardiac arrest when guided by electrophysiologic testing. Quinidine also can terminate atrial flutter or fibrillation in many patients, especially of recent onset and if the atria are not enlarged. Quinidine also has vagolytic effects that can enhance AV nodal conduction. In some patients, this can result in an increased ventricular rate with some atrial tachyarrhythmias, such as atrial flutter, unless an AV nodal blocking agent is also given. Typically, therapeutic levels range from 3 to 6 μg/mL.

Side Effects

Gastrointestinal side effects are common, with diarrhea and nausea the most bothersome. Quinidine may cause tinnitus, blurred vision, dizziness, lightheadedness, and tremor, a syndrome known as *cinchonism*. Rarely, severe antibody-mediated thrombocytopenia, pancytopenia, or hemolytic anemia may occur. Side effects may require cessation of therapy in as many as 30% of patients. Up to 3 to 4% of patients receiving quinidine may develop "quinidine syncope," a form of proarrhythmia usually caused by rapid polymorphic ventricular tachycardia associated with prolongation of the QT interval (torsades de pointes). Other cases have been attributed to sinus pauses or first-dose hypotension related in part to α-adrenergic receptor blockade. The risk of serious proarrhythmia is greatest during the first few days of dosing, during bradycardia or hypokalemia. Many advocate the initiation of quinidine therapy in the hospital with ECG monitoring, particularly in patients with cardiac dysfunction.

Interaction

Drugs that alter the kinetics of hepatic enzyme systems, such as phenobarbital, phenytoin, and rifampin, can increase hepatic metabolism of quinidine and reduce its concentration. Cimetidine, on the other hand, decreases hepatic metabolism of quinidine, increasing the plasma concentration. In addition, the concomitant administration of amiodarone increases the concentration of many antiarrhythmic drugs, including quinidine. Quinidine increases serum levels of digoxin by decreasing digoxin clearance, volume of distribution, and affinity of tissue receptors for digoxin and thus may contribute to digoxin toxicity. Digitoxin levels are also increased. Recently, quinidine has been shown to be a potent inhibitor of cytochrome P450db1, a genetically determined polymorphic enzyme responsible for oxidative metabolism of many drugs by the liver. Because of inhibition of this enzyme system, quinidine substantially decreases metabolism of some drugs, such as encainide and propafenone, decreasing the concentration of their metabolites while increasing the concentrations of the parent compounds.

Indications and Dosage

Quinidine is indicated for the treatment of incapacitating atrial, AV nodal, and ventricular tachyarrhythmias. The usual adult dose of quinidine sulfate is 200 to 400 mg four times daily or less frequently with longer-acting preparations. Intravenous quinidine gluconate is occasionally used in special situations such as the electrophysiology laboratory and may be given using a dose of 6 to 10 mg/kg at a rate of 0.3 to 0.5 mg/kg per minute with frequent checks of blood pressure and ECG parameters. In some patients, efficacy can be enhanced by the concomitant use of class Ib or class II antiarrhythmic drugs, such as mexiletine and propranolol.

Procainamide

Pharmacologic Description

Procainamide hydrochloride is an amide analogue of procaine hydrochloride, a local anesthetic agent. It was introduced in 1951 for the treatment of both supraventricular and ventricular arrhythmias.

Electrophysiologic Action

Procainamide is a class Ia antiarrhythmic agent. It decreases phase 0 of the action potential, decreases the amplitude of the action potential, and slows conduction velocity in atrial, ventricular, and Purkinje tissue. In addition, procainamide increases the effective refractory periods of atrial and ventricular cells. Its major electrophysiologic effects on myocardial tissues are similar to quinidine. Normal sinus node automaticity is not affected. Procainamide is less vagolytic than quinidine and does not induce α-adrenergic blockade. The major metabolite of procainamide, *N*-acetylprocainamide (NAPA), has different electrophysiologic effects, predominantly prolonging the action potential duration, a class III effect. Electrocardiographic effects of procainamide include prolongation of the QT, QTc, and QRS intervals.

Pharmacokinetics and Metabolism

Procainamide is currently available in parenteral (intravenous or intramuscular) as well as regular and sustained-release tablet and capsule formulations. The bioavailability of procainamide is approximately 83%. Following ingestion of regular-release tablets, peak plasma levels are obtained within 60 to 90 min. Approximately 15% of procainamide is bound to plasma proteins. In adults, the elimination half-life varies between 2.5 and 4 h. Elimination is more rapid in children, averaging 1.7 h. Approximately 50% of procainamide is excreted unchanged by the kidney. Of the remainder, a variable portion undergoes hepatic acetylation to NAPA, a cardioactive metabolite. Depending on a patient's genetically determined acetylator phenotype, 16 to 22% (slow acetylators) or 24 to 33% (fast acetylators) of procainamide is metabolized to NAPA. Elimination of NAPA is approximately 85% dependent on the kidney, with an elimination half-life of 7 to 8 h. Small amounts of NAPA may be deacetylated to procainamide.

Hemodynamic Effects

Procainamide can depress myocardial contractility but is usually well tolerated hemodynamically even in patients with moderately severe cardiac dysfunction. When given intravenously, hypotension may result from vasodilatation due to a mild ganglionic blocking action.

Antiarrhythmic Effects

Procainamide can effectively suppress a variety of atrial, AV nodal, and ventricular tachyarrhythmias, including 20 to 30% of patients with sustained ventricular tachyarrhythmias. It is a drug of choice in the acute medical treatment of wide-complex tachycardias including atrial fibrillation with ventricular preexcitation (Wolff-Parkinson-White syndrome). A mild vagolytic effect may result in an increased ventricular rate due to enhanced AV nodal conduction when given for supraventricular tachyarrhythmias such as atrial flutter. Suppression of ventricular arrhythmias has been shown to occur at plasma levels between 4 and 10 μg/mL of procainamide, but higher levels may be required for suppression of sustained ventricular tachyarrhythmias. In addition, the contribution of NAPA to efficacy cannot always be ascertained. Procainamide has been used extensively with electrophysiologic testing for life-threatening ventricular arrhythmias and cardiac arrest. Failure to respond to procainamide during electrophysiologic testing in these cases often predicts failure with other individual antiarrhythmic agents as well.

Side Effects

Major side effects of procainamide are gastrointestinal, with nausea, vomiting, anorexia, or diarrhea occurring in up to 30% of patients. A bitter taste, dizziness, mental depression, and psychosis also have been reported. Drug-induced fever, rash, and hepatitis may occur. Agranulocytosis, sometimes fatal, has been described. Most patients will develop a positive antinuclear antibody titer if exposed to the drug for prolonged intervals. Of these, up to 30% can develop a drug-induced systemic lupuslike syndrome. Slow acetylators may be at increased risk of procainamide-induced lupus due to increased production of a hydroxylamine metabolite, which appears to be important in the pathogenesis of this syndrome. Recently, procainamide-induced lupus anticoagulants have been described, which may increase the risk of thrombosis in some patients. Like quinidine, new onset polymorphic ventricular tachycardia in the setting of QT prolongation has been reported. Procainamide usually causes only minimal depression of cardiac function with chronic dosing, but hypotension is not uncommon with rapid intravenous infusions.

Interaction

Unlike quinidine, procainamide does not significantly alter the pharmacokinetics of digoxin. Trimethoprim and cimetidine decrease renal clearance of procainamide and NAPA, resulting in increased plasma levels of both. Concomitant administration of amiodarone also increases procainamide levels.

Indications and Dosage

Procainamide is indicated for the treatment of incapacitating atrial, AV nodal, and ventricular tachyarrhythmias. An average oral daily dose for patients under 50 years of age is 30 to 60 mg/kg, divided into equal doses given every 3, 4, or 6 h. Various sustained-release formulations facilitate dosing on a two, three-, or four-times-per-day basis with lower peak and higher trough levels. In addition, efficacy may be enhanced in some patients with concomitant use of other agents, including β blockers. Older patients or patients with renal insufficiency require smaller doses. Intravenous therapy can be initiated with loading infusion of up to 20 mg/kg given at a rate not to exceed 50 mg/min. Frequent blood pressure and ECG checks are required. A maintenance intravenous dose is approximately 30 to 60 μg/kg per minute in a patient with normal renal function.

Disopyramide

Pharmacologic Description

Disopyramide phosphate was first noted to have antiarrhythmic properties in 1962. It was subsequently released for clinical use in the United States in 1978. As currently available, disopyramide exists as a racemic combination of D and L enantiomers.

Electrophysiologic Action

The electrophysiologic effects of disopyramide are similar to those of other class Ia agents, such as quinidine and procainamide. It produces a rate-dependent decrease in the rate of rise of phase 0 of the action potential, slows conduction velocity, and prolongs the effective refractory period more than it prolongs the action potential duration. Disopyramide may prolong the action potential duration to a greater extent in normal cells than in cells from infarcted regions of the heart. The different enantiomers of disopyramide have differing electrophysiologic effects: the D enantiomer prolongs action potential duration, while the L enantiomer shortens it. The D enantiomer has approximately one-third the vagolytic properties as the L enantiomer. Disopyramide exerts strong anticholinergic effects that tend to counteract some of its direct electrophysiologic effects, particularly in the sinus and AV nodes. In humans, AV nodal conduction is minimally affected by disopyramide. However, in the denervated (transplanted) heart, AV nodal conduction is markedly depressed. Disopyramide can either increase or decrease the sinus rate, depending on prevailing cholinergic tone. Electrocardiographic effects of disopyramide include prolongation of the QRS, QT, and QTc intervals.

Pharmacokinetics and Metabolism

Disopyramide is available in regular and sustained-release capsule formulations. An intravenous preparation is undergoing clinical investigation. After an oral dose, disopyramide is almost completely absorbed, with peak plasma concentrations occurring within 2 h. Peak levels occur from 4 to 6 h after ingestion of sustained-release disopyramide capsules. The elimination half-life is 6 to 9 h, with 40 to 60% excreted unchanged by the kidney. Approximately 50% of disopyramide is excreted unchanged in the urine; an additional 20% is excreted as the mono-*N*-dealkylated metabolite, with another 10% excreted as other metabolites. Protein binding is highly variable, ranging from 40 to 90%, depending on plasma concentration. At higher doses, a greater concentration of drug is unbound, resulting in a greater pharmacologic effect than would be predicted based on the total plasma level. The clinical significance of this effect is unknown. α_1-Acid glycoprotein accounts for the majority of protein binding, with albumin accounting for only 5 to 10% of the total.

Hemodynamic Effects

Disopyramide causes significant depression of myocardial contractility, with reductions in systemic blood pressure, stroke index, and cardiac index. Systemic vascular resistance and right atrial pressure increase. Patients with left ventricular dysfunction tolerate disopyramide poorly. In a retrospective study among patients with preexisting congestive heart failure, 55% of patients given disopyramide had clinically significant worsening of their heart failure. In contrast, only 3% of patients without a history of congestive heart failure developed this complication during disopyramide therapy.

Antiarrhythmic Effects

Like other class Ia antiarrhythmic drugs, disopyramide is effective in a variety of supraventricular and ventricular tachyarrhythmias. Disopyramide can suppress premature ventricular contractions, with plasma concentrations in the range of 3 to 8 μg/mL, but is less effective with sustained ventricular tachycardia, as assessed by electrophysiologic testing. Disopyramide has been combined with other antiarrhythmic agents, such as mexiletine, for increased efficacy in treating ventricular arrhythmias with fewer side effects. Disopyramide has been used successfully for the treatment of atrial flutter and atrial fibrillation, including patients with the Wolff-Parkinson-White syndrome.

Side Effects

Disopyramide significantly depresses myocardial contractility and must be used with caution, if at all, in patients with left ventricular dysfunction. Anticholinergic side effects are frequent and in up to 10% of patients may necessitate discontinuation of the drug. These symptoms include dry mouth, blurred vision, and particularly in older men, urine retention. Disopyramide also can precipitate acute angle-closure glaucoma. Gastrointestinal symptoms are uncommon. As with other drugs that prolong ventricular repolarization and the QT interval, disopyramide can induce polymorphic ventricular tachycardia (torsades de pointes). Rare side effects include rash, cholestatic jaundice, psychosis, and agranulocytosis. Hypoglycemia occurs infrequently, apparently owing to increased pancreatic secretion of insulin.

Interaction

Drugs that induce hepatic enzymes, such as phenytoin and phenobarbital, increase hepatic metabolism of disopyramide and result in lower serum levels. Disopyramide does not induce hepatic enzymes, however. Disopyramide does not alter serum digoxin levels. Recently, erythromycin has been reported to increase disopyramide levels, with development of potentially fatal ventricular arrhythmias. The potent negative inotropic effects of disopyramide warrant additional caution in patients with possible cardiac dysfunction requiring therapy with β blockers or calcium channel blockers for indications such as ischemic heart disease.

Indications and Dosage

Disopyramide is indicated for the prevention or suppression of premature ventricular contractions and ventricular tachycardia. It also has been used to treat atrial arrhythmias but is not specifically approved for this indication in the United States. The usual adult oral dose is 300 to 1600 mg daily, divided into three or four equal doses. Dosage must be reduced in elderly patients and in patients with renal insufficiency. The controlled-release capsules may be given every 12 h.

CLASS IB AGENTS

Class Ib drugs also block sodium channels, but to a lesser degree than class Ia drugs. The association and disassociation kinetics are more rapid than in class Ia drugs, typically less than 1 s. In addition, repolarization tends to be mildly shortened. Class Ib drugs often suppress premature ventricular contractions but are only occasionally effective as monotherapy for life-threatening ventricular tachyarrhythmias. Class Ib drugs, as a class, are generally ineffective for atrial arrhythmias.

Lidocaine

Pharmacologic Description

Initially synthesized in 1943, lidocaine is widely used as a local anesthetic agent. Its antiarrhythmic properties were noted in the 1950s, but its use did not become common until the advent of coronary care units in the 1960s.

Electrophysiologic Action

Lidocaine is classified as a class Ib antiarrhythmic drug. The action potential duration and effective refractory period of Purkinje and ventricular tissues are shortened. At high concentrations, it depresses the rate of rise of phase 0 of the action potential and decreases conduction velocity in Purkinje fibers. Lidocaine has minimal effects on AV and intraventricular conduction except at high concentrations (above 30 μg/mL). In patients with severe His-Purkinje system disease, lidocaine may precipitate complete AV block. Lidocaine decreases phase 4 diastolic depolarizations in Purkinje tissue and decreases automaticity. Consequently, lidocaine may depress both the sinus node and potential subsidiary escape pacemakers, rarely causing asystolic pauses. Lidocaine increases the ventricular fibrillation threshold. In abnormal myocardium, the effects of lidocaine in depressing conduction may be more pronounced.

Pharmacokinetics and Metabolism

Lidocaine is almost completely absorbed after oral administration, but approximately 70% is rapidly metabolized by hepatic first-pass biotransformation. Less than 10% of an administered dose is recovered unchanged in the urine. For this reason, the drug is almost always given parenterally; however, rectal administration is feasible, as is intramuscular administration, particularly in the prehospital phase of acute myocardial infarction management. Lidocaine is approximately 60 to 80% protein-bound, depending on the concentration of α_1-acid glycoprotein in the serum. During acute myocardial infarction, serum levels of α_1-acid glycoprotein are increased, resulting in more drug bound to α_1-acid glycoprotein and less free (active) drug. Thus higher total lidocaine levels may be required during acute myocardial infarction. Lidocaine is almost completely cleared by the liver, with clearance proportional to hepatic blood flow. The mean elimination half-life of lidocaine in humans is 1.5 to 2 h, which is increased in the elderly, patients with reduced cardiac output, and patients with hepatic disease. Elimination is also delayed during prolonged infusions in patients with acute myocardial infarction, the mechanism of which is not understood. The two principal metabolites are glycinexylidide and monoethylglycinexylidide (MEGX), both of which have weaker antiarrhythmic effects in humans than does lidocaine but can contribute measurably to the central nervous system toxicity of lidocaine. Both metabolites are renally excreted, and glycinexylidide may accumulate in patients with renal failure.

Hemodynamic Effects

At usual doses, lidocaine causes minimal hemodynamic effects. Minimal decreases in cardiac output, arterial blood pressure, heart rate, and ventricular contractility have been reported.

Antiarrhythmic Effects

Lidocaine can be effective for the suppression of ventricular tachyarrhythmias. It is commonly used prophylactically to prevent ventricular tachyarrhythmias during acute myocardial infarction. It appears to reduce the incidence of ventricular fibrillation. Prophylactic lidocaine in the absence of so-called warning arrhythmias is currently used in a minority of institutions. Paradoxically, although thrombolytic therapy has reduced in-hospital infarct mortality, interest in the use of prophylactic lidocaine for suppression of reperfusion arrhythmias has renewed interest. Therapeutic plasma concentrations range from 2 to 5 μg/mL.

Side Effects

Adverse effects of lidocaine almost always involve the central nervous system. Early, transient effects include paresthesias, dizziness, and drowsiness, which can be managed by interrupting the drug temporarily. Later, more persistent effects include hallucinations, confusion, somnolence, and muscle tremor, which presage impending seizures and respiratory or cardiac arrest. Rarely, lidocaine can depress sinus node function or precipitate heart block in patients with severe His-Purkinje system disease; it also can inhibit escape rhythms from His-Purkinje tissue. Adverse effects of lidocaine are common when the plasma concentration exceeds 6 μg/mL.

Interaction

Lidocaine is highly dependent on hepatic metabolism for elimination. Drugs that alter hepatic metabolism cause marked changes in lidocaine pharmacokinetics. Propranolol, metoprolol, cimetidine, and halothane decrease lidocaine clearance.

Indications and Dosage

Lidocaine is indicated for the acute management of ventricular arrhythmias, such as those associated with acute myocardial infarction or cardiac surgery. It may be administered intravenously as a bolus of 0.7 to 1.4 mg/kg at a rate of 25 to 50 mg/min. If necessary, this dose may be repeated in 5 min followed by a continuous infusion of 0.014 to 0.057 mg/kg (1 to 4 mg/min). Alternative loading and maintenance infusion regimens also have been advocated, typically entailing a total of 2 to 4 mg/kg in divided doses over 30 min. Lidocaine may be given by intramuscular injection of 300 to 400 mg (4.3 mg/kg) for use during acute myocardial infarction. The deltoid muscle is the preferred injection site. Lidocaine also has been used in combination with other agents including procainamide, bretylium, and β blockers.

Tocainide

Pharmacologic Description

Tocainide hydrochloride is a primary amine analogue of lidocaine. Minor side-chain differences from lidocaine enable it to avoid substantial first-pass metabolism in the liver, thus allowing oral administration. Its antiarrhythmic effects were described in 1976, and it has been approved for oral use in the United States since 1984. As currently available, tocainide is supplied as a racemic mixture of enantiomers D-tocainide and L-tocainide.

Electrophysiologic Action

Tocainide produces dose-dependent decreases in sodium and potassium conductance, thus depressing myocardial excitability. It suppresses the amplitude and rate of depolarization of the action potential and may shorten the action potential duration and, to a lesser extent, the effective refractory period of Purkinje tissue. Tocainide increases the fibrillation threshold in normal and ischemic tissue. AV conduction and sinus node automaticity are usually unaffected by tocainide. Tocainide usually produces no significant changes on the electrocardiogram. However, the QT interval may decrease. The individual enantiomers of tocainide may be more effective for ventricular arrhythmias induced by programmed electrical stimulation than the racemic combination.

Pharmacokinetics and Metabolism

Following oral administration, the bioavailability of tocainide approaches 100%. Peak plasma concentrations appear between 0.5 and 2 h. Between 10 and 50% of tocainide is bound to plasma proteins. Approximately 40% is excreted unchanged in the urine. The elimination half-life averages 13 to 15 h in healthy subjects but can vary between 9 and 37 h. Elimination is delayed in the presence of renal insufficiency but only minimally changed in the presence of hepatic disease.

Hemodynamic Effects

Intravenous tocainide produces small degrees of left ventricular depression with no apparent change in cardiac output. Small increases in aortic and pulmonary artery pressures have been observed, probably secondary to increases in vascular resistance. In patients with moderate to severe left ventricular dysfunction, including those receiving β-blocking drugs, hemodynamic changes are often minimal, although more marked and additive effects may occur. In one study, congestive heart failure was precipitated by tocainide in approximately 1.5% of patients.

Antiarrhythmic Effects

Tocainide is a modestly effective agent for suppressing premature ventricular contractions in a number of patients, with approximately 90% suppression in some patients at plasma concentrations of 8.5 μg/mL. Typically, 30 to 75% of patients will have significant premature ventricular contraction suppression. Tocainide is at times effective in suppressing premature ventricular contractions in patients who are unresponsive to class Ia agents, and the response to lidocaine may be predictive of the response to tocainide. Response to lidocaine appears to be a sensitive but nonspecific predictor of efficacy with tocainide. Thus lidocaine failure is often predictive of tocainide inefficacy, while lidocaine efficacy does not necessarily predict tocainide success. Only a small percentage of patients with life-threatening ventricular arrhythmias will respond to tocainide when assessed by electrophysiologic testing. However, the drug may be synergistically effective when combined with class Ia drugs. Dosing tocainide at 600 mg orally twice daily produces levels effective in suppressing premature ventricular contractions in many patients (4 to 10 μg/mL).

Side Effects

Side effects are common with tocainide, having been reported in 20 to 40% of patients. Typically, gastrointestinal and central nervous system side effects occur, including nausea, dizziness, tremor, vomiting, paresthesia, tremor, ataxia, and confusion. These effects usually occur with high plasma concentrations and may be minimized by dividing doses and taking the medication with meals to delay absorption. Skin rash occurs not infrequently. Rarely, more serious adverse effects occur, such as pulmonary fibrosis, a lupus-like syndrome, or hematologic abnormalities, chiefly agranulocytosis.

Interaction

Tocainide has no significant effects on warfarin or digoxin. Concomitant use with β-blocking drugs is safe in most patients. Rifampin has been reported to increase elimination, resulting in reduced plasma levels of tocainide. Cimetidine, but not ranitidine, results in decreased bioavailability of tocainide.

Indications and Dosage

Tocainide is specifically indicated for the treatment of life-threatening ventricular tachyarrhythmias, although it is only infrequently effective for this purpose. It is also indicated for the treatment of some patients with symptomatic ventricular arrhythmias. Tocainide is available as tablets of 400 and 600 mg. Total daily doses of 800 to 2400 mg are usually administered as divided doses two to four times daily. The dosage should be reduced in the presence of renal insufficiency. Plasma levels above 3 μg/mL are associated with efficacy, while levels above 10 μg/mL are associated with increased side effects.

Mexiletine

Pharmacologic Description

Mexiletine hydrochloride is a drug closely related in structure to lidocaine. Initially developed as an anticonvulsant, mexiletine has been recognized to have antiarrhythmic properties since 1972. Used in Europe to treat ventricular arrhythmias since 1976, it became available in the United States in 1986.

Electrophysiologic Action

Mexiletine decreases the rate of rise of phase 0 of the action potential and shortens the action potential duration. The effective refractory period is decreased in Purkinje tissue but not in ventricular muscle. The slope of phase 4 diastolic depolarization is decreased. The electrophysiologic effects of mexiletine are similar to those of other class Ib agents. Usually, no significant changes occur in the PR, QRS, QT, or QTc intervals with either intravenous or oral mexiletine. In patients with normal His-Purkinje function, no significant changes are observed after mexiletine. Patients with His-Purkinje system disease may develop prolongation of conduction and rarely block, however. In addition, prolongation of QRS duration has been reported with mexiletine toxicity.

Pharmacokinetics and Metabolism

Mexiletine is highly bioavailable, with approximately 90% absorption. Absorption occurs in the alkaline environment of the proximal small bowel. Peak plasma levels occur in 2 to 3 h but may be delayed in clinical situations, such as acute myocardial infarction or diabetes mellitus, in which gastric emptying is delayed. Fifty to sixty percent of mexiletine is protein-bound. Mexiletine is extensively metabolized in the liver; only 10% is excreted unchanged by the kidney. Several metabolites have minor electrophysiologic activity, the most potent (*N*-methylmexiletine) having less than 20% of the effect of the parent compound. In healthy subjects, the average elimination half-life is 10 h, ranging from 8 to 12 h. Renal insufficiency has minimal effect on elimination half-life, whereas hepatic insufficiency or reduced hepatic blood flow reduces mexiletine clearance.

Hemodynamic Effects

Mexiletine generally has minimal negative inotropic effects at therapeutic levels. Small decreases in blood pressure and left ventricular contractility with increased left ventricular end-diastolic pressure have been observed in some studies. Administered orally, mexiletine produced no changes in left ventricular ejection fraction, blood pressure, heart rate, or exercise capacity.

Antiarrhythmic Effects

Mexiletine may be used to suppress frequent and high-grade ventricular arrhythmias, including those which have failed to respond to class Ia antiarrhythmic drugs. Used alone, mexiletine is only infrequently effective in suppressing life-threatening ventricular arrhythmias. Combination therapy with class Ia antiarrhythmic agents can be more effective than either agent alone, with potentially less toxicity. Mexiletine is effective in suppressing warning ventricular arrhythmias in a number of patients with acute myocardial infarction. The antiarrhythmic response to lidocaine may be used as a sensitive but nonspecific predictor of mexiletine efficacy. Thus failure to respond to intravenous lidocaine is a strong predictor of mexiletine inefficacy, while lidocaine efficacy only weakly predicts mexiletine efficacy. Similarly, the response to either tocainide or mexiletine is not necessarily predictive of the response to the other. Plasma concentrations of 0.5 to 2.0 μg/mL are associated with efficacy in many patients.

Side Effects

Side effects are common with mexiletine, occurring in up to 40 to 60% of patients in some series. The most frequent side effects are related to the central nervous system or the gastrointestinal tract and include nausea, vomiting, dizziness, tremor, ataxia, slurred speech, blurred vision, memory impairment, and personality changes. Skin rash and hepatitis occur infrequently. Rarely, seizures have been reported. Gastrointestinal side effects may be reduced by administering the drug with food or reducing the dosage. Adverse cardiac effects are rare, but worsening of congestive heart failure and proarrhythmic effects have been reported.

Interaction

No specific adverse effects have been reported to date from combining mexiletine with other cardiotonic agents, such as β-blocking drugs or other antiarrhythmics. Significant alkalinization of the urine by drugs may decrease renal clearance and result in elevated blood levels. Drugs such as phenobarbital or phenytoin, which induce hepatic enzymes, enhance mexiletine metabolism; cimetidine reduces metabolism and results in increased mexiletine levels.

Indications and Dosage

Mexiletine is indicated for the suppression of incapacitating ventricular arrhythmias, including ventricular tachycardia. Effective oral regimens usually require 200 to 400 mg every 8 h. Doses should be given with food to minimize side effects. Dosages may be increased or decreased by 50 to 100 mg at intervals of at least 2 to 3 days. An intravenous preparation is not available in the United States and is associated with a relatively high incidence of side effects. Intravenous therapy has been given as a loading dose of 400 mg over 40 min, with 600 to 900 mg/day for maintenance therapy.

CLASS Ic AGENTS

Class Ic drugs are potent sodium channel blocking agents. They have little effect on repolarization and have long half-time kinetics of channel association and dissociation, usually greater than 20 to 30 s. Thus drug effects are potentiated at moderate to rapid heart rates. They are effective for a variety of atrial and ventricular tachyarrhythmias. As a class, the Ic drugs are highly effective in suppressing chronic ventricular ectopy. Unfortunately, the marked slowing of conduction induced by these agents is an efficient mechanism to induce ventricular proarrhythmia. This effect is most marked in patients with significant structural heart disease but may occur in normal individuals, especially in the setting of rapid heart rates, such as those produced by exercise.

Moricizine

Pharmacologic Description

Moricizine is a phenothiazine derivative first synthesized in the Soviet Union.

Electrophysiologic Action

Intravenous moricizine (3 mg/kg) produces both a reduction in the upstroke velocity of phase 0 and a reduction in the action potential duration, effects similar to those of other class Ib antiarrhythmic agents. In contrast with class Ib agents, however, moricizine has prolonged sodium channel recovery kinetics, similar to class Ic agents. Moricizine does not decrease the slope of phase 4 depolarization in automatic Purkinje fibers, unless the fibers are ischemic. Voltage clamp experiments have shown that moricizine reduces the fast sodium current by decreasing maximal conduction of sodium ions. In humans, intravenous moricizine (1.5 to 2 mg/kg) lengthens the P wave to low-right-atrial (PA), atrial to His bundle (AH), and PR intervals. The sinus rate and QT and His bundle to ventricular (HV) intervals, as well as the effective refractory periods of the atrium, AV node, and ventricle, were not affected in early studies. The refractoriness of an accessory pathway or of the retrograde fast pathway of dual AV nodal pathways is increased by moricizine, however. Using an oral dose of 10 mg/kg, slight prolongation of the HV interval was noted, whereas at a higher dose of 15 mg/kg, the PR and QRS intervals were prolonged. In patients with sinus node dysfunction, moricizine given intravenously (2 mg/kg) has caused prolongation of the sinus node recovery time and second-degree sinus exit block. Although some properties are similar to those of other class Ib agents, in aggregate, moricizine behaves more like a class Ic drug.

Pharmacokinetics and Metabolism

Moricizine is well absorbed when given orally, with peak plasma concentrations occurring 1 to 1.5 h after dosing. The drug undergoes extensive metabolism, with less than 1% of the drug recovered in the urine and feces. Active metabolites have not been identified thus far. After a single oral dose, the elimination half-life is approximately 2 to 5 h. In patients with cardiac disease, the steady-state elimination half-life averages 10 h but may be prolonged up to 47 h in patients with renal insufficiency. Antiarrhythmic effects of the drug may not be noted for up to 24 h after dosing, an effect that is not completely understood. Therefore, plasma levels may provide little guidance for antiarrhythmic efficacy, and in fact, several studies have reported little correlation between plasma concentration and drug toxicity in the form of proarrhythmia.

Hemodynamic Effects

Hemodynamic data in humans are incomplete; however, moricizine appears to have minimal effect on most hemodynamic parameters. Moricizine does not appear to depress myocardial contractility in dogs. In patients with preexisting left ventricular dysfunction, moricizine may cause decompensation, however. In one study, the failure to increase cardiac index by 1.0 L/min per square meter or to increase stroke work during bicycle exercise not only predicted patients likely to decompensate, but also predicted those patients unlikely to have an antiarrhythmic response.

Antiarrhythmic Effects

Moricizine may be effective for the treatment of both supraventricular and ventricular arrhythmias. With doses ranging from 2.4 to 15 mg/kg per day, moricizine was effective in reducing premature ventricular contractions in 50 to 60% of patients, comparing favorably with disopyramide in one study. Moricizine appears less effective in the treatment of life-threatening ventricular tachyarrhythmias. Unlike other class Ib antiarrhythmic agents, moricizine, when given intravenously, has shown efficacy in terminating and preventing initiation of both AV nodal supraventricular tachycardias and reciprocating bypass tract tachycardias by slowing retrograde fast pathway conduction.

Side Effects

Moricizine appears to be a generally well tolerated antiarrhythmic agent. Nausea, vomiting, diarrhea, and dizziness as well as mild anxiety reactions have been reported. Nervousness, perioral numbness, vertigo, confusion, dry mouth, blurred vision, headache, and insomnia have occurred. Worsening of sinus node dysfunction may occur, and the drug may cause hypotension or worsening of congestive heart failure. Some patients have had transient elevation of hepatic transaminase enzyme levels. Rarely, diaphoresis and memory loss have been reported with long-term therapy. Proarrhythmia reportedly occurred in approximately 3.2% of patients in one review and was reportedly relatively unrelated to dose. Sinusoidal ventricular tachycardia, occasionally induced with exercise, has been reported.

Interaction

Serum digoxin levels may increase 10 to 15% during acute but not chronic dosing in cardiac patients with normal renal function. Other drug interactions have not been reported, but this has not been completely investigated.

Indications and Dosage

At doses of 150 to 250 mg every 8 h, moricizine appears effective for the treatment of atrial and ventricular ectopy. Doses may be given every

8 to 12 h. Therapeutic drug levels appear to be 0.2 to 1.5 μg/mL. The role of moricizine in the treatment of life-threatening ventricular arrhythmias remains undefined.

Flecainide

Pharmacologic Description

Flecainide acetate, a fluorobenzamide, is a derivative of procainamide first synthesized in 1972. Its antiarrhythmic effects were first reported in 1975, and it was released for the treatment of ventricular arrhythmias in the United States in 1985. Subsequently, it has been approved for the treatment of supraventricular tachyarrhythmias including atrial flutter and atrial fibrillation in patients with normal ventricular function.

Electrophysiologic Action

Flecainide exhibits potent sodium channel blocking action, depressing phase 0 of the action potential and slowing conduction in a frequency- and dose-dependent manner throughout the heart. His-Purkinje tissue and ventricular muscle are affected the most, followed by atrial muscle, accessory AV pathways, and AV nodal tissue. In most studies, the action potential duration is not significantly affected. Sinus rate, sinoatrial conduction, and sinus node recovery times are usually not affected by flecainide. However, patients with sinus node dysfunction may have significant increases in the corrected sinus node recovery time. Flecainide produces a concentration-dependent increase in PR, QRS, and intraatrial conduction intervals, as well as prolongation of the ventricular effective refractory period. An intravenous dose of 2 mg/kg (mean level 335 μg/L) produced a mean QRS increase of 23%. The QT interval increases, reflecting QRS prolongation, with minimal to no change in the JT interval.

Pharmacokinetics and Metabolism

Flecainide is well absorbed (95%), with peak plasma concentrations occurring 2 to 4 h after dosing. Flecainide is 30 to 40% bound to plasma proteins, independent of drug level over a range of 0.015 to 3.4 μg/mL. Clinically important drug interactions based on protein binding effects would therefore not be expected. In healthy subjects, 30% (range 10 to 50%) of flecainide is excreted unchanged in the urine. Approximately 70% of flecainide is metabolized in the liver. The major metabolite (meta-*O*-dealkylated flecainide) is approximately 20% as potent as the parent compound, while the minor metabolite (meta-*O*-dealkylated lactam of flecainide) is electrophysiologically inactive. The average elimination half-life is 20 h after repeated doses but is highly variable and ranges between 12 and 27 h. Steady-state levels are not obtained for 3 to 5 days. Since flecainide is extensively metabolized, the relationship between flecainide elimination and creatinine clearance is complex.

Reduced doses must be used in patients with renal insufficiency or hepatic insufficiency.

Hemodynamic Effects

Flecainide produces dose-dependent depression of cardiac contractility and cardiac output. Oral treatment is generally well tolerated, but patients with left ventricular dysfunction may develop new onset or worsening of congestive heart failure. Flecainide must be used cautiously in patients with left ventricular dysfunction.

Antiarrhythmic Effects

Flecainide is effective in suppressing both supraventricular and ventricular tachyarrhythmias and premature contractions. Flecainide is able to suppress chronic premature ventricular contractions by more than 75% and repetitive forms by more than 90% in most patients, including patients resistant to other antiarrhythmic drugs. Among patients with life-threatening ventricular tachyarrhythmias, flecainide is reported to prevent induction of ventricular tachycardia in 15 to 25%. Flecainide has shown efficacy in the prevention and treatment of atrial fibrillation and arrhythmias in patients with ventricular preexcitation or accessory pathways. Flecainide is most effective in suppressing chronic ectopy in patients with preserved left ventricular function without ventricular tachycardia. Patients with left ventricular dysfunction or clinically documented ventricular tachycardia are at increased risk for proarrhythmic side effects. Flecainide has been shown to increase cardiac mortality among patients with ventricular ectopy after acute myocardial infarction. Therapeutic levels of flecainide are 0.2 to 1.0 μg/mL; higher levels are associated with an increasing incidence of toxicity.

Side Effects

Most side effects of flecainide are neurologic and cardiac. Neurologic effects include blurred vision, headache, dizziness, paresthesias, and tremor. Skin rash, abdominal pain, diarrhea, and impotence have been reported. Cardiac effects are not uncommon and include worsening of arrhythmia, slowed conduction or heart block, and aggravation of congestive heart failure. Worsening of ventricular arrhythmias occurs in up to 10% or more of patients, more commonly in patients with left ventricular dysfunction and clinical ventricular tachycardia. Some episodes of ventricular tachycardia induced by flecainide have been resistant to electrical cardioversion. Acute and chronic elevations of the pacing threshold have been reported by some investigators.

Interaction

Small increases in serum digoxin concentrations have been noted with flecainide administration. Both flecainide and propranolol concentrations increase mildly with coadministration of both agents. No clinically important interactions have been reported. The concomitant administration of flecainide and a β blocker or calcium channel antagonist can be expected to have additive cardiac depressant effects.

Indications and Dosage

Flecainide is indicated for the treatment of life-threatening ventricular arrhythmias, such as sustained ventricular tachycardia, as well as resistant supraventricular arrhythmias in patients with normal ventricular function. In patients with normal renal and hepatic function, treatment may be begun with 100 mg every 12 h. Dose adjustments should be no larger than 50 mg per dose every 4 days to minimize toxicity. Total daily doses of 200 to 300 mg are associated with efficacy in most patients. Patients with left ventricular dysfunction or a history of ventricular tachycardia should have therapy initiated using smaller dosages with continuous electrocardiographic monitoring in a hospital environment.

Propafenone

Pharmacologic Description

Propafenone hydrochloride, an antiarrhythmic agent structurally similar to β-blocking drugs, was first synthesized in 1970. Commercially available since 1977 in Europe, propafenone is approved in the United States for the treatment of life-threatening ventricular arrhythmias. Propafenone exists as a racemic mixture of D-propafenone and L-propafenone.

Electrophysiologic Action

Propafenone blocks the fast inward sodium current in atrial, ventricular, and His-Purkinje tissue, decreasing the rate of rise of phase 0 of the action potential. The blocking effect is concentration-dependent, with ischemic tissue being more susceptible. In patients with ventricular preexcitation or bypass tracts, propafenone decreases conduction velocity and increases refractoriness of the accessory pathway. Sinus node automaticity may be depressed, especially in the presence of preexisting sinus node dysfunction. Propafenone possesses weak β-adrenergic and calcium channel antagonist activities. Both stereoisomers appear to have equal sodium channel blocking ability, while D-propafenone is responsible for the clinically observed β blockade. Propafenone suppresses delayed afterdepolarizations in ischemic Purkinje fibers. Endocardial pacing thresholds are increased. Electrocardiographic effects include prolongation of the PR and QRS intervals without significant change of the QT interval.

Pharmacokinetics and Metabolism

Absorption of propafenone is almost complete after oral dosing, with peak plasma levels obtained in 2 to 3 h, but extensive first-pass metabolism reduces systemic bioavailability to approximately 12%. The availability appears to vary with the dose, so higher doses have increased bioavailability, probably due to saturation of hepatic microsomal enzymes with larger doses. Seventy-seven to eighty-nine percent of propafenone is protein-bound, with α_1-acid glycoprotein being the major binding protein. The metabolism of propafenone is polymorphic and segregates with the debrisoquin metabolic phenotype. Extensive metabolizers form two major metabolites: 5-hydroxypropafenone and *N*-depropyl-propafenone. Each of these metabolites appears roughly comparable with propafenone in activity. Poor metabolizers have high levels of propafenone and minimal levels of active metabolites. Overall electrophysiologic effects appear similar in both groups given comparable doses, however. Elimination of propafenone is mostly hepatic; less than 1% is recovered intact in the urine. The average elimination half-life ranges from 3.6 to 7.2 h. In patients with hepatic disease, the elimination half-life is prolonged, averaging 14 h. Doses must be decreased in these patients.

Hemodynamic Effects

Propafenone has negative inotropic effects. In several studies, occasional patients with depressed cardiac function have had hemodynamic deterioration. Most patients experience no change in resting left ventricular ejection fraction, although ejection fraction may decrease with exercise. One study using intravenous propafenone (2 mg/kg) showed a slight depression of cardiac index with increased pulmonary vascular resistance but no change in systemic arterial pressure. Thus caution is necessary if propafenone is used in patients with left ventricular dysfunction.

Antiarrhythmic Effects

Propafenone appears effective in treating both supraventricular and ventricular arrhythmias. As other class Ic antiarrhythmic agents, propafenone is effective in suppressing frequent premature ventricular contractions, including complex forms. It is less effective in treating life-threatening ventricular arrhythmias, but even in this difficult population, up to 25% of patients may respond. Propafenone also has been shown to be effective in treating supraventricular tachyarrhythmias, such as atrial fibrillation or flutter, including patients with the Wolff-Parkinson-White syndrome. Propafenone should be used cautiously in patients with recent myocardial infarction in view of the recent CAST findings showing increased mortality in this population when treated with other class Ic drugs (flecainide or encainide).

Side Effects

Approximately 21 to 32% of patients experience adverse reactions to propafenone; 3 to 7% require discontinuation of the medication. Worsening of ventricular arrhythmias was reported to occur in 6.1% of 1579 patients in early clinical trials of propafenone. Patients at highest risk include those with left ventricular dysfunction and those with preexisting sustained ventricular tachycardia. Noncardiac side effects are predominantly gastrointestinal or related to the central nervous system. Dizziness, lightheadedness, nausea, vomiting, or a metallic taste occur most frequently. Central nervous system effects and effects related to β-adrenergic blockade may be more frequent in individuals with a poor metabolizer phenotype.

Interaction

Propafenone in a dose of 300 mg every 8 h orally increases digoxin levels an average of 83%; the magnitude of increase seems related to the dose of propafenone. Significant increases in plasma warfarin concentrations and prothrombin times have been reported. Propafenone concentrations may increase with concomitant cimetidine therapy. Propafenone also decreases metoprolol elimination, resulting in increased β-adrenergic blockade. Quinidine in low doses effectively stops hepatic metabolism of propafenone, converting rapid metabolizers to poor metabolizers. The clinical significance of this interaction is unknown.

Indications and Dosage

Propafenone is approved for the treatment of ventricular arrhythmias. Therapy for both supraventricular and ventricular arrhythmias may be initiated using a dosage of 150 mg three times a day; doses up to 900 mg (occasionally 1200 mg) daily have been used. Intravenous propafenone has been evaluated for supraventricular and ventricular arrhythmias at doses such as 2 mg/kg followed by a maintenance infusion, but this formulation remains investigational in the United States.

CLASS II AGENTS

Class II drugs are β-adrenergic blocking agents. Different β blockers will vary with respect to lipid solubility, membrane-stabilizing effect, relative specificity for the β_1 receptor (cardioselectivity), and partial agonist activity (intrinsic sympathomimetic activity). As a class, β blockers are useful in the treatment of many atrial or AV nodal arrhythmias. In addition, some β blockers may reduce ventricular ectopy. Several β-blocking agents have been shown to reduce mortality when administered after acute myocardial infarction and may be useful as primary or adjunctive agents in some patients with or at risk for life-threatening ventricular tachyarrhythmias. In general, the "cardioprotective" effects of β blockers appear to be proportionately less in β blockers with more marked intrinsic sympathomimetic activity.

Propranolol

Pharmacologic Description

Propranolol hydrochloride is a nonselective β-adrenergic receptor blocking agent. It is indicated in the United States for the treatment of supraventricular and ventricular arrhythmias. Itis also indicated for the treatment of hypertrophic cardiomyopathy, acute myocardial infarction, angina pectoris, hypertension, and numerous noncardiac conditions such as migrane headache and essential tremor.

Electrophysiologic Action

The electrophysiologic effects of propranolol relate primarily to its β-blocking activity, an effect almost entirely mediated by its L stereoisomer. Propranolol is a competitive nonselective β blocker. β_1 Receptors predominate in cardiac tissue, blockade of which produces an increase in the sinus node cycle length and slows AV nodal conduction. At high concentrations, propranolol depresses the inward sodium current in Purkinje fibers, the so-called membrane-stabilizing or quinidine-like effect. This effect generally occurs only at concentrations several times those required for β blockade and thus is probably insignificant clinically. Propranolol can shorten action potential duration acutely in Purkinje fibers and to a lesser extent in atrial and ventricular muscle. With chronic administration, the action potential may lengthen. Electrocardiographic effects include a slowing of sinus rate and an increase in the PR interval with minimal or no changes in QRS and QTc intervals. The effective refractory period is minimally increased.

Pharmacokinetics and Metabolism

Propranolol is almost completely absorbed after oral administration but undergoes extensive first-pass metabolism in the liver resulting in a bioavailability of approximately 30%. Peak clinical effects occur between 60 and 90 min after oral dosing. The average biologic half-life is 4 h. Elimination is hepatic and is proportional to hepatic blood flow. With oral dosing, a total of 160 to 240 mg daily is considered necessary for achieving effective β blockade, although smaller doses are often used in antiarrhythmic regimens. With intravenous dosing, a total dose of 0.2 mg/kg achieves effective β blockade, with activity almost immediately evident.

Hemodynamic Effects

Propranolol is a negative inotropic agent by virtue of its β-blocking action. It may precipitate or worsen congestive heart failure. By blocking β_2 receptors in the peripheral circulation, propranolol may increase vascular resistance.

Antiarrhythmic Effects

Propranolol is an effective agent for the treatment of supraventricular arrhythmias such as atrial tachycardia. Propranolol may help convert atrial fibrillation or flutter of recent origin to sinus rhythm, and it will slow the ventricular response to these arrhythmias. Propranolol may terminate arrhythmias requiring participation of the AV node, such as AV nodal reciprocating tachycardias and those associated with the Wolff-Parkinson-White syndrome and accessory pathways. Propranolol has a variable effect on the rapid ventricular response to atrial fibrillation due to accessory pathway conduction. Propranolol can be effective in treating arrhythmias due to digitalis toxicity, thyrotoxicosis, and anesthesia and as adjunctive therapy for pheochromocytoma. Ventricular premature contractions may be suppressed by propranolol, but it is infrequently effective as a single agent in the treatment of life-threatening ventricular tachyarrhythmias. Propranolol may be more effective in preventing rapid polymorphic ventricular tachycardias or ventricular fibrillation than monomorphic ventricular tachycardia when assessed by electrophysiologic testing. Propranolol can be an effective adjunctive agent in combination with other agents, with caution to avoid additive depressant effects on automaticity, conduction, and contractility. β Blockers also have been used successfully in some patients with congenital QT prolongation and associated ventricular tachyarrhythmias including torsades de pointes. Therapeutic plasma levels for propranolol are highly variable, but often range from 50 to 100 ng/mL.

Side Effects

Common side effects include bradycardia, hypotension, claudication, Raynaud's phenomenon, and AV block. Worsening of heart failure or asthma may occur. Propranolol is lipophilic and easily penetrates the blood-brain barrier, apparently contributing to central nervous system adverse effects such as vivid dreams, insomnia, mental depression, and possibly fatigue and impotence. Insulin-dependent diabetics may be at increased risk for hypoglycemia. Sudden discontinuation of β blockade may worsen angina pectoris and may even precipitate acute myocardial infarction.

Interaction

Negative inotropic drugs such as verapamil or disopyramide should be used cautiously with propranolol in patients with left ventricular dysfunction. Propranolol and verapamil in combination may occasionally precipitate AV block. Antacids containing aluminum hydroxide significantly reduce absorption of propranolol. Phenytoin, phenobarbital, and rifampin accelerate hepatic metabolism of propranolol, resulting in reduced serum concentrations; cimetidine increases serum concentrations of propranolol. Propranolol, by decreasing cardiac output, can reduce the systemic clearance of lidocaine, theophylline, and antipyrine.

Indications and Dosage

Arrhythmic indications for propranolol include supraventricular arrhythmias and arrhythmias associated with thyrotoxicosis or digitalis toxicity, as well as arrhythmias associated with increased catecholamine states. Propranolol may be effective for ventricular ectopy and some ventricular tachyarrhythmias. Propranolol, along with other β-blocking agents, has been shown to reduce cardiovascular mortality for at least 2 to 3 years after acute myocardial infarction. As a class, these drugs are the only antiarrhythmic agents shown to reduce mortality in patients following acute myocardial infarction. Intravenous doses should be given under electrocardiographic monitoring beginning with 0.25 to 1.0 mg using up to 0.2 mg/kg total dose. Oral dosages are highly variable, ranging from 20 to 240 mg daily or more, divided into three or four intervals for antiarrhythmic therapy. Longer-acting preparations may allow once- or twice-daily dosing. Doses of 180 to 240 mg daily in two or three divided doses are recommended to reduce mortality after myocardial infarction.

Acebutolol

Pharmacologic Description

Acebutolol hydrochloride is a relatively cardioselective β_1-adrenergic receptor antagonist with mild intrinsic sympathomimetic activity. It is available in the United States for the treatment of hypertension and ventricular arrhythmias.

Electrophysiologic Action

Electrophysiologic effects of acebutolol predominantly are related to its β_1-receptor blocking activity. At rest, the sinus cycle length increases minimally owing to intrinsic sympathomimetic activity. The sinus response to exercise is markedly blunted, however. Although acebutolol possesses membrane-stabilizing activity (sodium channel blocking ability) in high concentrations, this effect does not appear to be important clinically. Electrocardiographic effects consist of prolongation of the PR interval (AH interval) with minimal, if any, changes in the QTc interval. QRS duration is unchanged.

Pharmacokinetics and Metabolism

Following oral administration, acebutolol is well absorbed from the gastrointestinal tract but undergoes extensive first-pass metabolism, resulting in an absolute bioavailability of 40% (range 20 to 60%). The major metabolite, an *N*-acetyl derivative (diacetolol), is approximately equally active but is more cardioselective than the parent compound. Acebutolol is 26% bound to plasma proteins. Peak plasma concentrations of acebutolol are reached 2.5 h after oral ingestion, whereas peak levels of diacetolol occur at 3.5 h. The elimination half-life of acebutolol is 3 to 4 h, whereas the half-life for diacetolol is 8 to 13 h. Forty percent of acebutolol is eliminated by the kidneys; diacetolol is almost entirely renally excreted. In the presence of renal impairment, plasma concentrations of acebutolol are not significantly changed, but concentrations of diacetolol increase two- to threefold. Therefore, dose reduction is necessary with renal insufficiency. Acebutolol and diacetolol are hydrophilic; therefore, only minimal concentrations of these compounds are found within the central nervous system.

Hemodynamic Effects

As with propranolol, acebutolol decreases heart rate and cardiac contractility. The potential for heart rate slowing is somewhat less with acebutolol owing to its partial agonist activity. Blood pressure reduction typically is proportional to baseline pressure, but hypotension may occur in previously normotensive individuals.

Antiarrhythmic Effects

The β-blocking activity of acebutolol is approximately 25% that of propranolol on a milligram-to-milligram basis. Acebutolol can suppress premature ventricular contractions, including complex forms, in many patients. Patients with exercise-induced arrhythmias may respond favorably to acebutolol. Acebutolol is also effective for various supraventricular arrhythmias, especially those related to excess catecholamine states or those which require participation of the AV node, such as AV nodal and AV reciprocating tachycardias. Acebutolol, similar to other β-blocking drugs with partial agonist activity, is probably less effective than β blockers without this property in reducing mortality when used after myocardial infarction.

Side Effects

Side effects related to acebutolol are similar to those of other β-blocking agents. Patients with congestive heart failure, hypotension, severe peripheral vascular disease, brittle diabetes mellitus, or bronchospastic lung disease should not be treated with acebutolol, despite its partial agonist activity. Similarly, acebutolol may depress sinus node and AV nodal function. Fatigue, headache, reversible mental depression, skin rash, agranulocytosis, development of antinuclear antibodies, alopecia, and Peyronie's disease have been reported.

Interaction

Although specific interactions have not been reported with acebutolol, caution should be used if given with other drugs known to depress automaticity, conduction, or cardiac contractility or other drugs known to interact with β blockers.

Indications and Dosage

Acebutolol is indicated for treatment of ventricular premature contractions. It is also effective for some supraventricular arrhythmias. The initial antiarrhythmic dosage usually is 200 mg twice daily, with total daily doses up to 600 to 1200 mg necessary in some patients.

Esmolol

Pharmacologic Description

Esmolol hydrochloride, a phenoxypropanolamine, is a β_1-selective adrenergic receptor blocking agent. Esmolol is similar in chemical structure to the β blocker metoprolol but contains an ester linkage on the para position of the phenyl ring. Because of this ester linkage, esmolol has an ultrashort plasma half-life of 9 min. It has no appreciable intrinsic sympathomimetic or membrane-stabilizing activity. On a milligram-to-milligram basis, esmolol is approximately 1/50th as potent as propranolol.

Electrophysiologic Action

Electrophysiologic effects of esmolol are those typical of β blockade. Esmolol increases the sinus node cycle length and slows AV nodal conduction. AV nodal refractoriness is increased, as a result of decreased sympathetic tone. Thus esmolol may be effective when used to slow the ventricular response to atrial fibrillation or atrial flutter or when treating arrhythmias requiring participation of the AV node, such as reciprocating tachycardias. Electrocardiographic effects consist of prolongation of the PR interval with no significant changes in QRS or QTc duration.

Pharmacokinetics and Metabolism

Esmolol is rapidly metabolized by hydrolysis of the ester linkage, chiefly by esterases in the cytosol of red blood cells. The distribution half-life of esmolol is 2 min; the elimination half-life is 9 min, necessitating continuous infusion or repeated boluses for sustained effects. Metabolism of esmolol results in a negligible amount of methanol and an acid metabolite. Less than 2% of esmolol is recovered in the urine. The metabolite has about 1/1500th the β-blocking activity of esmolol and is eliminated with a half-life of 3.7 h in individuals with normal renal function. Unlike many other agents with ester groups, metabolism of esmolol is unaffected by plasma cholinesterase. With continuous high-dose infusion of esmolol, levels of methanol approximate endogenous methanol levels, with concentrations reaching only 2% of those associated with methanol toxicity. Esmolol is about 55% bound to plasma proteins, while the acid metabolite is only 10% bound.

Hemodynamic Effects

Esmolol produces a dose-dependent decrease in heart rate, cardiac contractility, cardiac output, and blood pressure. Recovery of these effects is nearly complete within 15 to 30 min after discontinuation of the infusion. In clinical trials, approximately 10 to 30% of patients (particularly those with borderline low or low normal pretreatment blood pressures) treated with esmolol developed transient hypotension, defined as a systolic pressure less than 90 mmHg or a diastolic pressure less than 50 mmHg. Twelve percent of patients were symptomatic.

Antiarrhythmic Effects

Esmolol has been used mainly in acute settings to control the ventricular response to supraventricular arrhythmias. In a multicenter double-blind, randomized study, esmolol was as effective as propranolol, resulting in at least a 20% reduction in ventricular rate in 72% of patients. Conversion to sinus rhythm occurred in 14%. In other studies, esmolol compared favorably with verapamil, with a significantly greater percentage of conversion to sinus rhythm. Esmolol has been shown to be particularly effective (nearly 50%) in converting new onset atrial fibrillation to sinus rhythm in postoperative open heart patients.

Side Effects

The principal side effect of esmolol is hypotension. Other side effects are typical of β blockers and include increased heart failure, dyspnea, bradycardia, decreased peripheral perfusion, nausea, vomiting, irritation at the infusion site, and headache. To avoid phlebitis, esmolol should not be infused using concentrations in excess of 10 mg/mL. For a typical patient requiring 50 to 150 μg/kg per minute, 20 to 60 mL per hour of fluid administration is required, necessitating attention to volume status.

Interaction

Esmolol can be very effective when used in combination with digoxin, and the effects on the AV node are additive. Concomitant administration of esmolol and morphine results in a 46% increase in steady-state levels of esmolol. Esmolol prolongs the metabolism of succinylcholine-induced neuromuscular blockade by 5 to 8 min. Esmolol should be administered with caution in patients prone to bradycardia, AV block, or hypotension or in patients on other medications likely to potentiate these effects.

Indications and Dosage

Esmolol is indicated for the acute management and rapid control of ventricular rate in patients with atrial fibrillation or atrial flutter and in some patients with noncompensatory sinus tachycardia. Therapy is usually initiated with a loading dose of 500 μg/kg per minute over 1 min, followed by a maintenance infusion of 25 to 50 μg/kg per minute. Dose titration can be performed after 5 min and consists of additional boluses of 500 μg/kg per minute over 1 min, followed by an increase in the maintenance infusion by 25 to 50 μg/kg per minute. Most patients are controlled with a maintenance infusion of 50 to 200 μg/kg per minute. Esmolol also may be useful in the management of acute myocardial ischemia or infarction, although this has not been studied extensively. The effects of prolonged infusions of esmolol (longer than 48 h) also have not been fully evaluated.

CLASS III AGENTS

Class III drugs prolong the action potential duration and refractoriness. The effect is often mediated by blockade of potassium channels during phase 2 or 3 of the action potential. Some newer agents prolong action potential duration by activation of sodium channels during the plateau phase.

Bretylium

Pharmacologic Description

Bretylium tosylate is a bromobenzyl quaternary ammonium compound introduced as an antihypertensive agent in 1959. The antiarrhythmic effects of bretylium were described in 1965. Bretylium is available in the United States for the treatment of ventricular fibrillation and ventricular tachycardia.

Electrophysiologic Action

Bretylium increases the action potential duration and effective refractory period of Purkinje fibers, ventricular, and atrial muscle. Thus it is classified as a class III antiarrhythmic agent. Bretylium decreases the disparity of action potential durations between normal and infarcted regions of the heart, possibly contributing to its antifibrillatory effects. Bretylium is concentrated in sympathetic ganglia and postganglionic nerve terminals, where it initially causes then subsequently prevents norepinepherine release. Bretylium does not interfere with the responsiveness of postganglionic adrenergic receptors. Bretylium increases the ventricular fibrillation threshold, and unlike most antiarrhythmic drugs, bretylium decreases the amount of energy required to defibrillate the heart. There is usually little to no effect on impulse conduction, QRS duration, or the AV node in humans.

Pharmacokinetics and Metabolism

Bretylium is erratically absorbed after oral administration (11 to 36% bioavailability) and is appproved only for parenteral use. Bretylium is not bound to plasma proteins and has no known metabolites. Elimination is almost entirely renal, with a half-life of 5 to 10 h. In renal failure patients, the elimination half-life is increased, necessitating a reduction in dose.

Hemodynamic Effects

Bretylium does not appear to depress cardiac contractility in the usual clinical doses. Initially the blood pressure increases, followed by a decrease in pressure due to blocking of the efferent limb of the baroreceptor reflex. Hypotension is most marked when patients are sitting or standing but may occur when supine, especially in volume-depleted patients. Orthostatic hypotension may persist for several days after discontinuing therapy with bretylium.

Antiarrhythmic Effects

Bretylium is effective in the treatment and prevention of life-threatening ventricular tachyarrhythmias. Initial norepinephrine release by bretylium may aggravate certain rhythms, such as those caused by digitalis toxicity or those occurring during acute myocardial infarction. Normally quiescent cells may become automatic. Onset of action after intravenous administration is rapid, but full antiarrhythmic effects may not occur for up to 2 h. In one study, bretylium was shown as effective as lidocaine in the management of out-of-hospital ventricular fibrillation, but since a placebo group was not included in this study, a direct assessment of absolute efficacy was not possible. In one report, bretylium at a dose of 300 to 400 mg delivered over 10 to 20 min defibrillated 10 of 17 patients while cardiopulmonary resuscitation was in progress. Three additional patients were able to be defibrillated by dc shock. Therapeutic concentrations of bretylium have been reported as 0.5 to 1.5 μg/mL.

Side Effects

The most common side effect of bretylium is hypotension, occurring in 50 to 75% of patients, but the fall in arterial pressure is usually mild. Orthostatic hypotension is common; patients receiving bretylium should remain supine. Protryptyline, a secondary amine antidepressant, can reverse bretylium-induced hypotension when given in doses of 5 to 10 mg orally every 6 to 8 h. Nausea and vomiting are common with rapid intravenous infusion of bretylium. Parotid swelling and pain have been reported with chronic oral therapy. Recently, severe hyperthermia (>108°C) has been reported with parenteral injection.

Interaction

Significant interactions have not been reported with bretylium, but experience is limited. Bretylium should be used with caution with other agents that cause hypotension. In addition, bretylium should not be used in patients with fixed cardiac outputs, such as critical aortic stenosis or severe pulmonary hypertension, since severe hypotension may result. Antidepressants such as protryptyline can decrease the hypotensive effects of bretylium.

Indications and Dosage

Bretylium is indicated for the prophylaxis and treatment of ventricular fibrillation. In addition, it may be used acutely for refractory ventricular tachycardia. The initial dose is usually 5 mg/kg administered rapidly. If necessary, this dose may be repeated. If possible, the drug should be diluted and administered over 30 min to minimize nausea. Bretylium may be administered as a continuous maintenance infusion of 1 to 2 mg/min or given as 5 mg/kg infusions every 6 h.

Amiodarone

Pharmacologic Description

Amiodarone hydrochloride, an iodinated benzofuran derivative, was developed initially as a vasodilating agent for the treatment of angina pectoris. Thirty-seven percent of its molecular weight is iodine. It was subsequently found to have potent antiarrhythmic properties in 1970. It has been used extensively for the treatment of supraventricular and ventricular arrhythmias, especially in Argentina, Israel, and Europe. Both oral and intravenous preparations are available in the United States for the treatment of life-threatening ventricular arrhythmias.

Electrophysiologic Action

Amiodarone has been shown to have class I, II, III, and IV effects. It is a weak, noncompetitive inhibitor of α- and β-adrenergic receptors. Its predominant action on cardiac tissue consists of prolongation of action potential duration and increases in refractoriness. Amiodarone has only slight effects on the rate of rise of phase 0 of the action potential. Conduction velocity is decreased, however, apparently owing to effects on resistance to passive current flow rather than effects on the inward sodium current. In automatic cells, amiodarone decreases the slope of phase 4 of the action potential, decreasing the depolarization rate of these cells. Electrocardiographic effects consist of a slowing of the sinus rate, and prolongation of the PR, QRS, and QT intervals. Amiodarone also prolongs the refractory period of accessory AV pathways in patients with bypass tracts or the Wolff-Parkinson-White syndrome. The time course of onset of antiarrhythmic effects varies, with effects on the sinus and AV nodes occurring within 2 weeks of therapy, whereas ventricular functional refractory period prolongation, QT prolongation, and ventricular antiarrhythmic effects are not maximal for up to 10 weeks.

Pharmacokinetics and Metabolism

Administered orally, absorption of amiodarone is slow and erratic. Bioavailability ranges from 22 to 65% in most patients. Peak plasma concentrations occur between 3 and 7 h after a single oral dose. Even with loading doses, maximal antiarrhythmic effects may not appear for several days to months. Amiodarone is 95% protein-bound and has a large but variable volume of distribution of approximately 60 L/kg. Amiodarone and its major metabolite, desethylamiodarone, are highly lipophilic and accumulate throughout the body, including liver, adipose tissue, lung, myocardium, kidney, thyroid, skin, eye, and skeletal muscle. Elimination is principally hepatic via biliary excretion. Enterohepatic recirculation may occur. The elimination of amiodarone is biphasic, with an initial one-half reduction of plasma concentration in 2.5 to 10 days; the terminal elimination half-life is 26 to 107 days, with most patients in the 40- to 55-day range. Desethylamiodarone has an elimination half-life averaging 61 days.

Hemodynamic Effects

With intravenous administration, amiodarone decreases heart rate, myocardial contractility, and systemic vascular resistance. Coronary vasodilatation also may occur. Rapid intravenous administration may produce profound hypotension, partly related to the vehicle Tween-80. Oral amiodarone usually does not worsen congestive heart failure, even in patients with severe left ventricular dysfunction, although caution is warranted, especially with high doses used during drug loading, since some patients may show hemodynamic deterioration.

Antiarrhythmic Effects

A large number of studies have documented the efficacy of amiodarone in suppressing ventricular arrhythmias even when other agents were ineffective. Although effective for many supraventricular arrhythmias, the drug is usually reserved for those patients with life-threatening ventricular tachyarrhythmias who are unresponsive to other antiarrhythmic agents. In a composite of 10 reports from the literature, amiodarone prevented recurrent sustained ventricular tachycardia or ventricular fibrillation in 66% of 567 patients during a mean follow-up of 13 months. The prognostic utility of electrophysiologic testing with amiodarone remains controversial. The ability to induce ventricular tachycardia using programmed ventricular stimulation during therapy with amiodarone does not preclude a good outcome. Patients rendered not inducible by amiodarone have a good outcome. Induction of a hemodynamically well-tolerated ventricular tachyarrhythmia apparently suggests a relatively favorable prognosis. Suppression of ventricular ectopy on ambulatory monitoring by amiodarone is an unreliable indicator of success, whereas failure to suppress ventricular ectopy appears to indicate a worse prognosis. Therapeutic plasma concentrations are usually between 1.0 and 2.0 μg/mL with chronic dosing. Recently, several trials have shown that amiodarone may improve mortality, or at least not worsen mortality, when used to treat patients after myocardial infarction or with left ventricular dysfunction. Whether amiodarone is superior in this regard to conventional β-blocking drugs is unknown. Intravenous amiodarone is at least as effective as bretylium for ventricular tachycardia or ventricular fibrillation and is associated with fewer hemodynamic side effects.

Side Effects

Almost every organ system is affected by amiodarone. Corneal microdeposits of brownish crystals are expected. They may result in blurred vision, halos, or a smokey hue, but reportedly disappear following cessation of therapy. Abnormal thyroid function tests are not uncommon, and in some cases, clinical hypothyroidism or hyperthyroidism becomes evident. A bluish-gray skin discoloration and photosensitivity may occur. Liver function abnormalities, neuropathy, and myositis have been reported. Occasionally severe hepatitis has occurred; two cases of fatal hepatic necrosis have been reported after rapid infusion of large intravenous doses. As many as 5 to 15% of patients treated with 400 mg/day will develop pulmonary toxicity. This usually resolves with discontinuation of therapy, but may be fatal. Therapy with corticosteroids may be beneficial. Cardiac side effects include bradycardia, AV block, worsening of congestive heart failure, and rarely, proarrhythmia. Torsades de pointes occurs only rarely, and a number of patients having this arrhythmia while on other drugs have not had this recur while on amiodarone. Intravenous amiodarone in concentrations of greater than 2.0 mg/mL should be infused only via a central venous catheter owing to a high incidence of peripheral vein phlebitis. Lower concentrations may be infused using a peripheral vein.

Interaction

Amiodarone interacts with many drugs, increasing the plasma concentrations of warfarin (100%), digoxin (70%), quinidine (33%), procainamide (55%), and NAPA (33%). Concentrations of phenytoin and flecainide also have been reported to increase. Appropriate caution should be exercised when using any of these agents along with amiodarone.

Indications and Dosage

The oral and newer intravenous formulations of amiodarone are indicated in the United States for the treatment of recurrent life-threatening ventricular arrhythmias that have not responded adequately to other agents. Because of the large volume of distribution, large loading doses are required initially. Typically, 1000 to 1600 mg is administered daily for 7 to 14 days, followed by 600 to 800 mg daily for the next 7 to 30 days. Long-term maintenance therapy usually requires 200 to 400 mg daily. Doses should be slowly reduced to the lowest level consistent with adequate arrhythmia control, since higher chronic doses are associated with an increased incidence of toxicity. Therapy with intravenous amiodarone is usually initiated with a bolus dose of 150 mg administered over 10 to 15 min, followed by a slower loading dose of 360 mg over 6 h (1mg/min). Maintenance therapy is given at a dose of 0.5 mg/min. Concomitant oral therapy may be started simultaneously. Given the favorable mortality results with amiodarone and its efficacy in treating almost any cardiac arrhythmia, clinical use of amiodarone has increased.

Sotalol

Pharmacologic Description

Sotalol is a nonselective β-adrenergic antagonist introduced in 1965 for the treatment of hypertension. It is without significant intrinsic sympathomimetic activity or membrane-stabilizing activity. Sotalol prolongs the action potential duration, however, accounting for its class III designation. The antiarrhythmic effects in humans were reported in 1970.

Electrophysiologic Action

Electrophysiologic effects of sotalol are those of β blockade and class III activity. Sotalol exists as a racemic mixture of D-sotalol and L-sotalol. The D-sotalol form has about 1/50th the β-blocking activity as L-sotalol, but both are equally responsible for class III effects. Sotalol causes an increase in the action potential duration and refractory period of human atria, ventricles, AV node, Purkinje fibers, and accessory pathways. Conduction velocity is reportedly not decreased by sotalol, except for the β-blocking effects on nodal tissues. Electrocardiographic effects consist of increases in the PR, QT, and QTc intervals. QRS duration and the HV interval are unchanged.

Pharmacokinetics and Metabolism

Sotalol is rapidly absorbed following oral administration, with bioavailability varying from 60 to nearly 100%. Sotalol is not bound to plasma proteins, and more than 75% of an administered dose is recovered unchanged in the urine. No metabolites have been detected. The elimination half-life averages 10 to 15 h, permitting twice-daily dosing. Sotalol will accumulate in patients with renal but not hepatic insufficiency.

Hemodynamic Effects

Prolongation of action potential duration allows more time for calcium ions to enter a cell, potentially increasing the inotropic state of the cell. Sotalol appears unique among β-blocking agents in this regard. Studies in isolated muscle preparations, animals, and humans suggest that sotalol may cause less depression of contractility than other β-blocking drugs. Nevertheless, sotalol can reduce blood pressure and precipitate or worsen congestive heart failure in some patients.

Antiarrhythmic Effects

Sotalol has been used effectively for the treatment of supraventricular and ventricular tachyarrhythmias, including patients with Wolff-Parkinson-White syndrome. Sotalol has been effective in terminating many supraventricular arrhythmias or slowing the ventricular response to atrial fibrillation or flutter. In one study, oral sotalol produced a beneficial response in 31 of 33 patients with atrial arrhythmias. Other studies have found sotalol effective in the treatment of life-threatening ventricular arrhythmias when assessed by electrophysiologic testing, including those refractory to class I antiarrhythmic agents. Polymorphic ventricular tachycardia (torsades de pointes) in the setting of a prolonged QT interval has occurred with sotalol, often in association with either hypokalemia or renal insufficiency (high sotalol levels).

Side Effects

Rates of bronchospasm, fatigue, impotence, depression, and headache are similar to those of other β-blocking drugs. Sinus node slowing, AV block, hypotension, and worsening of congestive heart failure may occur. Rare cases of retroperitoneal fibrosis have been reported. Polymorphic ventricular tachycardia is a potentially life-threatening adverse reaction to sotalol. Its incidence may be minimized by careful attention to electrolyte status, avoiding high serum concentrations or excessive bradycardia. Chronic oral therapy with sotalol can increase the serum level of cholesterol similar to other β blockers without partial agonist activity. The clinical significance of this effect is unknown.

Interaction

Significant drug interactions have not been reported. However, sotalol should be administered with caution with agents that produce hypokalemia or which prolong the QT interval. In addition, sotalol should be used cautiously with drugs that depress cardiac contractility, especially in patients with left ventricular dysfunction and in patients with contraindications to β blockers.

Indications and Dosage

Sotalol is potentially effective for supraventricular and ventricular tachyarrhythmias. Oral therapy is usually begun with 80 mg administered twice daily. Total daily doses greater than 480 mg rarely should be used. Dosage reduction is necessary in patients with mild to moderate renal insufficiency. Sotalol probably should not be used in patients with severe renal insufficiency. Intravenous doses of 0.2 to 1.0 mg/kg have been used in the acute treatment of arrhythmias.

The D stereoisomer of sotalol (D-sotalol) is currently undergoing clinical evaluation in the United States. One trial of D-sotalol found an increased mortality for treated patients after myocardial infarction compared with control patients.

Ibutilide

Pharmacologic Description

Ibutilide fumarate, a new antiarrhythmic agent that prolongs repolarization, was recently approved by the Food and Drug Administration for intravenous use in the United States. Ibutilide is structurally similar to sotalol but is devoid of any clinically significant β-adrenergic blocking activity.

Electrophysiologic Action

Ibutilide affects the action potential duration of atrial, ventricular, and His-Purkinje cells in a unique dose-dependent manner. At low concentrations (10^{-9} to 10^{-7} M), ibutilide prolongs action potential duration, whereas at higher concentrations (10^{-7} to 10^{-5} M), action potential duration decreases. Unlike other class III agents sotalol or *N*-acetylprocainamide, ibutilide prolongs action potential duration by activating an inward sodium current during the plateau phase of the action potential rather than blocking an outward potassium current (I_K). At higher concentrations, ibutilide appears to activate I_K, decreasing action potential duration.

Pharmacokinetics and Metabolism

Ibutilide is well absorbed after oral administration but, like lidocaine, is rapidly metabolized in the liver, such that oral bioavailability is small. Thus oral administration does not appear practical. Ibutilide has a large volume of distribution (10 to 15 L/kg), with a terminal elimination half-life of between 6 and 9 h.

Hemodynamic Effects

No significant effects on cardiac contractility have been seen in animal models. In addition, in preclinical studies to date, ibutilide does not appear to precipitate congestive heart failure, although large numbers of patients, including patients with existing congestive heart failure, have not been exposed to the drug.

Antiarrhythmic Effects

In animal studies and in phase 2 clinical trials, ibutilide has shown efficacy in prevention of induction of ventricular tachycardia during programmed electrical stimulation. Ibutilide appears to decrease the defibrillation threshold in dogs. In human studies, ibutilide has been investigated most extensively for its ability to terminate established atrial flutter or atrial fibrillation. Up to 80% of patients with atrial flutter and approximately 40 to 50% of patients with atrial fibrillation will revert to sinus rhythm with 0.035 mg/kg of ibutilide given intravenously.

Side Effects

To date, the most significant side effect observed in clinical trials of ibutilide is the development of polymorphic ventricular tachycardia (torsades de pointes) that has occasionally become sustained and required cardioversion. Rare episodes of advanced degree AV block and infra-His conduction block have been reported.

Interaction

Interactions of drugs with ibutilide are currently unknown. Agents that reduce hepatic blood flow, such as β blockers, would be expected to increase ibutilide plasma concentrations.

Indications and Dosage

Ibutilide is indicated for the acute treatment (cardioversion) of recent-nset atrial flutter or atrial fibrillation. Patients whose atrial arrhythmias were sustained longer than 90 days were not evaluated in preclinical trials. A dose of 1 mg is administered intravenously over 10 min. After an additional 10 min, the dose may be repeated if needed. Patients weighing under 60 kg should have the dose reduced.

CLASS IV AGENTS

Class IV antiarrhythmic drugs are calcium channel blocking agents.

Verapamil

Pharmacologic Description

Verapamil hydrochloride, a synthetic papaverine derivative, was the first calcium channel blocking agent to be used clinically.

Electrophysiologic Action

The principal electrophysiologic effect of verapamil is inhibition of the slow inward calcium current. Verapamil prolongs the time-dependent recovery of excitability and the effective refractory period of AV nodal fibers. It has little effect on fibers in the lower AV node (NH region) and no effect on atrial or Purkinje action potentials due to the rapid sodium current. Verapamil may be effective in suppressing triggered arrhythmias arising from ventricular or Purkinje tissue, however. Expected electrocardiographic changes consist of prolongation of the PR interval with no significant change in QRS or QT duration. Verapamil also may depress sinus node function (automaticity and conduction), particularly when it is abnormal.

Pharmacokinetics and Metabolism

Verapamil is almost completely (more than 90%) absorbed after oral administration but undergoes extensive first-pass metabolism. Absolute bioavailability ranges from 20 to 35%, with peak plasma levels occurring 1 to 2 h after dosing. Verapamil is 90% bound to plasma proteins. The L isomer of verapamil undergoes more rapid metabolism than the D isomer; the L-verapamil isomer is also more active electrophysiologically. Twelve metabolites of verapamil have been identified; the major one, norverapamil, can reach concentrations equal to the parent compound with chronic dosing. The cardiovascular activity of norverapamil is approximately 20% that of verapamil. After single oral doses, the elimination half-life of verapamil varies from 3 to 7 h; with multiple doses, the half-life ranges from 3 to 12 h. Elimination half-life is usually prolonged with increasing age. In one study, the elimination half-life in patients over the age of 61 years was 7.4 h compared with 3.8 h in individuals under 36 years of age. The elimination of verapamil also may be prolonged in patients with atrial fibrillation or with hepatic dysfunction.

Hemodynamic Effects

Verapamil produces negative inotropic, dromotropic (AV and SA nodes), and chronotropic (SA node) effects. However, it is well tolerated in most individuals, even in those with left ventricular dysfunction. Hypotension, bradycardia, AV block, and asystole have occurred on occasion. Simultaneous use of verapamil with a β blocker may result in significant hypotension and depression of cardiac function. This risk is more pronounced with intravenous administration of verapamil.

Antiarrhythmic Effects

Verapamil will slow the ventricular response with atrial fibrillation and flutter in patients with normal AV conduction. Patients with atrial fibrillation and accessory AV pathways may experience increases in ventricular rate after verapamil administration, related to either a reflex increase in sympathetic tone following vasodilation or decreased AV nodal conduction with less retrograde penetration of the bypass tract. Verapamil can slow and terminate most arrhythmias utilizing the AV node as part of the reentrant circuit, such as AV nodal reentry or AV reciprocating tachycardia using an accessory pathway. Oral verapamil is consistently less effective than intravenous verapamil in terminating these arrhythmias, a difference that may be explained in part by the differences in bioavailability and metabolism of the more active L isomer when the racemic mixture of D- and L-verapamil is given by these two routes. Verapamil can be effective monotherapy for long-term control of ventricular rate in patients with atrial fibrillation or as adjunctive therapy in combination with digoxin. Verapamil is generally ineffective in treating reentrant ventricular tachycardia but may be effective in certain ventricular tachyarrhythmias, usually seen in younger patients, presumedly due to triggered activity. Verapamil also may be used to suppress or reduce the ventricular rate in patients with multifocal atrial tachycardia.

Side Effects

Intravenous verapamil may produce hypotension, bradycardia, AV block, and occasionally, asystole. The risk of hypotension may be lessened by the prior administration of 1000 mg intravenous calcium chloride without interfering with the acute depressant effects of intravenous verapamil on AV nodal conduction. It should be avoided in patients with severe left ventricular dysfunction and in patients with wide QRS tachycardias in which ventricular tachycardia or atrial fibrillation with preexcitation are considerations. Oral therapy is most commonly associated with constipation, but some patients complain of dizziness, fatigue, or ankle edema. Rarely, increases in liver aminotransferases have been observed.

Interaction

Verapamil reduces the clearance of digoxin by 35%, with an increase in serum digoxin concentrations of 50 to 75% within the first week of verapamil therapy. Concomitant administration of verapamil and quinidine may result in significant hypotension, since both drugs antagonize the effects of catecholamines on α-adrenergic receptors. Other drugs with negative inotropic properties, such as disopyramide or flecainide, should be used cautiously with verapamil. Simultaneous administration of β blockers and verapamil may result in hypotension, bradycardia, or AV block. Verapamil appears to variably increase the bioavailability of metoprolol from 0 to 28%.

Indications and Dosage

Verapamil is indicated for the termination of supraventricular tachycardias involving the AV node. It is also indicated to control the ventricular rate in patients with atrial fibrillation or flutter and normal AV conduction. Intravenous doses of 5 to 10 mg given over no fewer than 2 min are often effective. The dose may be repeated if necessary in 30 min. Alternatively, smaller doses (e.g., 2.5 mg) repeated as indicated at more frequent intervals also may be effective. In contrast to β-blocking and certain class I antiarrhythmic agents, verapamil is rarely effective in converting atrial fibrillation or flutter to sinus rhythm. Oral therapy using doses of 160 to 480 mg per day, in three or four divided doses, can be effective for chronic control of ventricular response with atrial fibrillation or prophylaxis of paroxysmal supraventricular tachycardia. Sustained-release preparations may allow once or twice dosing in many patients.

Diltiazem

Pharmacologic Description

Diltiazem hydrochloride is a benzothiazepine derivative that blocks influx of calcium ions during cell depolarization in cardiac and vascular smooth muscle.

Electrophysiologic Action

The principal electrophysiologic effect of diltiazem is inhibition of the slow inward calcium current. It prolongs the time-dependent recovery of excitability and the effective refractory period of AV nodal fibers. Expected electrocardiographic changes consist of prolongation of the PR (AH) interval with no significant change in QRS or QT duration. Diltiazem also may depress sinus node function (automaticity and conduction), particularly when it is abnormal.

Pharmacokinetics and Metabolism

Diltiazem binds to both α_1-acid glycoprotein (40%) and serum albumin (30%). Diltiazem is extensively metabolized in the liver by the cytochrome P450 system. Little diltiazem is renally eliminated. As such, diltiazem doses do not need to be adjusted in the presence of renal insufficiency or failure. The elimination half-life of intravenous diltiazem is approximately 3.4 h.

Hemodynamic Effects

Intravenous diltiazem produces negative inotropic, dromotropic, and chronotropic effects. Administered acutely, diltiazem lowers both systolic and diastolic blood pressure and systemic vascular resistance. Coronary artery vascular resistance also decreases, increasing coronary blood flow.

Antiarrhythmic Effects

Diltiazem increases AV nodal conduction time and increases AV nodal refractoriness. The effects of diltiazem on the AV node demonstrate use dependence, being more pronounced at faster heart rates. In addition, diltiazem slows the rate of depolarization of the sinus node. AV nodal reentry and reciprocating tachycardia may be terminated by direct effects on the AV node. Increased AV nodal refractoriness also slows the ventricular response to atrial fibrillation and atrial flutter.

Side Effects

Hypotension is the most common side effect of diltiazem, occurring in approximately 4.3% of patients in preclinical trials. Although the sinus rate decreases with intravenous diltiazem, sinus bradycardia or high-grade AV block occurs rarely. Elevations of serum aminotransferase enzyme levels occur rarely.

Interaction

Drugs that produce hypotension or interfere with the sinus and AV nodal function would be expected to produce synergistic effects with coadministration of diltiazem. Agents that interfere with or induce the hepatic microsomal enzyme system would be expected to alter diltiazem levels. Diltiazem increases propranolol levels by 50%.

Indications and Dosage

Intravenous diltiazem is indicated for temporary control of rapid ventricular rate associated with supraventricular tachyarrhythmias such as atrial flutter, atrial fibrillation, atrioventricular nodal reentrant tachycardia, or reciprocating tachycardia utilizing an atrioventricular bypass tract. Diltiazem should not be used to treat patients with atrial fibrillation or flutter and atrioventricular bypass tracts. Initial therapy with intravenous diltiazem is usually administered as a bolus dose of 15 to 25 mg (0.25 mg/kg), followed by an infusion of between 5 to 15 mg/h. If ventricular rate control was not achieved after the first bolus, the bolus dose may be repeated in 15 min. An 11 mg/h infusion approximates the steady-state levels achieved with a 360-mg sustained-release preparation of diltiazem. Oral preparations are available in immediate-release tablets of between 30 to 120 mg used every 6 to 8 h and a sustained-release form of between 180 to 300 mg requiring only once-daily dosing. Although effective, oral forms of diltiazem are not approved for treatment of arrhythmias.

NEW AGENTS IN DEVELOPMENT

Dofetilide is a new class III antiarrhythmic agent being evaluated for its intravenous use as a converting agent in patients with atrial fibrillation. Azmilide is an orally active type III antiarrhythmic agent being evaluated for conversion of supraventricular tachyarrhythmias to normal sinus rhythm and for long-term antiarrhythmic maintenance therapy.

Studies with the antiarrhythmic drug bidisomide, a mixed type I orally active antiarrhythmic, were recently discontinued because of its lack of efficacy versus placebo in maintaining normal sinus rhythm in patients with paroxysmal supraventricular arrhythmias.

Ipazalide represents a new class of antiarrhythmic agent that is a member of the 4,5-diphenylpyrazolealkanamide series with both class I and class III properties. It is being developed as a therapy for severe arrhythmias.

UNCLASSIFIED ANTIARRHYTHMIC AGENTS

Adenosine

Pharmacologic Description

Adenosine is an endogenous compound found within every cell of the human body. It is approved by the Food and Drug Administration for use in the United States. Adenosine 5′-triphosphate (ATP), a nucleotide, has been used in Europe since 1929. Adenosine and ATP have short half-lives (less than 10 s), enabling multiple doses without danger of cumulative or long-lasting effects.

Electrophysiologic Action

Adenosine and ATP both exert negative chronotropic and dromotropic effects on the sinus and AV nodes. Both decrease the action potential duration and hyperpolarize atrial myocardial cells. No direct effect on ventricular tissue has been demonstrated; however, catecholamine-enhanced ventricular automaticity may be suppressed by adenosine. The electrophysiologic effects of ATP, and to a lesser extent adenosine, may be mediated in part by a vagal reflex. Electrocardiographic effects consist of slowing of the sinus rate and prolongation of the PR interval.

Pharmacokinetics and Metabolism

Both adenosine and ATP have half-lives less than 10 s. ATP is metabolized to adenosine by extracellular enzymes. Adenosine is degraded by extracellular deaminases as well as by intracellular deaminases after it is rapidly transported into cells, forming inosine.

Hemodynamic Effects

Adenosine and ATP are potent vasodilators that tend to reduce systolic blood pressure. Hemodynamic effects are transient following single-bolus doses of either agent and are usually well tolerated. Adenosine is also a potent coronary artery vasodilator.

Antiarrhythmic Effects

Both adenosine and ATP are extremely effective in terminating supraventricular tachyarrhythmias requiring participation of the AV node, such as AV nodal reentry or AV reciprocating tachycardia in patients with accessory pathways. In one study of 21 patients, ATP (100%) was more effective than verapamil (80%) in terminating paroxysmal AV nodal tachycardia. Compared with verapamil, adenosine may be more likely to unmask latent ventricular preexcitation after termination of AV reentrant tachycardia in patients with Wolff-Parkinson-White syndrome; it also may cause fewer hemodynamically significant arrhythmias after termination of AV reentrant tachycardia. Overall, adenosine has been effective in 60 to more than 90% of patients in different small series, in part reflecting dosing regimens, patient selection, and arrhythmia mechanism. Occasionally, transient atrial fibrillation has been reported following administration of adenosine or ATP, and therefore, caution is warranted in administering these agents to patients with preexcitation. In patients with various atrial tachyarrhythmias, including atrial flutter, adenosine will depress AV nodal conduction, which can be useful diagnostically. ATP and adenosine also can be effective for certain types of ventricular tachycardia in animal models and humans, including catecholamine-sensitive tachyarrhythmias in young adults. Further studies are required to determine the efficacy and utility of adenosine and ATP in the treatment of ventricular tachyarrhythmias, however.

Side Effects

Both adenosine and ATP produce transient flushing and dyspnea following intravenous administration. Additional side effects, apparently more prominent with ATP, include bronchospasm, dyspnea, vomiting, retching, cramps, headache, and rarely, cardiac arrest. The reported difference in side effects may be related in part to the fact that ATP has been in clinical usage for over 50 years, whereas adenosine has been studied for only a short time, but in addition, ATP triggers a more marked vagal reflex. Side effects with either compound are transient, and the potential for long-lasting adverse effects is minimal. Nevertheless, the possibility of profound bradycardia, AV block, or atrial fibrillation, especially in Wolff-Parkinson-White patients with accelerated accessory AV conduction, justifies appropriate caution.

Interaction

Numerous drugs affect adenosine transport or degradation in experimental models, often potentiating the effect of adenosine. Examples include dipyridamole, digitalis, verapamil, and benzodiazepines. Aminophylline and other methylxanthines antagonize the effects of both adenosine and ATP in humans. In one documented case, a patient receiving sustained-release theophylline failed to respond to high-dose adenosine.

Indications and Dosage

Adenosine and ATP are effective agents in the acute management of paroxysmal supraventricular and AV reciprocating tachycardias involving the AV node. Adenosine is usually administered in doses of 3 to 12 mg (3 mg/mL) by rapid intravenous bolus (mean effective dose 80 μg/kg). ATP, which remains investigational in the United States, has been given in doses of 2 to 20 mg. To be maximally effective, these agents must be given as rapid intravenous bolus injections, administered directly in a free-flowing intravenous line; effects are more marked with injection into a central line. Injection into a circuitous peripheral tubing line may be ineffective.

Digitalis

Pharmacologic Description

Digitalis glycosides are among the oldest antiarrhythmic agents still used today. Medicinal use of foxglove (digitalis) was mentioned by Welsh physicians as early as 1250. Used to treat heart failure and arrhythmias in patients in 1775, William Withering described his experiences with digitalis 10 years later in the classic monograph, "An Account of the Foxglove and Some of Its Medical Uses. . . ." Digitalis preparations are steroid glycosides mostly derived from the leaves of common flowering plants *Digitalis purpurea* (digitoxin) and *Digitalis lanata* (digoxin, lanatoside C, and deslanoside). Ouabain, a rapidly acting digitalis preparation, is derived from seeds of *Strophanthus gratus*. Digoxin and to a much lesser extent digitoxin are the most commonly used digitalis preparations.

Electrophysiologic Action

Digitalis glycosides produce electrophysiologic effects by a direct effect on myocardial cells as well as by indirect effects mediated by the autonomic nervous system. Digitalis preparations are specific inhibitors of a magnesium- and ATP-dependent, sodium-potassium ATPase enzyme. Inhibition of this enzyme indirectly promotes an increased concentration of intracellular calcium ions. Increased intracellular calcium results in an increased force of myocardial contraction and also appears to be responsible for many of the arrhythmic effects seen with digitalis toxicity. Indirect effects result from a vagomimetic action and include negative chronotropic and dromotropic (AV node) effects. At toxic levels, digitalis results in increased sympathetic activity. Effective refractory periods of atrial and ventricular muscle generally decrease, while those of the AV node and Purkinje fibers increase. Refractory periods of accessory AV pathways may decrease in some patients, which can increase the rate of AV conduction in these patients with atrial fibrillation. In most individuals, digitalis does not appreciably alter the sinus rate. Sinus rate may slow markedly in patients with heart failure treated with digitalis, however, owing in part to vagal effects and to withdrawal of sympathetic tone. Electrocardiographic effects include prolongation of the PR (AH) interval with various changes in the ST segment and T wave, characteristically with concave coving of downward sloping ST segments.

Pharmacokinetics and Metabolism

Digoxin is 60 to 80% bioavailable when administered orally in tablets. A capsule preparation of digoxin in solution is 90 to 100% bioavailable.

In as many as 10% of patients, intestinal bacteria may degrade up to 40% of digoxin to cardioinactive products such as dihydrodigoxin, resulting in reduced digoxin serum levels. Digoxin is 20 to 25% protein-bound. Elimination is mostly renal, with a half-life averaging 36 to 48 h in normal individuals. Severe renal insufficiency can prolong the elimination half-life up to 4.4 days.

Digitoxin is a less polar glycoside that constitutes the principal active ingredient of the digitalis leaf. Digitoxin is nearly completely bioavailable after oral administration and is approximately 95% bound to serum proteins. Elimination is predominantly hepatic, with an elimination half-life averaging 7 to 9 days.

Hemodynamic Effects

Digitalis produces positive inotropic effects in both normal and failing hearts (see Chapter 8). Cardiac output does not increase in normal individuals, however, owing to counteracting changes in preload and afterload. Digitalis increases arterial and venous tone, increasing systemic vascular resistance. Vascular resistance may increase prior to positive inotropic effects. Thus caution is required when digitalis is administered acutely in patients in whom rises in vascular resistance would be deleterious. Rapid administration increases coronary vascular resistance, an effect that may be avoided by slow administration. In addition, increased mesenteric vascular tone possibly may, on occasion, result in ischemic bowel necrosis.

Antiarrhythmic Effects

Antiarrhythmic effects result predominantly from conduction slowing within the AV node. Thus digitalis is most useful in controlling the ventricular rate in patients with atrial fibrillation. It is somewhat less effective in adequately slowing AV conduction in patients with atrial flutter or atrial tachycardia or in cases where sympathetic tone is high. Addition of a β blocker or calcium channel antagonist such as verapamil or diltiazem typically results in additive electrophysiologic effects. Whether digitalis can reduce the frequency of these arrhythmias or facilitate their conversion to sinus rhythm has not been clearly established. Digitalis also may be effective in the chronic prophylactic or acute management of patients with AV nodal reentrant tachycardia. Therapeutic plasma levels range from 0.8 to 2.0 ng/mL for digoxin and from 14 to 26 ng/mL for digitoxin.

Side Effects

Adverse reactions most commonly involve the heart, central nervous system, and gastrointestinal tract. Hypersensitivity reactions are rare, and gynecomastia occurs infrequently. Patients with abnormal AV nodal function may experience heart block in the absence of toxicity. Digitalis toxicity results in many cardiac and noncardiac manifestations. Noncardiac effects include nausea, vomiting, abdominal pain, headache, and visual disturbances, especially a yellow-green color distortion.

Ventricular premature contractions are perhaps the most common manifestation of cardiac toxicity; however, ventricular tachycardia or fibrillation may occur. In addition, advanced-degree AV block, atrial tachycardia, and accelerated junctional rhythms are seen commonly. Combinations of enhanced automaticity (or triggered activity) with AV block (e.g., paroxysmal atrial tachycardia with AV block) are suggestive of digitalis toxicity. Toxicity may be treated with potassium if serum concentrations of potassium are low or normal, with monitoring to avoid high-grade AV block. Magnesium, lidocaine, propranolol, and temporary cardiac pacing may be helpful in selected cases, when withdrawal of digoxin is not sufficient to resolve toxicity. In some patients with Wolff-Parkinson-White syndrome and accelerated AV conduction, digoxin may shorten the refractory period of the bypass tract, making rapid anomalous conduction more likely if atrial fibrillation occurs.

In cases of severe digoxin or digitoxin toxicity associated with life-threatening ventricular arrhythmias, hyperkalemia, and/or heart block, rapid reversal of toxicity is possible with the administration of ovine digoxin immune antibody binding fragments (Fab). Free levels of digoxin drop to undetectable levels within 1 min of administration, with favorable cardiac effects usually occurring within 30 min. Each vial of antibody fragments (40 mg) will bind approximately 0.6 mg of digoxin or digitoxin. The average dose of Fab used during clinical trials was 10 vials; however, up to 20 vials or more may be necessary in suicidal overdose situations. Antibody fragments are excreted mainly by the kidneys, with an elimination half-life averaging 15 to 20 h in patients with normal renal function. Patients with significant renal insufficiency must be observed closely for the reemergence of digitalis toxicity. The Fab fragments may not be excreted from the body in these patients but rather are degraded by other processes with subsequent liberation of previously bound digitalis.

Interaction

Concomitant administration of quinidine, verapamil, amiodarone, flecainide, or propafenone increases digoxin levels and may precipitate digitalis toxicity. Potassium-depleting diuretics and corticosteroids also may precipitate digitalis toxicity. Antibiotics may increase digoxin absorption by reducing metabolism of digoxin by intestinal bacteria. Antacids and resins such as cholestyramine may reduce digoxin absorption. Concomitant administration of calcium channel antagonists or β blockers may produce heart block when administered with digitalis preparations. Digitoxin metabolism may be enhanced by agents such as phenobarbital and phenytoin that enhance hepatic microsomal enzyme activity.

Indications and Dosage

Digitalis preparations are indicated as antiarrhythmic agents to control the ventricular rate in patients with paroxysmal or chronic atrial fibrillation and in patients with AV nodal reentrant or AV reciprocating. Complete digitalization of an adult typically requires 0.6 to 1.2 mg of digoxin administered in divided doses intravenously or orally; however, differences in bioavailability between preparations must be considered. Maintenance doses of digoxin usually range from 0.125 to 0.25 mg daily but must be substantially reduced in patients with renal insufficiency. When rapid digitalization is not required, therapy may be begun with maintenance therapy, with steady-state levels achieved in approximately 7 days in patients with normal renal function.

Digitoxin may be useful in patients with renal insufficiency, since its metabolism is not dependent on renal excretion. Digitalization may be accomplished by giving 0.2 mg digitoxin orally twice daily for 4 days. Maintenance therapy ranges from 0.1 to 0.3 mg daily.

Electrolytes

Although not traditionally considered antiarrhythmic agents, serum electrolytes can have a profound effect on many cardiac arrhythmias. Alterations in the concentration of sodium, potassium, magnesium, or calcium may exacerbate many cardiac arrhythmias. In some cases, arrhythmias may be entirely due to electrolyte imbalance, and correction of electrolyte imbalance may be all that is required to treat these patients. Electrolyte abnormalities may be particularly arrhythmogenic in the setting of hypoxemia, ischemia, high catecholamine states, cardiac hypertrophy or dilatation, altered pH, and in the presence of digitalis.

During myocardial infarction, hypokalemia increases the risk of ventricular tachycardia and fibrillation. In addition, hypokalemia diminishes the effectiveness of class I antiarrhythmic agents; it also may increase the risk of toxicity or proarrhythmia, especially with class Ia antiarrhythmic agents (torsades de pointes). Arrhythmias due to digitalis toxicity often may be treated successfully with potassium supplementation, provided the serum potassium concentration is not elevated, and with monitoring to avoid high-degree AV block. Hypokalemia, hypoxia, and high catecholamine states also may cause or exacerbate abnormal atrial tachyarrhythmias, especially multifocal atrial tachycardia. In some patients, hypokalemia may be refractory to oral repletion unless concomitant magnesium replacement is undertaken.

Magnesium

Pharmacologic Description

Magnesium is the second most abundant intracellular cation (after potassium). It is involved as a cofactor in many diverse intracellular biochemical processes, including cellular energy production, protein synthesis, DNA synthesis, and maintenance of cellular electrolyte composition (potassium and calcium). All enzymatic reactions involving ATP have an absolute requirement for magnesium. Use of magnesium to treat cardiac arrhythmias was first documented by Zwillinger in 1935. Until recently, its use in the treatment of arrhythmias has been largely ignored, with only occasional case reports published. Magnesium deficiency has become more common with the widespread use of thiazide and loop diuretics.

Electrophysiologic Action

Magnesium effects on the heart may be mediated via direct effects or indirectly via effects on potassium and calcium homeostasis. Magnesium increases the sinus cycle length, slows AV nodal conduction, and slows intraatrial and intraventricular conduction. The effective refractory periods of the atria, AV node, and ventricles increase. Hypomagnesemia often produces opposite effects, such as sinus tachycardia and shortening of effective refractory intervals. Magnesium is essential for the proper functioning of sodium-potassium ATPase; thus magnesium deficiency reduces the ability of a cell to maintain a normal intracellular potassium concentration, producing intracellular hypokalemia. These alterations increase automaticity and excitability while reducing conduction velocity, predisposing to arrhythmogenesis. In addition, magnesium is a physiologic calcium channel antagonist. Electrocardiographic effects of magnesium administration include prolongation of the PR and QRS intervals and a shortening in the QT interval. Magnesium deficiency may produce ST-segment and T-wave abnormalities; occasionally, a prolonged QT interval and U wave are seen. In general, however, hypomagnesemia cannot be recognized with certainty on the ECG, and many of these changes may reflect hypokalemia, which is a commonly associated abnormality.

Pharmacokinetics and Metabolism

Magnesium is mostly contained within bones and soft tissues. Only 1% of total-body magnesium is found in the serum. Thus serum concentrations may not accurately reflect total body magnesium content. Absorption of magnesium occurs in the small bowel, typically beginning within 1 h of ingestion and continuing at a steady rate for 2 to 8 h. The kidney is the principal organ responsible for the maintenance of magnesium homeostasis. In the presence of hypomagnesemia, urinary excretion decreases to less than 1 mEq/day. Parathyroid hormone and vitamin D also may be important in magnesium regulation. In the presence of normal renal function, hypermagnesemia is difficult to maintain.

Hemodynamic Effects

Administration of magnesium may cause an increase in stroke volume and coronary blood flow related to arterial dilatation, which also may result in mild blood pressure reduction. Cardiac output may decrease, however, owing in part to a decrease in heart rate.

Antiarrhythmic Effects

Antiarrhythmic effects of magnesium have been demonstrated for the treatment of both digitalis toxicity and polymorphic ventricular tachycardia associated with a prolonged QT interval (torsades de pointes). Accumulating evidence also suggests that magnesium may be beneficial in the treatment of ventricular fibrillation and ventricular tachycardia. Correction of magnesium deficiency has been shown to reduce the frequency of ventricular ectopy. Administration of magnesium sulfate in doses sufficient to double the serum magnesium concentration (65 mmol/day) significantly reduced the number of deaths and serious ventricular arrhythmias in patients with acute myocardial infarction in one study.

Side Effects

Elevation of serum magnesium concentrations above 2.0 mmol/L often results in symptoms. Progressive increases in magnesium concentration produces hypotension, PR and QRS interval prolongation, and peaked T waves. At concentrations greater than 5.0 mmol/L, areflexia, respiratory paralysis, and cardiac arrest may occur. Hypermagnesemia most commonly occurs in patients with renal insufficiency.

Indications and Dosing

Magnesium may be beneficial in the treatment of many arrhythmias; however, arrhythmias secondary to magnesium deficiency, digitalis toxicity, and torsades de pointes appear especially responsive. Acute treatment of arrhythmias may be accomplished by the administration of 2 g of magnesium sulfate intravenously. If necessary, an additional 2 g may be administered in 5 to 15 min. Doses should be administered over 1 to 2 min. Maintenance infusions may be used, with doses ranging from 3 to 20 mg per minute. Continuous electrocardiographic monitoring is required, and serum magnesium levels should be checked frequently, especially in patients with renal insufficiency. Oral therapy with magnesium chloride (e.g., two to six 500-mg tablets daily) or magnesium oxide (e.g., 400 to 800 mg daily) may be used to prevent or treat diuretic-induced magnesium depletion. Substitution or addition of potassium- and magnesium-sparing diuretics (e.g., spironolactone, amiloride, or triamterene) also may be beneficial.

SUGGESTED READINGS

Cavusoglu E, Frishman WH: Sotalol: A new β-adrenergic blocker for ventricular arrhythmias. *Prog Cardiovasc Dis* 37(6):423, 1995.

Daoud EG, Strickberger SA, Man KC, et al: Preoperative amiodarone as prophylaxis against atrial fibrillation after heart surgery. *N Engl J Med* 337:1785–1791, 1997.

Doval HC, Nul DR, Grancelli HO, et al., for Grupo de Estudio de la Sobrevida en la Insuficiencia Cardiaca en Argentina (GESICA): Randomised trial of low-dose amiodarone in severe congestive heart failure. *Lancet* 344:493, 1994.

Frishman WH, Cavusoglu E: β-Adrenergic blockers and their role in the therapy of arrhythmias, in Podrid PJ, Kowey PR (eds): *Cardiac Arrhythmias—Mechanisms, Diagnosis and Management*. Williams & Wilkins, Baltimore, 1995, pp 421–433.

Greene HL, et al., for the CASCADE investigators: Randomized antiarrhythmic drug therapy in survivors of cardiac arrest (the CASCADE study). *Am J Cardiol* 72: 280, 1993.

Hessen SE, Michelson EL: Antiarrhythmic drugs, in Frishman WH, Sonnenblick EH (eds): *Cardiovascular Pharmacotherapeutics*. New York, McGraw-Hill, 1997, pp 281–321.

Mason JW, for the Electrophysiologic Study versus Electrocardiographic Monitoring (ESVEM) investigators: A comparison of electrophysiologic testing with Holter monitoring to predict antiarrhythmic-drug efficacy for ventricular tachyarrhythmias. *N Engl J Med* 329:445, 1993.

Miura D, Frishman WH, Dangman KH: Class II drugs, in Dangman KH, Miura D (eds): *Electrophysiology and Pharmacology of the Heart*. New York, Marcel Dekker, 1991, pp 665–676.

Singh SN, Fletcher RD, Fisher SG, et al., for the Survival Trial of Antiarrhythmic Therapy in Congestive Heart Failure: Amiodarone in patients with congestive heart failure and asymptomatic ventricular arrhythmia. *N Engl J Med* 333:77, 1995.

Singh BN, Wellens HJJ, Hiroka M (eds): *Electropharmacological Control of Arrhythmias*. Mount Kisco, NY, Futura Publishing, 1994, pp 589–596.

Chapter 13 Antiplatelet and Other Antithrombotic Drugs

William H. Frishman, Michael D. Klein, Ira Blaufarb, Bryan Burns

Remarkable advances have taken place in the management of ischemic heart disease, with innovative antiplatelet, antithrombotic, and thrombolytic therapies leading the list of breakthrough drugs. In this chapter, antiplatelet drugs and antithrombotic drugs are reviewed, focusing on the management of cardiovascular diseases.

ANTIPLATELET DRUGS

The chief function of the blood platelets is to interact with the vascular endothelium and soluble plasma factors in the hemostatic process. Under normal physiologic conditions, platelets are mostly inert; their adhesion to the subendothelial matrix is prevented by an intact vascular wall. In response to vessel trauma, platelets spontaneously adhere to newly exposed adhesive proteins, forming a protective monolayer of cells. Within seconds, these platelets are activated by agonists such as thrombin, collagen, and adenosine diphosphatae (ADP), causing them to change shape and release stored vesicles. The constituents of the vesicles are mostly involved in the further activation of platelets and the propagation of the hemostatic process. Ultimately, these activated platelets aggregate to form a hemostatic plug—closing the lesion in the endothelium and preventing further loss of blood from the site. Under certain pathologic conditions (i.e., rupture of an atherosclerotic plaque), these platelet aggregates can form thrombi associated with multiple cardiovascular ischemic events, including unstable angina and myocardial infarction (MI).

Conventional Antiplatelet Therapy

The efficacy of acetylsalicylic acid, or aspirin, as an antiplatelet agent has been thoroughly investigated, and today it remains the most widely used and cost-efficient drug in the prevention of platelet aggregation. Ticlopidine and clopidogrel, alternative drugs with demonstrated antithrombotic properties in the prevention of strokes, are approved for use in aspirin-sensitive patients; however, their higher cost, additional adverse side effects, and the essentially similar results obtained with aspirin preclude their general use. Until recently, dipyridamole was regarded as an antiplatelet agent, but a significant antithrombotic benefit of the drug when used alone has not been demonstrated.

ASPIRIN

By virtue of aspirin's antiplatelet properties, it has become an essential part of the treatment of ischemic cardiac syndromes. Aspirin diminishes the production of thromboxane A_2 through its ability to irreversibly inhibit the platelet enzyme cyclooxygenase. As a result, platelets exposed to aspirin exhibit diminished aggregebility to thrombogenic stimuli. Aspirin's ability to inhibit cyclooxygenase is impressive, since only 30 mg/day is required to eliminate the production of thromboxane A_2 completely. Since the body's reservoir of platelets is renewed only every 10 days, one dose of aspirin exhibits antithrombotic effects for more than a week. Additionally, there is evidence that aspirin may reduce clotting ability by inhibiting the synthesis of vitamin K–dependent factors, by stimulating fibrinolysis, and by antagonizing the lipooxygenase pathway of arachidonate metabolism in platelets.

In addition to inhibiting platelet cyclooxygenase, aspirin also inhibits the production of prostacyclin by the vascular endothelium. Prostacyclin is a substance that promotes vasodilation and inhibits platelet aggregation. Since its inhibition would theoretically promote thrombosis, it has been postulated that the beneficial effects of aspirin are reduced because of reduced prostacyclin levels. Unlike platelets, however, prostacyclin production recovers within hours after aspirin administration. Various formulations of aspirin have been studied in an attempt to selectively inhibit thromboxane A_2 without inhibiting prostacyclin. It seems, however, that even low doses of conventionally formulated aspirin inhibit them both. Selective inhibition of thromboxane A_2 has been achieved using a low-dose (75 mg), sustained-release aspirin preparation. Platelets in the prehepatic circulation have their cyclooxygenase irreversibly inhibited. Since extensive first-pass metabolism occurs, however, the endothelium in the systemic circulation is exposed to insufficient drug to inhibit prostacyclin production. Whether this will translate into clinical benefit is not known.

Aspirin in Chronic Stable Angina

One arm of the Physician's Health Study examined 383 male physicians with chronic stable angina. The subjects were randomized either to 325 mg of aspirin every other day or to placebo. Treatment was over a 5-year period. No change in symptom frequency or severity was noted between the two groups, however, the occurrence of a first myocardial infarction was reduced by 87% in those treated with aspirin. It seems likely that although there was no change in disease progression (as noted by unchanged symptomatology), the addition of aspirin reduced the risk of thrombosis in the event of plaque instability. This conclusion has been supported by data from Chesebro et al., who noted that the use of aspirin and dipyridamole decreased the incidence of myocardial infarction and new atherosclerotic lesions without affecting the progression of old atherosclerotic plaques.

Unstable Angina

Unstable angina represents the midpoint of the spectrum of ischemic cardiac syndromes that spans chronic stable angina and myocardial infarction. Its pathogenesis lies in the rupture of an intracoronary plaque that promotes platelet aggregation, thrombus formation, and luminal compromise. Theoretically, since aspirin has potent antiplatelet properties, it should be beneficial in the treatment of unstable angina.

Numerous studies have examined the use of aspirin in patients with unstable angina, all of which have shown marked clinical benefit. The Veterans Administration study examined 1384 patients with unstable angina within 48 h of hospital admission. These patients were randomized either to 325 mg of aspirin per day or to placebo for 12 weeks. Death or nonfatal (MI) occurred in 11% of those treated with placebo compared with only 6.3% in the aspirin group ($p < .004$). Although treatment was limited to 12 weeks, 1-year mortality was reduced from 9.6% in the placebo group to 5.5% in those treated with aspirin ($p < .01$). Cairns et al. randomized 555 patients with unstable angina within 8 days of admission either to 325 mg of aspirin four times a day or to placebo. Treatment was for 48 h and nonfatal MI or cardiac death was reduced from 14.7 to 10.5% in those treated with aspirin ($p < .07$). Similarly, total mortality was reduced from 10% with placebo to 5.8% in the aspirin group ($p < .04$). Theroux et al. randomized 479 patients with unstable angina to 325 mg of aspirin two times per day or to placebo. The patients were enrolled on presentation to the hospital and were treated for 3 to 9 days. Nonfatal MI was reduced from 6.4% in the placebo group to 2.5% in those treated with aspirin ($p < .04$). Finally, the RISC study investigated the effects of a reduced dose of aspirin in unstable angina. In the aspirin-versus-placebo arm it enrolled 388 patients to receive either 75 mg of aspirin or placebo for 3 months. This study demonstrated a reduction in the rate of nonfatal MI or noncardiac death from 17% in the placebo group to 7.4% in those treated with aspirin ($p = .0042$).

It is clear from the preceding studies that aspirin is effective at reducing the morbidity and mortality of unstable angina with and without heparin. Specifically, nonfatal MI and cardiac death were reduced by 50 to 70%. This benefit seemed to occur across a broad spectrum of daily doses, from 1300 mg/day in the study by Cairns, to only 75 mg/day in the RISC trial. Since platelets are exquisitely sensitive to aspirin, this finding is not unexpected.

Primary Prevention of Myocardial Infarction

As mentioned earlier, most of myocardial infarctions are caused by the rupture of an intracoronary atheromatous plaque. This exposes subendothelial collagen to local blood products, which results in the attraction and activation of platelets. These activated platelets release growth factors and vasoactive compounds that produce vasoconstriction, further platelet aggregation, and ultimately the formation of an occlusive mural thrombus.

Although aspirin was shown to improve outcomes in patients with unstable angina, its benefit in primary prevention of myocardial infarction was largely unknown until the results of the U.S. Physicians' Health Study were reported. In this study, 22,071 male U.S. physicians were randomized either to 325 mg of aspirin every other day or to placebo. Ninety-eight percent of those involved were free of cardiac-related symptoms, and treatment took place over a 5-year period. Although the frequency of angina, coronary revascularization, or death was unchanged between the two groups, the incidence of myocardial infarction was impressively reduced in the aspirin-treated group. Specifically, the risk of fatal or nonfatal myocardial infarction was reduced by 44% ($p < .00001$).

The observations made in the U.S. Physicians' Health Study were challenged by a similar study from Europe. The British Physicians' Health Study was an uncontrolled trial that involved 5139 British male physicians, two-thirds of whom were treated with 500 mg of aspirin per day. In contrast to the U.S. study, there was no significant reduction in myocardial infarction or total mortality. Criticisms of this trial were many and included its uncontrolled design, its smaller sample size, the higher dose of aspirin, its older subjects with poorer compliance, and its high confidence intervals. Its results, however, were sufficient to cast some doubt on aspirin's utility in the primary prevention of myocardial infarction.

Any doubts as to aspirin's role in the primary prevention of myocardial infarction were largely put to rest by a large observational study of U.S. nurses' aspirin usage. In this study, aspirin usage by 87,000 U.S. nurses was analyzed over a 6-year period. All the nurses involved were free of cardiac-related symptoms. The study showed that in women over the age of 50 years, ingestion of one to six 325-mg tablets of aspirin per week was associated with a 32% reduction in first myocardial infarction ($p = .005$). This benefit was most striking in women with risk factors for coronary artery disease including tobacco use, hypercholesterolemia, and hypertension. In women who took more than seven tablets per week, however, there was no reduction in the rate of myocardial infarction. In addition, women who took more than 15 tablets per week were at a significantly increased risk of hemorrhagic stroke.

It appears from the preceding studies that 325 mg of aspirin every other day is effective at preventing a first myocardial infarction in asymptomatic individuals. The benefit of aspirin is most pronounced in patients who are at high risk for coronary artery disease, specifically older individuals with multiple cardiac risk factors. Higher doses of aspirin do not appear to confer any additional benefit and most likely impart additional risk of developing hemorrhagic stroke.

Secondary Prevention of Myocardial Infarction

There have been seven prospective, randomized, placebo-controlled trials examining the use of aspirin in the secondary prevention of myocardial infarction. As a cumulative total, these studies have enrolled over 15,000 survivors of MI whose treatment has consisted of various aspirin regimens, with doses ranging from 325 to 1500 mg/day. Patients were enrolled from 4 weeks to 5 years after MI. When each of these trials was examined individually, no statistically significant decrease in mortality was observed. Since the numbers of patients in each study may have been too small to provide adequate statistical power, a metaanalysis of six of these trials was performed. This metaanalysis contained 10,703 patients and showed that when aspirin was compared with placebo, cardiovascular morbidity was reduced by 21% ($p < .0001$). Cardiovascular mortality was similarly reduced by 16% ($p < .01$), as was total mortality ($p < .03$). In another metaanalysis from the Antiplatelet Trialists Collaboration, the risk of developing a nonfatal reinfarction was shown to be reduced by 31% ($p < .0001$), and death from vascular causes was reduced by 13% ($p < .005$) in those patients treated with aspirin during the 1- to 4-year follow-up period. Finally, in a 23-month follow-up of 931 patients with acute infarction or unstable angina, 80% of subjects were found to use aspirin on a regular basis. Their cardiac death rate was markedly reduced (1 to 6%) compared with nonaspirin users (5.4%) and was not explicable by imbalances in predictors of postinfarction risk, by concurrent drug therapy, or by preinfarction thrombolysis or angioplasty.

In addition to the cardiac benefits demonstrated by the preceding studies, aspirin also seems to reduce the risk of stroke in post-MI patients. In a subset of the Antiplatelet Trialists Collaboration, the risk of stroke in those patients treated with aspirin was examined. A 42% reduction in nonfatal strokes in the aspirin group ($p < .0001$) was demonstrated as compared with placebo. With these results in mind, treatment of post-MI patients with low-dose aspirin (perhaps 75 mg/day) seems reasonable. Although many of the preceding trials relied on pooled data and metaanalysis to demonstrate aspirin's benefit in the post-MI population, the data are compelling to that effect. Aspirin does not appear to increase the risk of nonfatal cerebrovascular accident (CVA) and will most likely reduce the risk of future cardiac events. The optimal dose of aspirin for long-term postinfarction prophylaxis is unclear at this time and will need to be determined with future studies.

Acute Myocardial Infarction

Localized coronary thrombosis due to the rupture of an unstable intracoronary atheromatous plaque is thought to be responsible for more than 90% of Q-wave myocardial infarctions. Although thrombolytic agents break down the primary clot responsible for the acute event, substances liberated during this process can themselves promote platelet aggregation and reocclusion. Although spontaneous recanalization may occur, thrombus re-formation is common and may perpetuate the ischemic process. By virtue of aspirin's potent antiplatelet properties, it has been shown to be an effective agent when used either alone or with thrombolytic agents at reducing the mortality from acute myocardial infarctions.

The Second International Study of Infarct Survival (ISIS-2) was a double-blind, placebo-controlled trial that defined aspirin's role in the treatment of acute myocardial infarction. ISIS-2 enrolled 17,187 patients with suspected acute myocardial infarction and randomized them to either IV streptokinase (1.5 million units over 60 min), aspirin (162 mg/day for 1 month), both, or neither. Five weeks after randomization, aspirin reduced the risk of nonfatal reinfarction by 51% and of vascular mortality by 23% when compared with placebo. The addition of IV streptokinase further reduced mortality in conjunction with aspirin. The study results indicated that aspirin reduced mortality to a similar degree as did streptokinase alone and that when the two were combined, a cumulative benefit was observed. Aspirin's reduction in mortality also extended to groups treated with various heparin dosages, ranging from no heparin (288 versus 347 deaths), to SQ heparin (338 versus 431 deaths), to IV heparin (178 versus 238 deaths; $p < .001$). Mortality benefits were similar in both men and women and remained present after 24 months of follow-up. Importantly, treatment with aspirin did not result in any increased incidence of major bleeds (31 versus 33 bleeds) and seemed to decrease the risk of nonfatal CVA by 46% ($p = .003$). It seems clear that aspirin, with or without thrombolytic therapy, is effective at reducing the mortality and morbidity of an evolving myocardial infarction.

Non-Q-wave MI results when an intracoronary occlusion is incomplete or occurs for only a short time. The pathophysiology of a non-Q-wave MI is similar to both unstable angina and to Q-wave-MI in that a ruptured atheromatous plaque results in acute intracoronary thrombus formation. Although it seems likely that aspirin would confer a benefit in evolving non-Q-wave myocardial infarctions, no adequate trials have been performed to date in this subgroup of patients.

Percutaneous Transluminal Coronary Angioplasty and Arterial Stenting

When percutaneous transluminal coronary angioplasty is performed, the intracoronary atheromatous plaque that is acted on is "cracked" or "fissured" by the destructive action of balloon inflation. This results in the exposure of underlying subendothelial collagen to circulating blood products, which activates platelets and promotes thrombogenesis. It has been shown that the magnitude of platelet deposition after angioplasty is related to the depth of arterial injury and that in animals, pretreatment with aspirin reduces the degree of thrombus formation.

There have been two randomized, prospective trials that have evaluated the role of aspirin in preventing abrupt closure after angioplasty. In these studies, aspirin (650 to 990 mg/day) and dipyridamole (225 mg/day) were started 24 h before angioplasty and continued indefinitely. They demonstrated that the incidence of abrupt closure was significantly reduced when compared with placebo. In another trial by Barnathan et al., it was noted that when the coronary angiograms of patients undergoing angioplasty were analyzed retrospectively, the incidence of coronary thrombosis was significantly lower in those patients treated with aspirin or aspirin plus dipyridamole. Finally, although aspirin does appear to lower the risk of acute thrombosis after angioplasty, it has not been shown to affect the rate of late restenosis. With regard to coronary artery stenting, aspirin remains an important prophylactic treatment in preventing acute thrombosis especially in combination with ticlopidine.

Coronary Artery Bypass Surgery

In coronary artery bypass grafting (CABG) surgery, native coronary arteries whose blood flow is compromised by atherosclerotic blockages are "bypassed" using either venous or arterial conduits. The arterial conduit usually consists of either the left or right internal mammary arteries, and the venous conduit is usually a reversed saphenous vein from the leg. Although this surgery is one of the mainstays of treatment for coronary artery disease, occlusion of the bypass vessels either acutely or over time is not uncommon. It has been noted, for example, that 40 to 50% of saphenous vein grafts occlude within 10 years of their implantation. Reasons for graft occlusion vary with the age of the conduit. *Acute* closure (less than 1 month after placement) is usually due to thrombosis, whereas *intermediate* closure (1 month to 1 year) is caused by accelerated intimal hyperplasia. Finally, *late* occlusion (greater than 1 year) results from atherosclerosis within the bypass graft.

Multiple studies have demonstrated a decreased incidence of early thrombosis when aspirin is used in the perioperative period. Goldman et al. randomized 50 groups of CABG patients to receive either (1) aspirin, 325 mg per day; (2) aspirin, 325 mg three times per day (tid); (3) aspirin, 325 mg tid, and dipyridamole, 75 mg tid; (4) sulfinpyrazone, 267 mg tid; or (5) placebo. This study demonstrated a significantly decreased risk of early thrombosis in all groups treated with aspirin [73% graft patency with placebo at 2 months versus 93% with acetylsalicylic acid (ASA); $p < .05$]. The addition of dipyridamole resulted in no additional benefit, and sulfinpyrazone was ineffective at reducing the risk of thrombosis. Although those patients treated with aspirin had increased blood loss and need for reoperation, perioperative mortality was unchanged. The benefits noted in this study remained present after 1 year of follow-up.

Aspirin, therefore, should be given to all patients undergoing bypass surgery, unless a clear contraindication exists. A dose of 325 mg/day is probably reasonable, since higher doses do not add any additional clinical benefit. The medication ideally should be started preoperatively or within 48 h postoperatively if preoperative administration is not possible.

Transient Ischemia Attack and Stroke

The capacity of aspirin in doses of 50 to 1500 mg/day either alone or in combination with other antiplatelet agents (dipyridamole, sulfinpyrazone) to reduce the risk of recurrent cerebrovascular events has been studied in 10 trials involving about 8000 patients with stroke or transient ischemic attacks (TIAs). Based on these studies, treatment of 1000 patients with aspirin for 3 years reduces fatal and nonfatal cardiovascular events, including recurrent CVA, by about one-fourth. Optimal daily dose of aspirin for secondary prophylaxis in cerebrovascular disease remains somewhat controversial, but doses between 300 and 1200 mg/day are the recommended dose range.

Atrial Fibrillation

Aspirin has been used to reduce the hazard of thromboembolic stroke in nonvalvular atrial fibrillation (NVAF) and compared with the efficacy of warfarin. Data from randomized trials support aspirin use for thromboembolism prophylaxis in younger NVAF patients (<60 years), especially in the absence of associated risk factors of hypertension, recent congestive heart failure, or remote thromboembolism. A slightly greater hazard for intracranial bleeding with warfarin might make aspirin a suitable alternative to warfarin in selected other patients. An ongoing clinical trial (SPAF III) is evaluating the relative efficacy and safety of aspirin as an adjunct to low-intensity fixed-dose warfarin in preventing thromboembolism in high-risk NVAF patients.

Adverse Effects

The most common side effect of aspirin treatment is gastrointestinal (GI) intolerance. In the Aspirin Myocardial Infarction Study, where patients with known peptic ulcer disease (PUD) were excluded, 24% of those treated with aspirin (1000 mg/day) reported GI intolerance compared with 15% in the placebo group. In the United Kingdom TIA Trial, GI symptoms were reduced by 30% when the dose of aspirin was decreased from 1200 to 300 mg/day. Finally, in the Physicians' Health Study (patients with known PUD were excluded), 325 mg of aspirin every other day resulted in only a 0.5% increase in GI symptoms when compared with placebo. GI intolerance due to aspirin therefore appears to occur in a dose-dependent manner, and treatment with 325 mg/day appears to be well tolerated. Recently, two forms of cyclooxygenase enzymes have been identified, one that produces the "good" prostaglandins that act in the stomach and other tissues (COX-1) and another (COX-2) that is involved in thromboxane formation. Agents are in development to inhibit COX-2 while sparing COX-1, which could provide a stomach-sparing aspirin. Bleeding complications are a common side effect of aspirin therapy. Specifically, the risk of developing a hemorrhagic event such as bruising, melena, and epistaxis are all increased with aspirin use. The Physicians' Health Study confirmed this by reporting that 27% of those treated with aspirin (325 mg every other day) experienced bleeding complications as compared with only 20% in the placebo group ($p < .0001$). In the United Kingdom TIA Trial, there was a significant increase in the risk of GI bleeding when the dose of aspirin was increased to 1200 mg/day. For these reasons, the risks and benefits of aspirin therapy need to be weighed against one another in patients who are at increased risk of bleeding. Furthermore, the dose of aspirin utilized should be as low as possible, since higher doses do not appear to confer additional benefits but do increase bleeding risk substantially.

DIPYRIDAMOLE

Dipyridamole is a pyramidopyrimidine compound that can act as both a vasodilator and an antithrombotic. The drug acts to inhibit platelet action in vitro only at doses higher than those commonly used in patients, but it has been clinically effective in reducing platelet adherence to prosthetic surfaces in vivo at lower doses when combined with other agents. A number of mechanisms for its antiplatelet activity have been proposed, including either the inhibition of phosphodiesterase or the indirect activation of adenylate cyclase through its effects on prostacyclin and/or the inhibition of adenosine uptake by the vascular endothelium. The exact mechanism of action still requires further definition, though the common pathway involves elevated levels of intraplatelet cyclic adenosine monophosphate, a platelet inhibitory substance. The usual dose of dipyridamole is 400 mg/day in three to four divided doses, and it is eliminated by the hepatobiliary system. It is also used as a provocative agent in patients undergoing diagnostic testing for coronary artery disease.

Clinical Studies

Its primary use in humans has been as an adjunct to anticoagulant therapy in the prevention of thromboembolic events in patients with prosthetic heart valves. While current American College of Chest Physicians' recommendations do not include dipyridamole as a first-line therapy in a patient with prosthetic heart valves, it has been shown to be a useful adjunct to anticoagulant therapy. It is recommended as part of the therapy in patients with a prosthesis-related thromboembolic event, especially in those patients with peptic ulcer disease, in whom aspirin may need to be avoided. Dipyridamole has not been associated with an excess of hemorrhage when combined with anticoagulant therapy. Dipyridamole also has been used as part of the therapy for patients with prosthetic grafts. Both experimental and clinical evidence suggests a superiority of an aspirin-dipyridamole combination to either drug used alone in terms of both platelet survival and graft patency.

Controlled trials comparing aspirin to dipyridamole in patients with stable angina are few. The limited data suggest no statistically significant difference between aspirin and dipyridamole used together as compared with aspirin alone. No trial has shown a definitive superiority of combination therapy over aspirin alone in either stable coronary disease, graft survival after coronary artery bypass, or the need for emergency revascularization after angioplasty.

Adverse Effects

The primary side effects of dipyridamole are gastrointestinal and consist of nausea and vomiting. In rare cases, angina has been provoked through what is believed to be a coronary steal phenomenon.

TICLOPIDINE

Ticlopidine is a thienopyridine compound that acts by blocking ADP receptors within the platelet membrane and acts independently of arachidonic acid pathways. Ticlopidine produces a thrombasthenia-like state with a resulting reduction in platelet aggregation, a prolongation of the bleeding time, a decrease in platelet granule release, and a reduction in platelet and fibrin deposition on artificial surfaces.

Clinical Trials

Cerebrovascular and Peripheral Vascular Disease

Ticlopidine has been tested thoroughly in the prevention of cerebrovascular disease. When compared with placebo in 1000 patients, as part of a study in secondary prevention after stroke, the administration of ticlopidine resulted in a 30% reduction in the relative risk of stroke, myocardial infarction, or vascular death. When compared with aspirin in the TASS study, ticlopidine was found to be superior in terms of all-cause mortality as well as nonfatal stroke. This benefit persisted throughout the 5-year duration of the trial.

In patients with peripheral vascular disease and claudication, treatment with ticlopidine was associated with a reduction in mortality, myocardial infarction, and cerebrovascular events. Patients with cerebrovascular and peripheral vascular disease appear to benefit from ticlopidine therapy in terms of stroke, myocardial infarction, and vascular events.

Cardiovascular Disease

Ticlopidine has been used in the therapy of patients after coronary artery bypass grafting. In a randomized trial involving 173 patients, ticlopidine therapy resulted in a reduction in vein graft closure at 1 year as compared with placebo. When used in the therapy of patients with electrocardiographic evidence of unstable coronary syndromes, the addition of ticlopidine to standard therapy was associated with a reduction in vascular death and nonfatal myocardial infarction as well as the composite end point of both fatal and nonfatal myocardial infarction. In those patients who undergo coronary stent implantation, ticlopidine and aspirin have demonstrated a superiority over anticoagulant therapy with heparin and phenprocoumon.

Adverse Events

Neutropenia can occur in up to 4% of patients receiving ticlopidine. It is generally reversible, although cases of agranulocytosis have been reported. It is recommended that during the first 2 months of therapy white blood cell counts should be checked. The most common side effects of the medication are gastrointestinal, occurring in about 12% of patients, and include nausea, vomiting, diarrhea, and dyspepsia. Lastly, a rash has been reported within the first 3 months of ticlopidine treatment.

CLOPIDOGREL

Clopidogrel is a thienopyridine antiplatelet drug in the same class as ticlopidine. Similar to ticlopidine, clopidogrel is a prodrug that is not active in vitro but active in vivo. It functions as an ADP-selective agent whose antiaggregating properties are several times higher than those of ticlopidine and are apparently due to the same mechanism of action (i.e., inhibition of ADP binding to its platelet receptor and triggering the release of thrombogenic factor–containing alpha granules). After a single oral or intravenous administration, clopidogrel inhibited ADP-induced platelet aggregation for several days and potently reduced thrombus formation in various experimental animal models.

Clopidogrel has been evaluated in a large phase III clinical trial, CAPRIE (Clopidogrel versus Aspirin in Patients at Risk of Ischemic Events), a randomized, blind clinical study comparing clopidogrel, 75 mg/day, with aspirin, 325 mg/day, in 19,000 patients who have suffered a recent ischemic stroke or myocardial infarction or who have symptomatic atherosclerotic peripheral vascular disease. A preliminary report from the study showed a more favorable effect on clinical outcomes with clopidogrel compared with aspirin and clopidogrel was approved by the FDA for clinical use.

THE GP IIb/IIIa INTEGRIN GLYCOPROTEIN RECEPTOR ANTAGONISTS

Platelet aggregation is mediated by the GP IIb/IIIa receptor, a member of the integrin superfamily of membrane-bound adhesion molecules. Integrins are defined as subunit receptors composed of an α subunit (i.e., GP IIb) and a β subunit (i.e., GP IIIa) capable of mediating adhesive interactions between cells or matrix. Although integrins are distributed widely throughout the vasculature, where they are expressed on endothelial, smooth-muscle cells and leukocytes, expression of the GP IIb/IIIa integrin is restricted to platelets. It is the chief receptor responsible for platelet aggregation by its ability to find soluble fibrinogen that forms bridges between platelets and leads ultimately to thrombus formation. GP IIb/IIIa is widely distributed on platelet surfaces (approximately 50,000 per cell) but remains unable to bind fibrinogen unless the platelet is first stimulated by agonists (such as ADP, thrombin, arachidonic acid) and undergoes a conformational change. It is believed that the adhesive binding pocket is somehow hidden until platelet activation, although this process is still unclear. Although fibrinogen is the peptide that mediates aggregation, mostly because of the large concentration of fibrinogen in plasma, GP IIb/IIIa is also capable of binding von Willebrand factor, fibronectin, and vitronectin. It has been demonstrated that aggregation can be supported by von Willebrand factor in the absence of fibrinogen. Therefore, these molecules also may play a role in aggregation at high shear rates, such as is found in the coronary arteries.

GP IIb/IIIa, a heterodimer of two subunits, was the first integrin to be identified and has served as a model for characterization of other integrins. It has been demonstrated by electron microscopy that the receptor is composed of a globular head and two flexible tails embedded in the platelet membrane. The GP IIb subunit has calcium-binding sites that have homology with calmodulin. In the presence of the calcium chelating agent ethylenediamine tetraacetic acid, the receptor function is lost and the integrin dissociates into its two individual subunits. Each subunit contains a portion of the head and a single tail.

The GP IIb/IIIa domains responsible for binding adhesive proteins have been identified and in general are characterized by their ability to recognize the peptide sequence RGD. The RGD recognition sequence was originally described for fibronectin but is now known to be present in fibrinogen, von Willebrand factor, vitronectin, and thrombospondin. Fibrinogen is a symmetric protein composed of two α chains, two β chains, and two γ chains. Both of its RGD sequences are located on the α chain at residues 95–97 and 572–574. Fibrinogen also contains a 12-amino-acid residue that possesses the ability to bind to the GP IIb/IIIa receptor. This dodecapeptide (HHLGGAKQAGDV) is located at 400 to 411 on the fibrinogen γ chain. It has been proposed that the RGD residues and the dodecapeptide competitively bind to GP IIb/IIIa. By initiating a conformational change in the receptor after binding, one recognition sequence on fibrinogen renders the other sequence inaccessible for binding. This alteration in receptor shape may be a self-regulatory mechanism of the GP IIb/IIIa receptor.

If two activated platelets with functional GP IIb/IIIa each bind to the same fibrinogen molecule, a fibrinogen bridge is created between the two platelets. When this process of aggregation is repeated thousands of times, a thrombus forms. Experiments have indicated that the RGD peptides bind to the GP IIIa subunit at residues 109 to 171. In contrast, the dodecapeptide binds to the GP IIb subunit at 294–314. Genetic defects in either of these two subunits can lead to the rare hemostatic disorder of Glanzmann's thrombasthenia. Patients with Glanzmann's thrombasthenia usually have a bleeding disorder during childhood. Although they have a normal platelet count, GP IIb/IIIa is either nonfunctional or absent. Platelet aggregation, in response to agonists such as thrombin, ADP, or arachidonic acid, is therefore completely absent.

The two subunits of GP IIb/IIIa are encoded by separate genes on the long arm of chromosome 17. Although each subunit is synthesized separately, the receptor heterodimer must be assembled within the megakaryocyte for either subunit to be expressed. Therefore, if there is a defect in GP IIb, GP IIIa is not expressed at the platelet surface, and the thrombasthenic phenotype results. Specific defects in GP IIb/IIIa subunit genes have been reported. A single point mutation that substituted tyrosine for aspartic acid within the RGD-binding domain of the GP IIIa gene has led to nonfunctional GP IIb/IIIa. A base-pair deletion in GP IIIa that resulted in a frame-shift mutation also has caused severe Glanzmann's thrombasthenia in a group of Iraqi Jewish patients. The severity of this disorder has helped to highlight the role GP IIb/IIIa plays in thrombus development during normal hemostasis.

GP IIb/IIIa Antagonists as Antiplatelet Agents

As discussed earlier in this chapter, aspirin is the most common antiplatelet drug in use today. It is a relatively weak drug, effective against only one of the many platelet activators, thromboxane A_2. Other drugs such as ticlopidine and hirudin, effective against ADP and thrombin, respectively, also are limited because of the platelet's ability to be activated by multiple agonists. Many patients with vascular disease take the current antiplatelet drugs and still sustain thromboembolic complications that often develop into ischemic conditions. Of importance, therefore, is the development of more effective antiplatelet agents. A drug able to inhibit platelet activation in response to all endogenous agonists would constitute a more effective therapy.

The binding of fibrinogen to activated platelets has been identified as the final step in platelet aggregation, and this binding is completely mediated by GP IIb/IIIa. Therefore, expression of the GP IIb/IIIa integrin is the final common pathway for platelet aggregation by *all* agonists. GP IIb/IIIa also is unique to platelets and is the most abundant platelet surface glycoprotein. These factors make GP IIb/IIIa an extremely favorable target for therapeutic pharmacologic blockade. A drug that could block the binding of fibrinogen to GP IIb/IIIa theoretically could abolish thrombosis resulting from vessel damage or atherosclerotic plaque rupture, regardless of the platelets' degree of activation. Discussed next are two potential therapeutic GP IIb/IIIa antagonists: monoclonal antibodies to the GP IIb/IIIa receptor and synthetic peptide and nonpeptide receptor antagonists capable of blocking fibrinogen binding to platelets.

Murine Monoclonal Antibodies

Many recent studies using the monoclonal antibody 7E3 against GP IIb/IIIa have shown it to be a highly effective antithrombotic agent, specifically in preventing arterial thrombi, in both canines and primates, including human beings. To eliminate the binding of fibrinogen to activated platelets, large doses of 7E3 must be given to block GP IIb/IIIa receptor function effectively on all circulating platelets. However, by blocking all GP IIb/IIIa receptors and consequently inhibiting platelet aggregation, the risk of concurrent hemorrhage is increased. This bleeding risk is increased when combining antiplatelet therapy with invasive treatments such as coronary angioplasty or bypass surgery.

The results of a larger study demonstrated the effectiveness of 7E3 in the prevention of postangioplasty restenosis. The Evaluation of 7E3 for the Prevention of Ischemic Complications (EPIC) highlighted the importance of the GP IIb/IIIa receptor in abrupt vessel closure after high-risk coronary angioplasty and atherectomy. A random population (2099 patients) scheduled to undergo these procedures received either a bolus and infusion of placebo, a bolus of 0.25 mg/kg 7E3 and a 12-h infusion of placebo, or a bolus and infusion of 7E3. Results were measured as the risk of experiencing a composite primary end point (which included death, nonfatal MI, or unplanned invasive revascularization procedures) by 30 days. Data indicated that compared with those given placebo, patients who received the bolus and infusion of 7E3 had a 35% risk reduction in the composite-event rate. Patients who received only a 0.25 mg/kg bolus of 7E3 (and placebo infusion) still showed a 10% reduction in the risk of experiencing a primary end point. On the basis of the results of the EPIC trial and other pharmacologic studies, the 7E3 antibody (ReoPro; Centocor, Malvane, PA) received a favorable review by the U.S. Food and Drug Administration Cardiovascular and Renal Drugs Advisory Committee and was approved for use in patients undergoing high-risk angioplasty. In addition, during a 6-month follow-up, the number of ischemic events was reduced by 26% in patients who received the 7E3 antibody, suggesting a long-term benefit against clinical coronary artery stenosis.

Although these results demonstrate the importance of pharmacologic blockade of GP IIb/IIIa as therapy for ischemic events, the use of Abciximab (7E3 monoclonal antibodies) results in several negative complications. In 14% of the patients in the EPIC trial who received both the 7E3 bolus and infusion, a significant amount of bleeding, twice the number of major bleeding episodes than the placebo group, occurred and often required transfusion. The bleeding usually occurred at the site of vascular puncture in the groin. The increased bleeding time is compounded because the antibodies are inherently long-lived and do not dissociate from platelets during the platelets' survival time in the plasma. Thus the inhibitory effect on systemic platelet aggregation is nonreversible and may last several days. This situation may prove to be deleterious for patients with unstable conditions that may require unplanned invasive procedures. Last, the use of large doses of monoclonal antibodies would stimulate the proliferation of neutralizing antibodies and, therefore may restrict 7E3 therapy to a single use. Despite these complications, the positive results obtained by monoclonal antibody blockade of GP IIb/IIIa receptors have furthered the development of high-affinity synthetic peptide antagonists.

The EPILOG trial (Evaluation of PTCA to Improve Longterm Outcomes by 7E3 GPIIb/IIIa Receptor Blockade Trial) evaluated the use of both high- and low-risk PTCA with 7E3. The original study design called for the enrollment of 4800 patients who were to be randomized to either placebo and high-dose heparin (ACT >300), 7E3 and high-dose heparin, or 7E3 and low-dose heparin (ACT 225–250). The trial was double-blind and placebo-controlled, with an interim analysis to be done after 1500 patients. After the interim analysis, the study was terminated prematurely for several reasons. In those patients treated with 7E3, a three-time decrease in creatine phosphokinase (CPK) levels was noted as well as a 68% reduction in the combined end point of MI and death ($p < .0001$). Additionally, in contrast to the results from the EPIC trial, bleeding complications in the 7E3 and low-dose heparin group were not significantly different from those with placebo (<2% with treatment, 3.1% placebo). These reductions in the rate of bleeding complications may have been due to the use of early sheath removal in the EPILOG trial.

Finally, the use of Abciximab (7E3) in patients who developed unstable angina with ECG changes before scheduled PTCA was evaluated in the CAPTURE trial (Chimeric c7E3 Antiplatelet Therapy in Unstable

Angina Refractory to Standard Therapy). In this trial, patients who were scheduled for PTCA the following day and who developed unstable angina and ECG changes the night before were randomized to standard therapy with or without 7E3. The medication was continued into the PTCA the next day; 1200 patients were to be enrolled. The trial was stopped prematurely after only 1050 patients because of strongly favorable results in those treated with 7E3. Specifically, the primary end points of MI, death, and recurrent PTCA were reduced from 16.4 to 10.8% in the treatment group. Additionally, the incidence of MI was reduced from 9.4 to 4.9%, and the secondary end points of emergent CABG, repeat PTCA, and emergent stent placement were all significantly reduced in those patients who received c7E3. No increased risk of intracranial bleeding was noted, although the incidence of major bleeding was increased from 1.7 to 2.8%.

Synthetic Peptide and Nonpeptide Antagonists

As an alternative to monoclonal antibodies, researchers have been attempting to develop small synthetic peptides with the ability to block fibrinogen from binding to the GP IIb/IIIa platelet receptor. The goal has been to create a peptide with the same affinity and specificity exhibited by monoclonal antibodies but without the negative side effects of prolonged bleeding time, immunogenicity, and irreversibility. In many cases, the synthetic peptides were modeled on the "disintegrin" or natural antiplatelet antagonists but were smaller and therefore less immunogenic. Using the RGD-binding sequence found in circulating adhesive proteins, researchers have developed a series of modified RGD analogues capable of binding to GP IIb/IIIa. One modification has included the addition of disulfide bonds for the creation of cyclic peptides. The cyclic conformation not only has rendered the peptides more stable in plasma but also has imparted a higher affinity for the integrin receptor. A more recent modification has been to substitute lysine (K) in the RGD sequence for arginine (R). This substitution creates a peptide similar to the disintegrin barbourin (discussed earlier in this chapter), which has absolute specificity for GP IIb/IIIa integrin. Recently a novel peptide, Integrelin (eptifibatide), was approved as a new platelet inhibitor for use after PTCA.

CONCLUSION

Antiplatelet therapy has proved to be effective treatment for patients with coronary and cerebral vascular diseases. Aspirin has proved effective in reducing mortality risk in survivors of acute MI, and aspirin and ticlopdine are useful in preventing strokes in persons at high risk. Most recently, the development of monoclonal antibodies and peptide and nonpeptide compounds that bind to the GP IIb/IIIa receptor in activated platelets has shown great potential for treating patients undergoing coronary angioplasty to prevent short- and long-term complications and for treating patients with unstable angina and myocardial infarction.

OTHER ANTICOAGULANTS

In this section the anticoagulant drugs heparin and warfarin are reviewed, along with a discussion of a new heparinoid, danaparoid.

Heparin

Mechanisms of Action

Heparin, a glycosaminoglycan, is composed of alternating residues of D-glucosamine, a uronic acid. Its principal anticoagulant effect depends on a pentasaccharide with high-affinity binding to antithrombin III (AT-III). Heparin catalyzes the inactivation of thrombin by AT-III (Fig. 13-1) by providing a template to which both thrombin (factor IIa) and the naturally occurring serine protease inhibitor AT-III can bind. Additionally, heparin catalyzes thrombin inactivation via a specific pathway involving heparin cofactor II, a mechanism requiring higher heparin doses but not involving the AT-III-binding pentasaccharide. In contradistinction to direct thrombin inhibitors, which impede thrombin activity, heparin indirectly inhibits not only thrombin activity but also thrombin generation; the heparin–AT-III complex also inhibits other anticoagulation proteases, including factors IXa, Xa, XIa, and XIIa.

The molecular weight of heparin ranges from 5000 to 30,000, with a mean value of 15,000, containing an average of approximately 50 saccharide chains. Heparin's pharmacokinetic properties in anticoagulant activity are heterogeneous for several reasons: Its plasma clearance is influenced by molecular size, with larger molecules being cleared more rapidly than smaller species, resulting in an increased antifactor Xa to antifactor IIa (thrombin) activity ratio; anticoagulant activity of heparin is also influenced by molecular chain length; only about one-third of standard heparin molecules in clinical usage are sufficiently long (containing >18 saccharides) to possess AT-III–mediated anticoagulant action.

Pharmacokinetics

Since it is not absorbed orally, heparin is given either subcutaneously or intravenously. When given in sufficient doses, the safety and efficacy of both routes are comparable for treating venous thrombosis, if the reduced bioavailability of subcutaneous heparin is taken into account. At clinically therapeutic doses, a substantial proportion of heparin is cleared via the dose-dependent rapid pathway. Hence the anticoagulant response to heparin is not linear but increases dispro-

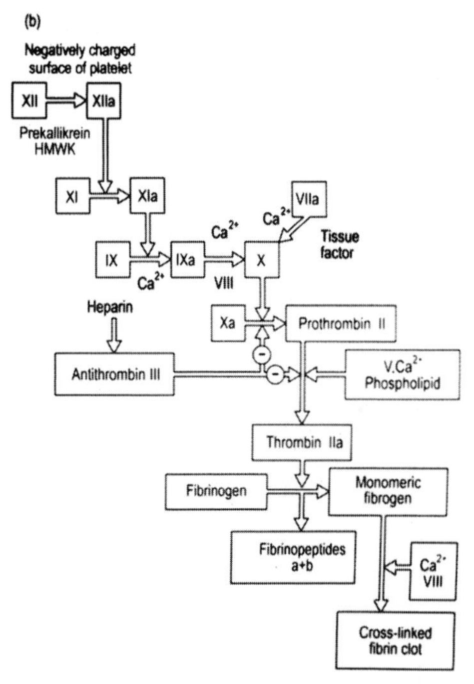

FIG. 13-1 Antithrombin III inactivates factors Xa and thrombin (IIa). This effect is enhanced by heparin.

portionately in both intensity and duration with larger heparin doses. The apparently biologic half-life of heparin increases from 30 to 60 to 150 min after bolus intravenous doses of 25, 100, and 400 U/kg, respectively.

Pharmacodynamics

The intensity of heparin anticoagulant effect is monitored by the activated partial thromboplastin time (APTT) test, which is sensitive to both antithrombin (antifactor IIa) and antifactor IXa and Xa effects. Experimental data have suggested than an APTT of 1.5 times control could prevent venous thrombus extension. When heparin is used clinically, however, consideration must be given to (1) interpatient variability in plasma and tissue binding, which alters heparin pharmacokinetics; (2) potential increases in factor VIII (occurring as part of an acute-phase reaction in seriously ill patients), which can blunt the APTT response to a given heparin level; and (3) variable potency of commercially employed APTT reagents. It has been recommended that the therapeutic range for each APTT reagent be calibrated to be the equivalent to a heparin level of 0.2 to 0.4 U/mL by protamine titration or to an antifactor Xa level of about 0.3 to 0.7 U/mL.

Clinical Usage—Venous Thrombosis

Randomized clinical trials have established the efficacy of heparin usage in venous thrombosis. Heparin should be given in an initial intravenous bolus of 5000 U followed by at least 30,000 U every 24 h by continuous infusion, with additional heparin dose adjustments to maintain a therapeutic APTT range. Heparin's effectiveness is dependent on using an adequate starting dose and maintenance infusion, which produce an adequate anticoagulant effect, measured either by APTT or by heparin levels, provided that the heparin level is >0.3 U/mL antifactor Xa activity.

Orthopedic and General Surgery

Heparin has been recommended for routine usage in the prevention of venous thromboembolism, especially in surgical patients undergoing elective hip or knee repair or replacement who are at high risk for perioperative venous thrombosis and pulmonary embolism. The prevalence of venous thromboembolism following total knee or hip replacement surgery has been summarized as between 45 and 84% and that following hip fracture surgery as being 36 to 60%, with a corresponding pulmonary embolism rate of 2 to 30% and 4 to 24%, respectively. A metaanalysis comparing the efficacy of low-molecular-weight heparin (LMWH) to low-dose unfractionated heparin (LDUH) indicated that LMWH was more effective in suppressing venous thromboembolism.

Elective neurosurgery and acute spinal cord injury patients also have a high risk for venous thromboembolism, averaging 24%. Though there has been concern regarding intracranial or intraspinal bleeding, recent studies have demonstrated the efficacy and safety of both LDUH and LMWH prophylaxis.

Acute Myocardial Infarction

Heparin has been used in acute myocardial infarction (AMI) patients to prevent venous thromboembolism, mural thrombosis, and systemic embolism. Among AMI patients not treated with antithrombotic agents, the incidence of deep vein thrombosis (DVT) is about 24%. Subcutaneous LDUH in doses of 5000 to 7500 U bid and high-dose intravenous heparin, 40,000 U/day, have been found to reduce DVT without adverse bleeding events. In the contemporary AMI patient, heparin anticoagulation has become a mainstay of treatment, coupled with aspirin as an antiplatelet therapy. In acute coronary syndromes, it has been used to reduce the frequency of unstable angina. It also has become a standard adjunct to thrombolytic drugs despite definitive proof of its efficacy, where it is used either concurrently with the tissue plasminogen activator (tPA) or anisoylated plasminogen streptokinase activator complex (APSAK) or subsequent to streptokinase, thereby minimizing thrombolytic drug activation of the coagulation system during fibrinolysis. The increased plasmin generated during fibrinolytic drug therapy mediates both platelet activation and plasmin-mediated prothrombinase activity, requiring ancillary antithrombotic drug treatment.

However, studies examining the efficacy of heparin therapy in the treatment of myocardial infarction in the thrombolytic era are few, and a brief historical perspective is therefore appropriate. The SCATI study examined 711 patients randomized to receive either subcutaneous heparin or no heparin as part of the therapy for myocardial infarction. Approximately half the patients received thrombolytic therapy with streptokinase. In the heparin plus thrombolytic group and the heparin alone group a reduction in mortality associated with heparin was noted. In addition, a trend toward a reduction in the number of postinfarction ischemic episodes was noted in those patients who received thrombolytic therapy plus heparin. Heparin therapy was clearly shown to be an effective either alone or as an adjunct to thrombolytic therapy in the treatment of acute myocardial infarction. In a larger trial, the GISSI-2 study, subcutaneous heparin therapy was not associated with a statistically significant difference in mortality, reinfarction, or unstable angina. It did, however, highlight an excess of bleeding. The International Study Group (which incorporated some of the GISSI-2 data) examined 20,891 patients who underwent thrombolytic therapy with either APSAC or streptokinase. The group that received subcutaneous heparin experienced an excess of bleeding episodes without the benefit of a reduction in reinfarction or stroke. In addition, the Third International Study of Infarct Survival examined 41,300 patients treated with thrombolytic therapy. The addition to aspirin of heparin resulted in an excess of transfused or major bleeding, with only a trend toward a reduction in reinfarction and with no differences in mortality or stroke. However, a metaanalysis of the data from the ISIS and GISSI trial supports a decrease in mortality during the treatment period. This mortality benefit came at the expense of increased bleeding. Taken together with a review of prior data on the use of heparin as adjuvent therapy for myocardial infarction published in 1985, heparin did not appear to significantly influence the rates of reinfarction or death.

A few trials using heparin have demonstrated an improved patency of the infarct-related artery up to 3 days after thrombolysis for acute myocardial infarction. The HART study, in which 205 patients received tPA plus either heparin or aspirin, demonstrated improved 18-h patency of the infarct-related artery associated with heparin therapy. There were no significant differences among the two groups in terms of patency at

7 days or in terms of hemorrhagic events. Examination of the data from either the TAMI or the GUSTO trial did not demonstrate an effect of heparin on mortality, reinfarction, major hemorrhage, infarct-related artery patency, or reocclusion. These angiographic trials highlight the fact that heparin may improve coronary patency in some patients, with improvement being greatest in those patients not treated or undertreated with aspirin.

In all, the data available with heparin as adjunctive therapy for myocardial infarction do not support its routine use with streptokinase. Anticoagulant therapy should be reserved for use in those patients who are at higher risk for further events, specifically those patients with atrial fibrillation, heart failure, or those who have suffered a large myocardial infarction. The data regarding the use of heparin with tPA are even more limited. However, the short duration of activity, the more specific fibrinolytic effect, and the angiographic data lend some support to its use with tPA

Randomized clinical trials have compared the effectiveness of intravenous heparin (an indirect thrombin inhibitor) with intravenous hirudin (a direct thrombin antagonist). In TIMI-9B, heparin (5000 U and 1000 U/h) and hirudin (0.1 mg/kg and 0.1 mg/kg per hour) were found to be equally effective and have similar major hemorrhagic side effects (4 to 5%) when used as adjuncts to tPA or streptokinase in preventing unsatisfactory thrombotic outcomes in AMI patients.

Dosing

Several methods for optimizing intravenous heparin dose adjustments have been developed. These nomograms have been utilized for the treatment of both venous thromboembolism and AMI patients. A weight-based heparin nomogram has been recommended in the treatment guidelines for unstable angina. Such algorithms are convenient to use, have been successful in achieving therapeutic APTT levels in an expeditious manner, and have demonstrated a reduction in thromboembolism.

Side Effects

Bleeding is the major side effect associated with heparin use and is in part a function of the drug's complex pharmacokinetics, its use in severely ill patients who are often on other antithrombotic or fibrinolytic agents, and the numerous other actions of heparin on a variety of processes besides anticoagulation.

Of special concern, however, is heparin-induced thrombocytopenia (HIT). Two mechanisms for HIT have been elucidated, an early reversible nonimmune thrombocytopenia, possibly related to weak platelet activation, and a late serious immune thrombocytopenia with IgG-mediated platelet activation in thrombotic complications. Immune-related HIT was seen in 1 and 3% of patients receiving LDUH for 7 and 14 days, respectively, but was not observed with LMWH. When present, HIT becomes manifest 5 to 15 days after initiating heparin therapy but may arise within hours in patients previously exposed to heparin within the prior 3 to 6 months. In vitro studies have suggested that LMWH can crossreact to activate platelets in serum from HIT patients.

Low-Molecular-Weight Heparins

Background

Low-molecular-weight heparins (LMWHs) are fragments of commercial-grade standard heparin produced by enzymatic or chemical depolymerization with a resultant molecular weight of 4000 to 6500 (Table 13-1). Since smaller heparin molecules (MW < 400) are not able to bind to thrombin (factor II) and antithrombin III (AT-III) simultaneously, LMWH has a diminished ability to accelerate the inactivation of thrombin by AT-III. However, LMWH retains its ability to catalyze the inhibition of factor Xa by AT-III. Therefore, as contrasted with standard heparin (average molecular weight 12,000 to 15,000) with an anti-Xa/anti-IIa inhibitory ratio of 1:1, commercial LMWHs have anti-Xa/anti-IIa ratios of 2:1 to 4:1 when tested in vitro. The persistence of anti-IIa activity by LMWH emanates from the larger oligosaccharide chains in its polydispersed spectrum.

Other properties that distinguish LMWH from standard heparin include lack of inhibition of activity by platelet factor IV (PF4), a potent inhibitor of standard heparin release during coagulation, persistence of inactivation of Xa bound to platelet membranes in the prothrombinase complex, a feature lacking in standard heparin, and lack of binding LMWH by plasma proteins, histidine-rich glycoprotein, fibronectin, vitronectin, and von Willebrand factor as opposed to the plasma binding of standard heparin, which partially neutralizes its anti-Xa inhibition.

Those features of LMWH that distinguished it from standard heparin can result in the following clinical advantages: (1) a more predictable

TABLE 13-1 Low-Molecular-Weight-Heparins

Generic name	Brand name	Mean and range molecular weight	Anti-Xa to anti-IIa ratio	Plasma half-life, min
Ardeparin	Normiflo	5000		
Certroparin	Sandoparin	6000 (5000–10,000)	2.0/1.0	270
Dalteparin*	Fragmin	5000 (2000–9000)	2.0/1.0	119–139
Enoxaparin*	Lovenox	4500 (3000–8000)	2.7/1.0	129–180
Naroparin	Fraxiparine	4500 (2000–8000)	3.2/1.0	132–162
Parnaparin	Flaxum	—	—	—
Reviparin	Clivarine	3900 (2000–4500)	5.0/1.0	—
Tinzaparin	Logiparin	4500 (3000–6000)	1.9/1.0	111

*FDA approved.

dose response with patient variability to a fixed dose, (2) a long half-life and reduced bleeding for equivalent antithrombotic effects, and (3) enhanced safety and efficacy in the treatment of patients with venous thrombosis.

Clinical Trials

A metaanalysis of the relevant randomized clinical trials comparing unfractionated heparin (UFH) with LMWH examined total mortality, pulmonary embolism mortality, rates of recurrent venous thromboembolism (RVTE), change in venography scores, and incidence of bleeding. LMWH significantly reduced short-term and pulmonary embolism mortality while causing less major bleeding as contrasted with UFH. Longer-term mortality and serious bleeding rates were influenced by case mix and efficacy of subsequent oral anticoagulation but were still favorably influenced by LMWH as compared with UFH with a relative risk of .30 (95% CI, .3 to .4; $p = .0006$) for mortality and 0.42 (95% CI .2 to .9; $p < .01$) for major bleeding. Further data favoring the safety of LMWH versus UFH were seen in a study of 3809 patients undergoing major abdominal surgery with heparin prophylaxis for 5 days or more perioperatively. Four-week incidence of major bleeding was reduced from 141 to 93% ($p < .058$) and moved hematoma from 2.7 to 1.4% by LMWH compared with UFH.

Unstable Angina

The use of antithrombotic agents for unstable angina, a process that results from platelet aggregation and thrombus formation, has been well studied. Gurfinkel et al. in a prospective, single-blind, randomized trial of patients with unstable angina, compared the effects of naroparin calcium, an LMWH (214 IU/kg anti-Xa SQ bid), and ASA versus UFH and ASA (200 mg/day) versus ASA (200 mg/day) alone in 211 patients. Primary outcomes were recurrent angina, acute MI, urgent revascularization, major bleeding, and death. There was a significant benefit with the use of LMWH and ASA versus UFH and ASA in the rate of recurrent angina, 21 versus 44%, respectively.

FRISC (Fragmin during Instability with CAD) is a multicenter study that randomized 1506 patients with unstable angina to LMWH (120 IU/kg SQ q 12 h) up to day 6 and then 7500 U qid at home until day 40 or placebo. At day 6, differences between the LMWH and placebo groups in the occurrence of new MI and were 1.8 and 4.7% for death and 7.8 and 13.9% for severe angina, respectively. The benefit continued at day 40. By day 150 no differences were noted between the two groups. Another multicenter, randomized study, FRIC, enrolled 1482 patients with unstable angina. Patients were randomized to unfractionated heparin (5000-U IV bolus, 1000 U/h infusion, then 1250 U SQ bid) versus LMWH (120 IU/kg q12h). Therapy was continued for

6 weeks. The initial data at 7 days indicate that there were no differences between groups in death, MI, urgent revascularization, non-Q-wave MI, or unstable angina.

In a recent study of thrombolytic therapy with enoxaparin plus aspirin versus unfractionated heparin plus aspirin, enoxaparin plus aspirin was more effective in reducing the incidence of ischemic events in patients with unstable angina or non-Q-wave myocardial infarctions in the early stage.

Leclerc et al. compared the use of the LMWH enoxaparin with placebo in patients undergoing knee replacement. The incidence of distal and proximal DVT in the placebo group was 45 and 20%. The LMWH group had only a 19% incidence of distal DVT and no proximal DVT. In a recent randomized, double-blind trial by Leclerc, enoxaparin and warfarin were compared. Patients undergoing knee replacement were randomized to enoxaparin (30 mg SQ q12 h) or warfarin (dose-adjusted to keep INR between 2.0 and 3.0). The primary end point was the incidence of DVT as per bilateral venography. The secondary end point was the incidence of hemorrhage. The incidence of DVT was 36.9% for the enoxaparin group and 51.7% for the warfarin group. There was no difference in the incidence of major bleeding, 1.8 versus 2.1%, respectively, or proximal DVT.

Other studies have been done, comparing LMWH to warfarin in patients undergoing knee arthroplasty. All but one of the studies also show that fixed-dose LMWH is more effective than adjusted-dose warfarin in preventing DVT postoperatively.

Acute Proximal Deep Vein Thrombosis

Acute proximal deep vein thrombosis has been associated with the risk of pulmonary embolism and recurrent thromboembolism. Management of this condition traditionally has required a hospitalization of 5 to 7 days for treatment with unfractionated heparin and initiation of oral anticoagulation with warfarin. Two recent studies compared the use of low-molecular-weight heparin in the outpatient setting to unfractionated heparin in hospital for the treatment of proximal DVT. Levine et al. randomized 253 patients to receive UFH intravenously and 247 patients to receive LMWH (enoxaprin 1 mg/kg SQ bid) for the management of acute proximal DVT. There was no statistically significant difference in recurrent thromboembolism or major bleeding between the two groups. There was a major difference in the average length of hospitalization, 1.1 days for the LMWH group and 6.5 days for the UFH group.

Danaparoid

The low-molecular-weight heparinoid danaparoid sodium is a mixture of sulfated glycosaminoglycans of porcine origin. Danaparoid consists of heparan sulfate ($\approx$84%), dermatan sulfate ($\approx$12%), and a small amount of chondroitin sulfate (≈4%). The drug has been approved by the FDA for prophylaxis of postoperative DVT in patients undergoing elective hip replacement surgery. In contrast to LMWHs, which have an 80% to 90% incidence of cross-reactivity in heparin-induced thrombocytopenia (HIT), danaparoid has a cross-reactivity rate of about 10%. Although danaparoid is effective for total DVT prophylaxis, it does not offer a significant advantage over comparators for prophylaxis of the more clinically important proximal DVT. For this reason, its high cost prohibits routine use for this indication. It is, however, a useful option in patients who have documented HIT and still require anticoagulation.

Warfarin

Mechanism of Action

Warfarin is a vitamin K antagonist that blocks the cyclic interconversion of vitamin K_{H2} and its 2,3 epoxide by inhibiting two regulatory enzymes, vitamin K epoxide reductase and vitamin K reductase. Vitamin K_{H2} is an essential cofactor for the carboxylation of glutamate residues on N-terminal portions of inactive coagulant proenzymes (factors II, VII, IX, X) in a reaction that is catalyzed by a vitamin K–dependent carboxylase. Since Y carboxylation of vitamin K–dependent coagulation enzymes is a requisite step in their ability to bind metals, undergo conformational changes, bind to cofactors, and become activated, warfarin impedes the activity of these essential ingredients in the coagulation pathway.

Pharmacokinetics

Warfarin, a racemic mixture of *R* and *S* isoforms, undergoes rapid and extensive GI absorption, reaching maximal plasma concentrations in 90 min. In the blood, it has a half-life of 36 to 42 h and is extensively bound to plasma proteins, principally albumin. Only about 1 to 3% of warfarin circulates in the free state, but it rapidly accumulates in the liver, where it is metabolized microsomally to inactive catabolites, the *R* isomers to warfarin alcohols and excreted in the urine and the *S* isomers oxidized and eliminated via the bile. Numerous drugs and disease entities that alter warfarin absorption, plasma protein binding, liver microsomal activity, or basal vitamin K levels can increase or decrease warfarin anticoagulant intensity. Since many of these agents may be prescribed concurrently with warfarin, adjustment in the daily anticoagulant dose will be necessary to avoid inadequate or excessive anticoagulation. A dietary inventory, including all drug and vitamin supplementation, is equally important; massive amounts of dietary vitamin K, which can increase warfarin resistance; dietary vitamin K deficiency; malabsorption problems; liquid paraffin laxatives; hypocholesterolemic bile binding resins, which can reduce warfarin absorption or increase warfarin excretion; and large doses of vitamin E, which are used as an antioxidant can antagonize vitamin K action. Moreover, variations in dose-response to warfarin can occur during extended periods of anticoagulation, variations that may have one or several patient, medication, or laboratory sources.

Laboratory Monitoring of Warfarin

Historically, the most commonly used test to monitor warfarin anticoagulation has been the prothrombin time. This test is sensitive to reduced activity of factors II, VII, and X but not to reduced activity of factor IX. Interpretation of the prothrombin time results, while satisfactory for individual patient measurement, has been complicated, however, because thromboplastin reagents in standard usage vary in their sensitivity to the reduction of vitamin K–dependent clotting factors. Hence, the prothrombin time result can reflect very different degrees of anticoagulation when different thromboplastins are utilized as reagents.

Efforts to resolve the problem of variability in thromboplastin sensitivity have led to the adoption of the International Normalized Ratio (INR) system, based on a World Health Organization International Reference Thromboplastin Reagent. The INR is the prothrombin time ratio obtained by testing a given anticoagulated patient plasma sample using the WHO Reference Thromboplastin. The INR for any prothrombin time ratio (PTR) measured with any thromboplastin reagent can be calculated if the International Sensitivity Index (ISI) of the reagent is known, where $\text{INR} = \text{measured PTR}^{\text{ISI}}$. The relationship between PTR and INR for thromboplastin reagents of differing ISI is shown in Fig. 13-2. The INR value has been the preferred method for expressing the degree of anticoagulation with warfarin, for comparing various results of clinical trials using warfarin, and for setting standard ranges of anticoagulation for specific clinical entities.

Certain caveats regarding the use of an INR measurement system should be kept in mind, however. First, during induction of warfarin anticoagulation, the prothrombin time (PT) may more accurately define warfarin effect, since the INR standard is based on ISI values derived from patients anticoagulated for at least 6 weeks, when factors II, VII, and X are all decreased in activity. During the initial 2 to 3 days of warfarin therapy, the PT increase is mainly attributable to decreased functional factor VII and, to a lesser extent, factor X. The impact of reduced factor II activity is not yet fully manifest. Second, individual thromboplastin reagents vary in their sensitivity to differing proportionate reductions in the activity of the three of four vitamin K–dependent procoagulant factors impeded by warfarin. Third, the calculated INR value is less accurate when the PT is measured with insensitive thromboplastin having high ISI values. Despite these limitations, expert panels continue to recommend the INR as a grading system for warfarin dosing during both induction and maintenance anticoagulation, especially

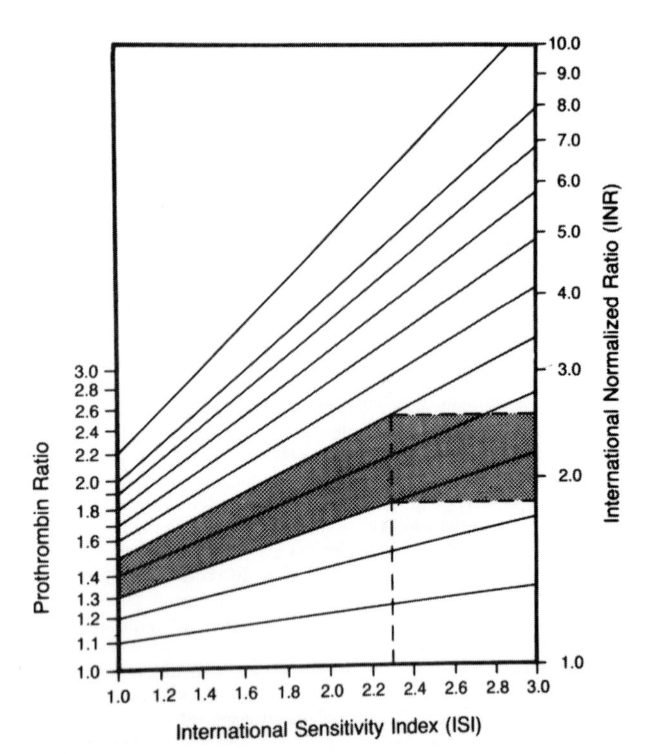

FIG. 13-2 Relation between the prothrombin time ratio and the INR for thromboplastin reagents over a range of ISI values. The example shown is for a prothrombin time (PT) ratio of 1.3 to 1.5 for a thromboplastin preparation with an ISI of 2.3. From the formula INR = PT^{ISI}, the INR is calculated as $1.3^{2.3}$ to $1.5^{2.3}$, or 1.83 to 2.54. (*Modified from Hirsh J, Polker L, Deykin D, et al: Optimal therapeutic range for anti-coagulants. Chest 95(Suppl 2):55, 1989.*)

when sensitive thromboplastin (INR $\leq$ 1.5) reagents are used, careful calibration of laboratory automated clot detectors is employed, and mean normal PT is calculated according to recommended guidelines.

Warfarin Dosing

Upon inception of warfarin, a measurable anticoagulation effect is delayed until circulating factors II, VII, and X are cleared and replaced by dysfunctional vitamin K–dependent factors with fewer carboxyglutamate residues. An initial anticoagulant effect will occur within 24 h as factor VII (half-time 6 to 7 h) is cleared. Peak anticoagulation action of warfarin is delayed for 72 to 96 h because of the longer half-times of factors II (50 h), IX (24 h), and X (36 h). Warfarin suppression of the anticoagulant activity of proteins C (half-time 8 h) and S (30 h) also may contribute to the initial delay in anticoagulant effect.

Selection of an initial warfarin dose depends on an appraisal of the age and nutritional status of the patient and concomitant medical conditions and drugs, which could alter warfarin impact on anticoagulation. Expeditious but safe anticoagulation is also an economic concern for hospitalized patients with decreased inpatient length of stay. For rapid effect, a dose of 10 mg warfarin can be given on day 1. If the INR is <1.5 on day 2, an additional 10 mg is given. If the INR is >1.5 on day 2, then a smaller warfarin dose may be given, 5.0 to 7.5 mg. By day 3, an INR of <1.5 suggests a higher than average maintenance dose (≥5 mg), an INR of 1.5 to 2.0 suggests an average maintenance dose (4 to 6 mg), and an INR of >2.0 suggests a lower than average maintenance dose is needed. When urgent anticoagulation is required, intravenous heparin should be utilized concurrently for 3 to 4 days.

When less urgent outpatient anticoagulation is desired, warfarin can be initiated at 5 mg/day. In many patients, an INR of 2.0 can be attained in about 4 to 5 days. Daily maintenance doses depend on the clinical condition being treated and the targeted INR range.

Warfarin Dosing—Maintenance Therapy

Chronic warfarin therapy is utilized in the prevention of venous and arterial thromboembolism. Specific clinical indications, generally recommended INR ranges, and duration of therapy are outlined in Fig. 13-3, summarized in greater detail in a consensus on antithrom-

Indication	INR	Duration of Therapy
Prophylaxis of venous thrombosis	2–3	Perioperative
Treatment of venous thrombosis		3–6 months
Treatment of pulmonary embolism		3–6 months
Treatment of systemic embolism		Variable
Tissue heart valves		
Atrial fibrillation		
Recurrent systemic emboli		
Post acute myocardial infarction	2.5–3.5	
Recurrent systemic embolism while on warfarin		
Mechanical heart valves*		Life
Aortic		
Bileaflet		
Caged-ball	3.5–4.5	
Tilting disk		
Mitral		
Mitral and Aortic		

FIG. 13-3 Therapeutic goals for warfarin therapy (*Adapted from *Chest* 108:2315; 1995. 371S–379S *N Engl J Med* 333:54; 1995.)

botic therapy and a detailed report of anticoagulation in patients with artificial cardiac valves. The use of specialized anticoagulation clinics can enhance the quality of care receiving warfarin treatment by ensuring that the INR remains within the desired range. Thromboembolic strokes arising from inadequate anticoagulation and serious bleeding adverse events stemming from excessive anticoagulation are thereby kept to a minimum.

Persistent questions regarding the optimal benefit-risk ratio of specific or combined drug therapy with warfarin and aspirin in the treatment of arterial thromboembolism have been addressed more recently. Three hundred and seventy cardiac surgical patients receiving a mechanical or tissue valve replacement were randomized to 100 mg delayed release enteric aspirin or placebo, in addition to warfarin adjusted to an INR of 3.0 to 4.5. Combined aspirin-warfarin therapy reduced total and cardiovascular mortality and major systemic and cerebral emboli, with an additional overall risk reduction of 61% (9.9% per year for placebo-warfarin, 3.9% per year for aspirin-warfarin), albeit with increased minor bleeding events. Averaged INR values in these patients were 3.0 to 3.1, averaged warfarin doses, 5.5 to 5.8 mg/day. Although further low-dose aspirin and low-dose warfarin studies have been proposed to test the efficacy and safety of such combinations, clinical experience with well-controlled adequate warfarin anticoagulation continues to be the mainstay of treatment for both prosthetic valve patients and nonrheumatic atrial fibrillation patients.

Further studies using a case control methodology indicate that among patients with nonrheumatic atrial fibrillation, warfarin anticoagulation prophylaxis is highly effective against ischemic stroke at an INR of ≥2.0. The adjusted odds ratio for ischemic stroke rose to 1.5 at INR 1.8 and more precipitously at lower INRs. Secondary stroke prevention in nonvalvular atrial fibrillation patients also was found to be effective at INR of ≥2.0, whereas hemorrhagic risk increased at INRs above 4.5. Although higher INRs were required for mechanical heart valves, adverse bleeding events also increase at INR levels of ≥4.5.

This system works quite well, with few exceptions. Initially, prolongation of the PT is a function of factor VII levels (which have the shortest half-life). The prolongation of the PT by the INR was based on long-term therapy, where the levels of all vitamin K–dependent factors are depleted. Thus the INR may be unreliable early in the course of therapy if the thromboplastin reagent used is relatively insensitive to factor VII levels. In addition, if relatively insensitive thromboplastin reagents are used (high ISI), the INR becomes less accurate and less precise. The reason for this phenomenon is that the PT ratio is raised to the power of the ISI. It has been recommended that reagents with an ISI of greater than 1.2 not be used. Lastly, the accuracy of the system as a whole depends on reliable ISI measurement and reporting by the manufacturers of reagents, as well as careful calculation and reporting of the PT control used for the PT ratio at the local level.

Clinical Recommendation for Myocardial Infarction

Data from the prethrombolytic era have demonstrated reductions in pulmonary embolism, stroke, and, in one case, mortality associated with anticoagulant use after myocardial infarction. A metaanalysis of several trials from this era revealed reductions in the combined end point of mortality and nonfatal reinfarction. More recently, the ASPECT trial demonstrated a 50% reduction in reinfarction and a 40% reduction in stroke associated with the use of warfarin after myocardial infarction. A number of studies from the thrombolytic era support the use of warfarin after myocardial infarction, particularly in the prevention of embolic events in those patients who are at high risk for thromboembolic phenomenon (anterior wall myocardial infarction, atrial fibrillation, significant left ventricular dysfunction). The Warfarin Aspirin Reinfarction Study (CARS) examined the effect of low-dose warfarin in combination with aspirin in the long-term treatment of the postinfarction patient. At doses of up to 3 mg/day, in combination with aspirin, 80 mg/day, warfarin did not improve mortality as compared with aspirin 160 mg/day. In fact, this group had a stroke rate that was higher than the aspirin group alone. At this juncture, the use of oral anticoagulants is recommended in those patients who have suffered an anterior myocardial infarction or have significant left ventricular dysfunction, atrial fibrillation, or a thromboembolic event.

Prosthetic Valves

There are clear indications for anticoagulation after the placement of prosthetic heart valves. For those patients with bioprosthetic heart valves in the aortic position, routine anticoagulation is not recommended. However, evidence exists for a high rate of embolic events in the first 3 months, and some recommend anticoagulants for the first 3 months postoperatively. The stroke risk ranges from 0.2 to 3% per year, a figure comparable with the stroke risk for those with mechanical prosthetics with anticoagulation, and when given just aspirin alone, there were no clear thromboembolic events during the course of a 3-year follow-up. For those patients with bioprosthetic valves in the mitral position, the rate of embolic events ranges from 0.4 to 1.9% per year without atrial fibrillation, without prior history of emboli, and without enlarged atria. However, given a thromboembolic rate of up to 80% within the first 3 months of replacement, all patients after mitral valve replacement should be anticoagulated for the first 3 months. However, it remains unclear whether these patients should be anticoagulated long term. If atrial fibrillation has become evident, left atrial thrombus is present, or there is a history of embolic events, these patients probably should be anticoagulated.

Those patients with mechanical heart valves should be anticoagulated regardless of location. Those patients with a prosthetic valve in the mitral position are more likely to have a thromboembolic event as compared with those patients with a prosthetic valve in the aortic position. Other risk factors for high rates of thromboembolic events include patients with prior thromboembolic events, atrial fibrillation, enlarged left atria, ball-and-cage-type valves, and dual valve replacement. Given that there are data for the different types of valves, each with its own optimal regimen, these recommendations are bound to be oversimplified. For those patients without a prior embolic event, a PT ratio of 2.5 to 3.5 is recommended, with a slightly higher INR for those patients with a ball-and-cage valve. For those patients with a prior embolic event, aspirin at an initial dose of 80 mg or dipyridamole at a dose of 400 mg/day should be added.

Atrial Fibrillation

There have been several randomized, placebo-controlled trials of anticoagulant therapy in atrial fibrillation. The current recommendations for anticoagulant therapy can be broken down into several major groups. Those patients with valvular atrial fibrillation should be anticoagulated. Those under the age of 75 years with nonvalvular atrial fibrillation, without structural heart disease, and without risk factors for heart disease can be managed without anticoagulant therapy and in many cases without aspirin. Those patients who are older than 75 years should be anticoagulated. However, the decision to treat should be balanced with an age-related increase in bleeds. For those patients who are older than 65 years and younger than 75 years, the presence of risk factors plays a major role in the decision to anticoagulate. Those with either a prior thromboembolic event, hypertension, diabetes, existing coronary disease, or reduced left ventricular function are at increased risk. Those with none of these risk factors are at a risk of thromboembolic events of 2 to 4% per year, and the benefit of therapy with oral anticoagulants as compared with aspirin is much reduced. In the Stroke Prevention in Atrial Fibrillation Trial II, there was no significant difference between aspirin therapy and warfarin therapy for some patients in this group. Lastly, patients with atrial fibrillation complicating thyrotoxicosis are at increased risk of thromboembolism and should be anticoagulated.

Adverse Effects

The main complication associated with warfarin therapy is bleeding. The risk of bleeding is directly related to the intensity of therapy, with higher anticoagulant levels being associated with the greatest risk of hemorrhage. The risk of bleeding also has been reported to be associated with advancing age, prior history of GI bleeding, prior stroke, concomitant use of aspirin, and use of other nonsteroidal anti-inflammatory agents.

Additional adverse events with warfarin have been described, the most important of which is warfarin-induced skin necrosis. The mechanism is still unclear; however, associations with both protein C and protein S deficiencies have been described. In addition, a similarity between these lesions and those seen in neonatal purpura fulminans (complicating homozygous protein C deficiency) has been noted. The lesion is caused by thrombosis of venules and capillaries in subcutaneous fatty tissue. In this group of patients, anticoagulation with warfarin must be overlapped with heparin, and warfarin therapy is begun at very low doses (0.03 mg/kg). Lastly, warfarin therapy should be avoided in pregnancy. Specifically, it has been associated with birth defects, central nervous system abnormalities, and fetal bleeding.

SUGGESTED READINGS

Armstrong PW: Heparin in acute coronary disease—Requiem for a heavyweight? (Editoral). *New Engl J Med* 337:492, 1997.

Cohen M, Demers C, Gurfinkel E, et al., for the Efficacy and Safety of Subcutaneous Enoxaparin vs Non-Q-Wave Coronary Events Study Group: A comparison of low-molecular weight heparin with unfractionated heparin for unstable coronary artery disease. *N Engl J Med* 337:447–452, 1997.

Coller BS: Platelets and thrombolytic therapy. *N Engl J Med* 322:33, 1990.

EPIC Investigators: Use of a monoclonal antibody directed against the platelet glycoprotein IIb/IIIa receptor in high-risk coronary angioplasty. *N Engl J Med* 330:956, 1994.

Frishman WH, Klein MD, Blaufarb I, et al: Antiplatelet and other antithrombotic drugs, in Frishman WH, Sonnenblick EH (eds): *Cardiovascular Pharmacotherapeutics*. New York, McGraw-Hill, 1997, pp 323–379.

Golino P, Ambrosio G, Villari B, et al: Endogeneous prostaglandin endoperoxides may alter infarct size in the presence of thromboxane synthase inhibition: Studies in a rabbit model of coronary artery occlusion-reperfusion. *J Am Coll Cardiol* 21(2):493, 1993.

Hirsh J, Polker L, Deykin D, et al: Optimal therapeutic range for anticoagulants. *Chest* 5(Suppl 2):5s, 1989.

Hirsh J, Raschke R, Warkentin TE, et al: Heparin: Mechanism of action, pharmacokinetics dosing considerations, monitoring, efficacy and safety. *Chest* 108: 258S, 1995.

Schafer A: Antiplatelet therapy. *Am J Med* 101:199, 1996.

Wilde MI, Markham A: Danaparoid: A review of its pharmacology and clinical use in the management of heparin-induced thrombocytopenia. *Drugs* 54(6): 903, 1997.

Chapter 14 Thrombolytic Agents

Robert Forman, William H. Frishman, and Brian Strizik

Thrombolytic agents are drugs administered to patients for dissolution by fibrinolysis of established blood clot by activating endogenous plasminogen. Although some of these agents have been available for more than 50 years, it was not until the 1980s that they became widely used for treatment of patients with acute myocardial infarction and other thrombotic states.

Thrombolytic agents act by converting the proenzyme plasminogen to the active enzyme plasmin (Fig. 14-1) by cleavage of the Arg-Val peptide bond. Plasmin lyses fibrin clot and is a nonspecific serum protease that is capable of breaking down plasminogen factors V and VIII. The action of plasmin is neutralized by circulating plasma inhibitors, primarily α_2-antiplasmin. Endogenous thrombolysis is also inhibited by plasminogen activator inhibitor (PAI-1). Thrombolytics affect platelet function in response to pathologic shear stress by inhibiting platelet aggregation in stenotic arteries.

SPECIFIC THROMBOLYTIC AGENTS

Streptokinase

Streptokinase is a single-chain polypeptide derived from β-hemolytic streptococci. It is not an enzyme and thus has no enzymatic action on plasminogen. It binds with plasminogen in a 1:1 ratio, resulting in a conformational change in the plasminogen, which thus becomes an active enzyme. This active plasminogen-streptokinase complex catalyzes the conversion of another plasminogen molecule to active plasmin. This activation of plasminogen is enhanced in the presence of fibrinogen but also other coagulation proteins, resulting in a systemic fibrinolytic state. In contrast to plasmin, the plasminogen-streptokinase complex is not rapidly neutralized by α_2-antiplasmin.

Anistreplase

Anisoylated plasminogen-streptokinase activator complex (APSAC) is a second-generation agent consisting of streptokinase bound in vitro to plasminogen by the insertion of an anisoyl group. This results in a much more stable enzyme complex protecting it from plasmin inhibitors and resulting in a prolonged half-life by permitting the agent to be administered as a single bolus.

Urokinase

Urokinase is available in both single- and double-chain forms. The double-chain form originally was isolated from urine and is commer-

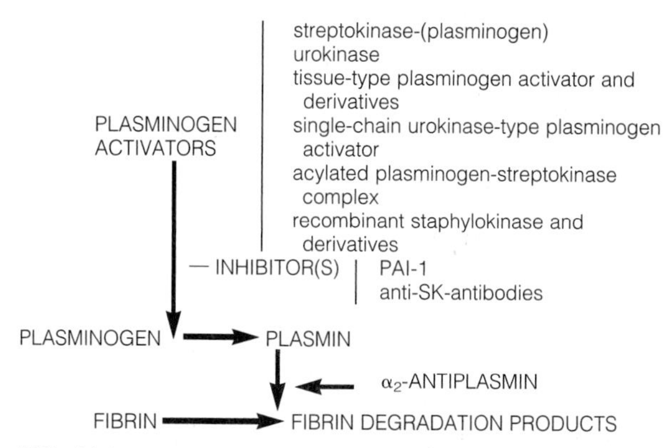

FIG. 14-1 Schematic representation of the fibrinolytic system. Plasminogen is a proenzyme and is activated by plasminogen activators into the active enzyme plasmin. Plasmin degrades fibrin into degradation products. Fibrinolysis may be inhibited at the level of plasminogen activators by PAI-1 (plasminogen activator inhibitor) and anti-SK (streptokinase) antibodies or the level of plasmin by α_2-antiplasmin.

cially available in the United States. Urokinase activates plasminogen directly and has no specific affinity for fibrin, activating both fibrin-bound and circulating plasminogen.

The single-chain form of urokinase is also known as *prourokinase* or *scu-PA* and *saruplase*. This single-chain form occurs naturally, and the agent is synthesized by recombinant DNA techniques and is considered fibrin-specific; that is, it is activated predominantly in the presence of fibrin.

Because urokinase is a naturally occurring product, it is not antigenic and is not neutralized by antibodies.

Tissue Plasminogen Activator

Single-chain tissue plasminogen activator (tPA) occurs naturally but is synthesized for commercial use using a recombinant DNA technique and is known as alteplase. A double-chain form of tPA, *duteplase*, also was synthesized and appeared to have similar activity when tested in vitro, but this form is not commercially available. The tPA molecule has a binding site enabling it to bind specifically to fibrin in thrombus. Thus it should theoretically be clot-specific and not result in activation of generally circulating plasminogen. PAI-1 is important, and under natural conditions it neutralizes endogenous tPA, but not with administration of therapeutic doses of tPA.

Reteplase (BM 06,022) is an unglycosylated recombinant plasminogen activator consisting of the kringle 2 and protease domains of tPA, with a three to four times longer half-life than tPA. Two open, nonrandomized pilot trials testing various dosages of reteplase in patients with acute myocardial infarction showed promising results. One recent study (RAPID I) showed that a double bolus of 10 + 10 MU of reteplase 30 min apart restored coronary blood flow more rapidly than r-tPA (alteplase). As a consequence, reteplase-treated infarction patients required fewer coronary interventions and had higher myocardial salvage than alteplase-treated patients.

The INJECT trial demonstrated that reteplase was at least as effective as streptokinase in reducing mortality but was associated with a significantly lower incidence of heart failure in patients than streptokinase. In a comparison trial with alteplase in patients with acute myocardial infarction (RAPID II), reteplase, when given as a double bolus of 10 + 10 MU, achieved significantly higher rates of early reperfusion of the infarct-related coronary artery, requiring fewer acute coronary interventions than front-loaded alteplase.

The safety profile of reteplase is similar to that of other thrombolytic agents, and the FDA approved reteplase for reduction of mortality, reduction of the incidence of congestive heart failure, improvement of ventricular function after acute myocardial infarction, and lysis of thrombi obstructing coronary arteries.

The currently available thrombolytic agents are listed in Table 14-1. The doses listed are for patients with acute myocardial infarction.

ACUTE MYOCARDIAL INFARCTION

Enthusiasm for the use of thrombolytic agents with the ensuing trials became popular only after the pathophysiology of acute myocardial infarction was understood. Davies and Thomas observed in pathologic specimens that most cases with acute myocardial infarction were due to sudden occlusion of a coronary artery by a thrombus at the site of a ruptured atherosclerotic plaque. DeWood and his colleagues confirmed this by demonstrating an occlusive thrombus in more than 85% of coronary angiograms performed in patients within the first 3 h of presentation of a transmural myocardial infarction. A decade earlier, it had been well established by Reimer that a "wave front" of myocardial infarction progressed from the subendocardium to the subepicardium with a longer duration of temporary occlusion of a circumflex coronary artery in dogs.

Rentrop and his colleagues in Germany demonstrated the use of intracoronary streptokinase with successful dissolution of the offending coronary thrombus. Subsequent trials utilizing intracoronary administration of streptokinase revealed significant improvement in survival,

TABLE 14-1 Thrombolytic Agents Currently Available

Characteristic	Streptokinase	Anistreplase	Urokinase	tPA	Reteplase
Molecular weight	47,000	131,000	31,000–55,000	70,000	
Plasma clearance time, min	15–25	50–90	15–20	4–8	11–19
Fibrin specificity	Minimal	Minimal	Moderate	Moderate	Moderate
Plasminogen binding	Indirect	Indirect	Direct	Direct	Direct
Potential allergic reaction	Yes	Yes	No	No	No
Typical dose	1.5 million units	30 units	2 million units	15 mg	10 units + 10 units after 30 min
Administration	1-h IV infusion	5-min IV infusion	1-million unit IV bolus, then 1 million units IV over 1 h	15-mg bolus, then 0.75 mg/kg over 30 min (max 5 days), then 60 min (max 35 mg)	IV bolus injection
Approximate cost, $	300	2000	2750	2200	

particularly in those patients in whom the thrombus was successfully lysed. However, it was not until intravenous thrombolytic agents were administered that large multicenter trials could be successfully undertaken.

Effect on Mortality

Intravenous administration of thrombolytic agents has been shown to significantly reduce the mortality rate of acute myocardial infarction by approximately 25%. The results of the larger multicenter randomized trials in which different intravenous thrombolytic agents were used are shown in Table 14-2.

The first large-scale trial conducted by the Gruppo Italiano per lo Studio della Streptochinasi nell'Infarcto Miocardico (GISSI) in 1986 convincingly showed that intravenous streptokinase administered within 6 h of acute myocardial infarction significantly reduced the 21-day mortality by 18%. A similar 25% reduction in vascular mortality with the use of intravenous streptokinase was shown in the Second International Study of Infarct Survival (ISIS-2). In this trial, patients were admitted with symptoms suggestive of acute myocardial infarction, and only 55% had significant ST-segment elevation. One smaller trial of Intravenous Steptokinase in Acute Myocardial Infarction (ISAM) showed no significant survival benefit despite improved ventricular function and smaller infarcts in the thrombolyzed group.

In the APSAC Interventional Mortality Study (AIMS), patients with acute myocardial infarction and ST-segment elevation were randomized within 6 h of onset of symptoms. The trial was terminated prematurely because of the significant 47.5% reduction in mortality in the actively treated group.

The effect of tPA on mortality was studied in the Anglo-Saxon Scandinavian Study of Early Thrombolysis (ASSET) using the then-standard 3-h dosing regimen and randomizing the patients within 5 h of the onset of symptoms. As with the ISIS-2 trial, no ECG criteria were required for enrollment, and consequently, only 72% were considered

TABLE 14-2 Early Mortality Following Thrombolysis*

Thrombolytic agent	Trial	*n*	Mortality, %		Survival benefit, %
			Control	Agent	
Streptokinase	ISAM	1,741	7.1	6.3	11 (NS)
	GISSI-1	11,806	13.0	10.7	18
	ISIS-2	17,187	12.0	9.2	25
APSAC	AIMS	1,004	12.2	6.4	47
tPA	ASSET	5,011	9.8	7.2	27

*n = number of patients randomized in trial; NS = not significant.

to have an acute myocardial infarction, yet there was a significant 26% reduction in mortality in patients receiving tPA.

Comparison of Thrombolytic Agents

The mortality rates comparing the three thrombolytic agents most frequently used are shown in Table 14-3. In the GISSI-2 and ISIS-3 trials, the mortality rates were similar in the groups of patients who received streptokinase and tPA. In the ISIS-3 trial, the mortality rate in the one-third of patients who also received APSAC was similar. However, in these two trials conducted predominately in Europe, heparin was administered subcutaneously and not intravenously, as is customary in the United States. In the Global Utilization of Streptokinase and Tissue Plasminogen Activator for Occluded Coronary Arteries (GUSTO) trial, there was a 14% relative and a 1% absolute reduction in mortality rate in patients assigned to receive tPA compared with those receiving streptokinase. In this trial, tPA was administered using an accelerated protocol in which a thrombolytic agent was administered over 1.5 h with two-thirds of the dose being given in the first 30 min rather than the conventional 3 h. The tPA utilized in the ISIS-3 trial was duteplase rather than the standard alteplase, but the 90-min patency rate is regarded as similar.

The Importance of Time on Efficacy

In the GISSI-1 trial, there was nearly a 50% reduction in mortality when streptokinase was administered within 1 h of the onset of symptoms, a 23% reduction in mortality when thrombolytic agent was administered within 3 h, and a 17% reduction in mortality between 3 and 6 h. There was no significant reduction in mortality when streptokinase was administered between 6 and 12 h after the onset of symptoms. However, in the AIMS trial, there was a similar reduction in mortality when the APSAC was administered within 4 h or between 4 and 6 h after the onset of symptoms, but the relatively small number of patients randomized in the trial makes these results less meaningful. In

TABLE 14-3 Early Mortality Comparing Different Thrombolytic Agents*

		Agent and mortality, %			
Trial	*n*	Streptokinase	tPA	APSAC	*P* value
ISIS-3	41,299	10.6	10.3	10.5	NS
GISSI-2	12,490	8.6	9.0	—	NS
GUSTO	41,021	7.3	6.3	—	0.001

*n = number of patients; NS = not significant; tPA = tissue plasminogen activator; APSAC = anisoylated plasminogen streptokinase activity complex.

the ASSET trial in which tPA was administered, there was a similar reduction in mortality in patients who received thrombolysis within 3 h or between 3 and 5 h. In the ISIS-2 trial, the greatest reduction in vascular mortality (35%) occurred when streptokinase was administered within 4 h of the onset of chest pain, yet there was still significant reduction in those patients who were randomized between 5 and 24 h. In the South American EMERAS trial, there was no improvement in survival when streptokinase was administered between 7 and 12 h or up to 24 h following chest pain.

The Late Assessment of Thrombolytic Efficacy (LATE) study was designed to prospectively randomize patients to receive tPA between 6 and 24 h after the onset of chest pain. However, only 55% of the patients had significant ST-segment elevation. There was a significant reduction (25.6%) in the 35-day mortality rate in patients randomized to receive tPA between 6 and 12 h compared with placebo (8.9 versus 12.0%, respectively). There was no significant difference in mortality when these patients were randomized between 12 and 24 h after the onset of symptoms. However, if patients whose thrombolysis was delayed more then 3 h after being initially assessed in the hospital were excluded from the study, patients who received their thrombolytic agents between 12 and 24 h after the onset of symptoms had a 22.4% reduction in mortality.

Thus it has become standard practice to administer thrombolytic agents up to 12 h following the onset of chest pain in patients with acute myocardial infarction. It is controversial whether patients should receive thrombolytic agents if they present 12 to 24 h after the onset of chest pain. However, patients who have continued chest pain beyond 12 h or patients who are at higher risk, for example, anterior wall or complicated inferior wall myocardial infarction, can be considered for late administration of thrombolytic agents.

It is not clear why patients benefit from late thrombolysis, since it is assumed that myocardial necrosis would have been completed within 6 h. Thus its benefits may be attributed to a reduction in postmyocardial infarction remodeling and ventricular arrhythmias. In addition, infarction may not have been completed if significant collateral blood flow is present to maintain viability beyond 6 h, or the occluded coronary vessel may have intermittently or partially spontaneously reperfused.

Patency

The mechanism whereby thrombolysis improves survival is by achieving and maintaining patency of the infarct-related artery. Early or 90-min patency has been shown to be an important determinant of survival following thrombolysis. The Thrombolysis in Myocardial Infarction trial (TIMI) grade classification is generally used to evaluate patency:

grade 0, no perfusion; grade 1, penetration without perfusion; grade 2, partial perfusion with a rate of entry or clearance of contrast material beyond the occlusion is impaired; grade 3, complete reperfusion.

The patency rates (TIMI grade 2, plus grade 3) at 90 min from grouped studies are shown in Table 14-4. Treatment with front-loaded or accelerated tPA regimen is associated with the highest patency rates, whereas streptokinase is associated with the lowest patency rates. However, by 24 h there is no difference in the patency rates between the different thrombolytic agents. By 2 to 3 h there was no significant difference in the patency rates between the different agents. Patency rates reported by Granger et al. are shown in Fig. 14-2.

Reocclusion and Reinfarction

Reocclusion and reinfarction following successful thrombolysis carry a significant increase in morbidity and mortality. For a diagnosis of reocclusion to be made, angiograms must be performed immediately following thrombolysis and at a later date, generally prior to hospital discharge. The diagnosis of reinfarction is often difficult, since it may immediately follow successful thrombolysis. In a metaanalysis combining the results of randomized trials, Granger et al. reported a reocclusion rate of 13.5% when patients received tPA and intravenous heparin compared with 8.0% when non-fibrin-specific thrombolytic agents (streptokinase, APSAC, and urokinase) were used. Thus it was somewhat surprising to observe the lower reported rates of reinfarction in those patients who received tPA with subcutaneous heparin compared with streptokinase in the GISSI-2 and ISIS-3 trials. Since more than 50% of the reocclusion occurs within 24 h, it is possible that these events were undetected in clinical trials. However, there was no difference in the reocclusion rates reported with streptokinase compared with tPA in the GUSTO and angiographic substudy.

TABLE 14-4 Patency Rates (TIMI Grades 2 and 3) at 90 Min and 1 Day after Thrombolysis with Different Agents*

Thrombolytic agent	90-min patency,		1-day patency,	
	%	*n*	%	*n*
Streptokinase	54	1365	84	551
APSAC	70	511	80	379
Urokinase	60	408	72	121
tPA	70	1648	84	1366
Accelerated tPA	83	615	86	427

**n* = number of patients randomized; tPA = tissue plasminogen activator; APSAC = anisoylated plasminogen streptokinase activator complex.

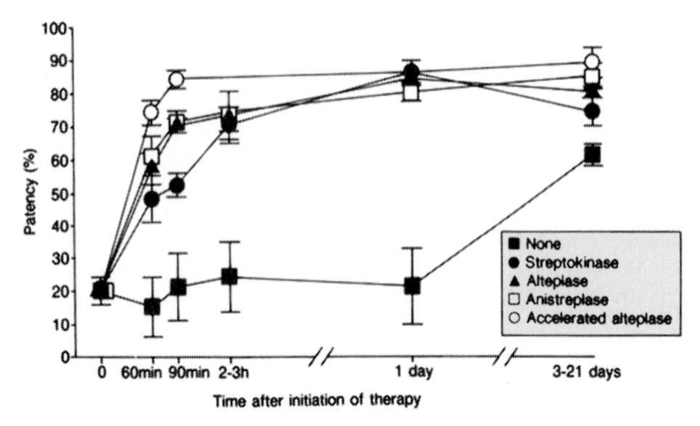

FIG. 14-2 Angiographic patency rates of the infarct-related coronary artery over time. The data are from pooled analyses of different thrombolytic agents or regimens.

Reocclusion after successful thrombolysis was recorded in 9.2% of patients in the Thrombolysis and Angioplasty in Myocardial Infarction (TAMI) 1, 2, and 3 trials but was 16.9% in those patients who required emergency angioplasty following thrombolysis. The reocclusion was clinically recognized in 58% of the patients and was associated with deleterious effects whether silent or clinically evident. The mortality rate was 4.5% if the infarct-related artery remained patent and 11.0% if the artery reoccluded.

Patients who developed recurrence of infarction while in the hospital are generally managed by performing immediate angioplasty without repeat administration of a thrombolytic agent. However, should performing an angioplasty not be feasible or appropriate, the patient can receive a second dose of a thrombolytic agent. Streptokinase resistance titers increase by the fifth day after administration of either streptokinase or APSAC and remain raised for at least 1 year. Therefore, for patients who have received either of these two agents in the past year and probably longer, it is advisable that they receive either tPA or urokinase. Recurrence of reinfarction after thrombolysis with tPA or streptokinase was successfully treated with tPA in 85% of patients (two-thirds within 1 h of completion of thrombolysis) without an increase in bleeding complications, but reocclusion occurred in more than half of these patients.

Completeness of Reperfusion

In the western Washington trial in which intracoronary streptokinase was administered, the 30-day survival was significantly improved in those patients receiving thrombolysis compared with control (3.7 versus 11.2%, respectively), but by 1 year there was no difference in the survival. However, when the survival was analyzed for completeness of reperfusion, there was a significant improvement in survival in those patients who had complete reperfusion (and presumably TIMI grade 3 flow) compared with patients with partial (presumably TIMI grade 2 flow) or no reperfusion (98 versus 77 versus 85%, respectively), suggesting that partial reperfusion could possibly be harmful.

The Thrombolysis Trial of Anistreplase in Acute Myocardial Infarction (TEAM-3) trial, in which APSAC or tPA were administered and the patients studied 30 h after administration of their thrombolytic agents, patients with TIMI grade 3 perfusion had better left ventricular systolic function and a trend toward lower mortality compared with patients with TIMI grade 2 and TIMI grade 0 or 1.

The angiographic substudy of the GUSTO trial reported the 24-h mortality was 2.93% and highest in patients who had TIMI grade 2 flow 90 min after thrombolysis. The survival was 0.89% and was the lowest in patients with TIMI grade 3 flow and 2.35% in patients with TIMI grade 0 or 1 flow. In this angiographic substudy in which 1210 patients were randomized to have a 90-min coronary angiogram, 54% of the patients who received tPA had TIMI grade 3 flow compared with 31% of patients who received streptokinase. However, irrespective of the treatment regimen the patient received, the 30-day mortality was 4% in patients with TIMI grade 3 flow and 8.4, 9.2, and 7.8% in patients with TIMI grades 0, 1, and 2, respectively. When the 90-min patency data and the corresponding 30-day mortality from the angiographic substudy were extrapolated to the 41,021 patients in the main GUSTO trial, they were able to accurately predict the mortality in the different subgroups of thrombolytic regimen.

Thus it appears that the 90-min patency rate following thrombolysis, and in particular the TIMI grade 3 flow, can accurately predict an improved survival compared with patients with TIMI grade 2 flow, who may have no difference in survival compared with patients who have TIMI grade 0 or 1 flow.

Thrombolysis in Clinical Subgroups

Anterior Wall Myocardial Infarction

The mortality rate of patients with anterior wall myocardial infarction has been reduced significantly by thrombolysis, with a 37% reduction in mortality in the ISIS-2 trial and a 21% reduction in the GISSI-1 trial. These reductions in rates were significantly greater with anterior than inferior wall myocardial infarctions. In the GUSTO-1 trial, it was shown that there was a significant 18% or a 1.9% absolute reduction in mortality in patients who received tPA compared with streptokinase in patients with anterior wall myocardial infarction, whereas the 11%

reduction in mortality in patients with inferior wall myocardial infarction who received tPA compared with streptokinase was of borderline significance.

Inferior Wall Myocardial Infarction

Inferior wall myocardial infarction is generally associated with a lower mortality rate because of the smaller mass of myocardium supplied by the right coronary artery. Thus it is not surprising that there was no statistical difference in the mortality in the individual trials in patients treated with thrombolysis compared with placebo. However, when the data were pooled, there was a significant 22% relative reduction in mortality from 8.7 to 6.8% with the use of thrombolytic agents. In a more recent overview, which included patients in the ISIS-3, EMERAS, and LATE trials, the reduction in mortality was only 11% in patients randomized to receive thrombolysis.

Patients with inferior wall myocardial infarcts with the highest mortality are most likely to derive the greatest benefit with thrombolysis and include patients with right ventricular infarction, accompanying anterior ST-segment depression, and heart block. Thus the use of thrombolytic agents should be considered in all patients with inferior wall myocardial infarctions, particularly those who are considered to be at the highest risk.

Non-Q-Wave Myocardial Infarction

Approximately 50% of patients presenting acute myocardial infarction do not have ST-segment elevation or left bundle branch block. Administration of thrombolytic agents to patients in the GISSI-1 and ISIS-2 trials who presented with ST-segment depression did not result in improvement in survival despite a significant mortality in these groups (16 to 20%). This question was specifically addressed in a prospective manner in the TIMI-3B trial, where patients who presented with non-Q-wave myocardial infarction or unstable angina with ST-segment depression or T-wave inversion were randomized to receive tPA or placebo. The mortality rate was not significantly different in the tPA versus placebo groups (10.9 versus 8.9%, respectively). It is possible that thrombolytic agents actually may be harmful in patients with non-Q-wave myocardial infarction, since thrombolytic therapy has a prothrombotic action by activating platelets and exposing thrombin, resulting in progression of the partially occluded coronary artery to complete occlusion. In a recent post hoc analysis of the LATE study, it was found that thrombolysis was beneficial to patients presenting 6 h after the onset of chest pain with non-Q-wave myocardial infarction. However, the authors themselves caution against accepting these results without further prospective testing in a larger number of patients.

Left Bundle Branch Block

The diagnosis of acute myocardial infarction in the presence of left bundle branch block may be masked, and even utilizing the criteria developed from the GUSTO-1 study, the sensitivity of diagnosis was as low as 36%. Unfortunately, relatively few patients with left bundle branch block have been randomized in the megatrials, and there was no difference in survival in the ISIS-2 trial, whereas the mortality was 27.7% in the patients receiving thrombolysis compared with 19.8% in the GISSI-1 trial, and the difference was of marginal significance. However, it has become standard practice to administer thrombolytic agents in all patients with presumed new left bundle branch block and typical symptoms of acute myocardial infarction.

Cardiogenic Shock

Patients with cardiogenic shock generally have been excluded from most of the thrombolytic trials. Thus there are limited data concerning the efficacy of these agents. In the GISSI-1 trial, there was no significant difference in survival of patients who presented in cardiogenic shock who receive thrombolysis or placebo. In the ISIS-2 trial, patients who were hypotensive with a systolic blood pressure of less than 100 mmHg had a 24% significant relative reduction in 5-week mortality of 28.5% in streptokinase compared with 37.5% in the control group. In an overview of the megatrials presenting with blood pressure less than 100 mmHg, the 35-day mortality was 28.9% in patients receiving thrombolysis compared with 31.5% of patients in the control group.

A problem in treating patients in cardiogenic shock with streptokinase is that the patients are already hypotensive before administration of a drug that itself may cause a decrease in blood pressure. However in the GUSTO-1 trial, patients treated with tPA were much less likely to develop cardiogenic shock, whereas patients who were in cardiogenic shock at the time of randomization and who received streptokinase with intravenous heparin had a better 30-day mortality of 54% compared with 59% in patients receiving tPA. The poor results with administration of thrombolytic agents in patients with cardiogenic shock are probably related to the low patency rates achieved even with the use of intravenous streptokinase. The low patency rate has been attributed to the poor delivery of thrombolytic agents to the occluded coronary vessel in the presence of cardiogenic shock, but this does not explain the poor results with administration of intracoronary thrombolysis. Because of the high mortality associated with thrombolysis and administration of thrombolytic agents, it has become common practice to not use thrombolytic agents and transfer these patients directly to the cardiac catheterization laboratory for immediate angioplasty. However, the true efficacy of this invasive approach has yet to be proven and is at present the objective of two ongoing international trials.

Elderly Patients

There is a general reluctance to use thrombolytic agents in elderly patients because of the perceived notion that the complication rate from their use is higher and that effectiveness is inferior in the elderly. In addition, a higher percentage of elderly patients either have contraindications to thrombolytic therapy, including severe hypertension, recent cerebrovascular accident, and bleeding disorders or arrive too late in the emergency room.

Streptokinase is the only thrombolytic agent that was administered to patients older than 70 years in these early trials. In the GISSI-1 trial there was a significant reduction in mortality in patients younger than 65 years treated with streptokinase compared with controls. Whereas the mortality rate was lower in patients older then 65 or 75 who were thrombolyzed, the reduction in mortality was not significantly different. However, the number of lives saved was more than 4 patients per 100 treated in the elderly and only 2 in the younger group. The Intravenous Streptokinase in Acute Myocardial Infarction (ISAM) trial was the only study in which a greater mortality in the elderly was reported, but the total number of patients in this age group was small and results were not statistically significant. By far the largest number of elderly patients were randomized in the ISIS-2 trial, in which the mortality rate was significantly reduced in the elderly but particularly when aspirin was combined with streptokinase. In the ASSET trial in which the patient received tPA or placebo, all patients were younger than 75. In this trial, a reduction in mortality for patients younger than 66 years was not significant but was highly significant for those older than 65 years. The results of the AIMS trial were similar to those of the ASSET trial in that the mortality rate was reduced in patients randomized to receive APSAC but was only significant in the older and not in the younger patients. In this trial all patients were younger than 70 years, and the numbers were relatively small.

Three large trials directly compared the outcome of streptokinase with tPA. In the GISSI-2 trial, 22.5% of the 12,490 patients were older then 70 years, but the results were not separately analyzed according to age. In the ISIS-3 trial, 26.1% of the 41,299 patients were 70 years or older. The results also were not separately analyzed according to age.

In the GUSTO-1 trial, in which 12% of the 31,021 patients were older then 75 years, there was no significant difference in the mortality of 19.3% in the patients receiving tPA compared with 20.6% with streptokinase. In the angiographic substudy, regional left ventricular dysfunction was greater in the elderly patients older than 75 years, and in contrast to the younger patients, this dysfunction was maintained at follow-up despite patency of the infarct-related artery. This has led the authors to speculate that a more rapid progression or impaired recovery of ischemic injury occurs in the elderly.

Thus elderly patients can benefit significantly from administration of thrombolytic agents with acute myocardial infarction, but it should be remembered that the incidence, albeit small, of intracerebral hemorrhage increases with age (see "Intracranial Hemorrhage"). Therefore, thrombolytic agents generally should be reserved for those patients who are at high risk who suffer anterior wall myocardial infarction and complicated inferior wall myocardial infarction.

ADJUNCTIVE ANTITHROMBOTIC THERAPY

Successful thrombolysis paradoxically results in conditions that favor rethrombosis. In the process of thrombolysis, thrombin bound to fibrin is exposed to reperfused blood on the thrombus surface. This clot-bound thrombus activates fibrinogen and platelets and is a major contributor to the rethrombosis and hence reocclusion of successfully thrombolyzed coronary arteries.

The objective of adjunctive treatment is to improve patency and reduce the high incidence of reocclusion following successful thrombolysis by inhibiting thrombin activity and platelet function. It is not clear whether adjunctive therapy can enhance thrombolysis itself.

Aspirin and Other Antiplatelet Drugs

Aspirin inhibits platelet aggregation by irreversibly inhibiting cyclooxygenase and the consequent production of thromboxane A_2. Aspirin has been convincingly shown to reduce mortality and presumably prevent reocclusion after successful thrombolysis. In the ISIS-2 trial, there was a 23% reduction in mortality in patients receiving aspirin alone, compared with placebo, and this was similar to the 25% reduction in mortality in patients who received streptokinase alone. When combined with streptokinase, there is an additional 19% reduction in mortality. Since aspirin administration following thrombolysis decreased the late but not the early mortality, it is postulated that the mechanism whereby it is beneficial is in preventing reocclusion and consequently reinfarction rather than by accelerating thrombolysis.

Thromboxane is one of the many activators of the IIb/IIIa receptors on the platelet surface that permit the binding of fibrinogen to platelets and the consequent aggregation. Thus aspirin is a relatively weak antiplatelet drug in comparison with the recently developed and more powerful IIb/IIIa receptor inhibitors. The latter prevent the binding of fibrinogen to these receptors, thereby inhibiting platelet aggregation irrespective of the pathway initiating the platelet aggregation. Currently, intravenous administration of IIb/IIIa receptor antagonists is being evaluated as an adjuvant with thrombolytic agents in the treatment of acute myocardial infarction.

Ticlopidine is an orally active antiplatelet agent that blocks adenosine diphosphate (ADP)–induced platelet activation, is more expensive, and has potential adverse effects on the bone marrow, but it can be used in patients who cannot tolerate aspirin.

Heparin and Other Antithrombin Drugs

The anticoagulant affect of heparin is primarily related to its antithrombin activity. Thus heparin has been administered to improve the patency, particularly following thrombolysis with tPA, but also is used with streptokinase. Heparin has been shown to improve the patency but has not been shown clearly to improve mortality and reduce reinfarction. In the TAMI study, patency at 90 min following thrombolysis with tPA was 79% whether the patients received heparin or not. This led the authors to conclude that heparin did not facilitate the fibrinolytic effect of tPA. In the Heparin Aspirin Reperfusion trial, the coronary artery patency in 205 patients who had been thrombolyzed was assessed at 18 h after patients had received either aspirin or heparin. The patency rate was 82% in the heparin group and significantly greater than the aspirin group, but a low dose of aspirin (80 mg) was used. In the European Cooperative Study Group-6 trial, patency rate at the mean of 81 h following thrombolysis with tPA was 80% in patients who received both aspirin and heparin and was significantly greater than that of the 75% of patients who received aspirin alone. It is concluded that intravenous heparin in doses of 5000-U bolus following by 1000 U/h increases the patency during the first few days following thrombolysis with tPA, probably by preventing rethrombosis.

The effect of heparin on mortality is less convincing. In the GISSI-2 study, patients received aspirin with either streptokinase or tPA and randomized either to 12-h delayed administration of subcutaneous heparin or placebo. It is surprising to observe that the mortality was improved with addition of heparin to streptokinase rather than tPA (GISSI International). Similar results were reported in the Studio sulla Calciparina nell'Angina e nella Trombosi Ventricoliare nell'Infarcto (SCATI) study. Addition of subcutaneous heparin 4 h following thrombolysis therapy in the ISIS-3 study resulted in a nonsignificant reduction in reinfarction and 35-day mortality. Addition of heparin to aspirin resulted in a small absolute excess of 0.16% cerebral bleeds and 0.2% of serious noncerebral bleeds. The data from these trials do not assess the benefit of intravenously administered heparin. In the GUSTO-1 trial there was no additional clinical benefit on mortality and patency when intravenous compared with subcutaneous heparin was added to streptokinase.

There are insufficient data from randomized trials to assess the efficacy of intravenous compared with subcutaneous heparin on mortality following thrombolysis with tPA. In the LATE trial where patients were randomized to tPA or placebo, intravenous heparin did not have a beneficial effect on the mortality, but the administration of heparin was not randomized.

The decision to use heparin in addition to thrombolysis is not clearly evident, though it is current practice. It is advised that heparin may be given concomitantly with tPA or delayed 2 to 3 h after streptokinase.

In recent trials, high doses of heparin were being used in conjunction with tPA and resulted in an excess of intracerebral hemorrhages (GUSTO-2A, TIMI-9A). An increase in intracerebral bleeding also has been recorded with the use of hirudin, an antithrombin agent that acts directly to inhibit thrombin independently of antithrombin III.

With the high incidence of intracerebral bleeding recorded in elderly patients weighing less than 70 kg, it is now recommended that heparin be given according to weight, particularly in smaller patients: 70 U/kg bolus followed by 15 U/kg per hour maintenance infusion.

COMPLICATIONS

Intracranial Hemorrhage

An intracerebral bleed is the most feared complication following administration of thrombolytic agents. Results are generally devastating, with the event usually occurring within 24 h of thrombolysis and carrying a high mortality of approximately 50%. However, it should be realized that the incidence of stroke in the prethrombolytic era was 1.7 to 2.4%. A metaanalysis of the major thrombolytic trials has shown that administration of thrombolytic agents is associated with a 0.4% absolute increase in the incidence of stroke (1.2% for patients receiving thrombolysis versus 0.8% in controls). This increase is attributed mostly to 0.4 to 0.5% incidence of intracerebral bleeding occurring on the first day. The 0.3% incidence of stroke is very significantly lower in patients under the age of 55, compared with 2.0% in patients 75 years and older (see Table 14-5).

TABLE 14-5 Incidence of Stroke Following Thrombolysis*

Age, years	Control, %	Thrombolytic, %	Excess per 1000 (SD)
<55	0.4	0.3	−1.7 (1.1)
55–64	0.6	1.1	5.1 (1.5)
65–74	1.0	1.4	4.8 (1.9)
>75	1.2	2.0	7.6 (3.7)

*SD = standard deviation.

It has been considered that patients admitted to thrombolytic trials are at lower risk for intracerebral bleeding, and thus it is important to note the results from two separate surveys that were conducted outside the trials. The incidence of intracerebral hemorrhage in a group of nonrandomized patients admitted to 61 hospitals in Holland over 18 months was 1.0% (95% confidence limits, 0.62 to 1.3%). Analysis of events from a Myocardial Infarction Triage and Intervention (MITI) study, where patients in the Seattle area with myocardial infarction were monitored, revealed an equal incidence of stroke in patients receiving thrombolysis (1.6%) compared with patients who did not (2.2%). The incidence of hemorrhagic stroke was 1.1% in the patients receiving thrombolysis compared with 0.4% in those who did not receive thrombolytic agents.

The incidence of intracranial hemorrhage was as high as 1.3% in the TIMI-II trial, in which patients were treated with 150 mg tPA. This was decreased to 0.4% when the dose of tPA was decreased to 100 mg, and thus the larger dose of tPA is no longer used.

Although hypertension is generally regarded as a significant risk factor in the development of an intracranial bleed following administration of thrombolytic agents, this has not been proved from the trials or general surveys. A multivariant logistic regression analysis found that only prior treatment with other anticoagulants, body weight less than 70 kg, and age greater than 65 were associated with a significantly greater incidence of intracerebral bleeding.

It was originally deemed that patients who had a prior cerebrovascular episode more than 6 months prior to the myocardial infarction would be at low risk for an intracerebral bleed. When such patients were randomized to receive tPA in the TIMI study, the incidence of cerebral hemorrhage remained very high at 3.4%, compared with 0.5% in the later part of the trial when such patients were excluded.

There appears to be a small difference in hemorrhagic stroke according to the thrombolytic agent used. A significant difference in intracerebral bleeding was found in the ISIS-3 trial between patients who received tPA (0.7%) and those who received streptokinase (0.3%). This difference has been attributed to a higher dose of duteplase compared with a lower dose of alteplase, which is currently the form of tPA used today. In the GISSI-2 trial, the incidence of hemorrhagic stroke was 0.3% in the tPA group and 0.25% in those patients receiving streptokinase. However, in the GUSTO trial, the incidence of hemorrhagic stroke was 0.7% and significantly greater than 0.5% in patients receiving streptokinase. In patients older than 75 years, the incidence of hemorrhagic stroke was 2.08% in patients treated with tPA and significantly greater than the 1.23% in patients receiving streptokinase. Thus it may be more judicious to use streptokinase in elderly patients presenting with acute myocardial infarction.

Noncerebral Hemorrhage

The incidence of major noncerebral bleeds that require blood transfusion occurred more frequently in patients who received thrombolysis with an excess of 7.3 per 1000 patients (1.1% in patients receiving thrombolysis and 0.4% in the patients in the control group).

Treatment of Bleeding with Thrombolysis

Massive bleeding accompanied by hemodynamic compromise, particularly if the bleeding site is incompressible, should be treated with coagulation factors and volume replacement. If the patient is receiving heparin, it should be discontinued and protamine administered. In the absence of heparin therapy, a prolonged partial thromboplastin time will identify patients with a persistent fibrinolytic state. The patient should immediately receive 10 U of cryoprecipitate. A fibrinogen level should be monitored only after the cyroprecipitate has been given, and if less than 100 mg%, the patient should receive an additional 10 U of cryoprecipitate. If bleeding persists after fibrinogen has been restored, 2 U of fresh frozen plasma should be given. If the bleeding continues to be uncontrolled, it is recommended that bleeding time be monitored. If this is longer than 9 min, the patient should receive 10 U of platelets; if the bleeding time is less then 9 min, it is suggested that the patient receive antifibrinolytic agents such as aminocaproic acid.

Cardiac Rupture

Myocardial rupture is a consequence of transmural myocardial necrosis and occurs in approximately 4% of patients admitted to the hospital with acute myocardial infarction. It has been reasoned that early administration of thrombolytic therapy will reduce cardiac rupture by preventing transmural necrosis, whereas late thrombolysis, which promotes hemorrhage into a transmural myocardial infarct, will increase the incidence of myocardial rupture. Honan et al., in a metaanalysis of placebo-controlled trials in which thrombolysis was administered to 1638 patients, considered that 58 patients had developed myocardial rupture. Regression-line analysis revealed that the incidence of myocardial rupture increased with the time interval between the onset of symptoms and the administration of the thrombolytic agent and that the odds ratio is greater than 1.0 of developing cardiac rupture when the thrombolytic agents were administered 11 h after the onset of symptoms. However, in the prospectively designed LATE study, the incidence of myocardial rupture was greater with thrombolysis between 6 and 12 h compared with 12 and 24 h after the onset of symptoms.

Thus it appears that the time course of rupture may be accelerated by thrombolysis but that the overall incidence may not be increased.

TABLE 14-6 Criteria for Thrombolysis in Acute Myocardial Infarction

Chest pain consistent with acute myocardial infarction lasting 30 min
Electrocardiographic changes
  ST-segment elevation in at least two contiguous limb leads of 0.1 mV
    V_1–V_3 of 0.2 mV
    V_4–V_6 of 0.1 mV
  ST-segment depression in V_{1-3} with tall RV_2 with diagnosis posterior infarction
  New or presumed left bundle branch block
Time from onset of symptoms

<6 h	Most beneficial
6–12 h	Intermediate benefit
>12 h	Least benefit; consider if chest pain present or stuttering pain course in high-risk patients

INDICATIONS AND CONTRAINDICATIONS TO THROMBOLYSIS

Indications for thrombolysis in patients with acute myocardial infarction are listed in Table 14-6 and the contraindications in Table 14-7. A more detailed discussion on the following items is provided in the earlier part of the text: time after myocardial infarction, site of myocardial infarction, non-Q-wave myocardial infarction, cardiogenic shock, elderly patients, and hypertension. The distinction between absolute and relative contraindications to thrombolysis becomes less important when a cardiac catheterization laboratory is available for the performance of immediate coronary angioplasty.

TABLE 14-7 Contraindications to Thrombolytic Therapy

Absolute contraindications
  Prior intracranial bleed
  Thromboembolic stroke within 2 months
  Neurosurgery within one month
  Active internal bleeding (excluding menstruation)
  Dissecting aortic aneurysm
Relative contraindications
  Persistent hypertension ≥ 180/110 despite therapy
  Recent puncture of noncompressible vessel
  Gastrointestinal and genitourinary bleeding within 1 month
  Bleeding diathesis
  Anticoagulant therapy
  Significant liver and renal disease
  Pericarditis
  Pregnancy
  Recent surgery or biopsy of internal organ within 2 weeks

THROMBOLYSIS FOR CONDITIONS OTHER THAN ACUTE MYOCARDIAL INFARCTION

Obstructive Mechanical Prosthetic Valve

The incidence of thrombosis of mechanical mitral prostheses is greater than that in the aortic position, with an annual incidence of less than 0.5%. The operative mortality has been reported to be 11 to 12% but significantly higher, 17.5%, in patients with class IV New York Heart Association symptoms. Roudaut and colleagues describe successful thrombolysis in 73% of 75 thrombotic events, with a 92% success rate in patients with functional classes I and II and 63% in patients with functional classes III and IV. Embolic events occurred in 12 of the 64 patients, 4 of which were major. Recurrence of thrombosis occurred in 11 patients in approximately 1 year. In a metaanalysis, thrombolysis was reported to be effective in 84%, and streptokinase appeared to be more effective than urokinase.

It has been recommended that patients who have obstructed prostheses with minimal clot seen on transesophageal echocardiography should receive thrombolysis, with an expected success rate of 92%. Should thrombolysis not be successful within 24 to 72 h, surgery is recommended. Surgery is also recommended for patients with large, substantial clots or patients who have class IV symptoms of obstructive prostheses.

Pulmonary Embolism

In the Urokinase Pulmonary Embolism Trial (UPET) conducted in the early 1970s, in which urokinase followed by heparin was compared with heparin alone in a total of 160 patients, there was a trend toward reduction in mortality and recurrent emboli in patients assigned to receive thrombolysis. However, there was a significantly more rapid and complete dissolution of thrombi but more bleeding complications in the patients receiving thrombolysis.

Unfortunately, the subsequent trials have utilized even fewer patients than has UPET. The PAIMS-2 trial in Italy showed that thrombolysis produced a more efficient dissolution of thrombus and more rapid reduction in pulmonary arterial pressure following 2 h of tPA infusion compared with heparin. When tPA was compared with urokinase in the European Cooperative Study Group, it was observed that there was a more significant and rapid reduction in pulmonary vascular resistance at 2 h, but the results were similar at 6 h.

In the series of trials carried out by Goldhaber, it was shown that after tPA infusion there was significantly greater clot lysis after 2 h when compared with urokinase administered over 24 h, but at 24 h there was no difference in the clot lysis between these two groups. Similar efficacy resulted when a condensed dose of urokinase was administered.

This group also demonstrated that there was significantly greater improvement in right ventricular systolic function as measured by echocardiography at 24 h when tPA was administered compared with heparin. It has been shown that tPA administered via a pulmonary catheter or a peripheral vein resulted in similar rate of thrombolysis of thrombi, and thus thrombolytic agents did not have to be administered via a pulmonary catheter infusion.

Approved FDA regimens for the treatment of pulmonary embolism are streptokinase, 2500-U loading dose over 30 min followed by 100,000 U/h for 24 h; urokinase, 4400 U/kg loading dose over 10 min, followed by 4400 U/h for 12 to 24 h; tPA, 100 mg over 2 h. It is recommended that heparin not be given simultaneously with a thrombolytic agent.

Ischemic Stroke

The use of thrombolytic agents in the treatment of ischemic stroke remains controversial. Earlier studies using streptokinase were stopped prematurely because of excess intracranial hemorrhage or were of no benefit when tPA was used. These trials treated patients up to 6 h after the onset of stroke. In a more recent study, patients were randomized to receive tPA or placebo within 3 h after the onset of stroke. After a computed tomographic scan had excluded intracranial hemorrhage, patients who received thrombolysis were 30% more likely to have minimal or no disability at 3 months.

Based on the preceding study, tPA was given FDA approval for the management of acute ischemic stroke in adults for improving neurologic recovery and reducing the incidence of disability. The drug needs to be used within 3 h of symptoms if patients do not show evidence of intracranial bleeding on CT scan.

Thrombotic Arterial Occlusion

Patients with acute arterial occlusion of the lower limbs and pelvis are potential candidates for intraarterial infusion of thrombolytic agents. With acute ischemia that threatens the viability of the limb, surgery primarily should be considered and thrombolysis only if surgery is not feasible or the limb not threatened. Thrombolytic therapy should be infused via an intraarterially directed catheter into the occluded artery. This has been performed successfully using streptokinase, urokinase, and tPA and has resulted in fewer lower limb amputations and a significant increase in clot lysis and recanalization. The dose of thrombolytic agents used was urokinase, 600,000-U bolus followed by 150,000 to 250,000 U/h; tPA, 0.5 to 0.1 mg/kg per hour for up to 12 h.

Arterial emboli are better removed by balloon catheter techniques or surgery, since thrombolysis has not been as successful.

SUGGESTED READINGS

ACC-AHA Guidelines for the Management of Patients with Acute Myocardial Infarction: A report from the American College of Cardiology/American Heart Assn. Task Force on Practice Guidelines (Committee on Management of Acute Myocardial Infarction). *J Am Coll Card* 28:1328, 1996.

Bode C, Kohler B, Smalling RW, Runge MS: Reteplase (r-PA): A novel recombinant plasminogen activator. *Fibrinolysis* 9(Suppl 1):97, 1995.

Collen D: Fibrin-selective thrombolytic therapy for acute myocardial infarction. *Circulation* 93:857, 1996.

Forman R, Frishman WH: Thrombolytic agents, in Frishman WH, Sonnenblick EH (eds): *Cardiovascular Pharmacotherapeutics*. New York, McGraw-Hill, 1997, pp 381–398.

Granger CB, Califf RM, Topol EJ: Thromobolytic therapy for acute myocardial infarction. *Drugs* 44:293, 1992.

Verstraete M, Fuster V: Thrombogenesis and antithrombotic therapy. In Alexander RW, Schlant RC, Fuster V: *Hurst's The Heart*, 9th ed. New York: McGraw-Hill, 1998, pp 1501–1551.

Chapter 15 Lipid-Lowering Drugs

William H. Frishman and Peter Zimetbaum

A direct relationship between elevated serum cholesterol levels, especially elevated low-density lipoprotein (LDL)-cholesterol levels, and the incidence of coronary artery disease (CAD) is well established. Lowering LDL-cholesterol levels by means of diet and/or drug therapy has been shown to reduce the progression of coronary artery lesions (Fig. 15-1) and the incidence of clinical coronary artery events. As predicted from the Framingham Study, a 10% decrease in cholesterol levels is associated with a 20% decrease in the incidence of combined morbidity and mortality related to CAD. Elevations in triglycerides and reductions in high-density lipoprotein (HDL)-cholesterol levels also may contribute to an increased CAD risk.

Advances in the understanding of lipid metabolism and the development of new drugs and dietary strategies for the treatment of lipid and lipoprotein disorders have made effective therapy of hyperlipidemia, and thus coronary heart disease risk intervention, an understandable and attainable goal.

In the following introductory section, a framework for understanding the treatment of lipid disorders is presented. Recommendations are provided, based on the second expert panel report of the National Cholesterol Education Program, regarding screening and dietary and drug interventions in human populations with hyperlipidemia at risk for premature CAD.

RATIONALE FOR THE TREATMENT OF HYPERLIPIDEMIA IN PREVENTION OF CORONARY ARTERY DISEASE

The premise for the treatment of hyperlipidemia is based on the hypothesis that abnormalities in lipid and lipoprotein levels are risk factors for CAD and that changes in blood lipids can result in decreased risk of disease and complications. Levels of plasma cholesterol and LDL-cholesterol have consistently been shown to be directly correlated with the risk of CAD.

The results of the clinical trials with cholesterol- and LDL-cholesterol-lowering interventions support the premise that cholesterol-lowering therapies aimed at reducing cholesterol by 20 to 25% produce clinically significant reductions in cardiovascular events in patients having preexisting vascular disease across a broad range of cholesterol values within 5 years of starting treatment. The greatest impact of cholesterol lowering still occurs in individuals with the highest baseline cholesterol levels. The absolute magnitude of these benefits would be even greater in those individuals having other risk factors for CAD, such as cigarette smoking and hypertension. These risk relationships are the basis for recommending lower cholesterol cut points and goals

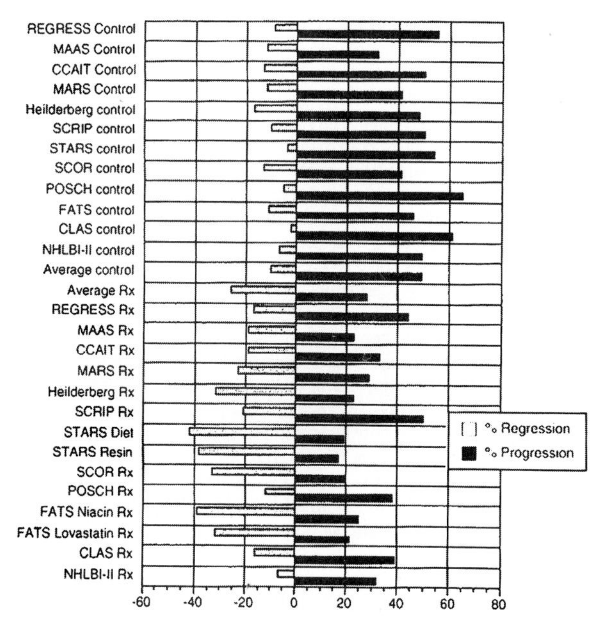

FIG. 15-1 Arteriographic CAD "regression" trials. The percents of subjects classified as regression are to the left, and those classified as progression are to the right. The control groups are listed on top of the figure, and the treatment groups are on the bottom. *(Modified from Superko HR, Krauss RM: Coronary artery disease regression. Convincing evidence for the benefit of aggressive lipoprotein management. Circulation 90:1056, 1994.)*

for those who are at high risk for developing clinical coronary heart disease.

Thus, taking into consideration the recommendations of the National Cholesterol Education Program (NCEP) and data from recently published trials, two general groups of patients that warrant aggressive therapy for hypercholesterolemia can be identified—those without evidence of CAD who are at high risk for developing coronary heart disease (primary prevention) and those with known coronary disease or other atherosclerotic process and high cholesterol (secondary prevention). In patients without coronary disease and moderately elevated serum LDL-cholesterol but no other risk factors, there is understable skepticism toward recommending pharmacologic therapy, although dietary modification would be appropriate. However, in patients with coronary heart disease (including the elderly and women), even mild elevations of LDL-cholesterol should be treated aggressively, targeting treatment to an LDL-cholesterol <100 mg/dL.

The evidence for elevated triglycerides as a risk factor for CAD is less clear. Several prospective studies have shown a correlation between levels of plasma triglycerides and CAD. Data from the Framingham Study, however, have indicated that when other risk factors, such as obesity, elevated serum cholesterol (or hypercholesterolemia), hypertension, and diabetes, were accounted for, triglycerides are not an independent risk factor for CAD. However, there is a select group of patients with hypertriglyceridemia who are at increased risk of coronary heart disease and who can be identified by a strong family history of premature CAD. Another important factor is that serum triglyceride levels are inversely related to HDL levels, and reductions in triglyceride levels are associated with a rise in HDL. Since HDL might be protective against CAD, this provides an additional rationale for the treatment of hypertriglyceridemia. However, as of yet, there is no evidence that lowering triglyceride levels or raising HDL levels will result in a diminished risk of CAD. A trial is in progress, Veterans Affairs Low HDL Intervention Trial (HIT), to see whether raising HDL-cholesterol with drugs as a primary target affects outcomes in post-myocardial infarction patients.

WHO SHOULD BE SCREENED FOR HYPERLIPIDEMIA?

The Expert Panel Report of the National Cholesterol Education Program on Detection, Evaluation and Treatment of High Blood Cholesterol in Adults suggests that total cholesterol be measured in all adults 20 years of age and older at least once every 5 years. A controversy was raised when the American College of Physicians recommended only general cholesterol screening for middle-aged men, a screening approach that has been vigorously challenged. A recent NCEP panel recommended that cholesterol screening should not be done routinely in children unless a history of familial hyperlipidemia exists or a family history of premature CAD is present. Cholesterol values in the general pediatric population may not always predict the future development of hypercholesterolemia in adults.

WHO SHOULD BE TREATED FOR HYPERCHOLESTEROLEMIA

Once the screening cholesterol values are obtained (Fig. 15-2), the NCEP recommends the following approach to clinical management in adults. The presence of a high cholesterol should always be confirmed with a second test and the fasting LDL-cholesterol measured in a lipoprotein analysis to make a more precise estimate of CAD risk. The standard deviation of repeated measurements in an individual over time

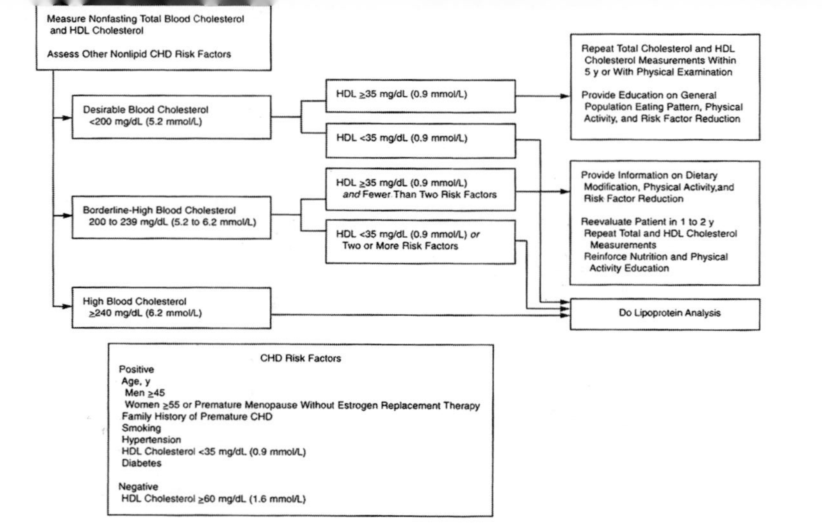

FIG. 15-2 Primary prevention in adults without evidence of coronary heart disease (CHD). Initial classification is based on total cholesterol and high-density lipoprotein (HDL) cholesterol levels. *(From Expert Panel on Detection, Evaluation and Treatment of High Blood Cholesterol in Adults: Summary of the Second Report of the National Cholesterol Education Program (NCEP), Expert Panel on Detection, Evaluation and Treatment of High Blood Cholesterol in Adults (Adult Treatment Panel II). JAMA 269:3015, 1993, with permission.)*

has been reported as 0.39 mm/L (15 mg/dL) for total cholesterol and 0.39 mm/L (15 mg/dL) for LDL-cholesterol. Patients should be maintained on the same diet during these initial determinations before therapy is instituted. Secondary causes of hypercholesterolemia (hypothyroidism, nephrotic syndrome, diabetes mellitus) also should be considered.

The NCEP recommends an approach in adults based on LDL-cholesterol, which is shown in Figs. 15-3 and 15-4 and Table 15-1. Management should always begin with dietary intervention, as outlined in Fig. 15-4. When response to diet is inadequate, the NCEP recommends the addition of pharmacologic therapy (Fig. 15-5). Specific drug therapies are discussed in subsequent sections of this chapter.

WHO SHOULD BE TREATED FOR HYPERTRIGLYCERIDEMIA

Interest in the link between serum triglyceride levels and coronary heart disease has grown in recent years. Triglyceride levels correlate positively with levels of LDL-cholesterol and inversely with HDL. Clinical trials with triglyceride-lowering drugs, nicotinic acid, and gemfibrozil have shown a benefit on coronary artery event frequency compared with placebo therapy. However, therapy in these trials was not targeted to patients with primary hypertriglyceridemia. The currently recommended approach to the problem of hypertriglyceridemia is presented in the report of the NCEP.

Much of borderline hypertriglyceridemia [2.82 to 5.65 mm/L (250 to 500 mg/dL)] is due to various exogenous or secondary factors, which include alcohol, diabetes mellitus, hypothyroidism, obesity, chronic renal disease, and drugs. Changes in lifestyle and/or treatment of the primary disease process may be sufficient to reduce triglycerides.

Patients with borderline hypertriglyceridemia due to familial hypertriglyceridemia (type IV) are not at risk of having premature CAD. Caloric restriction and increased exercise can be recommended for obese patients, but drug therapy is inappropriate.

Patients with familial combined hyperlipoproteinemia (type IIb) often have mild hypertriglyceridemia. Patients with this condition are at risk of premature coronary heart disease. These patients should have dietary treatment first and, if necessary, drugs. Patients with borderline hypertriglyceridemia with clinical manifestations of CAD can be treated as if they have familial combined hyperlipoproteinemia.

APPROACH TO LOW SERUM HDL-CHOLESTEROL

A low serum HDL-cholesterol level is emerging as a strong lipoprotein predictor of coronary heart disease. In one prospective study, after adjustment for other risk factors in predicting the risk of myocardial infarction, a change in one unit in the ratio of total to HDL-cholesterol was associated with a 53% change in risk. However, it is still not known

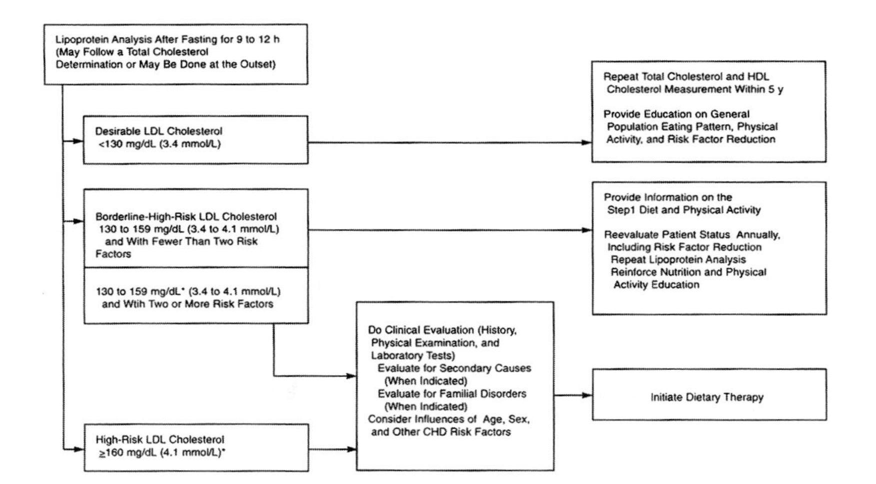

FIG. 15-3 Primary prevention in adults without evidence of coronary heart disease (CHD). Subsequent classification is based on low-density lipoprotein (LDL)-cholesterol levels. *On the basis of the average of two determinations. If the first two LDL-cholesterol test results differ by >30 mg/dL (0.7 mmol/L), a third test result should be obtained within 1–8 wks and the average value of the 3 tests used. *(From Expert Panel on Detection, Evaluation and Treatment of High Blood Cholesterol in Adults: Summary of the Second Report of the National Cholesterol Education Program (NCEP), Expert Panel on Detection, Evaluation and Treatment of High Blood Cholesterol in Adults (Adult Treatment Panel II). JAMA 269:3015, 1993, with permission.)*

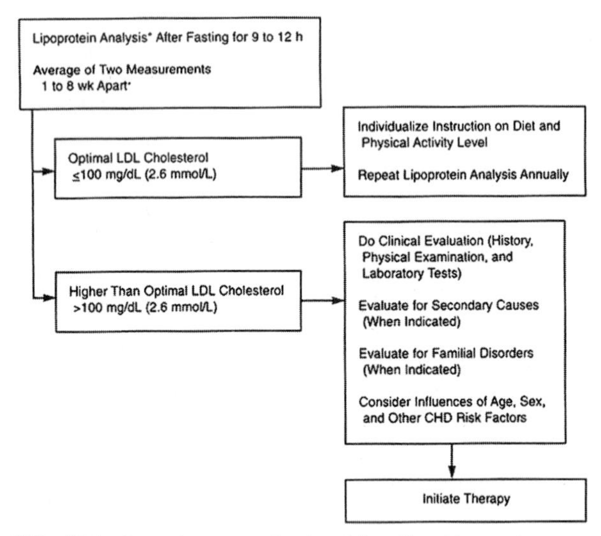

FIG. 15-4 Secondary prevention in adults with evidence of coronary heart disease (CHD). Classification is based on low-density lipoprotein (LDL)-cholesterol levels. *Lipoprotein analysis should be performed when the patient is not in the recovery phase from an acute coronary or other medical event that would lower the usual LDL-cholesterol level. †If the first two LDL-cholesterol test results differ by >30 mg/dL (0.7 mmol/L), a third test result should be obtained within 1–8 wks and the average value of the 3 tests used. *(From Expert Panel on Detection, Evaluation and Treatment of High Blood Cholesterol in Adults: Summary of the Second Report of the National Cholesterol Education Program (NCEP), Expert Panel on Detection, Evaluation and Treatment of High Blood Cholesterol in Adults (Adult Treatment Panel II). JAMA 269:3015, 1993, with permission.)*

how low HDL levels are linked to CAD and whether raising HDL levels can lower coronary disease risk. The major causes of reduced serum HDL-cholesterol are listed in Table 15-2. Clearly, attempts should be made to raise low HDL-cholesterol by hygienic means. When a low HDL is associated with an increase in very low-density lipoprotein (VLDL), the latter deserves consideration for therapeutic modification. However, when the HDL is reduced without associated risk factors, attempts to raise HDL levels by drugs cannot be justified because of a lack of clinical trial evidence showing benefit.

TABLE 15-1 Treatment Decisions Based on LDL-Cholesterol Level*

Patient category	Initiation level	LDL goal
	Dietary therapy	
Without CHD and with fewer than two risk factors	≥160 mg/dL (4.1 mmol/L)	<160 mg/dL (4.1 mmol/L)
Without CHD and with two or more risk factors	≥130 mg/dL (3.4 mmol/L)	<130 mg/dL (3.4 mmol/L)
With CHD	>100 mg/dL (2.6 mmol/L)	≤100 mg/dL (2.6 mmol/L)
	Drug treatment	
Without CHD and with fewer than two risk factors	≥190 mg/dL (4.9 mmol/L)	<160 mg/dL (4.1 mmol/L)
Without CHD and with two or more risk factors	≥160 mg/dL (4.1 mmol/L)	<130 mg/dL (3.4 mmol/L)
With CHD	≥130 mg/dL (3.4 mmol/L)	≤100 mg/dL (2.6 mmol/L)

*LDL = low-density lipoprotein; CHD = coronary heart disease.

BILE ACID SEQUESTRANTS

The bile acid binding resins cholestyramine and colestipol are among the drugs of first choice for hypercholesterolemia in patients without concurrent hypertriglyceridemia. Cholestyramine was used originally for treatment of pruritus caused by elevated concentations of bile acids secondary to cholestasis. However, attention has focused on the bile acid sequestrants' (BAS) ability to lower LDL-cholesterol plasma concentration. The resins have been tested extensively in large-scale, long-term follow-up clinical trials to explore their efficacy for such an application. These drugs are not absorbed in the gastrointestinal (GI) tract and, therefore, have a limited range of systemic side effects. For this reason, they are particularly useful for treatment of pregnant women with hypercholesterolemia and are the only drugs to be considered safe for use in children with heterozygous familial hypercholesterolemia. The disadvantage of the sequestrants lies in their mode of administration and the frequency of GI side effects.

Chemistry

Cholestyramine (Questran powder) is the chloride salt of a basic anion-exchange resin. The ion-exchange sites are provided by the presence

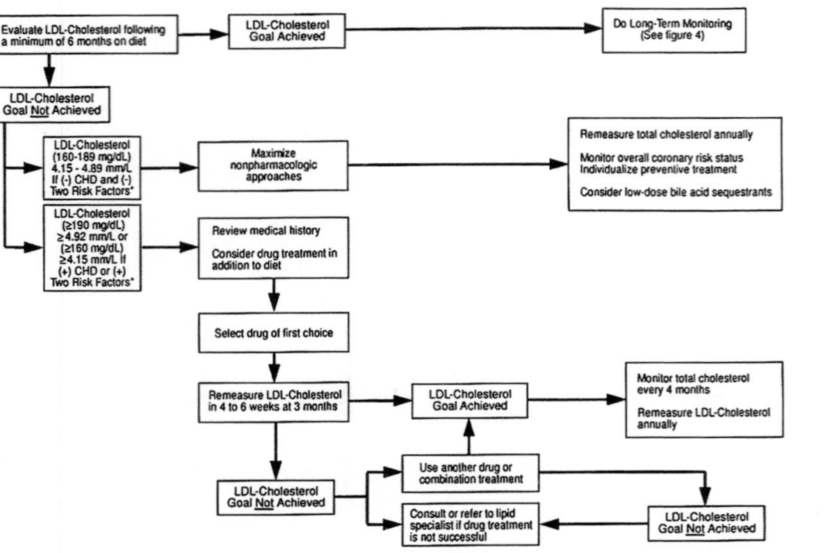

FIG. 15-5 Drug treatment (adults). *one of which can be male sex; LDL = low density lipoprotein; CHD = coronary heart disease. *(From Expert Panel on Detection, Evaluation and Treatment of High Blood Cholesterol in Adults: Summary of the Second Report of the National Cholesterol Education Program (NCEP), Expert Panel on Detection, Evaluation and Treatment of High Blood Cholesterol in Adults (Adult Treatment Panel II). JAMA 269:3015, 1993, with permission.)*

TABLE 15-2 Major Causes of Reduced Serum HDL-Cholesterol

Cigarette smoking
Obesity
Lack of exercise
Androgenic and related steroids
Androgens
Progestational agents
Anabolic steroids
β-Adrenergic blocking agents
Hypertriglyceridemia
Genetic factors
Primary hypoalphalipoproteinemia

of trimethylbenzylammonium groups in a large copolymer of styrene and divinyl benzene. Cholestyramine's average polymeric molecular weight is $>10^6$. The resin is hydrophilic yet insoluble in water. It is given orally after being suspended in water or juice. It is not absorbed in the GI tract, and it is not altered by digestive enzymes, permitting it to remain unchanged while traversing the intestines.

Colestipol (Colestid), supplied as the powder colestipol hydrochloride, is a basic anion-exchange copolymer made up of diethylenetriamine and 1-chloro-2,3-epoxypropane. It has approximately one out of its five amine nitrogens protonated (chloride form). Like cholestyramine, colestipol is not altered by digestive enzymes, nor is it absorbed in the digestive tract. It is supplied in powder form and is taken orally after it is suspended in liquid.

Pharmacology

Bile acids are synthesized in the liver from cholesterol, their sole precursor. They are then secreted into the GI tract, where they interact with fat-soluble molecules, thereby aiding in the digestion and subsequent absorption of these substances. Bile acids are absorbed along with the fat-soluble molecules and are subsequently recycled by the liver via the portal circulation for resecretion into the GI tract. The bile acids remain in the enterohepatic circulation and never enter the systemic circulation.

Both cholestyramine and colestipol bind bile acids in the intestine. The complex thus formed is then excreted in the feces. By binding the bile acids, the resins deny the bile acids entry into the bloodstream and thereby remove a large portion of the acids from the enterohepatic circulation. The decrease in hepatic concentrations of bile acids allows a disinhibition of cholesterol 7α-hydroxylase, the rate-limiting enzyme in bile acid synthesis. Also seen is an increase in activity of phosphatidic acid phosphatase, an enzyme responsible for the conversion of α-glycerol phosphate to triglyceride. The increased activity of this enzyme causes a shift away from phospholipid production and, ultimately, an increase in the triglyceride content and size of VLDL particles. There is also evidence to suggest that the BASs also cause an increase in the activity of 3-hydroxy-3-methyl glutaryl-coenzyme A (HMG-CoA reductase), the rate-limiting enzyme in the hepatic cholesterol synthesis pathway. Although cholesterol synthesis is increased when BASs are used, there is no rise in plasma cholesterol, presumably because of the immediate shunting of the newly formed cholesterol into the bile acid synthesis pathway. The apparent shortage of cholesterol causes the hepatocyte cell surface receptors for LDL particles to be altered either quantitatively by increasing in number or qualitatively by increasing their affinity for the LDL particle. By sequestering the cholesterol-rich LDL particles, the liver decreases the plasma concentration of cholesterol.

Pharmacokinetics

Cholestyramine and colestipol bind bile acids in the intestines, forming a chemical complex that is excreted in the feces. There is no chemical modification of the resins while in the GI tract; however, the chloride ions of the resins may be replaced by other anions with higher affinity for the resin. Colestipol is hydrophilic but is virtually insoluble in water (99.75%). Neither the high-molecular polymer of cholestyramine or colestipol is absorbed in the GI tract. Less than 0.05% of ^{14}C-labeled colestipol is excreted in the urine.

Since the resins are not absorbed into the systemic circulation, any interactions that occur between the resins and other molecules occur in the intestines and usually occur with substances ingested with or near the time of resin ingestion. Interaction between resins and fat-soluble substances, such as the fat-soluble vitamins, causes a decrease in absorption of these substances. Malabsorption of vitamin K, for instance, has been associated with a hypoprothrombinemia. It is therefore recommended that vitamins K and D be supplemented in patients on long-term resin therapy. Likewise, medications taken with or near the time of resin ingestion may be bound by the resin and not be absorbed. Drugs at risk include phenylbutazone, warfarin, chlorothiazide (acidic), propranolol (basic), penicillin G, tetracycline, phenobarbitol, thyroid and thyroxine preparations, and digitalis.

The dose-response curves for the bile acid resins are nonlinear, with increases in the antihypercholesterolemic effect minimal for doses $>$30 g/day. Furthermore, there tend to be compliance problems when large doses of resin are used, making doses $>$15 g two times daily inefficacious.

Since the BASs are polymeric cations bound to chloride anions, continued ingestion of the resins places a chloride load on the body. This chloride load may cause a decrease in the urine pH and also an increase in the urinary excretion of chloride, which can reach 60% of the ingested resin load. Furthermore, there may be an increase in excretion of calcium ions, which is dependent on the extent of chloride ion excretion. Because of this increase in calcium ion excretion, care should be taken, especially when treating a person at risk for osteoporosis, to limit the extent of calcium excretion by controlling the chloride dietary load.

Clinical Experiences

Numerous studies have shown the BAS cholestyramine and colestipol to be efficacious in lowering LDL and total cholesterol levels in the plasma. Studies have further correlated the decreased levels of LDL-cholesterol with the slowing of progression of coronary atherosclerosis and a lowered incidence of coronary events. Furthermore, studies of lipoprotein content in resin-treated individuals have detected a qualitative effect that may have a contributory role in the antiatherosclerotic effects of the drug. Sequestrants are limited to use in those patients with hypercholesterolemia not associated with severe hypertriglyceridemia. Therefore, unless bile acid resins are combined with other antihyperlipidemic drugs, their use is limited to treatment of individuals with type IIa hyperlipoproteinemia.

Clinical Use of Resins

Bile acid resins are indicated as adjunct therapy to diet for reduction of serum cholesterol in patients with primary hypercholesterolemia. Dietary therapy should precede resin usage and should address both the specific type of hyperlipoproteinemia in the patient and the body weight of the patient, since obesity has been shown to be a contributing factor in hyperlipoproteinemia. Since resin use can cause a 5 to 20% increase in VLDL levels, it should be restricted to hypercholesterolemic patients with only slightly increased triglyceride levels. The increase in VLDL seen with resin use usually starts during the first few weeks of therapy and disappears 4 weeks after the initial rise. It is thought that excessive increases in the VLDL particles may dampen the antihyper-LDL effect of the drug by competitively binding the upwardly regulated LDL receptors on the hepatocyte. The resins therefore should not be used in patients whose triglyceride levels exceed 3.5 mmol/L unless accompanied by a second drug that has antihypertriglyceride effects; some suggest not using resins if the triglyceride level exceeds 2.5 mmol/L. A general rule of thumb is that if the triglyceride level exceeds 7 mmol/L, the LDL concentration is seldom raised, and therefore, bile acid resin treatment would not be effective.

Both cholestyramine and colestipol are available as powders that must be mixed with water or fruit juice before ingestion and are taken in two to three divided doses with or just after meals. BAS can decrease absorption of some antihypertensive agents, including thiazide diuretics and propranolol. As a general recommendation, all other drugs should be administered either 1 h before or 4 h after the BAS. The cholesterol-lowering effect of 4 g of cholestyramine appears to be equivalent to 5 g of colestipol. The response to therapy is variable in each individual, but a 15 to 30% reduction in LDL-cholesterol may be seen with colestipol treatment 20 to 30 g/day or cholestyramine 16 to 24 g/day. The fall in LDL concentration becomes detectable 4 to 7 days after the start of treatment and approaches 90% of maximal effect in 2 weeks. Initial dosing should be 4 to 5 g of cholestyramine or colestipol, respectively, two times daily. The drugs are also useful if administered once daily. In patients who do not respond adequately to initial therapy, the dosing can be increased to the maximum mentioned above. Dosing above the maximum does not increase the antihypercholesterolemic effect of the drug considerably but does increase side effects and therefore decreases compliance. Since both resins are virtually identical in action, the choice of one over the other is based on patient preference, specifically taste and the ability to tolerate ingestion of bulky material.

To avoid some of the difficulties with use of the powders, colestipol is available in 1-g tablets that need to be swallowed whole. In comparative studies with colestipol powder, both formulations were equally effective and safe in reducing plasma cholesterol in hypercholesterolemic patients. In addition, colestipol is available in a flavored powdered form. Cholestyramine is also available in a low-calorie, low-volume formulation that has 1.4 cal per packet.

If resin treatment is discontinued, cholesterol levels return to pretreatment levels within a month. In patients with heterozygous hypercholesterolemia who have not achieved desirable cholesterol levels on resin plus diet therapy, the combination therapy of colestipol hydrochloride and nicotinic acid has been shown to provide further lowering of serum cholesterol, triglycerides, and LDL and cause an increase in serum HDL concentration. Other drug combinations are now being studied, and of particular promise is the combination therapy of bile acid sequestrants and HMG-CoA reductase inhibitors.

Adverse Effects of Resins

Since cholestyramine and colestipol are not absorbed in the body, the range of adverse effects is limited. A majority of patient complaints stem from the resin's effect on the GI tract and from subjective complaints concerning the taste, texture, and bulkiness of the resins. The most common side effect is constipation, which is reported in approximately 10% of patients on colestipol and 28% of patients on cholestyramine. This side effect is seen most commonly in patients taking large doses of the resin and most often in patients over 65 years of age. Although most cases of constipation are mild and self-limiting, progression to fecal impaction can occur. A range of 1 in 30 to 1 in 100 patients on colestipol and approximately 12% on cholestyramine experience abdominal distention and/or belching, flatulence, nausea, vomiting, and diarrhea. Peptic ulcer disease, GI irritation and bleeding, cholecystitis, and cholelithiasis have been reported in 1 of 100 patients taking colestipol but have not been shown to be purely drug-related.

Fewer than 1 in 1000 patients on colestipol experience hypersensitivity reactions such as urticaria or dermatitis. Asthma and wheezing were not seen with colestipol treatment but were reported with cholestyramine treatment in a small number of patients. In a small percentage of patients, muscle pain, dizziness, vertigo, anxiety, and drowsiness have been reported with both drugs. With cholestyramine treatment, hematuria, dysuria, and uveitis also have been reported. Resin therapy has been associated with transient and modest elevations of serum glutamic oxaloacetic transaminase and alkaline phosphatase. Some patients have shown an increase in iron-binding capacity and serum phosphorus, along with an increase in chloride ions and a decrease in sodium ions, potassium ions, uric acid, and carotene.

Case reports have described hyperchloremic acidosis in a child taking cholestyramine suffering from ischemic hepatitis and renal insufficiency, in a child with liver agenesis and renal failure, and in a patient with diarrhea due to ileal resection. For these reasons, those patients at risk for hyperchloremia should have serum chloride levels checked during the course of resin treatment.

In the LRC-CPPT study, the incidence of malignancy in the cholestyramine-treated group was equal to the control group, however, the incidence of GI malignancy in the treated group was higher than in the nontreated group (21 versus 11, respectively), with more fatal cases in the treated group (eight deaths in the treated group versus one in the control group). In animal studies, cholestyramine was shown to increase the mammary tumorigenesis capabilities of 7,12-dimethylbenzanthracene (DMBA) in Wistar rats. In the cholestyramine plus DMBA-treated rats, there was a fivefold increase in the incidence of mammory cancer over control. Stemming from the resin's ability to disrupt normal fat-soluble vitamin absorption in the gut, there have been a number of reports concerning the occurrence of hypoprothrombinemic hemorrhage secondary to vitamin K malabsorption. In both the previous cited cases, the patients responded to vitamin K adjunct therapy.

An early study showed that colestipol can bind T_4 in the gut and in vitro. This binding can theoretically upset the normal reabsorption of T_4 from the gut and thereby disrupt normal T_4 recycling, causing hypothyroidism. However, a subsequent study showed that for euthyroid patients, thyroid function tests remained normal throughout resin treatment. It is advisable that patients on thyroid replacement therapy avoid taking the replacement drug at the same time as ingesting the resin to avoid any malabsorption problems.

GEMFIBROZIL AND OTHER FIBRIC ACID DERIVATIVES

Fibric acid derivatives (FAD) are a class of drugs that have been shown to inhibit the production of VLDL while enhancing VLDL clearance, owing to stimulation of lipoprotein lipase activity. The drugs can reduce plasma triglycerides and concurrently raise HDL-cholesterol levels. Their effects on LDL-cholesterol are less marked and more variable.

This section reviews the clinical pharmacology of gemfibrozil, discusses the therapeutic experiences with this agent, and provides recommendations for its clinical use.

Pharmacokinetics

Gemfibrozil is well absorbed from the GI tract, with peak plasma levels seen 1 to 2 h after administration. The plasma half-life is 1.5 h after the single dose and 1.3 h after multiple-dose therapy. The plasma drug concentration is proportional to dose and steady state and is reached after 1 to 2 weeks of twice-daily dosing. Gemfibrozil undergoes oxidation of the ring methyl group in the liver, to form hydroxymethyl and carboxyl metabolites (in total, there are four major metabolites). No reports as yet have described distribution of the drug into human breast milk or across the placenta. Two-thirds (66%) of the twice-daily dose is eliminated in the urine within 48 h, 6% is eliminated in the feces within 5 days of dosing, and less than 5% of the drug is eliminated unchanged in the urine. Regardless of the dosing schedule, there is no drug accumulation with normal or impaired renal function.

In vitro, gemfibrozil is 98% bound to albumin at therapeutic levels. There have been reports that gemfibrozil, in vitro, when administered concurrently with warfarin, leads to a doubling of the unbound warfarin fraction. Similarly, clofibrate has been found to potentiate the anticoagulation activity of warfarin.

Mechanism of Action of Gemfibrozil

At this stage of knowledge, it is impossible to delineate one clear mechanism of action of gemfibrozil. However, observations have been made regarding the effects on the individual lipoprotein components and the cholesterol-triglyceride metabolic pathways.

One direct action of FADs appears to be an increase in the level of plasma lipoprotein lipase (LPL). LPL is deficient in type I hyperlipoproteinemia, types I and II diabetes mellitus, hypothyroidism, heart failure, and nephrotic syndrome. LPL is increased by insulin treatment of diabetes mellitus, aerobic exercise, and FADs. LPL is the rate-limiting enzyme governing the removal of triglycerides from lipoproteins in the plasma. It functions at the luminal surface of the vascular endothelium and depends on the presence of apo CII on chylomicrons, VLDL, and HDL to activate its hydrolytic capacity. The level of LPL has been found to be increased after the addition of gemfibrozil for reasons that are not yet understood. Enhancement of LPL also is found with fenofibrate therapy.

VLDL is produced in the liver and circulates in the plasma, where LPL hydrolyzes it to a VLDL remnant by removing triglyceride. The VLDL remnant is then either taken up by an apo E receptor-mediated process in the liver or converted to LDL. FADs have been shown to decrease the production of VLDL and to increase its fractional catabolic rate (FCR). An increased FCR means an increased production of VLDL remnants that are then taken up by the liver or converted to LDL.

Gemfibrozil has been studied predominantly in subjects with hypertriglyceridemia. In the hypertriglyceridemic state, there are alterations in the usual homogeneity of lipoprotein subtractions. For instance, much of the LDL of hypertriglyceridemic patients contains a smaller amount of cholesterol ester and a greater amount of triglyceride than is usual. Presumably, this aberration results from an exchange of triglyceride for cholesterol between VLDL and LDL. The triglyceride-enriched LDL is then hydrolyzed by hepatic triglyceride lipase, leading to further reduction in size and increase in density of the LDL molecule. Thus, in the hypertriglyceridemic state, there are LDL fragments of normal composition coexisting with triglyceride-enriched and triglyceride-depleted forms. The clinical consequences of this heterogeneous LDL population are not yet apparent.

In the hypertriglyceridemic state, the production and fractional clearance of LDL are also increased. Thus patients with isolated hypertriglyceridemia may have low to normal LDL levels. Correction of the hypertriglyceridemic state with gemfibrozil restores the normal LDL population, as well as reduces the production and catabolism of LDL. The result is often a slight increase in LDL levels. Similarly, with fenofibrate or bezafibrate, when there are normal or low LDL levels, treatment increases levels of LDL. Grundy and Vega offer the explanation that during fibrate therapy, the increased lipolysis of VLDL triglyceride promotes increased hepatic uptake of VLDL remnants, leaving fewer receptors for clearance of LDL and thus increased plasma LDL. Saku et al. suggest that the short-term result of FAD therapy is an increased production of LDL-cholesterol secondary to increased VLDL catabolism and resulting downregulation of hepatic LDL receptors. As the VLDL levels decrease, the LDL-cholesterol content increases, establishing a more normal LDL particle. Regardless of the mechanism for changes in LDL levels, the importance of inhibiting production of VLDL, as well as enhancing catabolism, has been well documented. Studies show that gemfibrozil, in the primary hypertriglyceridemic state, increases LDL less than clofibrate, a drug that enhances VLDL catabolism without altering production. Fenofibrate treatment of hypertriglyceridemic patients causes LDL levels to increase by 25%, as

VLDL levels decrease by 77%. The drug also increases the clearance rate of apo B and causes a decrease in apo B levels of approximately 35% Similar observations have been made with bezafibrate treatment of hypertriglyceridemia.

HDL composition is also altered in hypertriglyceridemia. Normally, HDL_{2a}, the cholesterol ester–rich subfraction, predominates in the circulation. HDL_{2a} is transformed to HDL_{2b} when it acquires triglyceride. HDL_3 is formed from the removal of triglyceride from HDL_{2b} by hepatic triglyceride (TG) lipase and LPL. HDL_3 then acquires new cholesterol ester via lecithin cholesterol acetyl transferase (LCAT) and forms HDL_{2a}. Hypertriglyceridemia markedly reduces HDL_{2a} concentration and increases HDL_{2b} concentrations. Essentially, hypertriglyceridemia decreases the cholesterol content of HDL. FAD therapy reverses this process, leading to increased cholesterol content of HDL. Gemfibrozil also has been found to stimulate the synthesis of apo AI, the major apoprotein on HDL without altering its catabolism. Similarly, fenofibrate and bezafibrate increase apo AI levels during treatment of hypertriglyceridemia. However, the levels of apo AI rarely increase to the extent that HDL rises.

Finally, the hypertriglyceridemic state is thought to be associated with an increase in cholesterol synthesis. One explanation for this is that hypertriglyceridemic LDL is altered and may present less cholesterol to the cells, thus leading to less effective downregulation of LDL receptors and less inhibition of HMG-CoA reductase. Consequently, cholesterol synthesis is increased. There is some evidence that FADs inhibit cholesterol synthesis. From comparison studies conducted by Hunninghake and Peters, it appears that the newer FADs, fenofibrate, bezafibrate, and ciprofibrate, are more effective than gemfibrozil and clofibrate in reducing cholesterol levels. The results of animal studies appear to confirm that these new agents inhibit HMG-CoA reductase. Although the older agents may have some minimal HMG-CoA reductase inhibition activity, the results of animal studies have shown much greater activity with the newer agent like bezafibrate versus clofibrate. In vivo, fenofibrate has been shown to decrease HMG-CoA activity on human mononuclear cells in type IIa and IIb patients. Similarly, bezafibrate has been found to inhibit HMG-CoA reductase activity from mononuclear cells of both normal and hypercholesterolemic patients. Other data suggest an increased peripheral mobilization of cholesterol from tissues with FADs and feedback inhibition of hepatic cholesterol synthesis.

FADs are also known to increase the secretion of cholesterol into bile and to decrease the synthesis of bile acids. This effect is modulated by LDL receptor activity, with FADs increasing hepatic uptake of cholesterol and subsequent secretion into the bile. In 1972, Grundy et al. first noticed this increased lithogenicity of bile accompanying clofibrate therapy. Since then, other investigators have reported decreased fecal bile acid secretion and increased fecal excretion of neutral steroid with gemfibrozil therapy. The net effect of decreased bile acid concentration and increased cholesterol concentration is a cholesterol supersaturation of bile, providing the potential nidus for gallstone formation. Studies with the newer FADs, especially fenofibrate, have shown variable results in terms of total bile acid synthesis and subsequent bile acid saturability. European and American studies so far have shown no increase in gallstone formation in patients on fenofibrate therapy. Thus the newer FADs may have less potential for gallstone formation.

Clinical Experience

The effects of FADs are largely dependent on the pretreatment lipoprotein classification of the patient. In short, most patients respond to therapy with a decrease in triglyceride levels and an increase in HDL levels. Hypertriglyceridemic patients without hypercholesterolemia often have a slight increase in cholesterol and LDL levels. However, patients with hypercholesterolemia often have a decrease in their cholesterol and LDL levels. The predominant difference between gemfibrozil and the newer FADs is that the newer FADs lower LDL to a greater degree than does gemfibrozil. As mentioned earlier, one explanation for this is that these new derivatives appear to inhibit HMG-CoA reductase as well as enhance the action of LPL.

The clinical data for FADs are best summarized according to their effect on hypertriglyceridemic patients, subjects with combined hypertriglyceridemia and hypercholesterolemia, and subjects with only hypercholesterolemia. Patients with type I chylomicronemia would not benefit from FADs because these individuals lack LPL, the enzyme upon which FADs presumably act.

Combination Drug Therapy

The principle of combination therapy is to combine drugs of different mechanisms to achieve an additive or synergistic effect in patients with hyperlipidemia while hoping to minimize adverse effects of the individual drugs used.

East et al. studied types II and IV patients to compare the combinations of gemfibrozil and colestipol with gemfibrozil and lovastatin. Overall, gemfibrozil plus lovastatin proved to be the superior combination. Both these combinations are theoretically sound because the mechanisms of action are all distinct. The combination of HMG-CoA reductase inhibitors and FADs is very efficacious. However, their use together is limited by an increased incidence of myositis and rhabdomyolitis. Bile acid resins are also a good choice; however, they are known to raise triglycerides, an unwanted effect in many of the patients for whom FADs are ideal. Furthermore, there may be a slight mitigation of the HDL-raising effect with the addition of a resin compared with gemfibrozil alone.

Tuomilheto et al. tested the combination of guar gum, a water-soluble fibric compound that functions like a bile acid resin, with gemfibrozil. They found that the addition of guar gum decreased total cholesterol values 13% more than gemfibrozil alone. LDL also was decreased significantly more with the combination; however, HDL levels were 5% lower with this dual therapy.

Clinical Use

It is well established that FADs are first-line therapy to reduce the risk of pancreatitis in patients with very high levels of plasma triglycerides. Results from the Helsinki Heart Study also have suggested that the hypertriglyceridemic patient with low HDL values can derive a cardioprotective effect from gemfibrozil. It is currently not recommended to treat isolated low HDL levels with pharmacologic intervention.

FADs, particularly the newer generation, decrease total cholesterol and LDL levels. However, in the absence of elevated triglycerides, they should not be first-line therapy for hypercholesterolemic patients. Type IIb patients are the subset most commonly seen in clinical practice that would benefit from FAD therapy. HMG-CoA reductase inhibitors combined with FADs are excellent therapy for severe type IIb disease; however, CPK values must be monitored closely. Bile acid resins plus gemfibrozil are also a reasonable combination for type IIb disease; however, HDL levels may drop slightly.

Gemfibrozil Dose

Gemfibrozil is approved for clinical use in the United States for the treatment of patients with very high serum triglycerides who are at risk of developing pancreatitis and for reducing the risk of clinical CAD in patients with type IIB hypercholesterolemia who are not symptomatic and who have low HDL-cholesterol and elevated LDL-cholesterol and triglyceride levels. The recommended dose for gemfibrozil is 600 mg before the morning meal and 600 mg before the evening meal. Some patients may respond to 800 mg/day, and in most instances the therapeutic benefit is augmented with an increase to 1200 mg daily. Some patients derive benefit from increasing the dosage of gemfibrozil to 1600 mg daily.

Clofibrate is available for clinical use in the United States. The recommended doses of 25 to 2000 mg are usually divided into three daily doses.

Adverse Effects

Clofibrate, one of the earliest FADs, became unpopular because of its causative association with cholelithiasis and cholecystitis in the Coronary Drug Project. The World Health Organization trial then reported a 29% increase in overall mortality in clofibrate-treated compared with placebo-treated subjects. The mortality was principally due to post-cholecystectomy complications, pancreatitis, and assorted malignancies. The Helsinki Heart Study reported a decrease in cardiovascular mortality but not overall mortality in gemfibrozil-treated subjects. The reason for the similarity of overall mortality rates with placebo and gemfibrozil remains a mystery at this time. Obviously, these findings have led to careful scrutiny of currently used and tested FADs.

The significant adverse effects noted in the Helsinki Heart Study included atrial fibrillation, acute appendicitis, dyspepsia, abdominal pain, and nonspecific rash. The review of the European clinical trials of fenofibrate with 6.5 million patient-years shows a 2 to 15% adverse reaction rate, the most common adverse reactions being GI disturbances, dizziness and headache, muscle pains, and rash. However, the only side effect significant in frequency was skin rash. In the United States multicenter study of 227 patients treated with fenofibrate, there was a 6% increase in side effects from fenofibrate, similar to the observations of the European studies. Three of four of the patients who withdrew from the United States fenofibrate study had skin rashes; the fourth had fatigue and impotence. Overall, the adverse experiences with bezafibrate have been similar to fenofibrate, with GI and neurologic disturbances, muscle aches, and rashes most commonly seen. After 4.5 years of treatment in 22 patients on bezafibrate, no side effects were reported by Olsson et al.

In the Helsinki Heart Study, there was a 55% excess incidence of gallstones and a 64% excess incidence of cholecystectomy in the drug-treated compared with placebo-treated groups. Although European studies of fenofibrate may show some increased lithogenicity of the bile, there has been no increase in the incidence of gallstone formation, either during the trials or during postmarketing surveillance. Olsson et al. found no increase in gallstone formation in 4.5 years of bezafibrate therapy. An increased incidence of malignancy has not been observed.

The manufacturer of gemfibrozil has reported mild depressions of hemoglobin, white blood cell count, and hematocrit with the drug. The Helsinki Heart Study did not find significant alterations in these parameters. Fluctuations of serum transaminase have been seen with fenofibrate therapy, as well as a decrease in alpha-gluconyl transferase and alkaline phosphatase, all without clinical significance. Also, uric acid is noted to decrease 10 to 28% on fenofibrate therapy. The clinical significance of this is unknown.

The combination of gemfibrozil and lovastatin has been shown repeatedly to predispose to rhabdomyolysis and, in some cases, renal failure. The Helsinki Heart Study did not report any cases of myopathy in patients treated with only gemfibrozil.

HMG-COA REDUCTASE INHIBITORS

In 1987 the FDA approved the marketing of lovastatin, a competitive inhibitor of 3-hydroxy-3-methylglutaryl coenzyme A reductase, the rate-limiting enzyme step in cholesterol synthesis in the body. The pharmacology and clinical efficacy of this cholesterol-lowering drug and other drugs in this class that also were approved for marketing are reviewed in this section.

Lovastatin

Chemistry

Lovastatin (Mevinolin) is a fermentation product of the fungus *Aspergillus terreus*. It is similar in structure to an earlier compound, mevastatin, a less potent inhibitor of HMG-CoA reductase, whose clinical development was limited by its possible cardiogenicity in animals.

Pharmacology

Lovastatin, as a competitive inhibitor of HMG-CoA reductase, interferes with the formation of mevalonate, a precursor of cholesterol. Mevalonate also is a precursor of ubiquinone and dolichol, nonsterol substances essential for cell growth. It initially was thought that the HMG-CoA reductase inhibitors might inhibit formation of these substances, but this is not the case. Nonsterol synthesis does not appear to be inhibited by HMG-CoA reductase.

Pharmacokinetics

Lovastatin is an inactive lactone (prodrug) that is hydrolyzed in the liver to an active α-hydroxyacid form. The prodrug was developed rather than the active hydroxyacid form because the prodrug undergoes more efficient shunting to the liver on first pass. The potential result of this enhanced liver uptake is lower peripheral drug concentrations and fewer systemic side effects. This principal metabolite is the inhibitor of the enzyme HMG-CoA reductase. The dissociation constant of the enzyme inhibitor complex (K_i) is approximately 10^{-9} mol/L.

An oral lovastatin dose is absorbed from the GI tract, with greater absorption at meals. The drug undergoes extensive first-pass metabolism in the liver, its primary site of action, with subsequent excretion of drug equivalents in the bile. It is estimated that only 5% of an oral dose reaches the general circulation as an active enzyme inhibitor. The drug is excreted via the bile (83%) and the urine (10%).

Lovastatin and its β-hydroxyacid metabolite are highly bound to human plasma proteins. Lovastatin crosses the blood-brain and placental barriers. The major active metabolites present in human plasma are the β-hydroxyacid of lovastatin, its 6′-hydroxy derivative, and two unidentified metabolites. Peak plasma levels of both active and total inhibitors are attained 2 to 4 h after lovastatin ingestion. The half-life of the β-hydroxyacid is approximately 1 to 2 h. This rapid metabolism would seem to necessitate multiple doses per day. Clinical trials, however, have indicated that once- or twice-daily dosing is optimum. With a once-daily dosing regimen, within the therapeutic range of 20 to 80 mg/day, steady-state plasma concentration of total inhibitors after 2 to 3 days was about 1.5 times that of a single dose. Single daily doses administered in the evening are more effective than the same dose given in the morning, perhaps because cholesterol mainly is synthesized at night (between 12 and 6 A.M.). A substantial clinical effect of lovastatin is noted within 2 weeks, a maximal effect at 4 to 6 weeks, and the effect completely dissipates 4 to 6 weeks after stopping the drug.

Clinical Experiences

Several investigators have demonstrated that lovastatin lowers the cholesterol levels of normal and hypercholesterolemic animals. These studies demonstrate that the increased LDL receptor activity and decreased LDL synthesis are responsible for the hypocholesterolemic effect of the drug. Several studies in humans have confirmed this observation. This increase in LDL receptor activity occurs in response to a decrement in cholesterol synthesis by HMG-CoA reductase inhibition. LDL may be reduced by either its increased clearance from the plasma or its decreased production.

Combination Therapy The rationale for using lovastatin in combination with other cholesterol-lowering drugs is to cause an additive or synergistic reduction in total and LDL-cholesterol through complementary effects on LDL receptor function and other mechanisms. One interesting combination is lovastatin with bile acid binding resins. Both drugs work to lower intracellular cholesterol and to maximize LDL receptor expression. The potential result is one of synergism without drug interaction.

Lovastatin (20 and 40 mg daily), when combined with nicotinic acid (3 g daily), was found to decrease LDL concentrations by 49%. Triglycerides also were reduced, making this combination particularly attractive for the treatment of type IIb hypercholesterolemia. However, this duo may retard lovastatin's excretion secondary to nicotinic acid's potential impairment of hepatic metabolism. This observation that nicotinic acid plus lovastatin has been associated with the development of myopathy is possibly explained by this interaction.

Although the combination of lovastatin and gemfibrozil may increase the risk of myopathy, this regimen has been shown to be very effective in the treatment of severe familial combined hypercholesterolemia, as well as marked hypertriglyceridemia, in patients with non-insulin-dependent diabetes mellitus.

Effects on Coronary and Carotid Artery Disease Progression In a recent report from the Familial Atherosclerosis Treatment Study (CATS), the combination of lovastatin, 40 mg daily, and colestipol, 30 g daily, was more effective than colestipol and diet alone in reducing LDL and raising HDL in patients with CAD and elevated apoprotein B levels. There were also fewer cardiovascular events, less progression of coronary lesions, and more regression.

In the Monitored Atherosclerotic Regression Study (MARS), patients whose cholesterol was 190 to 295 mg/dL and who were receiving lovastatin, 80 mg/day, and a cholesterol-lowering diet, showed a slower rate of progression and an increase in the regression in coronary artery lesions, especially in more severe lesions, compared with placebo plus diet. These anatomic changes on coronary angiography with lovastatin were associated with a significant reduction in total cholesterol, LDL-cholesterol, and apoprotein B levels, with a modest increase in HDL-cholesterol. In this study, lovastatin also was shown to reduce the progression of early, preintrusive atherosclerosis of the carotid artery evaluated by B-mode ultrasonography.

In the Canadian Coronary Atherosclerosis Intervention Trial (CCAIT), 331 patients with diffuse but not necessarily severe coronary atherosclerosis on coronary angiogram and cholesterol between 220 and 300 mg/dL were randomized to receive either diet plus lovastatin (20, 40, and 80 mg), titrated to achieve a LDL-cholesterol below 130 mg/dL, or diet plus placebo. Lovastatin treatment was shown to slow the progression of coronary atherosclerosis, especially of the milder lesions, and inhibited the development of new lesions. In a substudy analysis of female participants in CCAIT, lovastatin was shown to be effective in slowing the progression and neogenesis of coronary atherosclerotic lesions.

The effects of lovastatin on atherosclerotic lesions in the carotid arteries was assessed in The Asymptomatic Carotid Artery Progression Study (ACAPS). In this study, 919 asymptomatic men and women with early carotid atherosclerosis as defined by B-mode ultrasonography and LDL-cholesterol levels between 130 and 159 mg/dL were randomized to receive 20 to 40 mg of lovastatin or placebo. In addition, all patients received 80 mg aspirin daily, and one-half were treated with warfarin, 1 mg daily. Lovastatin reduced LDL-cholesterol levels and, after 3 years of follow-up, slowed the progression of mean intimal medial thickness of the common carotid arteries and decreased mortality and major cardiovascular events.

Similar to the findings in ACAPS, FATS, MARS, and CCAIT, reductions in cardiac event rates also were observed with lovastatin compared with placebo.

In a small study of 32 patients with ambulatory ECG ischemia, lovastatin was demonstrated to eliminate myocardial ischmic episodes compared with placebo.

There are primary prevention studies using lovastatin that are now in progress.

Effects on Triglycerides, HDL, and Other Lipoproteins Lovastatin appears to have variable effects, with most studies showing a reduction in triglycerides and an increase in HDL-cholesterol. There is an increasing interest in the effects of lovastatin on the lipoprotein profile. In a thorough study of this issue, Helve and Tikkanen found that the reduction of apoprotein B is similar to that of LDL-cholesterol. Further, a dose of 80 mg daily increased HDL_2-cholesterol by 10 to 18%. HDL_3-cholesterol levels, hepatic lipase, and lipoprotein lipase activity, all important components of the HDL pathway, were not significantly altered.

Another consideration is the effect of lovastatin on lipoprotein a [Lp(a)], an LDL-type molecule with an additional protein, apo A, bound to the apo B moiety. Apo A bears homology to plasminogen; it contains multiple copies of the kringle 4 domain of plasminogen, as well as single copies homologous to the protease and kringle five domains. While the physiologic role and metabolic pathway of Lp(a) are not known, many believe that an elevated Lp(a) may be an independent genetic risk factor for atherosclerotic disease. However, it also has been reported that the risk from Lp(a) can be eliminated by lowering LDL-cholesterol alone. Since HMG-CoA reductase inhibitors are known to upregulate LDL receptors, thereby lowering the plasma concentration of apo B particles, it is conceivable that Lp(a) would be similarly affected. Nevertheless, reports have generated conflicting results: One study of 24 patients and another of eight demonstrated a significant increase, yet another study of 30 patients found no change in serum Lp(a) levels.

Clinical Use

Lovastatin is approved as an adjunct to diet for the reduction of elevated total and LDL-cholesterol in patients with primary hypercholesterolemia (type IIa and IIb) when the response to a diet restricted in saturated fat and cholesterol has not been adequate. Lovastatin doses as low as 5 mg twice daily produce significant reductions in serum cholesterol.

Patients should be placed on a standard cholesterol-lowering diet prior to drug treatment. The recommended starting dose is 20 mg once daily given with the evening meal. The recommended dosing range is 20 to 80 mg daily in single or divided doses. Adjustments should be made at intervals of 4 weeks or more. A dose of 40 mg daily can be initiated in patients with cholesterol levels >7.76 mm/L (>300 mg/dL).

Twice-daily dosing appears to be the most effective treatment regimen, with daily evening doses being slightly less effective and daily morning doses least effective. Maximal and stable cholesterol reduction typically is achieved within 4 to 6 weeks of treatment initiation.

In patients with high cholesterol, diet and lovastatin may not reduce cholesterol to the desired level. Colestipol, in combination with lovastatin, may provide additional efficacy.

Studies have been done comparing lovastatin in doses of 40 to 80 mg daily versus cholestyramine, 12 g twice daily, and probucol, 500 mg twice daily, with greatest efficacy seen with lovastatin.

Adverse Effects

Several hypercholesterolemic agents are available, each having a significant side-effect profile. Lovastatin has an acceptable rate of adverse reactions but needs to be used with some caution.

In the published trials, approximately 2% of patients were withdrawn from treatment because of adverse reactions. Gastrointestinal side effects (diarrhea, abdominal pain, constipation, flatulence) are the most commonly reported adverse side effects. Marked, persistent, but asymptomatic increases (to greater than three times the upper limit of normal) in serum transaminases have been reported in 2% of patients receiving the drug for 1 year. The increases are predominantly in serum glutamate pyruvate transaminase (SGPT) and serum glutamic-oxaloacetic transaminase (SGOT), rather than alkaline phosphatase, suggesting a hepatocellular, not cholestatic, effect. These abnormalities rapidly return to normal after discontinuation of the drug, and no permanent liver damage has been reported with the drug. Symptomatic hepatitis in patients without underlying disease or other known hepatotoxic medications has been observed. It is recommended that liver function tests be performed before the initiation of treatment, at 6 and 12 weeks after initiation of therapy, or elevations of dose, and semi-annually thereafter.

The side effect of greatest concern with lovastatin is a myopathy, which appears to develop in three clinical patterns. The first, a moderate elevation in plasma creatinine kinase levels, is asymptomatic. Second, patients may develop muscle pain, primarily in the proximal muscle groups. CPK elevations may or may not be present. Finally, patients may develop a severe myopathy marked by extreme elevations in CPK, muscle pain with weakness, myoglobinuria, and rarely, acute renal failure. This finding most often occurs in the setting of concurrent immunosuppressive therapy (cyclosporine), particularly when gemfibrozil, erythromycin, or niacin is added. Similarly, the use of intraconazole, an antimycotic drug, has been shown to drastically increase plasma concentrations of lovastatin and lovastatin acid. Inhibition of CYP3A4-mediated hepatic metabolism probably explains the increased toxicity of lovastatin caused not only by intraconazole but also by cyclosporine, erythromycin, and other inhibitors of CYP3A4. Cases of myopathy have been identified as early as a few weeks and as late as 2 or more years after the initiation of therapy. CPK elevations appear to correlate little with the severity of the symptoms, but if CPK levels rise or muscle pain develops, it is recommended that lovastatin be reduced. If levels rise drastically (>10 times the upper limits of normal) with muscle pain, therapy should be discontinued.

Several reports of bleeding, increase in prothrombin time, or both have been observed in patients on concomitant warfarin anticoagulation. Although these accounts have not been attributed to lovastatin, it is recommended that prothrombin time be regulated carefully in these patients.

In addition to reports of rashes during the clinical trials, there have been several accounts of serious hypersensitivity reactions during prescription use; anaphylaxis, arthralgia, a lupus-like syndrome, angioedema, urticaria, hemolytic anemia, leukopenia, and thrombocytopenia have all been reported. Twenty-five cases were considered serious, but all recovered with discontinuation of lovastatin therapy. Since these adverse effects were never reported during the clinical trials, it is likely that the incidence is significantly less than 1 in 1000. Sleep disturbances, characterized by insomnia or shortening of the sleep period, also have been described.

Simvastatin

Simvastatin (Synvinolin) is a prodrug that is enzymatically hydrolyzed in vivo to its active form. In clinical trials since 1985, and approved in 1992, simvastatin is synthesized chemically from lovastatin and differs from lovastatin by only one methyl group. Like lovastatin, it has a very high affinity for HMG-CoA reductase, but on a milligram-per-milligram basis, simvastatin is twice as potent. Peak plasma concentrations of active inhibitor occur within 1.3 and 2.4 h.

Effect in Coronary Artery Disease

Similar to lovastatin and pravastatin, simvastatin was shown to slow the progression of coronary atherosclerosis assessed by coronary angiography. In the Multicentre Anti-Atheroma Study (MAAS), simvastatin, 20 mg daily, was compared with placebo in 381 patients with CAD receiving a similar lipid-lowering diet. Patients on simvastatin had a 23% reduction in total cholesterol, a 31% reduction in LDL-cholesterol, and a 9% increase in HDL-cholesterol compared with placebo over 4 years. Patients on simvastatin had less progression and more regression of existing lesions and a lower rate of new lesion development.

In a landmark secondary prevention study, The Scandinavian Simvastatin Survival Study (4S), simvastatin was shown to reduce mortality and morbidity in patients with known CAD and hypercholesterolemia. In this study, 4444 patients with prior angina pectoris or myocardial infarction and elevated total serum cholesterol levels (220 to 320 mg/dL or 5.5 to 8.0 mm/L) were randomized in double-blind fashion to receive either simvastatin, 10 to 40 mg, or placebo and were followed for a median of 5.4 years (Fig. 15-6). All patients were on a cholesterol-lowering diet. Compared with placebo, simvastatin reduced total cholesterol 25% and LDL-cholesterol 35% and increased HDL-cholesterol 8%. Compared with placebo, all fatal coronary events were reduced by 42% with simvastatin, all fatal cardiovascular events were reduced by 35% (Fig. 15-7), and all-cause mortality was reduced by 30%. There was a nonsignificant trend showing less cerebrovascular morbidity with simvastatin. Patients over 60 years had a 27% reduction in mortality. There was no difference in noncardiovascular mortality comparing placebo and simvastatin treatment. Based on this study, subsequent pharmacoeconomic analysis has demonstrated the cost-effectiveness of simvastatin in secondary prevention.

From experimental studies, there is information to suggest that simvastatin may reduce cardiovascular events beyond the effect on lipid lowering. Simvastatin and other HMG-CoA reductase inhibitors have

FIG. 15-6 Kaplan-Meier curves for all-cause mortality. Number of patients at risk at the beginning of each year is shown below the horizontal axis. *(From Scandinavian Simvastatin Survival Study Group: Randomised trial of cholesterol lowering in 4444 patients with coronary heart disease: The Scandinavian Simvastatin Survival Study (4S). Lancet 344: 1384, 1994, with permission.)*

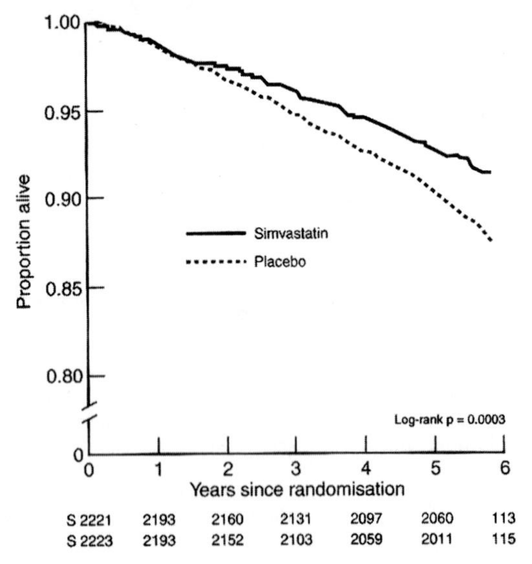

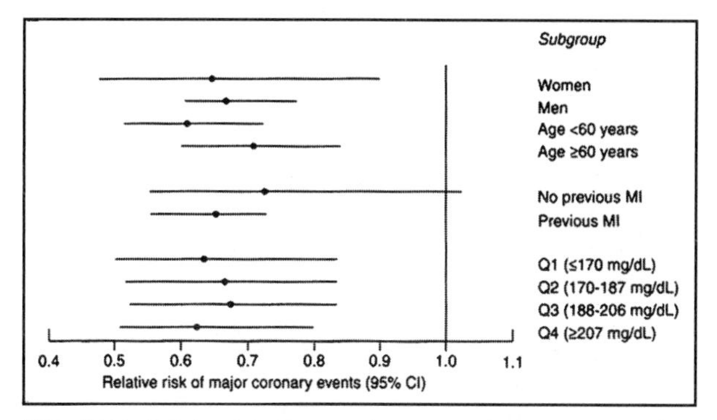

FIG. 15-7 Relative risks [95% confidence interval (CI)] by age, gender, history of myocardial infarction (MI), and baseline low-density lipoprotein (LDL)-cholesterol quartile (Q1–Q4). The quartile limits were ≤4.39, 4.40–4.84, 4.85–5.34, and ≥5.35 mmol/L. Risk reduction = (1 − relative risk) × 100%. *(From Kjekshus J, Pedersen TR, for the Scandinavian Simvastatin Survival Study Group (4S): Reducing the risk of coronary events: Evidence from the Scandinavian Simvastatin Survival Study. Am J Cardiol 76:64C, 1995, with permission.)*

been shown to reduce factor VIIc activity and inhibit platelet activation, while reducing the propensity of LDL to oxidation.

Clinical Use

Similar to other marketed HMG-CoA reductase inhibitors, simvastatin is approved for use in patients with primary hypercholesterolemia. In addition, based on the results of the 4S study, the drug also has been approved as long-term treatment for reducing morbidity and mortality in patients with known CAD (angina pectoris and survivors of acute myocardial infarction) and hypercholesterolemia.

Simvastatin is administered orally as a single dose in the evening. The recommended starting dose is 5 to 10 mg daily, which is then titrated according to the individual patient's response at 4-week intervals to a maximum 40-mg daily dose. To achieve the morbidity and mortality benefits achieved in the 4S trial, simvastatin should be used in doses of 20 to 40 mg daily. In patients with severe renal insufficiency or in those receiving cyclosporine, the recommended starting dose is 5 mg daily and close monitoring is required.

Adverse Effects

The side-effect profile of simvastatin is similar to that of lovastatin and other HMG-CoA reductase inhibitors. The rare occurrence of a lupus-like syndrome has been reported recently with both lovastatin and simvastatin.

Pravastatin

Pravastatin (Pravachol CS 514, SQ 3100, epstatin) is the 6α-hydroxy acid form of compactin. It has been approved for marketing by the FDA. It is the first HMG-CoA reductase inhibitor to be administered in the active form and not as a prodrug. In vitro studies by Tsujita et al. demonstrated that pravastatin has a greater specificity for hepatic cells than lovastatin. In vivo animal studies comparing pravastatin with lovastatin and simvastatin, however, found that the concentration of pravastatin in the liver was only half that of the latter two, whereas the concentrations in peripheral tissues were three to six times greater.

In a recent study, pravastatin was found to be a specific inhibitor of hepatic HMG-CoA reductase in humans. Other enzymes involved in cholesterol metabolism [α-hydroxylase, which governs bile acid synthesis and acyl-coenzyme A; cholesterol *O*-acetyltransferase (ACAT), which regulates cholesterol esterification] were not affected by treatment. Inhibition of hepatic HMG-CoA reductase activity by pravastatin results in an increased expression of hepatic LDL receptors, which explains the lowered plasma levels of LDL-cholesterol.

Effects on Coronary and Cerebral Artery Disease

The benefit of using pravastatin to reduce morbidity and mortality in patients with CAD was first established in the Pravastatin Multinational Study. In this 6-month trial, pravastatin treatment was demonstrated to reduce the incidence of serious cardiovascular events including myocardial infarction and unstable angina.

Four vascular regression trials using pravastatin have been completed, with the results reported on two of the trials. PLAC-I (Pravastatin Limitation of Atherosclerosis in the Coronary Arteries) and REGRESS (Regression Growth Evaluation Statin Study) included patients with CAD to assess by serial angiography the effects of pravastatin on CAD. PLAC-II was designed to evaluate the ability of pravastatin to retard the ultrasonographic 3-year progress of extracranial carotid artery in patients with known CAD. The KAPS (Kuopio Atherosclerosis Study) was a 3-year ultrasonographic study that evaluated the effects of pravastatin on the progression of carotid and femoral artherosclerosis.

All the studies were placebo-controlled, and pravastatin doses of 20 to 40 mg were used as monotherapy. Patients receiving pravastatin in PLAC-I had a 40 to 50% reduction in coronary lesion progression, a 28% reduction in LDL-cholesterol, and fewer nonfatal and fatal myocardial infarctions compared with placebo. In PLAC-II, pravastatin-treated patients showed a 35% reduction of atherosclerosis in the common carotid artery and a 80% reduction in fatal and nonfatal infarctions compared with placebo. In KAPS, there was a significant reduction in the progression of carotid atherosclerosis compared with placebo. In REGRESS, there was a significant reduction in the progression of coronary atherosclerosis with pravastatin and a reduced rate of adverse cardiovascular events compared with placebo, including fewer myocardial infarctions, sudden deaths, strokes, and invasive coronary procedures.

In these four studies, a total of 1891 patients had been evaluated, and although the major objective was to assess regression of atherosclerosis with agressive lipid lowering with pravastatin, a metaanalysis was performed to assess the impact of treatment on clinical cardiovascular events compared with placebo. The risk of fatal plus nonfatal myocardial infarctions was reduced by 62%, the risk of strokes reduced by 62%, and total mortality by 46%.

On the basis of these findings, the U.S. FDA approved pravastatin for two new secondary indications: to slow the progression of coronary atherosclerosis and to reduce the risk of acute coronary events in patients with hypercholesterolemia and clinically evident CAD, including prior myocardial infarction. These studies also provide convincing evidence for the benefit of agressive lipoprotein management in patients with atherosclerotic disease and suggest the potential for greater use of noninvasive treatment of patients with known CAD. Mechanisms of HMG-CoA reductase benefit in reducing risk of cardiovascular events may extend beyond their direct lipid-lowering effects.

Pravastatin also was used in one recently completed primary prevention and one secondary prevention study with reported benefit on clinical cardiovascular outcomes. In the West of Scotland Prevention Study (WOSCOPS), 6595 middle-aged men with no history of myocardial infarction and average plasma cholesterol values above 252 mg/dL (upper quartile) were randomized to receive either placebo or 40 mg pravastatin and followed for an average of almost 5 years. Pravastatin decreased LDL-cholesterol by 26% and increased HDL-cholesterol by 5%. Pravastatin treatment also significantly reduced the incidence of myocardial infarction and death from cardiovascular causes without adversely affecting the risk of death from noncardiovascular causes (Fig. 15-8). On the basis of this study, pravastatin also has been approved for use in patients having cholesterol values above 25 mg/dL, to reduce the risk of myocardial infarction

The Cholesterol and Recurrent Events Study (CARE) was designed to assess whether pravastatin treatment (40 mg daily) could reduce the sum of fatal CAD and nonfatal myocardial infarctions in patients who have survived a myocardial infarction yet have a total cholesterol below 240 mg/dL, a population different from that studied in 4S. Preliminary results suggest a benefit of pravastatin therapy on cardiovascular out-

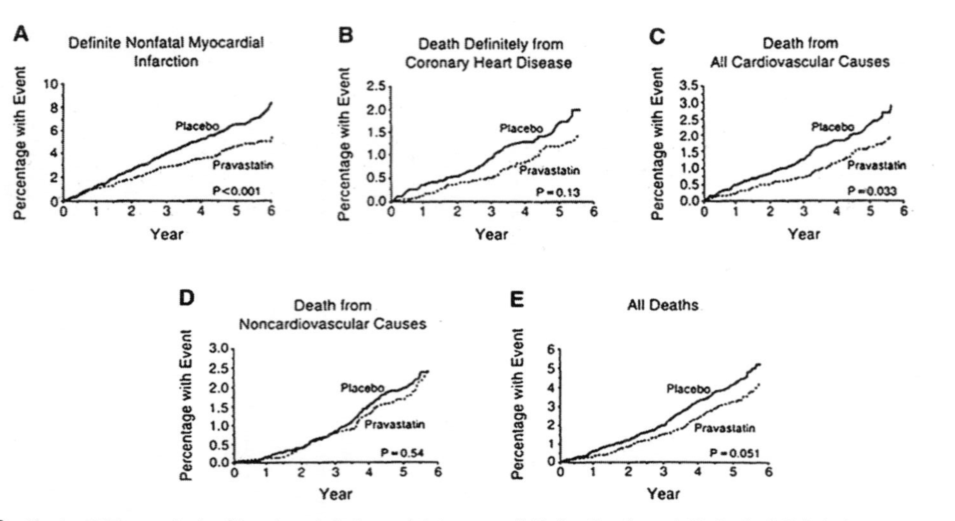

FIG. 15-8 Kaplan-Meier analysis of time to a definite nonfatal myocardial infarction (panel *A*), death definitely from coronary heart disease (panel *B*), death from all cardiovascular causes (panel *C*), death from noncardiovascular causes (panel *D*), and death from any cause (panel *E*) according to treatment group. *(From Shepherd J, Cobbe SM, Ford I, et al: Prevention of coronary heart disease with pravastatin in men with hypercholesterolemia. N Engl J Med 333:1301, 1995, with permission.)*

comes compared with placebo, especially in patients having a baseline LDL-cholesterol above 125 mg/dL.

Finally, there are two major ongoing secondary prevention studies with pravastatin. The first, Long-term Intervention with Pravastatin in Ischemic Heart Disease trial (LIPID) is evaluating placebo versus pravastatin, 40 mg, in more than 9000 patients who had either an acute myocardial infarction or an unstable angina episode and who have cholesterol values of 155 to 271 mg/dL. This study, which should be concluded this year, is looking at the effects of treatment on CAD mortality as the primary end point. The final results from this project will be evaluated as part of a prospective metaanalysis (Prospective Pravastatin Pooling Project) that also will include results from the CARE and WOSCOPS.

An additional pravastatin study is evaluating the use of HMG-CoA reductase inhibitors with or without vitamin E and marine polyunsaturated fats (fish oil) in 6000 patients with a history of myocardial infarction (Gruppo Italiano per lo Studio del Sopravivenza nell'Infarto Miocardico, GISSI Prevention). The results from this study, when concluded, will be combined with those from LIPID, CARE, and WOSCOPS as part of an even larger prospective metaanalysis (Cholesterol Treatment Trialists Collaboration, CTT).

Clinical Use

Pravastatin has a similar approval for treatment of cholesterolemia as other HMG-CoA reductase inhibitors and, in addition, is approved for both the primary and secondary prevention of the complications related to CAD. The recommended starting dose is 10 to 20 mg once daily at bedtime for primary hypercholesterolemia, with a usual dosing range of 10 to 40 mg daily. A 40-mg dose may be necessary to achieve the clinical benefits observed in the primary and secondary prevention trials done with the drug.

Similar to other HMG-CoA reductase inhibitors, the drug may be combined with other classes of lipid-lowering drugs. When combined with cholestyramine, pravastatin should be administered 1 h before or 4 h after the bile-acid resin is given.

Adverse Effects

The adverse effect profile is similar to other HMG-CoA reductase inhibitors in use. Since the drug does not cross the blood-brain barrier, it has been observed to cause a lower incidence of sleep disturbances than either lovastatin or simvastatin. However, this finding needs to be confirmed. A rare peripheral neuropathy complication with both lovastatin and pravastatin has been described recently.

Fluvastatin

Fluvastatin is the first synthetic HMG-CoA reductase inhibitor, and it is structurally distinct from the fungal derivatives lovastatin, simvastatin, and pravastatin. It was approved for clinical use in the United States for the treatment of primary hypercholesterolemia (type IIa and IIb). The drug also recently received approval as the fourth statin to slow the progression of coronary arteriosclerosis in patients with coronary heart disease, as part of a treatment to lower total and LDL-cholesterol to target rates.

Fluvastatin is well absorbed after oral administration and, like other HMG-CoA reductase drugs, undergoes extensive first-pass metabolism. Its side-effect profile is similar to other HMG-CoA reductase inhibitors, and it may cause less myopathy and risk of rhabdomyolysis when used alone or with gemfibrozil, nicotinic acid, cyclosporine, and erythromycin.

The drug has been combined with other lipid-lowering therapies to achieve greater lipid-lowering effects, including cholestyramine, bezafibrate, and nicotinic acid. It also has been used safely in diabetic and hypertensive patients.

Use in Patients with CAD

Although many patients with known CAD have received fluvastatin, there are as yet no published morbidity and mortality studies with the drug. Two large secondary prevention trials with fluvastatin are in progress. One study is designed to assess the efficacy of high-dose fluvastatin (80 mg daily) in preventing restenosis after balloon angioplasty. The other study, known as the Lipoprotein and Coronary Atherosclerosis Study (LCAS), is assessing the effects of fluvastatin versus placebo on long-term atherosclerosis progression in patients with known CAD using serial angiographic procedures. Results from the LCAS demonstrate a benefit of fluvastatin treatment on the progression and regression of atherosclerosis.

Clinical Use

Fluvastatin is an effective and safe drug for reducing LDL-cholesterol. Although not as potent, on a milligram-to-milligram basis, as the other HMG-CoA reductase inhibitors, it is now available to patients at a less expensive price.

The recommended starting dose is 20 to 40 mg once daily at bedtime. The recommended dosing range is 20 to 80 mg daily. The 80-mg dose should be divided. Similar to other HMG-CoA reductase inhibitors, it takes at least 4 weeks to achieve the maximal effect.

If fluvastatin is combined with cholestyramine, fluvastine plasma levels drop considerably. Fluvastatin needs to be given at least 4 h after a cholestyramine dose.

Atorvastatin

Atorvastatin is a new synthetic HMG-CoA reductase inhibitor with a long half-life that is similar in structure to fluvastatin; atorvastatin is twice as potent on a milligram-to-milligram basis as simvastatin and much more potent than fluvastatin in reducing total cholesterol and LDL-cholesterol. In addition, atorvastatin is unique in its ability to reduce triglycerides. It is not a prodrug.

The results of recent randomized, placebo-controlled studies of 56 patients with hypertriglyceridemia (average 603 mg/dL) demonstrated that atorvastatin in doses of 5, 20, and 80 mg at 4 weeks reduced triglycerides up to 45.8%, LDL-cholesterol up to 41.7%, VLDL-cholesterol up to 57.7%, and VLDL triglycerides up to 47.3%. The drug did not cause a redistribution of triglycerides but consistently lowered triglycerides in all lipoprotein fractions.

It was proposed by the investigator that the mechanism by which atorvastatin reduces triglycerides more than other available HMG-CoA reductase inhibitors may relate to its ability to lower cholesterol synthesis to a much greater degree, thereby depleting the liver of cholesterol and causing a decrease in the synthesis and secretion of VLDL. Perhaps potent agents such as simvastatin might achieve the same triglyceride-reducing effect if it were used in higher doses than currently recommended.

The drug was approved for clinical use in 1997. Its side-effect profile appears to be similar to other HMG-CoA reductase inhibitors in doses up to 80 mg daily used once daily. The drug is being investigated currently as an adjunctive anti-ischemic agent.

Cerivastatin

Cerivastatin is a potent synthetic HMG-CoA reductase inhibitor that has been studied in controlled trials and shown to be effective in reducing plasma total cholesterol and LDL-cholesterol in patients with heterozygous familial and nonfamilial forms of hypercholesterolemia, and in mixed hyperlipidemia. Similar to other drugs in the class, it was recently approved for clinical use as an adjunct to diet for the reduction of elevated total and LDL-cholesterol levels in patients with primary hypercholesterolemia and mixed dyslipidemia (Fredrickson Types IIa and IIb) when the response to dietary restriction of saturated fat and cholesterol and other nonpharmacological measures alone has been inadequate. It is recommended that the drug be administered once daily in the evening using a 0.3 mg tablet. The drug can be combined with bile acid resins, but should be administered at least 2 hours after the resin. Patients with moderate or severe renal dysfunction should use a starting dose of 0.2 mg. The side effect profile of cerivastatin is similar to other HMG-CoA reductase inhibitors.

NICOTINIC ACID

Nicotinic acid (NA, pyridine-3 carboxylic acid, or niacin) is a water-soluble B-complex vitamin that is used for the prophylaxis and treatment of pellagra. The substance functions in the body after conversion to either nicotinamide-adenine dinucleotide (NAD) or nicotinamide-adenine dinucleotide phosphate (NADP).

Pharmacokinetics

NA is readily absorbed from the intestinal tract after oral administration of pharmacologic doses. The level of free NA in plasma reaches a peak value between 30 and 60 min after ingesting a single dose of 1 g. Because NA is rapidly eliminated, the doses necessary to achieve pharmacologic effects (2 to 8 g daily) are much greater than the amount needed for its physiologic function as a vitamin. When large doses of the vitamin were given to rats by intraperitoneal injection, the half-life of the compound was found to be approximately 1 h in blood. The half-life of NA seems to be determined primarily by the rate of renal clearance of the unchanged compound when given in high doses. At lower doses, NA is mainly excreted as its metabolites.

The metabolic fate of NA is complex and varies with the dose. Under normal conditions, metabolites of NA found in the urine are mainly the products of catabolism of the pyridine nucleotides, the stored forms of the vitamin. The primary route of metabolism is via methylation to *N*-methyl-nicotinamide, which is further oxidized to *N*-methyl-2- and 4-pyridone carboxamides. With pharmacologic doses, the excretion of nicotinuric acid, produced by the conjugation of NA and glycine, is enhanced and seems to play a role as a detoxification product at these higher doses. Once the dose is large enough to overcome the production rate of nicotinuric acid, NA is mostly excreted unchanged.

Pharmacologic Action

NA in large doses lowers total plasma cholesterol and has been found to have beneficial effects on the levels of the major serum lipoproteins. Specifically, it decreases the levels of VLDL triglyceride (VLDL-Tg) and LDL-cholesterol and causes an increase in the levels of HDL-cholesterol. This lipid-altering activity is not shared by nicotinamide and seems to be unrelated to the role of NA as a vitamin in the NAD and NADP coenzyme systems. Pharmacologic doses of NA result in a rapid decrease in plasma triglyceride levels, in part by lowering VLDL-Tg concentrations by 20 to more than 80%. The magnitude of the reduction is related to the initial VLDL levels. Within 1 week of initiation of therapy, concentrations of LDL-cholesterol decrease. Typically, a 10 to 15% reduction in LDL-cholesterol is observed within 3 to 5 weeks of attaining full dosage. The magnitude of the drop is also related to the dose of NA. In addition to these lipid-lowering effects, NA raises HDL-cholesterol concentrations. Mobilization of cholesterol from peripheral tissues seems to occur after prolonged therapy, as evidenced by the regression of eruptive, tuboeruptive, tuberous, and tendon xanthomas.

Clinical Experience

As outlined above, NA has been shown to have beneficial effects on all plasma lipoprotein fractions and was identified as one of the drug choices for the treatment of hypercholesterolemia by the Adult Treatment Panel of the National Cholesterol Education Program. Studies of the clinical efficacy of NA fall into two main groups: those which examine the use of NA in patients with known coronary heart disease (CHD) and those which test its efficacy, often in combination with other lipid-lowering agents, in altering plasma lipoprotein levels in patients with various types of hyperlipoproteinemias.

Coronary Heart Disease

The Coronary Drug Project, a long-term, nationwide, double-blind, placebo-controlled study, looked at a number of lipid-altering regimens including NA and clofibrate in male survivors of MI. In particular, the investigators assessed whether the various regimens could prevent new CHD events or prolong life in patients with clinical CHD. The subjects were men, aged 30 through 64 years, with electrocardiogram-documented evidence of one or more previous MIs. Each subject was free of evidence of recent worsening of his CHD and had his last MI at least 3 months prior to entering the study. These men were randomized to either a control group, which included 2789 subjects who received 3.8 g of lactose placebo daily, or to one of the treatment groups. The NA group included 1119 men who received 3 g of the drug each day for 5 to 8.5 years, with a mean of 6 years, 2 months. The primary end point for determining drug efficacy was total mortality. Other end points included cause-specific mortality (especially coronary mortality and sudden death) and nonfatal cardiovascular events. Subjects also were monitored for adverse effects.

Over the follow-up period, NA effected mean decreases in total serum cholesterol of 9.9% and in total triglycerides of 26.1%. However, the incidence of all deaths in the follow-up period (8.5 years) was insignificantly lower than that in the placebo group (24.4 versus 25.4%). In contrast to the findings on total mortality, the incidence of definite, nonfatal MI over the total follow-up period was 27% lower in the treatment group than in the control group (10.1 versus 13.9%). Also, during this period, the treatment group showed a 24% lower incidence of fatal or nonfatal cerebrovascular events than the placebo group.

There was also a lower incidence of bypass surgery in the group receiving NA (0.9 versus 2.7%).

Investigators in the Coronary Drug Project conducted a follow-up study nearly 9 years after termination of the original trial. With a mean total follow-up of 15 years, total mortality in the NA group was found to be 11% lower than in the placebo group (52 versus 58.2%). The men in the study had presumably stopped taking the drug after the original mean follow-up of 6.2 years. The decreased mortality is primarily due to a decrease in CHD mortality, with smaller decreases in death due to cerebrovascular causes, other cardiovascular events, cancer, and other noncardiovascular and noncancer causes.

The Cholesterol-Lowering Atherosclerosis Study (CLAS) employed a colestipol-NA combination to test the hypothesis that aggressively lowering LDL-cholesterol and raising HDL-cholesterol reverses or retards the progression of atherosclerotic lesions. The subjects, chosen to minimize the effects of other major nonlipid risk factors for atherosclerosis, included 162 normotensive nonsmoking men aged 40 to 59 years with previous coronary bypass surgery and fasting total cholesterol levels in the range of 4.78 to 9.05 mm/L (185 to 350 mg/dL).

Subjects underwent coronary angiography and were then randomly assigned to either the treatment group or the placebo-control group. Both groups were instructed to follow a diet restricting the intake of cholesterol and saturated fat. The diets differed in that the control group followed a more lenient diet "to enhance the differential in blood cholesterol responses between the two groups." Subjects in the treatment group also took 30 g of colestipol plus 3 to 12 g of niacin daily. Follow-up visits included nutritional counseling and measurement of fasting blood lipids and lipoprotein levels. A repeat angiogram was performed on each subject after 2 years of treatment.

Changes in lipid values from baseline after drug treatment were as follows: decreases in total cholesterol (26%), triglycerides (22%), and LDL-cholesterol (43%) and an increase in HDL-cholesterol (37%). These results were all statistically significant and differed from the control group changes of −4, −5, −5, and 2%, respectively.

The results of these readings show that the treatment group score distribution was significantly shifted toward lower scores than that of the control group, indicating less disease progression with colestipol-NA treatment. In fact, 61% of the treatment group subjects improved or remained the same, and 16.2% showed regression of atherosclerotic lesions at 2 years. This differs from the results in the placebo control group of 39 and 2.4%, respectively. Regarding native vessels, treatment reduced the average number of lesions that progressed per subject and the percentage of subjects with new lesions. Similarly, with respect to bypass grafts, the percentage of subjects either with new lesions or showing any adverse change in preexisting lesions was significantly lower in the treatment group. Recently reported were the results of a 7-

year follow-up of a subpopulation from CLAS. These new data substantiate the benefit of lipid-lowering therapy on the progression and regression of coronary artery lesions. These findings from CLAS suggest that following coronary artery bypass surgery patients should receive intensive interventions to beneficially alter blood lipid and lipoprotein levels.

The results of the Familial Atherosclerosis Treatment Study (FATS) were reported, which demonstrated a favorable effect of NA plus colestipol on the progression of coronary atherosclerotic disease. Patients with disease, a family history of premature cardiovascular events, and elevated levels of apoprotein B (≥3.23 mm/L or ≥125 mg/dL) were counseled on diet and assigned to three treatment regimens: NA, 4 g/day plus colestipol 30 g/day; lovastatin, 40 mg/day plus colestipol; or colestipol alone (control). The combination regimens caused the greatest reductions in LDL and the greatest elevations in HDL. Bimonthly visits spanned 2.5 years between coronary angiograms. Favorable changes in clinical course and lesion severity appeared with the combination regimens. With the NA-colestipol combination, 25% of patients showed progression of coronary lesions, 39% showed regression, and only two cardiovascular events occurred. In contrast, 10 cardiovascular events occurred in the control group, 46% of patients showed region progression, and 11% regression of coronary lesions.

Lp(a) Elevations

Patients with heterozygous familial hypercholesterolemia (FH) with serum cholesterol levels ranging from 300 to 500 mg/dL are markedly predisposed to premature coronary artery disease. However, since not all patients with FH have CAD, other factors must affect the atherogenicity of elevated LDL-cholesterol levels.

Lp(a) is a lipoprotein fraction that is similar to LDL and believed to be an atherogenic lipoprotein. Lp(a) has an apoprotein (apoprotein a) that has a close structural relationship to plasminogen. It has been suggested that Lp(a) might block the availability of true plasminogen to the blood vessel wall, thereby predisposing individuals to atherosclerosis and thrombotic events. Individuals with high Lp(a) levels appear to be at increased risk for CHD and for clinical recurrence after coronary balloon angioplasty.

The drugs usually used to treat high LDL-cholesterol, such as the bile acid binding resins and the HMG–coenzyme A reductase inhibitors, do not affect Lp(a) levels. However, niacin is effective in lowering elevated Lp(a) levels, as is plasmapheresis.

These findings have clinical significance and present with management questions. Should Lp(a) levels be measured, and if they are elevated, should drugs such as NA be used instead of, or in addition to, other drugs used to lower LDL-cholesterol?

Clinical Use

Single-Drug Therapy

NA, through its beneficial effects on VLDL-Tg, LDL-, and HDL-cholesterol levels, is indicated in most forms of hyperlipoproteinemia and for patients with depressed HDL. This includes patients with types II, III, IV, and V hyperlipoproteinemia. It is particularly useful in patients who have elevated plasma VLDL-Tg levels as a part of their lipid profile. It is important to remember that a diet that is low in cholesterol and saturated fats is the foundation of therapy for hyperlipoproteinemia.

NA is available in 100-, 125-, 250-, and 500-mg tablets, as well as in a time-release form. The typical dosage of NA is 3 to 7 g daily given in three divided doses. Therapeutic effects of the drug usually are not manifested until the patient reaches a total daily dose of at least 3 g. A greater response may be attained with periodic increases in doses up to a maximum of 7 to 8 g daily, although the incidence of adverse effects also increases with higher doses. In general, it is best to use the lowest dose that is necessary to achieve the desired alterations in plasma lipoprotein levels. Unfortunately, many patients cannot tolerate therapeutic doses of NA, the primary side effects being cutaneous flushing and GI disturbance. However, certain steps can be taken to minimize these untoward effects.

NA therapy should be initiated with a low-dosage regimen (100 mg daily), gradually increasing the dose every few days over a period of several weeks until the patient attains a dosage level of 3 g daily given in three divided doses. If, while increasing the dose, the patient develops any adverse effects, the dose should be cut back and then resumed at a more gradual pace. Taking the doses with meals decreases gastric irritation and cutaneous flushing. Further, cutaneous flushing can be reduced or avoided by taking one aspirin tablet daily (more frequent administration is unnecessary because one tablet will inhibit cyclooxygenase for up to 2 weeks). It is interesting that tachyphylaxis to the flushing phenomenon often occurs within a few days, although the bothersome episodes may recur if the patient misses two or three doses. Once the initial maintenance dose is reached, it is important to evaluate for therapeutic effects by measuring plasma lipoprotein values. If the therapeutic effects are unsatisfactory, the dose should be increased by a further 1.0 to 1.5 g/day, with periodic increases to a maximum of 7 to 8 g daily as needed. Usually when doses of 4 g daily are achieved, another lipid-lowering drug is added.

Regardless of the dose, it is important to make several laboratory evaluations for potential adverse effects at regular intervals. These include assessment of liver function (bilirubin, alkaline phosphatase, and transaminase levels), uric acid levels, and serum glucose levels.

NA is contraindicated in patients with active peptic ulcer disease. The drug also may impair glucose tolerance and is contraindicated in patients with diabetes that is difficult to control. NA is also associated with reversible elevations of liver enzymes and uric acid and should not be used in patients with hepatic disease or a history of symptomatic gout.

A time-release form of NA was developed after noting that the incidence of cutaneous flushing is reduced by taking the drug with meals, suggesting that this side effect is related to the rate of GI absorption. In fact, patients taking the time-release preparation do have a lower incidence of flushing than patients with unmodified NA. However, this is outweighed by the far greater incidence of GI and constitutional symptoms experienced by patients on the time-release form, including nausea, vomiting, diarrhea, fatigue, and decreased male sexual function. In addition, the time-release preparation may be associated with more hepatotoxicity, even with low doses, including greater alkaline phosphatase and transaminase elevations. This preparation was implicated as the cause of fulminant hepatic failure requiring liver transplant in a patient who, 2 months previously, began taking 6 g daily of time-release NA. Prior to this time, he had taken 6 g daily of unmodified NA for 1 year without side effects.

A clinical experience was reported on describing the use of a new form of NA that employs a wax-matrix vehicle for sustained-release drug delivery. Patient groups receiving 2000 and 1500 mg of NA in this formulation demonstrated significant reductions in values of LDL-cholesterol and total cholesterol when compared with diet- and placebo-treated controls. Smaller improvements were seen in HDL-cholesterol and triglycerides. A favorable side-effect profile was reported with this NA formulation, perhaps related to the lower daily dose of NA used. A larger, long-term clinical experience with this formulation is still needed to confirm these safety and efficacy results.

Combination Therapy

The employment of combined drug therapy is beneficial in patients who are inadequately controlled on restricted diet and NA monotherapy. This is often the case in patients with heterozygous FH (type IIa) or familial combined hyperlipidemia (type IIb). One such regimen combines NA with a bile acid binding resin, such as colestipol. This treatment takes advantage of the synergistic mechanism of action of the two agents. The resin promotes LDL catabolism and cholesterol excretion, while secondarily increasing hepatic synthesis of cholesterol and VLDL, thus achieving a new steady state with limited reduction of LDL. The addition of a drug such as NA, which reduces the synthesis of VLDL (and LDL), would be expected to add further therapeutic benefits to those achieved by diet and resin alone. In fact, the use of colestipol (30 g daily) in combination with NA (3 to 8 g daily) consistently decreases plasma levels of total cholesterol by 34 to 45% and LDL by 45 to 55% in patients with heterozygous FH. Further, this combination has been associated with the regression of atherosclerotic lesions, as well as the prevention of new lesion formation in native coronary vessels and coronary bypass grafts. The addition of NA also adds the beneficial effects over diet and resin alone of increasing HDL levels and decreasing VLDL levels, particularly useful in familial combined hyperlipidemia.

The decrease in hepatic cholesterol synthesis that occurs with HMG-CoA reductase inhibitors is thought to induce an increased rate of receptor-mediated uptake of LDL from the plasma as well as a decrease in LDL production, thus lowering LDL levels. The combination of lovastatin and NA might be expected to have additive and synergistic effects, given their mechanisms of action. In fact, Lees et al. found that when lovastatin (20 to 40 mg daily) was combined with NA (3 g daily), LDL concentrations decreased by 49%, a 14% greater drop than with lovastatin alone. Triglyceride levels also were reduced, making this combination especially useful in patients with concurrent elevations in LDL-cholesterol and triglycerides (type IIb hyperlipoproteinemia). However, caution must be taken when using lovastatin and NA in combination, since NA may adversely affect liver function and thereby impair the hepatic metabolism of lovastatin. This interaction possibly explains the increased risk of myopathy associated with this regimen over that of monotherapy.

Patients with severe heterozygous FH who inadequately respond to the use of two drugs may benefit from triple-drug combinations. One such therapy with proven efficacy is NA with lovastatin and resin. In fact, this triple-drug regimen decreases LDL levels by as much as 69%, making it more effective than resin-NA, resin-lovastatin, or lovastatin-NA. The triple-agent combination also results in increases in HDL with moderate reductions in triglycerides. Further, this regimen may allow for lower doses of NA and resin to achieve therapeutic changes in plasma lipoprotein levels, thus possibly reducing the incidence of adverse effects.

Adverse Effects

Despite NA's efficacy in beneficially altering serum lipoprotein levels, its use is limited by a variety of troublesome and sometimes serious side effects. Some studies have experienced as much as a 50% dropout rate as a result of drug-related side effects.

The Coronary Drug Project, with 1100 subjects on NA therapy, reported the common occurrences of cutaneous flushing and pruritus. Other dermatologic side effects include dryness of skin, rash, and acanthosis nigricans, all reversible with cessation of therapy. The mechanism of the flushing is presumed to be related to the effect of NA on vasodilatory prostaglandins and is frequently attenuated by pretreatment with aspirin. This vasodilatory effect, in combination with antihypertensive therapy, may potentially result in postural hypotension. The Coronary Drug Project also described an increased incidence of atrial fibrillation, and other transient cardiac arrhythmias were noted. In addition, elevations in uric acid levels associated with an increased incidence of acute gouty arthritis were observed.

GI symptoms including diarrhea, nausea, vomiting, and abdominal pain also were frequent complaints encountered in the Coronary Drug Project. Activation of peptic ulcer disease by NA is a potential adverse effect but was not observed in this large-scale study.

Liver function tests are frequently abnormal during NA therapy. Generally, there is elevation in alkaline phosphatase and hepatic transaminases. Some studies also have noted elevations in bilirubin occasionally leading to jaundice. The elevations in transaminases are generally transient and reverse with decrease in dosage or cessation of therapy and can be minimized by increasing the dosage in gradual increments when initiating therapy. Unlike the elevations in hepatic enzymes associated with HMG-CoA reductase inhibitors, the elevations that occur with the use of NA may be symptomatic. Several cases of "niacin hepatitis" progressing to fulminant hepatic failure have been described, most frequently with the time-release formulation, with biochemical, clinical, and histologic evidence of hepatocellular injury. This seems to be a dose-related hepatotoxicity rather than a hypersensitivity, occurring in almost all cases at doses greater than 3 g daily. In most cases, cessation of therapy leads to eventual resolution of abnormalities, although there is one reported case of a patient on time-release NA who required liver transplantation.

Hyperglycemia and impaired glucose tolerance may occur with NA therapy and often necessitates adjustments in diet and hypoglycemic therapy in diabetic patients.

The Coronary Drug Project noted a statistically significant increase in CPK levels with NA therapy, and there have been reports of associated reversible myopathy. The combination of lovastatin and NA has been causally implicated in at least one case of rhabdomyolysis.

PROBUCOL

Probucol was first introduced in the early 1970s and was advocated for its LDL-cholesterol–lowering properties and favorable side-effect profile. However, it was soon noted that, in most instances, this drug lowered HDL-cholesterol more than it lowered LDL-cholesterol. Probucol also was challenged for its potential to prolong the ECG QT interval, leading possibly to ventricular arrhythmias in nonhuman primates. Nonetheless, this agent has enjoyed fairly widespread popularity for the treatment of patients with elevated cholesterol who are unable to tolerate the side effects of the other hypocholesterolemic medications. Probucol has enjoyed a resurgence in interest because of its antioxidant properties, and the potential, through this mechanism, to possibly halt the progression of atherosclerosis and postangioplasty restenosis despite its HDL-lowering activity.

Chemistry

The chemical name for procubol is 4,4′-[(1-methyl-ethyldene)-bis(thio)]bis[2,6-bis(1,1-dimethyl-ethyl)phenol]. The structure is two butylated hydroxytoluenes connected by a sulfur-carbon-sulfur bridge. The butylated hydroxytoluene groups are potent antioxidants, and the sulfur-containing bis phenol is unrelated in chemical structure to any other cholesterol-lowering drug. Probucol is also very hydrophobic.

Pharmacokinetics

Probucol is poorly absorbed from the GI tract, with only 2 to 8% of the dose reaching the circulation. Probucol is transported from the gut within chylomicrons and VLDL. In the plasma it is carried predominantly by LDL, VLDL, and HDL; however, Polachek et al. note that there is no absolute correlation between the plasma levels of probucol and the degree of serum cholesterol lowering.

Mechanisms of Action

The actions of probucol appear to be multifold but, as of yet, have not all been clearly delineated. It is believed that probucol causes an increased uptake of LDL by the liver. This increased concentration of cholesterol is then converted into bile acids and excreted in the feces. This increased bile acid formation leads to a depletion of hepatocyte cholesterol and an increase in cholesterol turnover. In essence, a new steady state is achieved where LDL formation is equal to LDL breakdown.

The final proposed mechanism of probucol's action relates to its antioxidant properties and possibly its effects on atherosclerotic lesions. Many animal studies had shown that probucol could inhibit the progression and may cause regression of atheromas, independent of its effect on total cholesterol and despite reducing HDL levels. However, in a prospective, placebo-controlled study evaluating the effects of probucol on femoral atherosclerosis, the Probucol Quantitative Regression Swedish Trial (PQRST), the addition of the drug to diet and cholestyramine provided no benefit on the progression of atherosclerosis. After 3 years, the probucol-treated patients had 17% lower serum cholesterol, 12% lower LDL-cholesterol, and 24% lower HDL-cholesterol.

Clinical Experience

Monotherapy

Miettinen et al. conducted a 5-year multifactorial primary prevention trial in middle-aged men. Patients were treated with either probucol or clofibrate, with or without diuretic or β blocker. They noted an increase over the placebo group in coronary events for those treated with a β blocker or with clofibrate but not with probucol or diuretics. The incidence of cerebrovascular events was reduced in all groups compared with placebo. Miettinen reports that the probucol-treated group had a reduction in HDL in greater proportion than the reduction in LDL. However, despite this lowered HDL, the incidence of new cardiac events was lowest in the probucol-treated group. There is no clear explanation for this finding in light of the understanding that HDL varies inversely with coronary heart disease. Thus either probucol's LDL-lowering effect or some other property, such as its antioxidant activity, confers protection.

Combination Therapy

Several studies have identified probucol's additive hypocholesterolemic effects when combined with other lipid-lowering drugs, including colestipol, cholestyramine, and lovastatin. Furthermore, many lipid-lowering drugs other than probucol have an HDL-elevating effect that might partially counteract probucol's HDL-lowering effect.

Use in Preventing Angioplasty-Induced Restenosis

In various experimental models, probucol was shown to reduce neointimal thickening after vascular balloon injury in rabbits and swine and in preventing postangioplasty restenosis in humans. Various clinical studies with probucol for this indication also have shown benefit.

Adverse Effects

Side effects are few, mild, and most often GI in origin. Common side effects include diarrhea, loose stools, and flatulence. These side effects generally resolve after a few months of treatment. A major concern with probucol was raised when it was found to induce ventricular fibrillation in dogs sensitized with epinephrine. Monkeys taking probucol were then found to have a prolonged ECG QT interval that often evolved into torsades de pointes. Miettinen et al. conducted a 5-year prevention trial with probucol and found that there were small but significant prolongations in the QT interval with the drug. However, there was no observed increase in the incidence of cardiac arrhythmias during the 5 years of the trial or during the 5 years of follow-up after completion of probucol treatment. Naukkarinen et al., in a review of the above-mentioned study, noted that hospital admissions secondary to arrhythmias were more frequent in the placebo group than in the probucol-treated group.

Clinical Use

Probucol has too many disadvantages to be a practical treatment for managing patients with FH, despite its serum cholesterol-lowering effects and its ability to cause regression of xanthomas.

There is no question that probucol consistently depresses HDL-cholesterol levels, in many cases to a greater degree than it lowers LDL-cholesterol levels, and has the ability to induce ventricular tachyarrhythmias in susceptible patients.

SUGGESTED READINGS

ACC/AHA Guidelines for the Management of Patients with Acute Myocardial Infarction: A report from the American College of Cardiology/American Heart Association Task Force on Practice Guidelines (Committee on Management of Acute Myocardial Infarction). *J Am Coll Cardiol* 28:1328, 1996.

Expert Panel on Detection, Evaluation and Treatment of High Blood Cholesterol in Adults: Summary of the Second Report of the National Cholesterol Education Program (NCEP), Expert Panel on Detection, Evaluation and Treatment of High Blood Cholesterol in Adults (Adult Treatment Panel II). *JAMA* 269:3015, 1993.

Frishman WH, Patel K: Lipid-lowering drug, in Frishman WH, Sonnenblick EH (eds): *Cardiovascular Pharmacotherapeutics*. New York, McGraw-Hill, 1997, pp 399–479.

Haria M, McTavish D: Pravastatin: A reappraisal of its pharmacological properties and clinical effectiveness in the management of coronary heart disease. *Drugs* 53:299, 1997.

Jones PH, Grundy SM, Gotto AM Jr: Assessment and management of lipid abnormalities, in Alexander RW, Schlant RC, Fuster V (eds): *Hurst's The Heart*, 9th ed. New York, McGraw-Hill, 1998, pp 1553–1581.

Kjekshus J, Pedersen TR, for the Scandinavian Simvastatin Survival Study Group (4S): Reducing the risk of coronary events: Evidence from the Scandinavian Simvastatin Survival Study. *Am J Cardiol* 76:64C, 1995.

Lea AP, McTavish D: Atorvastatin: A review of its pharmacology and therapeutic potential in the management of hyperlipidaemias. *Drugs* 53:828, 1997.

Opie LH, Frishman WH: Lipid-lowering and antiatherosclerotic drugs, in Opie LH, Chatterjee K, Frishman W, et al. (eds): *Drugs for the Heart*, 4th ed. Philadelphia, Saunders, 1995, pp 288–306.

Sacks FM, Pfeffer MA, Moye LA, et al: The effect of pravastatin on coronary events after myocardial infarction in patients with average cholesterol levels. *N Engl J Med* 335:1001, 1996.

Shepherd J, Cobbe SM, Ford I, et al: Prevention of coronary heart disease with pravastatin in men with hypercholesterolemia. *N Engl J Med* 333:1301, 1995.

Scandinavian Simvastatin Survival Study Group: Randomised trial of cholesterol lowering in 4444 patients with coronary heart disease: The Scandinavian Simvastatin Survival Study (4S). *Lancet* 344:1384, 1994.

Superko HR, Krauss RM: Coronary artery disease regression: Convincing evidence for the benefit of aggressive lipoprotein management. *Circulation* 90:1056, 1994.

Witzum J: Drugs used in the treatment of hyperlipoproteinemias, in Hardman JG, Limbird LE (eds): *The Pharmacologic Basis of Therapeutics*, 9th ed. New York, McGraw Hill, 1996, pp 875–897.

Chapter 16 Combination Drug Therapy in Hypertension

Michael A. Weber, Benjamin E. Zola, and Joel M. Neutel

Drug combinations have been used traditionally to treat many cardiovascular conditions such as congestive heart failure, angina pectoris, and hypertension. But the historical development of using multiple medications has differed for each condition. For example, digitalis was first used in the eighteenth century to provide clinical benefits for patients with congestive heart failure. Then, recently in this century, diuretics were shown to produce symptomatic and functional advantages when used in addition to digitalis. Most recently, physicians also have added an angiotensin converting enzyme (ACE) inhibitor and an α-β-adrenergic blocker to digitalis and diuretic treatment to improve clinical findings and prolong survival, thereby completing a logical triad of drugs, each of which contributes in a separate, but meaningful, fashion.

Hypertension therapy, which is the main focus of this chapter, almost always has required drug combinations. Usually, more than one drug was required because earlier classes of drugs either were not effective alone or doses that produced efficacious decreases in blood pressure, unfortunately, also produced unacceptable adverse side effects or events. Indeed, 30 years ago the pooling of low doses of as many as three separate agents into a single fixed-dose product was quite commonplace. Serapes, for example, brought together reserpine, hydralazine, and hydrochlorothiazide; this fixed-combination product was popular with physicians, reasonably well tolerated by patients, and quite effective for reducing blood pressure.

The first attempt at a systematic method for treating hypertension was termed the *stepped-care* approach. Very simply, it recommended that treatment of all hypertensive patients begin with a diuretic—albeit in higher doses than would be customary now. If the diuretic was not efficacious, then a second-step drug, typically a sympatholytic agent, could be added. If success still was not achieved, then a third-step drug, usually a vasodilator, would be superimposed on the previous drugs. Yet further agents could be added, as necessary, to bring the blood pressure under control. At each step, the added medication usually would be increased to the maximum dose, often limited by side effects or adverse reactions.

EVOLUTION OF CARE

The stepped-care approach, employing separate drug prescriptions or the use of fixed combinations, became standard practice by the early

1970s. Almost immediately, though, conceptual challenges to this method of treatment began to appear. The most visible challenge came from the volume-vasoconstriction hypothesis advanced by Laragh and his colleagues. They postulated that essential hypertension was a heterogeneous condition where each patient had a different combination of both volume excess and vasoconstriction as the pathophysiologic cause of the high blood pressure. Thus, ideally, some patients should be treated with diuretics to reduce the volume-excess component, whereas other patients, whose excess vasoconstriction might be due largely to increased activity of the renin-angiotensin system, should be treated with drugs to inhibit renin release or to inhibit angiotensin II.

Laragh's group suggested that a simple measurement of plasma renin activity could guide the selection of a single agent from the drug class most likely to be beneficial. For instance, low plasma renin levels would suggest volume excess (treatable with diuretics) and high plasma renin levels would suggest increased activation of the renin-angiotensin system (treatable with ACE inhibitors or β blockers). Of course, for the patients whose plasma renin levels fell into the middle range, presumably indicating the presence of both volume and vasoconstriction factors, it might be necessary to use a combination of these drugs. Also, at the time, it was reported that patients with different demographic backgrounds had different renin profiles and had a tendency to respond preferentially to certain drug types. For example, patients who were white or relatively young tended to respond well to such agents as β blockers, whereas African-American patients and the elderly tended to respond well to diuretics.

As diagnostic and therapeutic strategies evolved, innovative new drug classes were created. Later-generation β blockers, the calcium channel blockers, the ACE inhibitors, and angiotensin II receptor blockers were all effective and produced relatively few adverse events or side effects. For these reasons, the Fourth Joint National Committee (JNC-IV) recommended individualizing therapy and encouraged physicians to search for the single agent that would best suit the needs of each patient. Diuretics, β blockers, calcium channel blockers, and ACE inhibitors were all considered appropriate drugs with which to initiate the treatment of hypertension.

Despite this progress, however, the overall treatment of hypertension still has not progressed satisfactorily. The National Health and Nutrition Examination Survey (NHANES 3) revealed that only 21% of hypertensive patients in the United States had their blood pressures reduced below 140/90 mmHg. The growing number of drug classes and individual agents for the management of hypertension suggests that, as yet, there are no fully adequate solutions. Drug combinations, therefore, remain a staple of antihypertensive therapy for now and for the foreseeable future.

A MATTER OF DEFINITION

Combination therapy involves multiple doses of multiple medications. Most commonly, physicians start with a single agent, and, after making adjustments to its dose, add further drugs while adjusting the doses as necessary. Most of the discussion in this chapter assumes this approach. However, from the very origins of antihypertensive therapy, manufacturers have made available a variety of fixed combinations. The intent of these products has been to provide a more simple and convenient way of taking more than one agent. By and large, these fixed-dose combinations have been only moderately successful in the marketplace. For example, it is estimated that fixed formulations of an ACE inhibitor and a diuretic are prescribed only 10% as frequently as the primary ACE inhibitor. The main objection to these products has been that they do not allow physicians to titrate separately the dose of each drug but rather compel physicians to prescribe the use of the two agents in a prefixed ratio. This objection has been particularly popular in academic medical centers, where physicians usually have not allowed fixed combinations on their formularies. The attitude of the Food and Drug Administration (FDA) toward these combinations also has not encouraged their use. The regulatory agency has insisted that physicians first titrate each separate component to an appropriate level and then switch to the combination product only if the doses correspond to an available fixed combination. In reality, though, these products have gone through rigorous testing to ascertain the optimal doses of each agent within the combination. Apparently, most physicians find this a tedious approach and tend to construct their own multidrug combination regimens.

There have been exceptions to this rule. Combinations of two diuretics, hydrochlorothiazide and triamterene, with the trade names of Dyazide and Maxzide, have been widely accepted. Likewise, Ziac, which contains a diuretic and a β blocker, and Lotrel, Teczem, Lexxel, and Tarca, which contain an ACE inhibitor and a calcium channel blocker, have received attention because of the unusual nature of their dosing or their components.

Manufacturers recently have selected names for these fixed combinations that differ totally from those of the individual components to create the impression of what they call "new types of dual-acting single entities." Recent market research data seem to confirm the success of these strategies. For example, in the United States during the 1993–1994 and 1994–1995 business years, the growth rates of total prescriptions for single-agent antihypertensives were 6 and 7%, respectively, whereas for fixed combinations they were 8 and 20%.

RATIONALE FOR COMBINATION THERAPY

Treating hypertension with combination therapy provides more opportunity for creative solutions to a number of problems. Five issues in combined therapy—some practical, some speculative—are listed in Table 16-1.

The most obvious benefit of drug combinations is the enhanced efficacy that fosters their continued widespread use. Theoretically, some drug combinations might produce synergistic effects that are greater than would be predicted by summing the efficacies of the component drugs. More commonly, combination therapy achieves a little less than the sum of its component-drug efficacies. In contrast, some combinations of drugs produce offsetting interactions that weaken rather than strengthen their antihypertensive effects—as previously seen with agents affecting peripheral-neuronal actions. For instance, guanethidine and reserpine produced this offsetting interaction, but since these agents are used now only rarely, this issue need not be considered further.

A second benefit of combination therapy concerns the avoidance of adverse effects. When patients are treated with two drugs, each drug can be administered in a lower dose that does not produce unwanted side effects but still contributes to overall efficacy. A third issue concerns convenience. Obviously, the multiple drugs of a combination regimen could be confusing and distracting to patients and could lead to poor treatment compliance. On the other hand, a well-designed combination pill that incorporates logical doses of two agents could enhance convenience and improve compliance.

Further potential value of combination treatment may result from the effects that two drugs have on each other's pharmacokinetics. Although this has not been studied well, there might be situations where the clinical duration of action of the participating drugs becomes longer when used in combination than when they are administered as monotherapies. Finally, it is interesting to consider the attributes of such agents as ACE inhibitors, angiotensin receptor blockers, and calcium channel blockers, which exhibit antigrowth or antiatherosclerotic actions in addition to their blood pressure lowering properties. Is it possible that combinations of these newer agents may provide even more powerful protective effects on the circulation? Each of these five potentially important attributes of antihypertensive combination therapy is considered in more detail below.

TABLE 16-1 Rationale for Combination Drug Therapy of Hypertension

Increased antihypertensive efficacy
Additive effects
Synergistic effects
Reduced adverse events
Low-dose strategy
Drugs with offsetting actions
Enhanced convenience and compliance
Prolonged duration of action
Potential for additive target organ protection

EFFICACY OF COMBINATION THERAPY

The most common motivation for administering more than one antihypertensive agent is to increase overall efficacy. Most of the time, the effects of the two agents being used are approximately additive, although it is likely—in view of the theories of hypertension heterogeneity reviewed earlier—that one drug plays a predominant role in reducing the blood pressure. Sometimes, a form of synergy can be achieved.

The principal antihypertensive drug classes in modern use are diuretics, β blockers, calcium channel blockers, ACE inhibitors, angiotensin II receptor antagonists, selective α blockers, centrally acting sympatholytic agents, and direct-acting vasodilators. This wide array of drug classes offers an enormous number of potential combinations. In reality, most fixed combination products on the market employ a diuretic, mirroring the clinical practice of most physicians. Therefore, this chapter first discusses diuretic-containing formulations and then briefly discusses some nondiuretic combinations of interest.

COMBINATIONS INVOLVING A DIURETIC

Before considering their role in combination therapy, it is helpful to define the way in which diuretics are now used most commonly. In general, the popularity of this class of agents has diminished during recent years. This is largely because of a perception among physicians that unwanted metabolic side effects with diuretics, including changes in plasma lipids, glucose, uric acid, and potassium, might adversely increase the risk of cardiovascular events despite the antihypertensive efficacy of these agents. On the other hand, physicians have realized that alternative drug choices, while avoiding these metabolic effects, often are not successful in controlling blood pressure. Diuretic use, therefore, remains widespread, though often as a supplement to other drugs. Moreover, the diuretics are used mostly in doses far lower than when they were first used; 12.5 mg has become quite typical, especially when used as part of a combination, and doses as low as 6.25 mg can be effective when used in combinations. Most of the modern, fixed-dose products that include diuretics have employed these lower doses.

Combination with ACE Inhibitors

Combining a diuretic with an ACE inhibitor is one of the most logical approaches to the treatment of hypertension. Diuretics work primarily by increasing renal clearance of sodium and water, thereby reducing intravascular volume. For many patients, a diuretic alone is an effective way to reduce blood pressure. For example, monotherapy with diuretics is effective often in African-American patients and in the elderly. The renin-angiotensin system of patients in these two groups often exhibits less of a reactive response to volume depletion and thus generates less compensatory angiotensin-mediated vasoconstriction. In contrast, ACE inhibitors are effective often in white hypertensive patients and in other settings where renin activity is relatively high. From a clinical perspective, diuretics and ACE inhibitors appear to have complementary properties. These attributes appear to be maximized when the two drug classes are used together, especially since the ACE inhibitors effectively prevent the counterproductive stimulation of the renin-angiotensin system produced by the diuretics.

Clinical trials have confirmed that these complementary properties are highly effective. In patients whose blood pressures have responded only partly to initial treatment with an ACE inhibitor, addition of even a very small dose of diuretic is more effective in reducing blood pressure than major increases in the dose of the ACE inhibitor.

Of practical importance, the combination of a diuretic with an ACE inhibitor appears to be effective in as many African-American patients as white patients. This has strong clinical implications beyond blood pressure itself; as discussed elsewhere in this book, ACE inhibitors are believed now to have powerful renal and cardiovascular protective properties, and the thoughtful use of diuretic-ACE inhibitor combinations will make it possible for African-American patients—who are particularly vulnerable to hypertensive renal disease—to benefit from these target-organ actions.

Finally, it should be stressed again that only small doses of diuretics are required in this type of combination treatment. In fact, most currently available fixed-dose combinations of ACE inhibitors and diuretics employ a dose of 12.5 mg of hydrochlorothiazide. It is possible, too, that the ACE inhibitors and diuretics may have offsetting metabolic effects. These are discussed briefly later in this chapter.

Combination with Angiotensin Receptor Antagonists

Most of the theory underlying the successful pairing of diuretics with ACE inhibitors also should apply to diuretics with angiotensin receptor antagonists. Available agents work by selectively blocking the angiotensin II receptor (AT_1), thereby interrupting most of the known hemodynamic, endocrine, and growth effects of the renin-angiotensin system. At this time, losartan is the only agent of this class available for prescribing, although several other agents should be approved for use within the next 2 to 3 years.

Clinical trials with losartan have shown that the addition of hydrochlorothiazide in a dose of 12.5 mg can increase the antihypertensive response rate from approximately 50% to almost 80%. Clearly, the effects of the AT_1 blocker and the diuretic in combination are additive. An example of this efficacy is shown in Table 16-2. These data show that the addition of 12.5 mg of hydrochlorothiazide in patients receiving either placebo or a variety of losartan dosing regimens produces

TABLE 16-2 Effects on Systolic and Diastolic Blood Pressures of Monotherapy with Placebo or Various Dosages of Losartan Followed by Combination Therapy with Hydrochlorothiazide

Treatment	No. of patients	Mean (SD*) systolic/diastolic blood pressure		
		Baseline	After 4 weeks of monotherapy	Additional decrease after 2 weeks of combination therapy with hydrochlorothiazide, 12.5 mg/day
Placebo	26	148.5 (14.7)/100.5 (3.8)	150.8 (12.9)/99.9 (5.9)	8.7 (11.4)/4.0 (6.4)
Losartan, 50 mg once per day	21	159.3 (16.6)/101.0 (4.9)	148.9 (16.5)/96.2 (7.9)	5.5 (14.0)/5.1 (7.8)
Losartan, 100 mg once per day	16	150.9 (14.0)/102.3 (4.7)	140.9 (15.7)/95.6 (7.6)	6.0 (7.5)/4.0 (6.1)
Losartan, 50 mg twice per day	20	155.2 (13.8)/101.7 (4.1)	146.2 (12.6)/95.6 (6.4)	7.3 (10.4)/4.0 (6.9)

*SD = standard deviation.

Source: From Weber MA, Byyny RL, Pratt JH, et al: Blood pressure effects of the angiotensin II receptor blocker losartan. *Arch Intern Med* 155:405, 1995, with permission.

consistent beneficial effects. Indeed, the blood pressure decrements observed when the diuretic is added to the losartan treatments are virtually identical with those observed when the diuretic is added to placebo—suggesting that these two drugs have a true additive effect when given in combination. A very low dose of 6.25 mg of hydrochlorothiazide in combination with losartan was tested in only one study, and the results indicated that this dose may not be adequate to optimize efficacy.

Combination with β Blockers

The combination of diuretics with β blockers is highly efficacious and shares mechanisms in common with the ACE inhibitor–diuretic combinations. Earlier the combination of hydrochlorothiazide with metoprolol was discussed, pointing it out as an example of a synergistic relationship between two agents. Although illustrative, that particular example may not be typical of more modern diuretic usage, where doses are lower and stimulation of the renin system is less extreme.

β Blockers, as monotherapy, appear to be effective often in white patients and the young, although they can be effective in older patients as well. These agents, however, do not appear to be very effective in low-renin hypertension. In fact, investigators have previously noted a paradoxical increase in blood pressure in low-renin patients treated with propranolol, perhaps reflecting the unmasking of vasoconstrictor, α-adrenergic activity resulting from the blockade of the β receptors.

Because β blockers were introduced into widespread clinical use several years before the ACE inhibitors, most of the experience with β blocker–diuretic combinations, especially fixed combinations, had been with relatively higher diuretic doses. Typically, hydrochlorothiazide was used in 25-mg doses. There is one unique and exciting recent exception to this rule: the fixed combination of a very low dose of the β blocker bisoprolol with a dose of only 6.25 mg of hydrochlorothiazide. The implications of this special case are discussed later in this chapter.

Combination with Calcium Channel Blockers

Unlike the ACE inhibitors and the β blockers, the calcium channel blockers have been theorized to be poor choices for combination with a diuretic. Since both the calcium channel blockers and diuretics are thought to work best in similar populations, such as the elderly and African-Americans, and to be most effective in low renin hypertension, they might be too similar to provide additive effects. Acute administration of calcium channel blockers also has been shown to produce measurable natriuresis, further suggesting that these two classes would not have complementary actions. Experiences with different states of sodium loading have reinforced these prejudices. Dietary sodium restriction may attenuate the antihypertensive efficacy of calcium channel blocker monotherapy, whereas sodium loading actually may enhance it. In experimental rat models, sodium loading has been shown to increase the number of dihydropyridine receptors on cell membranes; under these circumstances, the calcium channel blockers appear to have increased effectiveness in blocking sympathetic stimulation.

However, in practice, the combination of calcium channel blockers and diuretics has worked very well in the clinical setting. All three major types of calcium channel blockers currently available—verapamil, diltiazem, and the dihydropyridines—have each been shown to produce additive effects when combined with a diuretic. Indeed, some authors have shown that the addition of a calcium channel blocker to a diuretic produces antihypertensive effects similar in amplitude to those observed when either β blockers or ACE inhibitors were added to a diuretic.

Some of the pivotal studies of the effects of calcium channel blockers and diuretics employed an innovative study design; the efficacies of a matrix of differing calcium channel blocker and diuretic doses were compared with each other and with placebo so as to define the optimal composition of the combinations. The results of a study using this factorial design to evaluate diltiazem and hydrochlorothiazide are shown in Fig. 16-1. Each of the drugs is more efficacious than placebo, and it is clear that their effects are additive when used in combination. It is also interesting that the low 6.25-mg diuretic dose contributes usefully to the combined effect, especially when used with the higher diltiazem doses.

Combination with Sympatholytics

A relatively large array of antihypertensive drugs, especially in the earlier days of antihypertensive drug development, were targeted primarily at the sympathetic nervous system. Some, such as clonidine and methyldopa, worked centrally to reduce sympathetic outflow. These agents could be effective as monotherapy but were more efficacious when combined with a diuretic. Newer members of this class, most recently guanfacine, actually were designed to supplement a diuretic. Sympatholytic agents with more peripheral sites of action, including reserpine and guanethidine, benefited similarly from working in combination with a diuretic. It should be remembered that most of these drugs were developed and became popular during the era when the stepped-care approach was the standard and when the therapy of most hypertensive patients started with a diuretic. Methyldopa, clonidine, and reserpine, among others, were formulated in fixed combinations with diuretics as well as being available as monotherapies. The newer, selective α_1 blockers, notably prazosin, terazosin, and doxazosin, also can have their efficacy enhanced when combined with a diuretic agent.

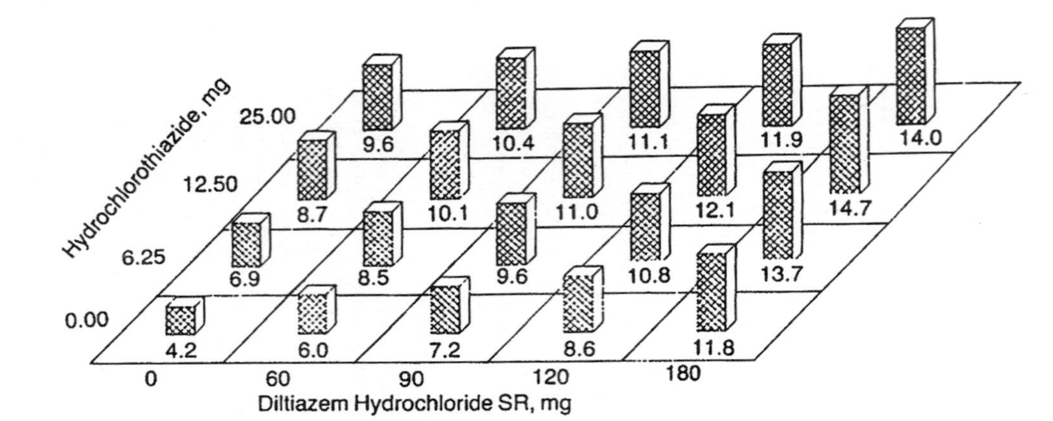

FIG. 16-1 Estimated mean supine diastolic blood pressure reduction (in mmHg) in response to therapy. Each dose was administered twice a day. SR indicates slow release. (*From Burris JF, Weir MR. Oparil S, et al: An assessment of diltiazem and hydrochlorothiazide in hypertension: Application of factorial trial design to a multicenter clinical trial of combination therapy. JAMA 263:1507, 1989, with permission.*)

Combination of Two Diuretics

It is rarely necessary to prescribe two diuretics at one time. This need usually occurs in the presence of renal insufficiency where refractory fluid retention might not respond adequately to usual or higher doses of a single diuretic. Under these circumstances, a loop diuretic or an agent such as metolazone might be combined with one of the more conventional thiazides.

The use of the combination of hydrochlorothiazide with the potassium-sparing diuretic triamterene has become ubiquitous. The two most common proprietary diuretic formulations in wide use are Dyazide, which contains hydrochlorothiazide, 25 mg, and triamterene, 50 mg; and Maxzide, which contains hydrochlorothiazide, 50 mg, and triamterene, 75 mg. Dyazide is provided as a capsule, whereas Maxzide comes as a tablet that can be halved to provide a lesser dose. These products are so well accepted that they are, in effect, often considered to be single entities. The confidence of physicians in these formulations may be well placed, for there has been recent evidence that diuretics that are not combined with a potassium-sparing component may be associated with an increased risk of sudden cardiac death in hypertensive patients.

OTHER ANTIHYPERTENSIVE COMBINATIONS

There is almost no limit to the number of ways in which different drug classes and individual agents can be combined effectively in the management of hypertension. This chapter considers some of the more interesting examples of such combinations.

Hydralazine, the direct-acting vasodilator, is effective during chronic treatment almost only when used as part of a combination. Although it is a powerful arterial vasodilator, this drug stimulates two powerful reactive mechanisms: It produces marked fluid retention, and it causes tachycardia, renin release, and other responses of sympathetic activation. Therefore, for hydralazine to work effectively, it must be combined with both a diuretic and a sympatholytic agent. For this reason, the stepped-care approach had always listed hydralazine as a third-step drug; it would be futile to administer it without a diuretic and sympatholytic drug already in place. It is interesting that the historical three-part fixed-dose combination, Serapes, contained all three of these ingredients: hydrochlorothiazide, reserpine, and hydralazine. Despite its efficacy, this product is now rarely prescribed.

The newer drug classes have prompted innovative new combinations, and pharmaceutical manufacturers have been studying formulations pairing two nondiuretic drugs. Three current combination formulations are worth exploring. The first combines calcium channel blockers with β blockers. Since they have complementary actions, at least in terms of the patient demographics in which they work best, β blockers and calcium channel blockers should work well together. One combination that already has completed pivotal early clinical trials couples felodipine, the calcium blocker, with metoprolol, the β blocker. This product (brand name Logimax) is significantly more efficacious than either of its component drugs used alone.

The development of Logimax highlights another issue in formulating fixed combinations: Because each component drug is formulated to maximize its own constant delivery and duration of action, the marrying of the two agents requires rigorous engineering and testing to ensure that their essential pharmacokinetic properties are maintained.

The second nondiuretic combination explored here involves the coupling of a calcium channel blocker with an ACE inhibitor. Fixed combinations of amlodipine and benazepril (brand name Lotrel), diltiazem and enalapril (Teczem), felodipine and enalapril (Lexxel), and verapamil and trandolapril (Tarka) were recently released for hypertension therapy and currently are the only available nondiuretic, fixed-dose, combination antihypertensives. Their mechanistic logic is similar to that of an ACE inhibitor–diuretic combination. The calcium channel blocker works best in low-renin hypertension, works in a large percentage of African-Americans and the elderly, and appears to be effective in blocking actions of the sympathetic nervous system. The ACE inhibitor works best in high-renin hypertension, succeeds in a large percentage of white patients and the young, and obviously is effective at interrupting the renin-angiotensin system. Moreover, unlike a diuretic, the calcium channel blocker should not cause any unwanted metabolic effects. The effects of amlodipine alone, benazepril alone, their combination, and placebo were compared. This study employed ambulatory blood pressure monitoring and demonstrated that benazepril and amlodipine each provide consistent antihypertensive efficacy during a 24-h dosing interval. The combination clearly provided additive efficacy throughout the day. The experience obtained during the development of this fixed-dose combination showed that its response rate, defined as either a reduction in diastolic blood pressure to less than 90 mmHg or a fall of at least 10 mmHg, exceeded 80% in patients with mild to moderate hypertension.

The third combination, at first sight rather illogical, couples an ACE inhibitor with an angiotensin receptor antagonist. Since each of these agents appears to work primarily by interrupting the renin-angiotensin system, their effects should not be additive. Nevertheless, clinical trials with a combination of an ACE inhibitor and an angiotensin receptor antagonist are currently under way in patients with congestive heart failure, and possibly will be expanded to hypertension. To understand why these drugs might work well together, their respective actions must be delineated in more detail.

ACE inhibitors prevent the conversion of angiotensin I, which is functionally inactive, into angiotensin II, the effector hormone. During chronic treatment with ACE inhibitors, however, it has been observed that plasma concentrations of angiotensin II, which are largely suppressed during the early stages of treatment, tend to rise toward their baseline values after several months. Despite this, the ACE inhibitors appear to retain much of their antihypertensive efficacy or, in the case of congestive heart failure, to sustain their beneficial hemodynamic and symptomatic effects and to reduce clinical events such as myocardial infarction. One possible explanation for this apparent discrepancy is that measurements of angiotensin II in the plasma are not an accurate reflection of the overall activity of angiotensin II at its sites of action within the circulation. Alternatively, the ACE inhibitors are known to interrupt the action of the kininase enzyme that breaks down kinins; thus ACE inhibitor treatment results in increased concentrations of bradykinin. Bradykinin has vasodilatory properties and also stimulates endothelial nitric oxide—which itself has vasodilatory and antigrowth properties. This bradykinin pathway stimulation may be a crucial part of ACE inhibitor efficacy.

In contrast to the ACE inhibitors, angiotensin II antagonists produce powerful and sustained blockade of the effects of angiotensin II at its receptors. For this reason, it could be conjectured that ACE inhibitors, with their recruitment of kinin and nitric oxide mechanisms, and angiotensin antagonists, with their powerful blockade of the renin-angiotensin system, could produce additive cardiovascular effects. No clinical data are yet available, but the results of current studies are awaited with interest.

COMBINATION THERAPY: REDUCTION IN SIDE EFFECTS

For many antihypertensive drugs there is a difference between their dose/efficacy relationships and their dose/adverse events relationships. In treating hypertension, the dose-response curve for efficacy often flattens early; low doses can achieve a large fraction of the potential maximum effect. On the other hand, adverse symptomatic complaints most often become a major problem with doses in the middle to upper end of the range. Low doses, for this reason, are attractive when they provide a moderate level of efficacy while minimizing unwanted effects. If two drugs have additive efficacies, then putting them together at low doses should produce a powerful therapeutic response without inducing adverse effects.

The Food and Drug Administration went so far as to publish an opinion on how this approach could be translated into new therapeutic formulations. In particular, it argued that there could be a basis for approving a low-dose fixed combination for the initial treatment of hypertension. Previously, the FDA had indicated combinations as later-step therapy, only to be used after monotherapies had proved inadequate.

To make a first-step approach valid, the FDA required that the two drug components must be drawn from classes known to have a dose-dependent increase in side effects, and where the use of very low doses could thus be anticipated to provide better tolerated therapy. By this reasoning, combinations of diuretics and β blockers would be appropriate, whereas combinations of ACE inhibitors and calcium channel blockers, both of which generally do not have dose-dependent side effects, would not qualify. A second criterion for approving the low-dose fixed combination was that each of the drugs involved, when tested as monotherapy in its proposed combination dose, should exhibit efficacy that would not differ meaningfully from placebo. Thus a clinically useful antihypertensive effect would be achieved only if the two drugs were used in combination.

Low-Dose Strategy for Reducing Side Effects

The most successful development of such a combination has been with hydrochlorothiazide, in a dose of 6.25 mg, and bisoprolol, the long-acting cardioselective β blocker. This combination product has the trade name of Ziac. The data used to justify the approval of this agent are shown in Table 16-3. It is evident that the combinations of the low-dose components produce meaningful decreases in blood pressure, whereas the individual components have only small effects. The JNC-VI report recommends a low dose combination treatment as an alternative first-line approach to hypertension management.

In a further study, this formulation was compared, in double-blind fashion, with full doses of the ACE inhibitor enalapril and the calcium channel blocker amlodipine. The combination decreased blood pressure at least as well as the full-dose monotherapies. Even more important,

TABLE 16-3 Multifactorial Trial with Bisoprolol, Hydrochlorothiazide, Placebo, and Combination: Mean Reduction (in mmHg) from Baseline Sitting Diastolic Blood Pressure at 3 to 4 Weeks*

	Bisoprolol, mg/day			
HCTZ, mg/day	0	2.5	10	40
0	3.8	8.4	10.9	12.6
6.25	6.4	10.8	13.4	15.2
25	8.4	12.9	15.4	17.2

Based on additive model with the factors bisoprolol dosage and hydrochlorothiazide dosage.
*Entry criteria: sitting diastolic blood pressure 95 to 115 mmHg
HCTZ = hydrochlorothiazide.
Source: Adapted from Frishman WH, Bryzinski BS, Coulson LR, et al: A multifactorial trial design to assess combination therapy in hypertension. *Arch Intern Med* 154:463, 1994, with permission.

especially in support of the underlying rationale for this type of formulation, mild and serious clinical adverse events tended to occur less commonly with Ziac than with the other agents. Quality-of-life measurements confirmed that the low-dose combination performed at least as well as enalapril or amlodipine.

Pharmacologic Interactions That Reduce Side Effects

From a practical point of view, most of the adverse effects of antihypertensive treatment can be divided into two main groups: those which cause symptomatic complaints and those which produce metabolic abnormalities in clinical test results—most commonly routine biochemistries. However, during combination therapy, even with full drug doses, it is possible that one agent could modify the adverse metabolic effects produced by the other agent, while at the same time contributing to overall antihypertensive efficacy.

One of the best examples of complementary metabolic effects is produced when ACE inhibitors are given together with diuretics. The diuretics are known to produce hypokalemia, hyperuricemia, and hyperglycemia, and possibly to increase plasma concentrations of LDL-cholesterol. However, concomitant administration of an ACE inhibitor moderates these changes enough to obviate the need to discontinue diuretic therapy or to introduce additional treatments to manage the unwanted metabolic effects. More recently, the angiotensin-receptor antagonist losartan also was noted to modify metabolic consequences of treatment with hydrochlorothiazide.

A good example of how one drug attenuates a clinical finding produced by another is given in Table 16-4. This study with the calcium

TABLE 16-4 How Combination Formulations Attenuate the Adverse Effects Produced by Individual Drugs

Adverse experience	Lotrel ($n = 760$)	Amlodipine ($n = 475$)	Benazepril ($n = 554$)	Placebo ($n = 408$)
Edema*	2.1	5.1†	0.9	2.2
Cough	3.3‡	0.4	1.8	0.2
Headache	2.2	2.9	3.8	5.6§
Dizziness	1.3	2.3	1.6	1.5

*Edema refers to all edema, such as dependent edema, angioedema, facial edema. Adverse experiences not statistically significant unless noted.

†Statistically significant difference between Lotrel and amlodipine ($p < .01$).

‡Statistically significant difference between Lotrel and amlodipine and between Lotrel and placebo ($p < .001$).

§Statistically significant difference between Lotrel and placebo ($p < .01$).

Source: Data on file, Ciba-Geigy, Geneva Pharmaceuticals, Summit, NJ

channel blocker amlodipine and the ACE inhibitor benazepril examined their individual and combined effects on common adverse experiences, most importantly edema. It is well known that calcium channel blockers can produce peripheral edema, which for some patients—most frequently women—can be bothersome. It is evident from this study, however, that when patients receive Lotrel, the fixed combination of amlodipine with benazepril, the frequency of edema is no different from that observed with placebo. The ACE inhibitor prevents the edema produced by the calcium channel blocker. The best explanation for this finding is that calcium channel blockers may produce edema because they primarily dilate the arterial side of the circulation. They have relatively minimal venous effects, thereby allowing plasma to pool peripherally. ACE inhibitors dilate both the arterial and venous circulations and thus are able to facilitate the central return of peripheral fluid accumulation. It is interesting, therefore, that the combination of a calcium channel blocker with an ACE inhibitor not only enhances efficacy but also has a beneficial effect on the side-effect profile.

COMBINATION TREATMENT: CONVENIENCE AND INCONVENIENCE

Persuading patients to continue taking their antihypertensive medications on a long-term basis is one of the more difficult tasks in clinical medicine. Compliance with treatment tends to be poor, and nearly 50% of patients started on drug therapy are lost to follow-up within a year. Explanations for this poor outcome include inadequate instructions to the patient, denial and other psychological responses, the side effects of the drugs, the cost of the drugs, and the burden of taking medications on a regular basis—often multiple drugs multiple times a day.

Combination treatment of hypertension, especially where more than two drugs are concerned, might easily have a deleterious effect on patient compliance. Clearly, such an approach may add to cost, complexity, and the likelihood of side effects. Patients find it discouraging to be dependent on this type of regimen when they may not have been taking any medications previously.

Fixed combinations potentially have some advantages. If efficacy can be achieved by two agents that happen to be part of a standard combined formulation, it is possible that this formulation alone might provide a satisfactory remedy for the hypertension. Combinations that pair an ACE inhibitor or a β blocker with a diuretic appear to be efficacious in a majority of patients. More innovative products, including the low-dose formulation of bisoprolol with hydrochlorothiazide or the calcium channel blocker–ACE inhibitor combination of amlodipine and benazepril, might be yet further examples of approaches that could enhance treatment compliance. The instructions for using the newly available angiotensin antagonist losartan also exploit this approach.

Physicians are recommended to start treatment of their patients with a single 50-mg dose of losartan; if this does not adequately control blood pressure, the recommendation is to switch immediately to the losartan-diuretic combination Hyzaar. The goal is to facilitate efficacy without intimidating the patient with multiple monotherapy titration steps or with a need for multiple drugs. Finally, manufacturers of the fixed combinations have understood that one of the advantages of these formulations is that they can be priced competitively and be made available at a cost only minimally higher than that of the primary monotherapy.

EFFECTS ON DURATION OF ACTION

During the development of new antihypertensive agents or formulations it is necessary to study pharmacokinetic interactions between the new drug and other drugs that might be used in the same patients. In general, drug-drug interactions among the antihypertensive classes are relatively minimal, and there has been no compelling need to alter doses or frequency of administration of the commonly prescribed agents.

This does not preclude the possibility that coadministration of two agents might sufficiently affect their biologic duration of action to justify altering their clinical use. The short-acting ACE inhibitor captopril is a notable example. This drug typically must be given two or three times daily as monotherapy, but adding hydrochlorothiazide changes this. Compared with placebo, the captopril-hydrochlorothiazide combination produced sustained reduction of blood pressure throughout the 24-h dosing interval when administered once daily. There was slightly greater efficacy with twice-daily administration, but it is clear that this combination, despite captopril's short duration of action, can provide true day-long efficacy. Indeed, if data in this study were considered only from those patients who were effective responders to the therapy, there was virtually no difference between once-daily and twice-daily treatment.

The mechanism of this prolonged effect is not clear, but it is possible that captopril retains sufficient ACE-inhibitory capacity, even in its low serum levels toward the end of the dosing interval, to moderate the diuretic-related stimulation of the renin-angiotensin system. In response to research with this combination, the FDA has granted once-daily labeling for the fixed combination of captopril with hydrochlorothiazide.

Another attempt to exploit this type of relationship was far less successful. A collaboration between the manufacturers of captopril and the calcium channel blocker diltiazem was undertaken to evaluate the efficacy of a fixed combination of the two drugs. At the time this venture was undertaken, diltiazem was still made only in its original, immediate-release, short-acting formulation and was typically administered three times daily. There was hope of an interaction between these two short-acting agents that might make their combination effective when administered just once daily, but study results did not support this expectation. Although the formal findings were not published in the medical literature, preliminary data on the efficacy of the combination, as judged by blood pressure reduction at the end of the 24-h dosing interval, demonstrated no differences between combination therapy and monotherapy. Of course, this failure of the combination to demonstrate either pharmacokinetic or clinical advantages does not detract from the logic of an ACE inhibitor–calcium channel blocker combination. As discussed earlier, the long-acting drugs benazepril and amlodipine are an example of how this approach to combination therapy can be highly effective.

ADDITIVE VASCULOPROTECTIVE ACTIONS

The chief goals of antihypertensive therapy include preventing major cardiovascular events, (such as myocardial infarction, arrhythmia, angina) and strokes. Although controlling the blood pressure and reducing other known cardiovascular risk factors are pivotal in achieving these goals, additional strategies also are needed to provide optimal protection against cardiovascular disease. A variety of endocrine and paracrine factors, including the renin-angiotensin system, the sympathetic system, endothelin, and other proteins and substances having effects on vascular growth and function, have become the targets of therapeutic intervention.

Both the ACE inhibitors and the calcium channel blockers have been shown to have strong vasoprotective actions in animal models of atherosclerosis. It is likely that other drug classes already available or in development also will perform in this fashion. It is not yet proved that data from the laboratory will translate into human clinical benefits, but already a number of studies have reported significant reductions in myocardial infarctions when patients with a variety of cardiovascular conditions are treated with ACE inhibitors. Calcium channel blockers also can exhibit antiatherosclerosis effects in humans, although recent controversies involving nifedipine and isradipine have raised clinical questions. Experiences with newer, long-acting agents appear promising.

If each of these drug classes has apparently beneficial actions on the vascular wall, is it possible that their use in combination could provide an additional measure of atherosclerosis prevention? In the same way that combining drugs from two classes produces additive antihypertensive actions, could they also produce additive effects within vascular tissue? No clinical data now exist, but there is speculation that combination therapies might produce clinical effects that differ from those produced with single-agent treatment.

DUAL-ACTING MOLECULES

Traditionally, combination therapy has been regarded as the concomitant use of two or more separate agents, but clinicians have learned that there are some molecules that can produce two separate actions, each of which can complement the other. Currently, there are at least two such agents, labetalol and carvedilol, that have been approved for the treatment of hypertension.

Labetalol is a molecule that possesses both α-adrenergic and β-adrenergic blocking properties. As described earlier, β blockade is an effective approach to blood pressure reduction, and agents with this property work particularly well in white patients, the young, and hypertensives with higher plasma renin values. α Blockers are efficacious across all age groups and in African-American patients. For this reason, the α-β blocker labetalol has been found to be efficacious in similar numbers of both white and African-American patients, whereas the β blocker propranolol tends to be most effective in white patients. Of more interest, β-blocker monotherapy produces a somewhat adverse effect on the lipid profile, decreasing plasma concentrations of HDL cholesterol. In contrast, α blockers have a slightly beneficial effect on the lipid profile. During treatment with labetalol, these offsetting actions result in a neutral effect on lipid measurements. Thus this single molecule provides complementary benefits of α and β blockade both on blood pressure reduction and on adverse outcomes.

Carvedilol similarly has β- and α-blocking activity. Its clinical effects are weighted more toward the α-blocking effect, and the drug appears to produce vasodilatory actions. As with labetolol, this newer agent provides antihypertensive efficacy across all ages, including the elderly, and all racial groups. Moreover, it has clear antianginal properties. Of note, carvedilol appears to provide hemodynamic benefits in patients with congestive heart failure, and it can decrease the incidence of new cardiovascular events in these patients.

SUGGESTED READINGS

Burris JF, Weir MR, Oparil S, et al: An assessment of diltiazem and hydrochlorothiazide in hypertension: Application of factorial trial design to a multicenter clinical trial of combination therapy. *JAMA* 263:1507, 1990.

Fenichel RR, Lipicky RJ: Combination products as first-line pharmacotherapy. *Arch Intern Med* 154:1429, 1994.

Frishman WH (ed): Antihypertensive fixed-drug combinations, in *Current Cardiovascular Drugs*, 2d ed. Philadelphia, Current Medicine, 1995, pp 276–288.

Frishman WH, Bryzinski BS, Coulson LR, et al: A multifactorial trial design to assess combination therapy in hypertension. *Arch Intern Med* 154:1463, 1994.

Joint National Committee: The fourth report of the Joint National Committee on Detection, Evaluation and Treatment of High Blood Pressure (JNC IV). *Arch Intern Med* 148:1023, 1988.

Joint National Committee: The fifth report of the Joint National Committee on Detection, Evaluation and Treatment of High Blood Pressure (JNC V). *Arch Intern Med* 153:154, 1993.

Joint National Committee: The sixth report of the Joint National Committee on Prevention, Detection, Evaluation and Treatment of High Blood Pressure (JNC VI). *Arch Intern Med* 157:2413, 1997.

Opie LH, Messerli FH (eds): *Combination Drug Therapy for Hypertension*. New York, Lippincott-Raven, 1997.

Packer M, Bristow MR, Cohn JN, et al: Effect of carvedilol on morbidity and mortality in chronic heart failure. *N Engl J Med* 334:1349, 1996.

Weber MA, Byyny RL, Pratt JH, et al: Blood pressure effects of the angiotensin II receptor blocker losartan. *Arch Intern Med* 155:405, 1995.

Weber MA, Priest RT, Ricci BA, et al: Low-dose diuretic and a beta-adrenoceptor blocker in essential hypertension. *Clin Pharmacol Ther* 28(2):149, 1980.

Weber MA, Zola BE, Neutel JM: Combination drug therapy: Focus on hypertension, in Frishman WH, Sonnenblick EH (eds): *Cardiovascular Pharmacotherapeutics*. New York, McGraw-Hill, 1997, pp 481–496.

Chapter 17 Selective Dopamine Receptor Agonists; Fenoldopam

William H. Frishman and Hilary Hotchkiss

Dopamine, the endogenous precursor of both norepinephrine and epinephrine, is used predominantly in intensive care unit settings as an intravenous pharmacotherapy for patients with ventricular dysfunction and various forms of shock. Dopamine acts at low doses by stimulating specific peripheral dopaminergic receptors, which are classified into two major subtypes (Fig. 17-1): D_1 receptors that, when stimulated, mediate arterial vasodilation in the coronary, renal, cerebral, and mesenteric arteries; and D_2 receptors, which are located in presynaptic areas, that mediate the inhibition of norepinephrine release when stimulated. At increasingly higher doses, dopamine also selectively activates the β_1-adrenergic receptors, leading to both a positive inotropic and a chronotropic effect on the heart. Next, the α_1- and α_2-adrenergic receptors are activated, leading to an increase in systemic vascular resistance and blood pressure due to vasoconstriction (Table 17-1).

Fenoldopam is an intravenous dopamine agonist that has specificity for the D_1 receptor, and has been used in treatment of congestive heart failure (CHF) and hypertensive crises. Fenoldopam's pharmacologic action is to dilate selected arteries while having the advantage of maintaining renal perfusion. Problems with oral bioavailability have limited the drug's use to parenteral treatment of severe hypertension.

In this chapter, the clinical pharmacology of the dopaminergic agonists are reviewed following a discussion of the peripheral dopaminergic receptors.

DOPAMINE RECEPTORS

Molecular pharmacologists have divided the dopaminergic receptors into various subtypes. The peripheral dopaminergic receptors, D_1 and D_2, have been the target of various cardiovascular pharmacotherapies in order to avoid drugs that could cross the blood-brain barrier and affect the central nervous system dopaminergic receptors.

A number of distinct dopamine receptors in the central nervous system have been found, and have been broken down into two groups: D_1-like and D_2-like. The D_1-like group includes the specific receptors, D_{1A}, D_{1B}, and D_5. These are G-protein-linked receptors that stimulate adenyl cyclase, causing an increase in intracellular cAMP. The D_2-like group includes D_2, D_3 and D_4. These are also G-protein-linked receptors, but they inhibit adenyl cyclase and thus

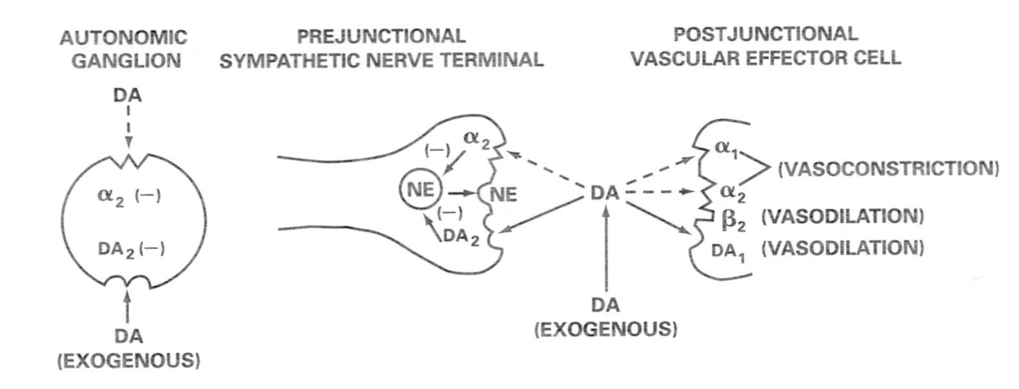

FIG. 17-1 Location of α_2 and D_2 receptors on the autonomic ganglion and prejunctional sympathetic nerve terminal to inhibit release of norepinephrine. α_1 and α_2 receptors are located on the postjunctional vascular effector cell to cause vasoconstriction. D_1 receptors and β_2 adrenoreceptors also are located on the postjunctional vascular effector cell and induce vasodilation. When dopamine is injected exogenously, it acts on D_1 and D_2 receptors at lower doses and on α_1 and α_2 adrenoreceptors at higher doses. Dopamine has little or no action on β_2 adrenoreceptors. Dopamine also acts on β_1 adrenoreceptors on myocardial cells to increase cardiac contractility. *(From Goldberg LI, Murphy MB: Dopamine, in Messerli FH (ed): Cardiovascular Drug Therapy. Philadelphia, WB Saunders, 1990, pp 1083–1089, with permission.)*

TABLE 17-1 Adrenergic and Dopaminergic Receptors: Location, Roles, and Agonists

Receptors	Location	Roles	Agonists
α_1	Postsynaptic	$\uparrow$ Vascular contraction & cardiac inotropism	PE, NE, E, EP, DA
α_2	Presynaptic	$\uparrow$ Vascular (vein) cont.	
	Postsynaptic	$\downarrow$ NE & renin release	E, NE, EP, DA
		$\downarrow$ H_2O, Na^+ reabsorption	
β_1	Postsynaptic	$\uparrow$ Cardiac inotropism and chronotropism	I, NE, EP, DA
		$\uparrow$ Lipolysis	
β_2	Presynaptic	$\uparrow$ Vasodilation (artery)	
	Postsynaptic	$\uparrow$ NE and renin release	I, EP
		$\uparrow$ Cardiac chronotropism and inotropism	
DA_1	Postsynaptic	$\uparrow$ Vasodilation	Fenoldopam, EP, DA
		$\downarrow$ H_2O, Na^+ reabsorption	
DA_2	Presynaptic	$\downarrow$ Ganglionic transmission	Bromocriptine, EP, DA
		$\downarrow$ NE and aldosterone release	

PE = phenylephrine; NE = norepinephrine; E = epinephrine; EP = epinine, DA = dopamine; I = isoproterenol; $\uparrow$ = increase; $\downarrow$ = decrease.

Source: Reproduced from Itoh H: Clinical pharmacology of ibopamine. *Am J Med* 90(Suppl 5B):36S, 1991, with permission.

inhibit the formation of cAMP. The D_1-like and D_2-like receptors are all distinct, however, they are currently grouped based on their similarities.

The peripheral dopamine receptors have a different nomenclature and are classified into two distinct families, D_1 and D_2 receptors. Recent studies have found the D_1 receptors to be similar to the D_1-like central receptors and the D_2 receptors to be similar to the D_2-like central receptors. However, additional study is required before a firm conclusion can be made regarding the significance of these similarities. The remainder of this chapter concentrates solely on the peripheral dopamine receptors and their activation.

D_1 receptors are located postsynaptically on the smooth muscle of the renal, coronary, cerebral and mesenteric arteries. Their activation results in vasodilation through an increase in cAMP production via increase in adenyl cyclase. The vasodilatory effect tends to be strongest in the renal arteries where blood flow can be increased up to 35% in normal arteries and up to 77% in patients with unilateral renal disease (dopamine doses were 1 μg/kg per min). Recent evidence points to additional D_1 receptors located in the tubule of the kidney that seem to be directly responsible for the natriuresis which also is seen with dopamine administration. Although their exact role in renal tubular physiology has not been established, the receptors have been shown to regulate both the Na^+/K^+-ATPase pump and the Na^+/H^+-exchanger. Bertorello and Aperia have demonstrated that dopamine agonists inhibit the Na^+/K^+-ATPase pump; however, Lee recently has pointed out the difficulty in dissecting the natriuretic influence of dopamine from other interacting factors under normal physiologic circumstances. The main point is that while the exact mechanism of D_1 receptor activation in the kidney may be unknown, the existence of D_1 receptors in the kidney that modulate natriuresis seems clear. Abnormalities in the renal D_1 receptors may, in fact, contribute to the etiology of some cases of systemic hypertension.

Based on the combined effects of activated D_1 receptors, research on selective D_1 agonists has focused on their use as a treatment for systemic hypertension and for hypertensive crises, particularly in patients with impaired renal function. The advantage of this pharmacologic approach over currently available antihypertensive medications is the maintenance of renal perfusion combined with natriuretic and diuretic effects. In addition, some research on D_1 agonists has focused on the possibility of increased myocardial blood flow with this treatment. Since currently available vasodilators often exhibit "coronary steal," where the coronary arteries end up receiving less blood, a D_1 agonist might correct this problem. Finally, the potential use of D_1 agonists for CHF is attractive based on the reduction in afterload caused by the selective vasodilation.

DOPAMINE RECEPTOR AGONISTS

Fenoldopam

Fenoldopam is a selective D_1 agonist, which is available in intravenous formulation. It is a potent vasodilator that is six to nine times as potent as dopamine itself (Fig. 17-2). Fenoldopam may have some α_1-adrenergic activity, but does not interact with D_2 or β receptors (Table 17-2). When taken orally, the serum half-life of fenoldopam is about 10 min; however, the effects are sustained up to 4 h after ingestion. The bioavailability of oral fenoldopam is low, with measurements ranging from 10 to 35%.

In the past, research concerning fenoldopam had focused predominantly on its potential use as an orally active chronic therapy for CHF and hypertension. The hope was that a selective D_1 agonist would result in vasodilation of the renal, coronary, cerebral, and mesenteric arteries, thus reducing ventricular afterload. In addition, a D_1 agonist would cause a natriuretic and diuretic effect because of

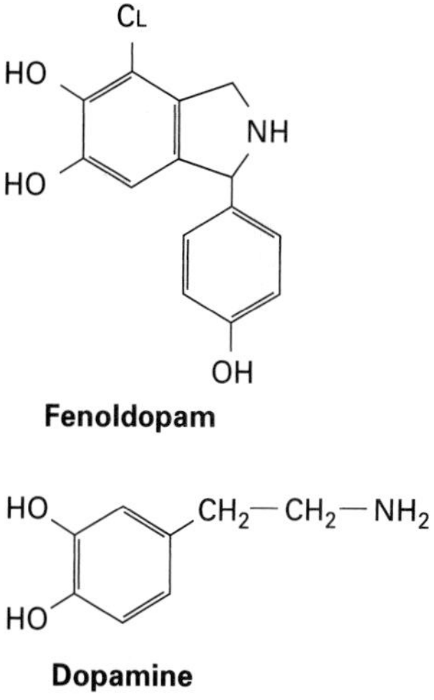

Fenoldopam

Dopamine

FIG. 17-2 Chemical structure of the dopamine receptor agonist fenoldopam compared with dopamine.

TABLE 17-2 Actions of Dopaminergic Agonists*

	Dopamine	Fenoldopam
DA_1 (vasodilation)	+++	+++
DA_2 (vasodilation, emesis, inhibits prolactin)	+++	−
α (vasoconstriction)	++	−
β_1 (inotropic, chronotropic)	+++	−
β_2 (vasodilation)	+	−
Oral availability	−	minimal

*+++ = major action; ++ = moderate action; + = minimal action; − = no action.

increased renal plasma flow and stimulation of specific D_1 receptors in the tubules of the kidney. Results of clinical trials, however, were inconclusive. Murphy et al. found that intravenous fenoldopam increased renal plasma flow 42%, glomerular filtration rate 6%, and sodium excretion 202% during free water diuresis. They also found, however, that plasma renin and norepinephrine levels increased significantly although aldosterone levels did not change. Ventura et al. evaluated oral administration of fenoldopam in hypertensive patients and found that fenoldopam was associated with a significant reduction in mean arterial blood pressure and a significant increase in renal plasma flow. These patients also exhibited a significant increase in cardiac index and stroke volume. In contrast to the above studies, Francis et al. found that both a single oral dose (100 mg) and a 3-day oral fenoldopam regimen (100 mg four times daily) resulted in a significant reduction in renal blood flow, but failed to produce diuresis and natriuresis. These effects were accompanied by activation of the renin-angiotensin-aldosterone system. Girbes et al. conducted a study of fenoldopam in normal healthy volunteers. They found that intravenous infusion of fenoldopam induced systemic and renal vasodilation. They also found a natriuretic effect, however, they noted that this effect seemed to be partially counteracted by a rise in the renin-angiotensin-aldosterone system.

These varied results with fenoldopam therapy in clinical trials, combined with the recent knowledge of its poor bioavailability, seem to have changed the focus of research concerning this selective D_1 agonist. In recent years, research has focused instead on its intravenous use in the acute management of severe hypertensive crises. Hypertensive crisis is a condition that affects 2.4 to 5.2% of hypertensive patients in the United States. This condition, associated with a diastolic blood pressure >115 mmHg, requires immediate care to prevent organ damage and even death. Sodium nitroprusside traditionally has been the preferred agent to treat these patients. It is a potent venous and arterial dilator with a rapid onset of action, a short half-life, a low incidence of tolerance, and a high predictability of response. However, sodium nitroprusside has some disadvantages, which include thiocyanate toxicity, a possible deterioration in renal function, and a possible coronary steal due to its potent vasodilation of both arteries and veins. Intravenous fenoldopam therapy, an alternative to this therapy, offers potentially fewer side effects and the additional advantage of providing improved renal function. Shusterman et al. found that severely hypertensive patients with impaired renal function who were treated with fenoldopam had improved blood pressure and renal function. Also, with fenoldopam, they found that there is no buildup of thiocyanate, a side effect seen with nitroprusside. Pilmer et al. reported on close to 200 patients who had been evaluated in various multicenter trials with intravenous fenoldopam. Overall, it was found that fenoldopam was as effective as nitroprusside in treating hypertensive crisis, but that fenoldopam was associated with fewer side effects such as hypotension and tachycardia. However, another recent study with 183 patients found that fenoldopam and nitroprusside were equivalent in terms of efficacy and acute adverse events. On the basis of the available studies, the Food and Drug Administration has just approved intravenous fenoldopam for use in hypertensive emergencies. One study did report that intraocular pressure increased with fenoldopam in hypertensive patients, an effect not seen with nitroprusside. Thus, at this point, additional studies are warranted before strong conclusions can be made regarding the first-line use of fenoldopam in hypertensive crisis.

CONCLUSION

Fenoldopam is a selective D_1 agonist that has been used to treat patients with CHF and hypertension. Since there are bioavailability problems with the oral formulation, only the intravenous form is available for use in patients with severe hypertension.

Dopexamine is an intravenous D_1 and β_2-receptor agonist that is being studied in patients with CHF and low cardiac output states.

Selective D_2 agonists are available that can inhibit the release of norepinephrine from sympathetic nerve terminals, thereby resulting in the reduction of systemic blood pressure. However, many of these drugs cross the blood-brain barrier and affect the nigrostriatal and mesolimbic central dopaminergic systems. Carmoxirole and ropinirole appear to have less central nervous system activity and may become useful drugs for treating systemic hypertension.

SUGGESTED READINGS

Brogden RN, Markham A: Fenoldopam. *Drugs* 54(4):634, 1997.

Frishman WH, Hotchkiss H: Selective and nonselective dopamine receptor agonists: An innovative approach to cardiovascular disease treatment. *Am Heart J* 132:861, 1996.

Frishman WH, Hotchkiss H: Selective and nonselective dopamine receptor agonists, in Frishman WH, Sonnenblick EH (eds): *Cardiovascular Pharmacotherapeutics*. New York, McGraw Hill, 1997, pp 727.

Post JB IV, Frishman WH: Fenoldopam: A new dopamine agonist for the treatment of hypertensive urgencies and emergencies. *J Clin Pharmacol* (in press).

Chapter 18 Prostacyclin in Cardiovascular Disease

William H. Frishman and Andrew N. Fink

Prostacyclin is found in all tissues and body fluids and is the major metabolite of arachidonic acid in the vasculature. Arachidonic acid is metabolized by cyclooxygenase to prostaglandin G_2 (PGG_2) and then by PG hydroperoxidase into PGH_2. These compounds are converted into prostacyclin by PGI_2 synthetase. Prostacyclin is produced predominantly in the endothelium and also by smooth muscle, and has interesting physiologic activity in relation to the cardiovascular system. It is the most potent vasodilator known and affects both the pulmonary circulation and the systemic circulation. Prostacyclin also has been noted to prevent smooth-muscle proliferation and causes vasorelaxation by increasing intracellular cAMP. Platelet aggregation and adhesion are also inhibited by the increase in intracellular cAMP induced by prostacyclin. An interesting note is that platelet aggregation is inhibited before adhesion.

These features have made it a very attractive substance in the attempt to treat many different cardiovascular diseases. Patients with primary pulmonary hypertension (PPH), congestive heart failure (CHF), myocardial ischemia, Raynaud's phenomenon, and peripheral vascular disease have all been treated with epoprostenol and its more stable analogues.

EPOPROSTENOL

Epoprostenol is the first synthetic prostacyclin to become commercially available and is currently approved for use in patients with PPH. It has the same structure as prostacyclin and is a very unstable molecule; its in vitro half-life at physiologic pH is approximately 6 min and is noted to be longer in alkaline solutions. It is also degraded by light. The product must be freeze-dried and stored at temperatures between 15 to 25°C. The drug must be reconstituted just prior to administration in a glycine buffer with a pH of 10.5 and must be protected from exposure to light during reconstitution and infusion. At room temperature, a single infusion should be completed within 8 h after the medication is reconstituted. Epoprostenol must be administered intravenously because it is degraded by the gastrointestinal (GI) tract before it can be absorbed.

Epoprostenol's in vivo half-life in humans is not measurable. In animal models, the half-life of epoprostenol is 2.7 min. It is hydrolyzed to 6-ketoprostaglandin $F_{1\alpha}$ in vitro, but in vivo, PGI_2 undergoes catalyzed oxidation to 15-*keto*-PGI_2. It has been noted that apolipoprotein (APO

A-I), a molecule associated with high-density lipoproteins (HDL), can prolong the half-life of prostacyclin.

Clinical Use

Studies done with epoprostenol usually have initiated infusion at a dose ranging from 1 to 2 ng/kg per minute with increases in the infusion rate at 5 to 15 min at increments of 1 to 2 ng/kg per minute until the appearance of side effects or the desired long-term infusion dose is obtained. The manufacturer of the drug recommends initiating the infusion with epoprostenol at 2 ng/kg per minute and increasing it at 2 ng/kg per minute increments every 15 min. The drug is titrated until the appearance of side effects, including systemic hypotension, or until the desired long-term infusion dose is obtained. The infusion rate can be lowered easily to a dose in which there are no side effects, and if severe systemic hypotension develops, the infusion can be stopped with the patient returning to baseline hemodynamic status quickly. This method can be used in both acute hemodynamic testing and long-term infusion. With long-term infusion, the dosage can be readjusted easily to meet the patient's changing needs.

There are several side effects noted with the drug. The most commonly noted are flushing, headache, nausea and vomiting, anxiety, and systemic hypotension. Other less common side effects are chest pain, dizziness, bradycardia, abdominal pain, musculoskeletal pain, dyspnea, back pain, sweating, dyspepsia, hyperesthesia, paresthesia, tachycardia, headache, diarrhea, flulike symptoms, and jaw pain (Table 18-1). These

TABLE 18-1 Adverse Events with Epoprostenol Infusion

During acute dose ranging*	
Adverse events in ≥1% of patients	Epoprostenol† (% patients, n = 391)
Flushing	58
Headache	49
Nausea/vomiting	32
Hypotension	16
Anxiety, nervousness, agitation	11
Chest pain	11
Dizziness	8
Bradycardia	5
Abdominal pain	5
Musculoskeletal pain	3
Dyspnea	2
Back pain	2
Sweating	1
Dyspepsia	1
Hypesthesia/paresthesia	1
Tachycardia	1

TABLE 18-1 (*continued*)

	Epoprostenol (% patients, $n = 54$)	Standard therapy (% patients, $n = 52$)
Occurrence more common with epoprostenol		
General		
Chills, fever, sepsis, Flulike symptoms	25	11
Cardiovascular		
Tachycardia	35	24
Flushing	42	2
Gastrointestinal		
Diarrhea	37	6
Nausea/vomiting	67	48
Musculoskeletal		
Jaw pain	54	0
Myalgia	44	31
Nonspecific musculoskeletal pain	35	15
Neurologic		
Anxiety/nervousness, tremor	21	9
Dizziness	83	70
Headache	83	33
Hypesthesia, hyperesthesia, paresthesia	12	2
Occurrence more common with standard therapy		
Cardiovascular		
Heart failure	31	52
Syncope	13	24
Shock	0	13
Respiratory		
Hypoxia	25	37

*Interpretation of adverse events is complicated by the clinical features of primary pulmonary hypertension which are similar to some of the pharmacologic effects of epoprostenol (dizziness, syncope). Adverse events probably related to the underlying disease include dyspnea, fatigue, chest pain, right ventricular failure, and pallor. Several adverse events, on the other hand, can clearly be attributed to epoprostenol, including headache, jaw pain, flushing, diarrhea, nausea and vomiting, flulike symptoms, and anxiety/nervousness. In an effort to separate the adverse effects of the drug from those of the underlying disease, the following lists adverse events that occurred at a rate at least 10% different in the two groups in controlled trials.

†Thrombocytopenia has been reported during uncontrolled clinical trials in patients receiving epoprostenol.

Source: Reproduced from package insert for Flolan.

unwanted effects are easily reversed by discontinuing the medication.

Most problems with long-term administration of the drug are related to the need for continuous intravenous delivery. These conditions include sepsis, line occlusion secondary to thrombosis, and pump failure—problems that can result in fatalities. Long-term studies have shown that most patients are able to reconstitute and properly administer their medications safely at home.

Primary Pulmonary Hypertension

Primary pulmonary hypertension is an idiopathic disease that is divided into three groups based on pathology: plexogenic arteriopathy, venoocclusive disease, and capillary hemangiomatosis. All three conditions also can be complicated by thrombosis in situ. Plexogenic arteriopathy is the most common form and is characterized by abnormalities in the intima and media of precapillary vessels that can range from mild neointimal proliferation to intimal fibrosis, plexiform lesions, and necrotizing arteritis. Pulmonary venoocclusive disease is less common and is characterized by fibrosis of the endovascular walls of small and medium-sized veins. The least common form, pulmonary capillary hemangiomatosis, is characterized by proliferation of the capillary network leading to changes in the arterial bed.

Although the mechanisms behind the disease are not completely elucidated, it does appear that there are definite features of the disease process. There is an imbalance of endothelial mediators of vascular tone characterized by an unfavorable balance between thromboxane A and prostacyclin predisposing the vasculature to thrombosis and constriction. There is also an increase in the production of endothelin by the pulmonary vasculature and an increase in circulating endothelin levels in patients with PPH, which causes further vasoconstriction. It also seems that there is a cycle involving vascular injury from an unknown cause in susceptible individuals, which leads to smooth-muscle invasion of the endothelium and a further disruption of the normal balance of vascular tone and coagulation mediators, further predisposing the endothelium to thrombosis, and obstruction. Presenting symptoms of the disease are dyspnea on exertion, syncope, and chest pain.

This disease has a poor prognosis. The results of a national registry of patients with PPH published in 1991 found that patients had a mean survival of 2.8 years after diagnostic catheterization was performed. In this study, the 1-year survival rate was 68%, the 3-year survival rate was 48%, and the 5-five year survival rate was 34%. In this registry, 39% of the patients had been diagnosed with PPH before being entered into the registry, but there was no significant difference between their survival rates and the survival rates of those who had not been previously diagnosed.

Traditionally, this disease has been treated with strong arterial vasodilators, such as calcium channel blockers, anticoagulation, and supplemental oxygen when needed. Nitrates also have been used as treatment, and rarely, cardiac glycosides and diuretics are used, and then only with extreme caution. Heart and lung transplantation and lung transplantation also have been used successfully in patients with PPH. However, there are always a number of patients who fail to respond to medical treatment.

Epoprostenol recently has been approved by the U.S. Food and Drug Administration for use in patients with PPH and seems to be useful in two ways. First, epoprostenol use appears to provide a safe method to screen patients with PPH for responsiveness to drug therapy. Second, epoprostenol has been shown to prolong survival in patients with New York Heart Association (NYHA) class III and class IV heart failure secondary to PPH.

There are well-defined goals for screening responsiveness to drug therapy in PPH. Not all patients respond to medication, and some will have an unfavorable response. An ideal response to administration of medication in patients with PPH would be a 20% decrease in pulmonary vascular resistance (PVR) or a decrease in PVR with a 20% decrease in pulmonary artery pressure (PAP) with or without an increase in cardiac output. An unfavorable response would be the development of symptomatic systemic hypotension or an observed decrease in cardiac output. A nonresponder to therapy would be a person who does not show any significant change in pulmonary vascular resistance or pulmonary artery pressure without the development of adverse side effects.

Epoprostenol seems to be an ideal screening agent for identifying responsiveness to medical therapy in patients with PPH. Advantages of this medication are its easy titratability, its potency, and its short half-life. Other medications that are used for screening responsiveness to therapy in patients with PPH are acetylcholine, adenosine, nitric oxide, and sublingual nifedipine. Epoprostenol is more potent than acetylcholine, giving it an advantage in this respect. Adenosine causes a decrease in pulmonary pressure, but it is suggested that this result is secondary to its actions on cardiac output and not because of its effects on the pulmonary vasculature. Nitric oxide seems to be comparable with epoprostenol in many of its hemodynamic actions. It has a short half-life and causes a decrease in pulmonary vascular resistance. Nitric oxide also does not cause systemic hypotension. However, it is not clear at this time if nitric oxide will replace epoprostenol as a screening agent for assessing the responsiveness to medical treatment in PPH. Sublingual nifedipine also has been shown to have similar effects on the pulmonary circulation and the systemic circulation when compared with epoprostenol. However, nifedipine is limited by its longer half-life.

If the patient has a favorable drop in pulmonary vascular resistance with epoprostenol without experiencing systemic hypotension, then there is a good indication that the patient will have a favorable response to longer-acting vasodilators such as nifedipine.

The other use for prostacyclin is in severely ill PPH patients who do not seem to be responding to other medical therapy. Recent studies have shown that long-term infusion of epoprostenol can improve survival in patients with PPH.

In 1990, Rubin et al. published the result of a small randomized trial looking at the effect of epoprostenol in patients with PPH who had not been responding to traditional therapy or had adverse reactions to therapy. They studied 24 patients with PPH with NYHA classes III and IV failure for 8 weeks and found that patients who received epoprostenol improved symptomatically and had improved hemodynamic function. Acutely, epoprostenol caused no change in PAP, a decrease in PVR of 27 to 32%, a decrease in systemic blood pressure, and an increase in cardiac output of 40%. At 2 months, there were no statistically significant changes in the hemodynamics of either group when compared with the beginning of therapy; however, there was a decrease in PVR from 21.6 to 13.9 units in the epoprostenol group, which approached statistical significance. Perhaps more interesting is that all the epoprostenol patients had an improvement in their NYHA functional class compared with two patients receiving conventional therapy. Both groups also had improvement in the distance walked during a 6-min encouraged walk, with the epoprostenol group showing a larger increase in distance walked.

Seventeen of these patients were followed from 37 to 69 months in an open, uncontrolled trial. When compared with historical controls, this group showed a decrease in mortality, with a 3-year survival rate of 63.3% compared with 40.6% in the control group (Fig. 18-1). These patients also had an improvement of approximately 100 m in a 6-min encouraged walk after 6 and 18 months of treatment with epoprostenol and showed some improvement in their hemodynamic variables (Table 18-2).

Recently, Barst et al. published the results of the largest epoprostenol trial in patients with PPH. In this study, 81 patients were randomized to receive epoprostenol or standard therapy for 12 weeks. Again, there was a dramatic improvement in exercise capacity and a decrease in mortality with epoprostenol. Patients who received epoprostenol were able to walk farther during a 6-min encouraged walk after 12 weeks of epoprostenol infusion. The control group showed a 29-m decrease in the distance walked in 6 min. Functional class improved in 40% of the epoprostenol group in this study. Forty-eight percent did not have any change in functional class, and 13% worsened. In the control group, 3% improved in functional class, whereas 87% remained unchanged and 10% worsened. It should be noted that only survivors who did not

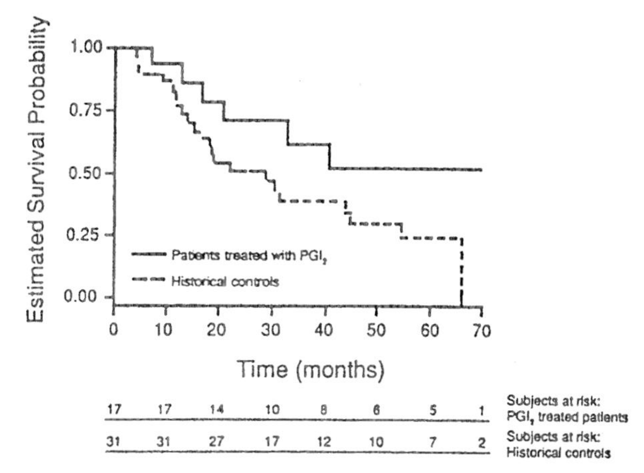

FIG. 18-1 In patients with PPH, a comparison of survival probabilities between patients treated with prostacyclin and historical controls. Kaplan-Meier observed survival probability curves for NYHA classes III and IV patients treated with prostacyclin (n = 17) and historical controls from the NIH Registry [NYHA classes III and IV patients receiving standard therapy including anticoagulant agents (n = 31)]. Survival function was calculated at 6-month intervals for 5 years. Survival was significantly improved in the patients treated with prostacyclin (p = 0.045). The 1-, 2-, and 3-year predicted survival rates estimated by the NIH Primary Pulmonary Hypertension Registry equation for the patients treated with prostacyclin were 63.2%, 50.4%, and 41.1%, respectively; for the historical controls, the predicted survival rates were 65.2%, 52.1%, and 42.4%, respectively. *(From Barst RJ, Rubin LJ, McGoon MD, et al: Survival in primary pulmonary hypertension with long-term continuous intravenous prostacyclin. Ann Intern Med 121:409, 1994, with permission.)*

undergo transplant were included in the above figures and that there were no deaths in the epoprostenol group and eight in the control. Cardiac parameters also improved with epoprostenol treatment. Patients treated with epoprostenol also reported improvement using the Nottingham health profile.

Although epoprostenol does not constitute a cure for PPH, it provides a substantial improvement as a palliative treatment for the disease. Higenbottam has been studying patients with PPH in England since the early 1980s and looked at the effect of epoprostenol use on heart and lung transplantation. His group studied 44 patients, 25 of whom received epoprostenol, and measured the time to transplantation and the success of transplantation. In this study, they noted that epoprostenol doubled the time on the waiting list for transplant or until death. They

TABLE 18-2 Hemodynamic Effects of Continuous Epoprostenol Infusion in Patients with Primary Pulmonary Hypertension after 6 and 12 Months of Follow-Up*

	Baseline ($n = 18$)	6 Months ($n = 16$)	12 Months ($n = 14$)
Mean right atrial pressure, mmHg	11 ± 7	7 ± 5	8 ± 6
Mean pulmonary arterial pressure, mmHg	61 ± 15	55 ± 11	54 ± 16
Mean systemic arterial pressure, mmHg	91 ± 13	90 ± 14	84 ± 11
Cardiac index, L/min/m^2	1.9 ± 0.6	2.3 ± 0.6	2.5 ± 0.8
Heart rate, bpm	81 ± 13	81 ± 13	89 ± 13
Mixed venous saturation, %	59 ± 12	67 ± 7	64 ± 12
Arterial oxygen saturation, %	93 ± 6	93 ± 6	92 ± 10
Stroke volume, mL/beat	41 ± 18	53 ± 18	51 ± 23
Total pulmonary resistance, U	22 ± 11	15 ± 6	14 ± 6
Total systemic resistance, U	31 ± 11	25 ± 11	22 ± 10

*Data are expressed as the mean ± SD.

Source: Reproduced from Barst RJ, Rubin LJ, McGoon MD, et al: Survival in primary pulmonary hypertension with long-term continuous intravenous prostacyclin. *Ann Intern Med* 121:409, 1994, with permission.)

also noted that epoprostenol was the one factor that influenced longevity the most. However, it should be noted that a total of only 10 patients were transplanted, and that 7 of these patients received epoprostenol.

SUGGESTED READINGS

Barst RJ, Rubin LJ, McGoon MD, et al: Survival in primary pulmonary hypertension with long-term continuous intravenous prostacyclin. *Ann Intern Med* 121:409, 1994.

Barst RJ, Rubin LJ, Long WA, et al: A comparison of continuous epoprostenol (prostacyclin) with conventional therapy for primary pulmonary hypertension. *N Engl J Med* 334:296, 1996.

Fink AN, Frishman WH: Uses of prostaglandins and prostacyclin in cardiovascular disease, in Frishman WH, Sonnenblick EH (eds): *Cardiovascular Pharmacotherapeutics*. New York, McGraw-Hill, 1997, pp 557–570.

Rubin LJ, Mendoza J, Hood M, et al: Treatment of primary pulmonary hypertension with continuous intravenous prostacyclin (epoprostenol): Results of a randomized trial. *Ann Intern Med* 112:485, 1990.

SPECIAL TOPICS SECTION

Chapter 19 | Pharmaceuticals in Noninvasive Cardiovascular Diagnosis

Jay S. Meisner, Jamshid Shirani, Joel A. Strom, and William H. Frishman

Pharmacologic agents have been used in cardiac diagnosis for years to bring out abnormalities that would not otherwise be detected. Nitrates, pressors, ergonovine, atropine, and more recently, dipyridamole, adenosine, and dobutamine have been utilized during diagnostic procedures that include physical examination, cardiac catheterization, and stress testing. In this chapter we emphasize those drugs used for detecting coronary artery disease during electrocardiographic (ECG) stress testing, radionuclide examinations, and echocardiographic study.

PROVOCATIVE TESTING IN CARDIAC AUSCULTATION

Because of its wide availability and accuracy, echocardiography has largely supplanted the need to augment auscultation of the heart by administration of the vasodilator amyl nitrate or the vasoconstrictors phenylephrine and methoxamine.

Amyl Nitrate

Administered by inhalation, amyl nitrate initially induces vasodilatation, a decrease in left ventricular size, and relative hypotension. These effects are followed by reflex tachycardia and an increase in cardiac output. The increased cardiac output augments the murmurs of valvular aortic stenosis, pulmonic stenosis, hypertrophic obstructive cardiomyopathy, and tricuspid regurgitation. Relative hypotension reduces the intensity of murmurs of mitral and aortic regurgitation, ventricular septal defect, and patent ductus arteriosus. The click and murmur of mitral valve prolapse occurs earlier because of reduction in mitral annular diameter, but like all mitral regurgitation murmurs, it is reduced in intensity.

Methoxamine and Phenylephrine

These agents are administered intravenously, with phenylephrine the preferred agent owing to its shorter duration of action. They are vasoconstrictors and affect murmurs by increasing arterial pressure, increasing heart size, and decreasing cardiac output. The murmurs of aortic and mitral regurgitation, ventricular septal defect, and patent ductus arteriosus are intensified by increasing arterial pressure. An increase in mitral annular diameter delays the click and murmur of mitral valve prolapse. A reduction in cardiac output decreases the intensity of the murmurs of aortic and mitral stenosis as well as functional murmurs.

RADIONUCLIDE TESTING AND STRESS ELECTROCARDIOGRAPHY FOR DETECTING MYOCARDIAL ISCHEMIA

ECG exercise-stress testing combined with myocardial perfusion imaging by nuclear scintigraphy is commonly used to assess known or suspected coronary artery disease (CAD) (Table 19-1). This method relies on exercise to induce autoregulatory vasodilation of the coronary arterioles. The coronary arterioles distal to a hemodynamically significant stenosis have a limited reserve of vasodilatory ability. With maximal exercise, these vessels achieve a smaller increase in perfusion than normal vessels, and the dependent myocardium may become ischemic. ECG changes are used to detect myocardial ischemia. Administration and scanning of a radionuclide with perfusion-dependent myocardial uptake detects regional inhomogeneity of perfusion. Perfusion imaging is most commonly performed with intravenous administration of ^{201}Tl-chloride or ^{99m}Tc-sestamibi, a potassium and a calcium analogue, respectively. Use of ECG and perfusion imaging yields a sensitivity and specificity of approximately 85% for hemodynamically significant CAD. Use of computer-assisted tomographic imaging techniques [single photon emission computed tomography (SPECT)] can boost sensitivity to almost 90% without loss of specificity.

Unfortunately, the technique is of limited utility in 20 to 30% of patients who have either abnormal ECGs, especially left bundle branch block, or are unable to reach the level of exercise required to attain a diagnostic heart rate. The latter includes patients on β blockers, patients who have just suffered after a myocardial infarction, and those with neuromuscular, vascular, orthopedic, or pulmonary disease. In these groups, exercise may fail to induce sufficient coronary vasodilatation to delineate those regions supplied by normal versus stenotic beds, leading to false-negative studies. Patients with orthopedic or vascular disease are a particular problem, since preoperative stress testing is often performed to determine their risk of a perioperative ischemic event. Patients with a left bundle branch block frequently demonstrate perfusion defects, most often in the interventricular septum, because of the aberrant sequence of depolarization. False-positive studies result. Dipyridamole and adenosine perfusion imaging and dobutamine stress echocardiography can address the need to detect CAD in selected patients in these groups.

Dipyridamole

Mechanism of Action

Dipyridamole produces arterial vasodilatation by inhibiting adenosine deaminase and by blocking reuptake of adenosine. Both these effects lead to greater agonist effects at adenosine A_2 receptors. Dipyridamole

TABLE 19-1 Some Noninvasive Methods of Assessing Coronary Artery Disease

	Standard ECG exercise stress test	Exercise perfusion imaging	Dipyridamole or adenosine perfusion imaging	Dobutamine stress echocardiography
Sensitivity	75%	85%	85%	85%
Ischemia localization	Poor	Good	Good	Good
Accuracy with LBBB	N/A	False (+) septal ischemia	Good	Good
Accuracy with resting wall motion abnormality	Poor	Good	Good	Fair
Detection of hibernating myocardium	N/A	Possible*	Possible*	Possible
Other information provided	Arrhythmia	Wall motion† rest EF,† lung uptake, infarct size, LV size	Wall motion† rest EF,† lung uptake, infarct size, LV size	Wall motion, LV/RV volume/function, wall thickness, valve function, ejection fraction
Technical problems	Unable to exercise; on digoxin	Unable to exercise, large breasts	Bronchospasm, obesity, large breasts	Inadequate acoustic window
Cost	1+	3+	3+	2+

*With delayed or reinjection thallium 201 scan.
†^{99m}Tc-sestamibi

Source: Adapted from Mayo Clinic Cardiovascular Working Group on Stress Testing: Cardiovascular stress testing: A description of the various types of stress tests and indications for their use. *Mayo Clin Proc* 71:43, 1996.

induces a small increase in heart rate of 5 to 10 beats per minute and a small decrease in systolic blood pressure of 10 to 15 mmHg.

Dipyridamole Perfusion Imaging

Test Development

Although initially developed as a coronary vasodilator to treat angina pectoris, dipyridamole was found to provoke myocardial ischemia in some patients. Based on its ability to induce ischemia, Tauchert et al. in 1976 proposed the dipyridamole ECG stress test for diagnosis of coronary artery disease. The sensitivity of this test, even with high doses of dipyridamole, was only 44 to 62%, with low specificity as well. In 1978, Gould proposed that dipyridamole-induced differences in perfusion of normal and stenotic coronary beds could be detected with radionuclide perfusion imaging. It was noted subsequently that dipyridamole induces a greater increase in coronary blood flow than can be achieved by exercise alone. Intravascular Doppler guidewire studies also have confirmed that dipyridamole produces flow inhomogeneity in humans with coronary stenoses, causing perfusion defects on imaging studies. Thus dipyridamole perfusion imaging has the advantage over exercise perfusion imaging of increasing the ratio of heart to lung counts and improving the resolution of radionuclide images. The ability to detect differences in perfusion has been enhanced by the development of SPECT.

Procedure

Standard-dose intravenous dipyridamole is administered at 0.56 mg/kg over 4 min by hand or with a Harvard pump. Submaximal handgrip and submaximal exercise can be used to further increase the degree of coronary vasodilatation. The radioisotope is injected 4 min after completion of the dipyridamole infusion. Heart rate, blood pressure, and 12-lead electrocardiograph are monitored continuously until 6 min after completion of the dipyridamole infusion or until symptoms resolve. When desired to quickly relieve symptoms caused by dipyridamole, aminophylline is administered intravenously in 50- to 100-mg slow boluses every 5 min to a maximum dose of 400 mg. Methylxanthine-containing substances are discontinued for 24 h prior to testing because they prevent vasodilation by dipyridamole.

In attempts to improve radionuclide image quality and test accuracy, the following have been proposed: use of high-dose dipyridamole (0.7 to 0.84 mg/kg), combination of exercise and usual-dose dipyridamole perfusion imaging, and combination of exercise and high-dose dipyridamole perfusion imaging.

Accuracy of Test

The accuracy of dipyridamole perfusion imaging has been assessed for each of its indications:

1. *Detection of CAD.* Numerous studies have demonstrated that oral or intravenous dipyridamole administration with perfusion imaging is comparable in sensitivity with submaximal exercise with perfusion imaging for single- or multiple-vessel disease. When compared with coronary angiography, dipyridamole perfusion imaging had, on average, 71% sensitivity and 71% specificity for identification of stenoses of greater than 50%. The detection of single-, double-, and triple-vessel disease in a study of 100 patients was 85%, 90%, and 100%, respectively. Dipyridamole is superior to exercise stress in avoiding false-positive septal perfusion defects in patients with left bundle branch block.

2. *Preoperative assessment before noncardiac surgery.* Dipyridamole perfusion imaging is the test most widely used to assess cardiovascular risk of noncardiac surgery. Several studies have demonstrated that patients without evidence of ischemia on dipyridamole perfusion imaging are at low risk of perioperative cardiac events. Those with ischemia on testing had a higher risk, but not more than 20 to 40% had a cardiac event. Patients with more than one ischemic bed were at greater risk than those with only one ischemic territory. Addition of clinical factors is required to identify a patient population at sufficiently high risk of perioperative myocardial infarction or death to warrant more invasive testing and intervention. Thus the role of dipyridamole perfusion scanning in the preoperative risk assessment of patients requires further clarification.

3. *Early postmyocardial infarction risk stratification.* Patients at high risk of further ischemic events after myocardial infarction can be identified by the presence of dipyridamole-induced ischemia within and remote from the area of primary infarction. Although several studies have confirmed this, sensitivity and specificity have varied with patient populations. In a study of 51 subjects for 19 months after myocardial infarction, Leppo et al. found ischemia on imaging in 11 of 12 patients who died or experienced reinfarction and noted that cardiac events occurred in only 6% of patients without ischemia. Gimple et al. reported a sensitivity of 63% and specificity of 75% for the ability of remote ischemia to predict cardiac events. The specificity of any area of ischemia for prediction of cardiac events was only 29%. Pirelli et al. found that postinfarction angina occurred in 7 of 11 patients with ischemia and in 2 of 24 patients without ischemia on perfusion imaging.

Dipyridamole Echocardiography

The sensitivity of echocardiographic wall motion abnormalities or changes in left ventricular function induced by dipyridamole for single-vessel coronary disease has been relatively low (52 to 74%) in several studies. More recently, in an angiographically confirmed comparison of dobutamine versus dipyridamole (up to 0.84 mg/kg), both plus atropine, there was comparable accuracy in detection of CAD. The sensitivity and specificity of dipyridamole-atropine stress echocardiography was 82 and 94%, respectively.

Dipyridamole Perfusion Imaging with Limited Exercise Stress

In a series of 397 tests, Daou et al. reported that in patients unable to achieve 85% of maximal predicted heart rate by exercise, the combination of dipyridamole plus exercise stress testing is superior to dipyridamole perfusion imaging alone and is comparable with maximal exercise testing.

Adverse Effects

A multicenter study of adverse effects of standard-dose dipyridamole in 3911 patients reported 2 deaths, 2 nonfatal myocardial infarctions, and 6 cases of bronchospasm. One of the patients who died and both those with nonfatal infarctions had unstable angina prior to the test. This study reported an incidence of 20% for chest pain, 12% for headache, and 12% for dizziness. Heart rate increased 22%, whereas systolic and diastolic blood pressure decreased by 5 and 8%, respectively. Aminophylline was administered in 12%, averaging 137 mg (range 10 to 600 mg). Although dipyridamole may produce bronchospasm and is contraindicated in patients with severe reactive airway disease, all episodes of bronchospasm responded to administration of aminophylline.

In a study of 1000 patients given standard-dose dipyridamole, 30% had chest pain, 5% dyspnea, 3% flushing, and 20% headache. Atrioventricular block did not occur. Aminophylline was used in 16% of patients. Use of aminophylline within the first 2 min after dipyridamole infusion was required in 2% of patients. Such use may reverse coronary vasodilatation before the isotope is completely absorbed by the myocardium.

The safety of dipyridamole administration in the early postinfarction patient has been demonstrated. It also has been shown to be safe in the elderly. However, dipyridamole testing should be avoided in patients with unstable angina.

In a multicenter safety study of high-dose dipyridamole (up to 0.84 mg/kg) in combination with two-dimensional echocardiography in more than 9000 subjects, major adverse reactions, including 1 death, occurred in 0.07%. Their analysis indicated that high-dose dypyridamole is safe when used selectively in patients in whom the usual dose did not induce either echocardiographic evidence of ischemia or limiting side effects.

Adenosine

Mechanism of Action

Adenosine is a naturally occurring nucleoside (6-amino-9-β-D-ribofuranosyl-9H-purine, $C_{10}H_{13}N_5O_4$) present in all body cells. It is produced in small amounts as part of the normal cellular metabolism and in large amounts during myocardial ischemia. Adenosine possesses a wide range of physiologic properties, among which is coronary vasodilation during ischemia and hypoxia. The cellular mechanism(s) of this vasodilator effect of adenosine is not completely understood. It may, however, be due to smooth-muscle cell relaxation resulting from the inhibition of slow inward calcium current and/or activation of adenylate cyclase through one of the two classes of adenosine receptors designated A_2. Adenosine also is a powerful inhibitor of atrioventricular node conduction and is used in urgent treatment of supraventricular tachycardia. The effects of adenosine on atrioventricular node are mediated through adenosine A_1 receptors present in the proximal portion of the node.

When injected intravenously, adenosine is rapidly taken up by cells (primarily erythrocytes and endothelial cells) and is either deaminated to inosine by the enzyme adenosine deaminase or phosphorylated to adenosine monophosphate by adenosine kinase. Consequently, the half-life of intravenously injected adenosine is less than 10 s. Both theophylline and caffeine are competitive blockers of the adenosine receptors and antagonize its physiologic effects.

Adenosine Myocardial Perfusion Imaging

The coronary vasodilator property of adenosine allows the use of this agent for pharmacologic stress testing, especially in individuals unable to perform exercise. Verani et al. demonstrated the utility of adenosine during thallium 201 myocardial perfusion imaging in 89 adults. The sensitivity and specificity of adenosine myocardial perfusion imaging for detection of CAD was calculated as 83 and 93%, respectively. False-negative studies occurred in patients with one-vessel CAD, and no patient had serious side effects. Subsequent studies have confirmed the findings of Verani et al. and have shown an average overall sensitivity of 90% and specificity of 91% for adenosine myocardial perfusion imaging, which are similar to values reported for exercise thallium 201 studies. In a multicenter study of 175 patients, Nishimura et al. also have shown good agreement between thallium 201 images performed with exercise or adenosine infusion (83% by visual estimation, 86% by quantitative analysis). Two multicenter trials have compared exercise thallium 201 and adenosine thallium 201 myocardial scintigraphy with coronary angiography in a total of 244 patients. The sensitivity, specificity, and overall accuracy of exercise and adenosine tomography were found to be similar in both studies. Adenosine specifically improves the sensitivity of thallium 201 scintigraphy in patients unable to perform adequate exercise; it also may be an appropriate substitute for exercise thallium 201 study in patients with left bundle branch block because of the increased frequency of false-positive results with the latter findings. Adenosine infusion also has been used in combination with submaximal exercise, in which case the side effects of adenosine are shown to be minimized while thallium 201 redistribution and heart-to-background ratios are improved. Direct comparison of adenosine and dipyridamole myocardial perfusion has not been done.

Adenosine Stress Echocardiography

Experience with pharmacologic stress echocardiography using adenosine infusion has been limited. Nguyen et al. compared thallium 201 myocardial perfusion and two-dimensional echocardiography in a subgroup of 25 in a study of the feasibility, safety, and diagnostic accuracy of thallium 201 imaging during adenosine infusion. New wall motion abnormalities were seen in 2 of 20 patients with CAD, 16 of whom had reversible thallium defects. The authors concluded that thallium 201 myocardial perfusion has higher sensitivity than echocardiography in detection of CAD. A subsequent study has shown better concordance between wall motion abnormalities detected by echocardiography and perfusion defects found on thallium 201 using SPECT during adenosine infusion. An overall agreement of 79% has been reported in this study, with an overall sensitivity of 89% for adenosine echocardiography that exceeded that of adenosine thallium imaging (83%). The lower sensitivity for the latter was believed to be a result of several false-negative tests in patients with ischemia limited to the inferior wall. One study of 40 patients, however, has shown superior accuracy of adenosine technetium 99m sestamibi tomography compared with adenosine stress echocardiography. Adenosine also has been compared with dipyridamole and dobutamine pharmacologic stress echocardiography in 40 patients who underwent all three tests. Significant CAD was present in 25 (68%) patients by angiography. Adenosine was shown in this study to be the least sensitive (40% compared with 76% for dobutamine and 56% for dipyridamole) but the most specific (93% compared with 60% for dobutamine and 67% for dipyridamole) agent. From the available information, it can be concluded that adenosine stress echocardiography is reasonably accurate in diagnosis of CAD in patients with multivessel disease, has lower sensitivity than perfusion testing in patients with single-vessel disease unless ischemia is limited to the inferior myocardial segment, and may improve diagnostic accuracy of noninvasive testing for myocardial ischemia when combined with thallium 201 imaging.

Dosage and Administration

Most studies of adenosine myocardial perfusion imaging have used a protocol of continuous adenosine infusion at a rate of 140 μg/kg per minute for 6 min. This is based on the observation by Wilson et al. that such an adenosine infusion rate results in near-maximal coronary vasodilation in most patients. Higher infusion rates may result in high frequency of undesirable side effects. When thallium 201 perfusion imaging is used, the tracer is injected 3 min after the onset of adenosine infusion, and images are obtained within 5 min of the termination of infusion and are repeated 4 h later. A similar infusion protocol is used for adenosine stress echocardiography.

Adverse Effects

Minor side effects are frequently encountered during adenosine infusion for myocardial perfusion testing or pharmacologic stress echocardiography. However, these adverse reactions are, for the most part, transient and typically subside within 1 or 2 min of discontinuation of the infusion, without a need for administration of aminophylline in most patients. The adverse reactions to adenosine infusion during perfusion imaging have been reported in a large, prospective, multicenter study of 9256 patients. At least one adverse reaction was reported in 81% of the patients. The most frequently encountered side effects were flushing (36.5%), shortness of breath or dyspnea (35.2%), chest pain (34.6%), gastrointestinal discomfort (14.6%), headache (14.2%), and throat, neck, or jaw pain (11.6%). Other adverse reactions occurred in less than 10% of the patients and included lightheadedness, atrioventricular block, ST-T changes, arrhythmias, and upper extremity discomfort. The adenosine dose had to be decreased in 13%, and the infusion had to be terminated in 7% of the patients. Only 0.8% required administration of aminophylline for reversal of the adverse effects of adenosine. Compared with dipyridamole, adenosine is associated with a higher frequency of adverse reactions; however, because of the short half-life of adenosine, these side effects are transient and well tolerated and require no specific therapy. Thus, at the adenosine doses recommended for coronary vasodilation during pharmacologic stress testing, serious adverse reactions are rare. It is important, however, to bear in mind that adverse reactions to adenosine infusion may occur with an anticipated higher frequency and severity in certain populations of patients such as those with unstable angina, asthma, chronic obstructive lung disease, sinus node dysfunction, high-grade atrioventricular block, aortic stenosis, pericardial effusion, hypovolemia, and carotid artery disease. Administration of adenosine should be avoided in such patients.

DOBUTAMINE STRESS ECHOCARDIOGRAPHY

Dobutamine, (±)4-{2-[[3-(*p*-hydroxyphenyl)-1-methylpropyl]amino]-ethyl}-pyrocatechol, is a synthetic catecholamine commonly used to transiently increase myocardial contractility in patients with congestive heart failure. It is a relatively selective β_1-adrenergic agonist that primarily increases myocardial contractility and, to a lesser extent, heart rate. It has mild β_2- and α_1-adrenergic agonist activity with the net effect of mild vasodilation of the peripheral circulation largely due to reflex withdrawal of sympathetic tone. The onset of action after intravenous administration is 1 to 2 min, reaching peak effect within 10 min.

The plasma half-life of dobutamine is approximately 2 min owing to hepatic conversion to inactive metabolites.

Dobutamine stress testing is a well-tolerated alternative to exercise-stress testing for detection of CAD and for risk stratification after myocardial infarction and before noncardiac surgical procedures in patients unable to exercise maximally and for detection of viable myocardium. Employing much the same mechanism of action as exercise, dobutamine produces greater autoregulatory vasodilatation of normal vascular beds than of ischemic beds of the heart where vasodilatory reserve is reduced. The heterogeneity of flow associated with significant CAD can be demonstrated by radionuclide perfusion imaging or by echocardiographic assessment of regional wall motion. Virtually all studies of the ability of dopamine stress testing to detect coronary disease have employed such assessments of wall motion. Although dobutamine stress testing with perfusion imaging should be as efficacious as exercise stress testing with perfusion imaging, this combination has not been as actively investigated. The lack of interest stems from the observation that dipyridamole produces greater flow heterogeneity than does dobutamine. This has led to the belief that dipyridamole should be coupled with perfusion imaging, whereas dobutamine is best used with a method of assessment of wall motion. However, a recent study has documented the absence of wall motion abnormalities associated with reversible perfusion defects on dobutamine stress testing. This was seen more frequently at low stress rate-pressure products and in women and raises the confounding issue of mechanically silent ischemia.

Development

In 1984, Mason et al. first reported that dobutamine infusions up to 20 μg/kg per minute with perfusion imaging detected coronary disease with sensitivity of 94% and specificity of 87%. Succeeding investigators increased the maximal dosage and confirmed that dobutamine echocardiography was equally efficacious.

Procedure

Performance of the test requires trained personnel to record and to interpret immediately heart rate, blood pressure, 12-lead ECG, and two-dimensional echocardiogram from parasternal long- and short-axis and apical four-chamber and two-chamber views. Dobutamine is infused at rates of 5, 10, 20, 30, and 40 μg/kg per minute, or until one or more of the following stop criteria are met: attainment of target heart rate, peak infusion rate, development of wall motion abnormalities in one or two myocardial segments, ECG ST-segment criteria for ischemia, sustained fall in blood pressure, excessive hypertension (systolic pressure >220 mmHg or diastolic pressure >110 mmHg), ventricular tachycardia, or supraventricular tachycardia. Two-dimensional echocardiographic views are recorded immediately before each increase in rate of dobutamine infusion. Some laboratories infuse dobutamine at a maximal rate of 50 to 60 μg/kg per minute. Many laboratories administer atropine in 0.5-mg intravenous boluses to a maximum of 1 to 2 mg if a heart rate equal to 85% of predicted maximum is not achieved at the maximal rate of dobutamine infusion. Esmolol, a short-acting β_1-selective agonist, can be administered intravenously at 0.5 mg/kg over 1 min to rapidly block the β_1-adrenergic agonist effects of dobutamine. Sublingual nitroglycerin can be administered for treatment of ischemia refractory to β-adrenergic blocking agents. Lidocaine is available for treatment of ventricular arrhythmias.

In addition, atropine also has been used to increase the sensitivity of both dobutamine and dipyridamole stress ECG. Atropine increases myocardial oxygen demand mainly through additional chronotropic stress. Atropine in divided doses up to 1 mg is given while continuing the dobutamine infusion, when no end point is reached with dobutamine alone.

Development of hypotension in 14 to 38% of patients is generally unrelated to ischemia, left ventricular outflow tract obstruction, or vasodepressor reflex. However, hypotension may be more common in patients with resting systolic hypertension. This phenomenon is likely multifactorial in etiology and requires further study.

The indications for dobutamine stress testing are those of exercise stress testing (detection of hemodynamically significant CAD, risk stratification post-myocardial infarction, and risk stratification of candidates for noncardiac surgery) as well as assessment of segmental myocardial viability. Although it is indicated as a substitute for exercise stress testing, dobutamine stress testing is often applied primarily to patients with a relative contraindication to administration of dipyridamole or adenosine: symptomatic cerebrovascular disease, bronchospasm, or prior reaction to dipyridamole or adenosine. It may provide more useful information than exercise echocardiography alone in patients with left main CAD. The procedure has been used safely for detection of coronary artery stenosis in children with Kawasaki disease.

The contraindications to dobutamine stress testing are identical with those of exercise-stress testing. In addition, hypokalemia should be corrected prior to dobutamine infusion, which induces extracellular to intracellular potassium shift through β_2-adrenergic agonism. The effects of dobutamine may be prolonged by liver failure. Atropine should be used with caution in patients with glaucoma or with a history of urinary retention. β-Adrenergic receptor blockade in dogs lowers the magnitude and slows the increase in peak heart rate and coronary flow during dobutamine stress echocardiography. Induction of ischemia and wall motion abnormalities by dobutamine is delayed or eliminated by the presence of beta blockade in the canine model. The effect of such blockade on the predictive value of the test in humans has not been studied.

Accuracy

Detection of Coronary Artery Disease

Several studies have compared the accuracy of dobutamine stress echocardiography with coronary angiography. Using either 50 or 70% stenosis in any artery as the criterion for hemodynamic significance by angiography and development of a new segmental wall motion abnormality as the criterion for a positive test, these studies demonstrated sensitivities from 76 to 96% and specificities from 66 to 95% over a wide range of patient populations.

Preoperative Assessment before Noncardiac Surgery

The presence of new or worsening wall motion abnormalities during dobutamine echocardiographic testing identifies the subset of patients who are subject to coronary events during noncardiac surgery. As is true for stress perfusion imaging for this purpose, the predictive value of a negative result far exceeds that of a positive test. Poldermans et al. performed dobutamine-atropine stress echocardiography on 302 patients presenting for vascular surgery and reported perioperative cardiac events in 27 of 72 with a positive test. They further identified intermediate and high-risk groups based on the "ischemic threshold"—the heart rate at which wall motion abnormalities occurred divided by maximum predicted heart rate. Using a threshold value of 70%, all patients with a fatal outcome and 8 of 12 with a nonfatal myocardial infarction were in the high-risk group. This method of quantifying the dobutamine echocardiography test increases the information obtainable but requires further verification.

Early Postmyocardial Infarction Risk Stratification

Most of the studies of dobutamine echocardiography performed soon after myocardial infarction have attempted to identify areas of reversible dysfunction (see below) rather than to stratify the risk of another cardiac event. However, there is a need to determine both the degree of residual stenosis of the culprit artery and the status of the uninvolved arteries. The latter was addressed in an early, limited study by Berthe et al., who reported no new wall motion abnormalities outside the infarct zone with dobutamine infusion in 15 of 17 patients without multivessel disease. In 11 of 13 patients with multivessel disease, appropriate new wall motion abnormalities were observed. More recently, Takeuchi et al. addressed the former concern and reported a sensitivity of 93% and a specificity of 91% when using worsened or unchanged wall motion at the infarct zone with dobutamine infusion as a predictor of greater than 50% stenosis of the culprit artery.

Detection of CAD in Patients with Idiopathic Dilated Cardiomyopathy

Smart et al. performed dobutamine echocardiography and coronary angiography on 54 patients with dilated cardiomyopathy. Using a change in global wall motion as the criterion for a positive dobutamine test, they reported overall sensitivity and specificity of 83 and 71% and sensitivity of 100, 83, and 69% for triple-, double-, and single-vessel disease, respectively.

Assessment of Myocardial Viability

Noncontractile myocardium may be viable in the setting of acute and chronic ischemia. In the former case, reversible ischemia induces a temporary state of "stunning" that may last for several months. In the latter case of "hibernation," residual myocardial perfusion is sufficient to support viability but not contractility. Low-dose dobutamine echocardiography may permit detection of these states. In this test, dobutamine is infused at increasing dose intervals of 2.5 to 5.0 μg/kg per minute, and the myocardial segments are observed for signs of contractility (contractile reserve). Typically, in "hibernating" myocardium, contractility again diminishes at higher doses (biphasic response), whereas sustained improvement is more consistent with permanent myopathy.

Detection of Stunned Myocardium

Low-dose dobutamine echocardiography performed during the first week after anterior myocardial infarction correlated with PET scanning in differentiating stunned from infarcted myocardium in 17 patients. Similarly, the results of low-dose dobutamine stress after thrombolysis compared with follow-up echocardiography yielded a sensitivity of 83% and specificity of 86 to 93% for detection of viability.

Detection of Hibernating Myocardium

Presence of any contractile reserve yielded a sensitivity of 82% and specificity of 86% for improved segmental contractility after coronary revascularization surgery in 25 patients. In a study of 20 patients, presence of contractile reserve followed by diminished contractility at increasing doses of dobutamine (biphasic dose response) had a predictive value of 72% for recovery of segmental function after coronary angioplasty. Improvement in function in the biphasic group occurred at a dobutamine dose of 5.0 to 7.5 μg/kg per minute and was followed by worsening usually seen with doses greater than 20 μg/kg per minute. In

18 patients, Perrone-Filardi et al. found that 91% of myocardial segments with improved contractility after angioplasty or bypass-graft surgery had contractile reserve on preoperative dobutamine stress testing. Only 18% of segments without postoperative improvement had preoperative contractile reserve. Of note, this study relied only on contractile reserve and did not require a biphasic dose response to dobutamine.

In a canine model, presence of a β blocker prevented the wall motion changes used to assess viability. In a comparison of dobutamine echocardiography with PET in patients with chronic ischemic left ventricular dysfunction, dobutamine echocardiography less reliably identified viable dysfunctional myocardium. Further controlled clinical trials will determine if dobutamine stress testing can reliably detect stunned and hibernating myocardium.

Adverse Effects

Although patients complain of chest pain, palpitations, tremor, headache, and nausea, dobutamine stress testing is generally well tolerated. Serious side effects may be due to the adrenergic effects of dobutamine or to induced myocardial ischemia. Four cases of sustained ventricular tachycardia and one case of ventricular fibrillation were treated successfully without mortality in a series of studies of more than 3000 patients.

Dobutamine echocardiography has been shown to be safe within days to weeks after myocardial infarction, in dilated cardiomyopathy in the elderly, and in patients with abdominal aortic aneurysms.

ARBUTAMINE STRESS TESTING

Addendum

Arbutamine was recently approved by the FDA for use in CAD in conjunction with radionuclide myocardial perfusion imaging and echocardiography in patients with suspected CAD who cannot exercise adequately. Arbutamine was approved only for delivery through a closed-loop computer-controlled drug delivery system (GenESA System) which is designed to elicit acute cardiovascular responses similar to those produced by exercise. The agent increases cardiac work through its positive chronotropic and inotropic actions.

ERGONOVINE ECHOCARDIOGRAPHY

Ergonovine is a vasoconstricting agent used to induce coronary artery vasospasm during coronary angiography. Song et al. have used the drug during echocardiographic examination for making the diagnosis of coronary vasospasm before angiography in patients with chest pain syndromes who have negative treadmill or normal stress myocardial perfusion scans, using a bolus of ergonovine until either ischemia or a total dose of 0.7 mg was administered. These investigators observed that ergonovine echocardiography could diagnose coronary vasospasm with a sensitivity of 91% and specificity of 88%. Of 53 patients showing regional wall motion abnormalities during the test, characteristic ST-segment elevation in the simultaneously recorded ECG was observed in only 20 (38%). There were no complications during myocardial infarction or fatal arrhythmia during the test. Pepine, in an accompanying editorial, suggests that ergonovine be utilized in the catheterization laboratory where rapid administration of nitrates may be given to counteract ergonovine-induced vasospasm. Pepine believes ergonovine provocation testing is too dangerous a procedure to be used outside the catheterization laboratory.

ULTRASONIC CONTRAST AGENTS DURING PHARMACOLOGIC STRESS ECHOCARDIOGRAPHY

The major limitation of stress echocardiography is the failure of left ventricular endocardial border delineation in as many as 15 to 20% of patients studied. Intravenously injected albumin microbubbles produced by high-speed sonication of 5% human albumin (Albunex) has been shown to cross the pulmonary capillary bed and opacify the left ventricular cavity. Left ventricular opacification by Albunex can improve endocardial resolution, wall motion analysis, and measurement of chamber volumes during dobutamine stress echocardiography. Left ventricular opacification following intravenous injection of Albunex may, however, be suboptimal in patients with low output states such as those with left ventricular systolic dysfunction, significant mitral or tricuspid regurgitation, atrial fibrillation, or pulmonary hypertension. Sonicated albumin microbubbles have thus been modified to improve their stability while crossing the pulmonary circulation. Porter et al. have shown that serial dilution of sonicated albumin in 50% dextrose can improve left ventricular endocardial border resolution during dobutamine stress echocardiography. It is also shown that the gas diffusivity and solubility of sonicated dextrose microbubbles can be further reduced by their exposure to perfluoropropane gas. Such exposure is shown to result in improved transpulmonary stability of the microbubbles, enhanced left ventricular chamber opacification and endocardial border resolution, and detectable myocardial uptake of the microbubbles. Several other ultrasonic contrast agents with improved transpulmonary microbubble stability are under investigation, and preliminary results with saccharide-based and fluorocarbon-based microbubbles have been promising. Most recently, second harmonic processing of the signal reflected from contrast agents has shown promise in enhancing the effect of contrast and in visualization of coronary arteries and measurement of coronary flow velocity. In conclusion, ultrasonic contrast agents have been shown to improve left ventricular endocardial border detection during dobutamine stress echocardiography. Further improvement in the stability of these microbubbles during pulmonary transit and understanding of the techniques to enhance wall motion analysis are expected to increase the accuracy of pharmacologic stress echocardiography for detection of CAD.

SUGGESTED READINGS

Afridi I, Kleiman NS, Raizner AE, Zoghbi WA: Dobutamine echocardiography in myocardial hibernation. *Circulation* 91:663, 1995.

Cigarroa CG, deFilippi CR, Brickner E, et al: Dobutamine stress echocardiography identifies hibernating myocardium and predicts recovery of left ventricular function after coronary revascularization. *Circulation* 88:430, 1993.

Kiat H, Iskandrian AS, Villegas BJ, et al: Arbutamine stress thallium-201 single-photon emission computed tomography using a computerized closed-loop delivery system. *J Am Coll Cardiol* 26:1159, 1995.

Mayo Clinic Cardiovascular Working Group on Stress Testing: Cardiovascular stress testing: A description of the various types of stress tests and indications for their use. *Mayo Clinic Proco* 71:43, 1996.

Meisner JS, Shirani J, Strom JA: Use of pharmaceuticals in noninvasive cardiovascular diagnosis, in Frishman WH, Sonnenblick EH (eds): *Cardiovascular Pharmacotherapeutics*. New York, McGraw-Hill, 1997, pp 975–988.

Weissman NJ, Levangie MW, Guerrero JL, et al: Effect of β-blockade on dobutamine stress echocardiography. *Am Heart J* 131:698, 1996.

Chapter 20 | Drug Treatment of Orthostatic Hypotension and Vasovagal Syncope

William H. Frishman and Tracy Shevell

Orthostatic hypotension is a term that is used to describe a fall in blood pressure after assuming an upright position that leads to symptoms referable to cerebral hypoperfusion. Controversy exists as to the numerical markers responsible for symptomatology. Most authors believe a drop in systolic blood pressure in the range of 20 to 30 mmHg within 3 min of standing with resulting complaints common to the disorder point toward orthostatic hypotension. In normal individuals, after rising to a standing position, systolic blood pressure usually drops only 5 to 10 mmHg and diastolic pressure rises in tandem with an increase in pulse rate from 10 to 25 beats per minute; in patients with orthostatic hypotension, such a rise will not occur. Many believe that avoiding absolute values to describe this condition is more cautious, since a wide range of pressure changes may be tolerated by each patient. Furthermore, when orthostatic hypotension is due to a primary condition such as autonomic failure (described in detail later), many are able to accommodate to blood pressure falls of up to 50 mmHg without significant symptoms. In studies done by Thomas and Bannister, cerebral autoregulation, or the capacity to maintain constant cerebral blood flow despite perfusion pressure changes, was maintained in normal subjects until mean arterial pressure fell to 60 to 70 mmHg. In patients with autonomic failure, however, autoregulation occurred until the mean arterial pressure was as low as 40 mmHg. Therefore, to demarcate absolute values for diagnostic criteria may exclude patients for consideration and for therapeutic intervention.

To define orthostatic hypotension appropriately, the most useful measure is to assess associated symptomatology in tandem with blood pressure fall. Patients typically present with lightheadedness and presyncopal or syncopal complaints. Functional activity is often greatly compromised by these symptoms, which also include dimming of vision and visual blurring, neck pain (often the only symptom present), weakness or buckling of the legs, cognitive slowing, headache, seizures (usually clonic jerks), and postprandial angina pectoris. Both visual changes and neck pain are most likely due to ischemia of the retinal or occipital lobe and the neck muscles, respectively. Focal neurologic findings may or may not be present; if they are, this may suggest concomitant cerebrovascular disease. If syncope occurs, patients typically awaken without postictal confusion or drowsiness almost immediately after a horizontal position is assumed. In contrast to the most common cause of syncope, which is neurally mediated (vasovagal syncope), patients with autonomic failure or other causes of orthostatic hypotension do not complain of associated pallor, nausea, vomiting, or diaphoresis. Other major findings or complaints may include mild anemia, hypohidrosis, a parkinsonian-like syndrome, recurrent urinary tract infections and/or bladder dysfunction, sleep apnea, hoarseness, nasal stuffiness, impotence, and constipation or diarrhea. All symptoms are relieved within 1 min of lying down.

Symptoms and the likelihood of syncope are most commonly reported in the morning or in the hour following meals, since food is a strong hypotensive stimulus. They are also worse after sudden postural changes, prolonged standing, in hot environments (i.e., a hot bath or shower or summer weather), when febrile, and after consuming alcohol. Exercise and hyperventilation also may provoke symptoms, as will activities that involve straining, including heavy lifting, coughing, or straining at stool. Patients are often more likely to tolerate their symptoms as the day progresses; this is indicative of a gradual rise in blood pressure. Although this is somewhat beneficial for a short time, by day's end it can result in a problematic situation for many whose orthostatic hypotension is secondary to autonomic failure—namely, supine hypertension. Supine hypertension may be most pronounced just after a patient retires at night and also may be accompanied by a significant nocturia as a result of pressure natriuresis.

Orthostatic hypotension is a common problem estimated in the general population to occur in 5 of every 1000 individuals, but in an acute setting incidence may be as high as 7 to 17% of all patients. When it leads to dizziness or syncope, frequency may then be considered to account for up to 21% of patients presenting to the emergency room. Furthermore, when dealing with elderly patients, orthostatic hypotension may be even more prevalent than evidenced by these statistics. Baroreceptor sensitivity decreases with aging, and increased drug intake and other causes may lead to greater than 20% of all elderly patients dropping their systolic pressure more than 20 mmHg on standing. The combination of side effects from medication, physiologic changes, and a greater incidence of chronic illnesses has an additive effect. Thus, in the primary care evaluation of dizziness in older patients, multiple sensory deficits and orthostatic hypotension play a greater role than other conditions more common in younger persons such as peripheral malfunctions and cerebrovascular disorders. In a study done by Sloane and Blazer, up to 18% of persons over the age of 60 were found to have symptomatology severe enough to interfere with activities of daily living; the presence of these complaints was associated with self-perceived depression, poor health, and other negative findings. With the increasing number of geriatric patients in our society, orthostatic hypotension may become a greater diagnostic possibility than ever before.

PHYSIOLOGY AND PATHOPHYSIOLOGY

As humans evolved into bipedal animals in an erect position from quadripeds maintaining a horizontal stance, the cardiovascular system was subsequently challenged to maintain cerebral blood flow in an adequate fashion. Assuming upright posture results in upward of 500 mL of blood pooling in the lower extremities, which then results in decreased venous return, decreased cardiac output, and thus decreased blood pressure. These changes provoke a compensatory reflex by arterial baroreceptors that is mediated by the central nervous system (CNS) and effected by peripheral efferent autonomic outflow. Lowered arterial pressure decreases tonic inhibition, which produces less vagal nerve activity and an increase in sympathetic efferent activity. An increase in heart rate and contractility and an increased constriction of vasculature results. Therefore, compensation manifests as increased peripheral resistance, increased venous return, and increased cardiac output, modifying blood pressure changes; should this mechanism fail, orthostatic hypotension results. Furthermore, plasma volume contraction recently has been found to contribute to symptomatology. Hormones also may have an effect, as evidenced by the renin-angiotensin system that leads to systemic constriction, aldosterone that affects sodium and volume, and endothelin and nitric acid that affect local vasoconstiction and vasodilation, respectively.

DIFFERENTIAL DIAGNOSIS

Many diverse disorders can give rise to orthostatic hypotension (see Table 20-1). Classification into specific categories becomes more and more important as treatment is becoming increasingly individualized; hypoadrenergic patients are exquisitely sensitive to pressor agents, whereas hypovolemic patients may benefit greatly from mineralocorticoids. Furthermore, there are several conditions that, once diagnosed, can be treated easily, including removal of offending medications from a patient's pharmaceutical regime and others, such as dopamine β-hydroxylase (DBH) deficiency, a cause of primary autonomic failure that has uniquely effective medical treatment available.

The most crucial step in management is to seek what can be treated; potentially reversible causes must first be considered along with nonautonomic causes (primary autonomic disorders are reviewed later). Up to 50% of reported cases of orthostatic hypotension have been found to be due to drug usage; most common offenders include antihypertensive agents, diuretics, antianginal agents, and antidepressants. Although it may seem paradoxical, antihypertensives are often used in patients with orthostatic hypotension because supine hypertension often coexists. Supine hypertension often unmasks hypotension during the day, once medical therapy has been employed. Alcohol, nitrates, narcotics, major and minor tranquilizers, marijuana, and nasal sprays are often reported as offending agents. Patients with autonomic failure are sensitive to the hypertensive effects of over-the-counter preparations (i.e. cold remedies), and problems also may result from the use of topical ophthalmic

TABLE 20-1 Causes of Conditions Producing Orthostatic Hypotension

Autonomic neuropathies
Primary
- Bradbury-Eggleston syndrome
- Shy-Drager syndrome
- Riley-Day syndrome
- Dopamine β-hydroxylase deficiency

Secondary
- Diabetes mellitus
- Uremia
- Guillain-Barré syndrome
- Amyloidosis
- Porphyria
- Idiopathic

Transient neurogenic (autonomic) syncope
Micturition syncope
Carotid sinus syncope
Vasovagal syncope
Bezold-Jarisch reflex activation
Glossopharyngeal neuralgia

Endocrinologic disorders
Pheochromocytoma
Hypoaldosteronism
Renal artery hypertension

Vascular insufficiency/vasodilatation
Varicose veins
Arteriovenous malformations
Absent venous valves
Carcinoid
Mastocytosis
Hyperbradykininism

Hypovolemic disorders
Anemia
Decreased plasma volume
Hemorrhage
Anorexia nervosa
Diarrhea
Overdialysis
Overdiuresis

Miscellaneous causes
Drugs (antihypertensives, diuretics, antidepressants, etc)
Pregnancy
Space flight

Source: Adapted from Robertson D: Treatment of cardiovascular disorders: Orthostatic hypotension, in Melmon KL, Morelli HF, Hoffman BB, et al (eds): *Clinical Pharmacology*: *Basic Principles of Therapeutics,* 3d ed. New York, Macmillan, 1992, pp 84–103, with permission.

solutions owing to increased intraocular pressure. Other potentially reversible causes fall under the rubric of hypovolemia; volume depletion from hemorrhage, dehydration, anorexia nervosa, diarrhea, diuresis, or vomiting should be evidenced from history, and subacute causes secondary to endocrinologic disorders may include pheochromocytoma, renovascular disease, Addison's disease, and excessive dialysis. The mitral valve prolapse syndrome resulting in orthostatic hypotension also may be considered hypovolemic in nature; many patients may have up to an 8% reduction in blood volume. Vascular insufficiency may result from varicose veins or other malformations, and symptoms of carcinoid, mastocytosis, or hyperbradykininism may all be gathered from a thorough history. Other miscellaneous causes include prolonged bed rest that was a result of probable baroreceptor desensitization, pregnancy, or weightlessness after space flight. Secondary causes also should be readily apparent from history and physical examination. It is also important to note chronicity of symptoms—nonautonomic causes of orthostatic hypotension tend to present in an abrupt fashion (in less than 1 month), whereas autonomic failure can evoke symptoms that progress over a period of 2 to 5 years.

Once orthostatic hypotension has been diagnosed, the key to management includes nonpharmacologic and pharmacologic modalities and target improvement of functional capacity rather than any specfic blood pressure. Although many measures do ease symptoms, current approaches remain deficient, and in the case of autonomic disorders, little can be done to stabilize or reverse the disease process. Changes can be evaluated by increase in blood pressure, increase in length of standing time, and subjective feelings of improvement.

PHARMACOLOGIC TREATMENT

Certain patients have been found to derive great benefit from drugs that are currently available; however, most are only slightly beneficial to the great majority when used alone. Most commonly, treatment is limited by the development of supine hypertension up to 200/120 or by other drug-specific side effects. Currently, researchers have found promise in an approach that combines three highly beneficial agents, fludrocortisone, midodrine, and erythropoietin alfa, that allows the orthostatic hypotension of autonomic failure to be well controlled. A listing of agents is found in Table 20-2; although many of these are used for primary autonomic dysfunction, they are also employed in secondary cases. The most commonly used drugs are discussed here in more detail. Caffeine, as mentioned previously, is also frequently used in therapy and is considered pharmacologic therapy by many, but others believe it falls under the rubric of nonpharmacologic intervention.

TABLE 20-2 Pharmacotherapeutic Agents Used in Orthostatic Hypotension

Agent
Fludrocortisone*
Erythropoietin (epoetin alfa)
Sympathomimetic amines
Midodrine
Phenylpropanolamine
Ephedrine
Somatostatin analogues
Somatostatin
Octreotide
Nonsteroidal anti-inflammatory agents
Ibuprofen
Indomethacin†
Antihistamines
Other agents
Caffeine†
Vasopressin agonists
Yohimbine
Clonidine
Hydralazine
Ergotamine
Pindolol

*Denotes volume-increasing agents.
†Denotes nonspecific pressors to prevent postprandial hypotension.

Fludrocortisone

Fludrocortisone (9-α-fluorohydrocortisone, Florinef) is a potent mineralocorticoid with little glucocorticoid effect. It is the most important agent for therapy of chronic orthostatic hypotension because of its wide availability, low cost, and demonstrated efficacy. This drug increases blood volume, increases sodium retention, and increases sensitivity of vasculature to circulating catecholamines. It requires 1 to 2 weeks for full action, and patients will gain between 5 and 8 lb when effects are maximum. Dosage begins at 0.1 mg (tablet form) once a day and is increased at 1- to 2-week intervals, which allows for titration up to 1 mg/day. Most require 0.3 to 0.4 mg to derive greatest benefit.

Common side effects include decreased levels of potassium within 2 weeks of therapy; often magnesium levels are reduced as well. Correction of hypokalemia with potassium supplementation often results in a secondary adjustment of hypomagnesemia. Since fluid retention is crucial to the beneficial effects of the drug, supine hypertension may develop and limit use or preclude use altogether in patients with CHF. Headache is a commonly noted side effect, but the problem fortunately is more common in younger patients and those with milder disease versus those who are in desperate need of therapy. Drug interactions may occur, and patients who receive warfarin may require a substantial increase in their dose to maintain the same protime. Patients often note improvement in their standing time and their quality of life using this drug, and it is rare that side effects are serious enough to discontinue treatment.

Sympathomimetic Agents—Agonists

Although increases in blood pressure may indicate a functional benefit, this is not often the case in patients treated with pressor agents such as ephedrine, pseudoephedrine, and phenylpropanolamine (direct and indirect effects) phenylephrine (direct effects), and dextroamphetamine sulfate (indirect effects). Some benefits have been shown with the use of phenylpropanolamine (as demonstrated by Biaggioni et al.), with a significant increase in blood pressure seen in patients with autonomic failure and orthostatic hypotension; this medicine is available in the United States without a prescription.

The most promising agent of late is another α_1 agonist, midodrine, which was approved for clinical use by the FDA for treatment of patients with orthostatic hypotension. The drug appears to have highly predictable blood pressure responses, appears to be well tolerated, and is shown to stimulate both arterial and venous systems without direct CNS or cardiac effects; there is no increase in heart rate. Its use is also remarkable in that benefits were noted not only in patients with primary failure but also in patients with diabetic neuropathy; one study found an average of a 22 mmHg increase in standing systolic blood pressure for both groups. The same increase was found in a second study by Jankovic et al. at the same dose (10 mg). Furthermore, both groups reported improvement in symptoms including presyncopal/syncopal prodrome, low energy level, feelings of depression, and standing time with only mild side effects reported. All these improvements, especially the ability to stand, were more significant than previously noted with ephedrine.

Midodrine is a prodrug that is activated to the actual agonist deglymidodrine after absorption; it is best used to raise pressure in the daytime. Dosage usually begins at 2.5 mg at breakfast and lunch and is increased in 2.5-mg increments or until a maximum dose of 30 mg has been reached. Side effects include piloerection, pruritus, and tingling of the scalp, all related to muscle contraction of integumentary hairs. Supine hypertension is also slightly problematic, but it is widely believed that midodrine is a safe and effective new addition to the myriad of available drugs for orthostatic hypotension.

Sympathomimetic Agents—Antagonists

Yohimbine is an α_2-adrenoceptor antagonist that has been found to be especially beneficial by antagonizing central and presynaptic receptors (or both). It has been found to improve systolic and diastolic blood pressure, heart rate, and plasma norepinephrine in seated patients and is most beneficial in Shy-Drager syndrome or mild Bradbury-Eggleston syndrome. It essentially enhances the patient's own nervous system, but unwanted side effects include anxiety, nervousness, and diarrhea. Other sympathomimetic agents that have been tried include clonidine and ergotamine. None of these agents has enjoyed tremendous success when used alone.

Erythropoietin

Frequently, patients with autonomic neuropathy resulting in orthostatic hypotension have a decreased red cell mass. This anemia is usually proportional to the degree to which the plasma norepinephrine levels are also abnormal. There is an inadequate response of erythropoietin as well, and this leads to decreased effective blood volume aggravating the preexisting hypotension. It has been shown that this anemia responds dramatically to recombinant erythropoietin (epoetin alfa, Epogen) administered intravenously or subcutaneously. Blood pressure also rises an average of 10 mmHg, although the mechanism is unclear and not entirely thought to be due to an increased blood volume or increase in viscosity. In a study performed on patients with different categories of diseases including diabetes and primary autonomic failure, epoetin alfa was shown to increase hematocrit, increase blood pressure, and improve symptoms of orthostasis, especially dizziness. Epoetin alfa is administered in 25 to 75 U/kg doses three times per week until the hematocrit is in the normal range for gender.

Side effects are minimal; iron deficiency that often develops as the hematocrit is increasing is easily treated with supplementation, and doses of epoetin alfa usually can be tapered to maintenance doses as low as 25 U/kg thrice weekly. Patients often report improvement in symptomatology, an increased appetite, and a tremendously improved sense of well-being. Although still a novel therapy tried on low numbers of patients, this strategy appears to be very effective and will continue to be refined.

Miscellaneous Agents

A number of other agents have been used in therapy of orthostatic hypotension. Indomethacin blocks the synthesis of prostaglandins, which help mediate vasodilatation and natriuresis while augmenting norepinephrine release. Somatostatin and octreotide (a somatostatin analogue) have been used to attenuate the secretion of vasodilatory peptides to reduce postprandial hypotension. Antihistamines are employed in mastocytosis and occasionally in diabetic dysautonomia. Dihydroxyphenylserine is a unique, effective treatment to replace absent norepinephrine in dopamine β-hydroxylase deficiency. β Blockers occasionally have been recommended (pindolol in particular), but efficacy is not uniformly shown.

Agents for Treatment of Vasovagal Syncope

Once the diagnosis of vasovagal syncope has been ascertained (i.e., via tilt table testing), patients must be counseled to avoid any known triggers and be sensitive to prodromal symptoms as well as mildly increasing salt intake. However, this is often not enough to suffice, and drug therapy needs to be employed (Table 20-3). No double-blind, controlled studies exist regarding currently used medications; thus any treatment must be approached cautiously. Low-dose β blockers (i.e., metoprolol, 50 mg bid) are often found to be effective via prevention of excessive stimulation of ventricular mechanoreceptors and by preventing excessive vasodilatation of arteries. In a smaller study, fludrocortisone was effective when given for 10 days at a dose of 0.1 mg/day. This agent is thought to be important in vasovagal syncope not just because of volume increase but also because of increased vasoconstriction via sensitization of vascular adrenergic receptors to norepinephrine. Disopyramide also has been used in an attempt to benefit from its negative inotropic effects and its anticholinergic properties; however, results are mixed. Verapamil, fluoxetine, and α agonists also have met with limited success.

As the roles of adenosine and nitric oxide in recurrent vasovagal events are becoming more evident, therapy may be directed toward this end. The actions of adenosine, both direct and indirect, are antagonized at the receptor level by theophylline. Thus this treatment, not currently first-line, may become more commonplace as the trigger to the vasovagal cascade focuses more on adenosine. Adenosine also may be responsible for the diminished postural change in plasma renin activity in the elderly, which is abated after theophylline administration. This may have important therapeutic implications regarding the increased problem of orthostasis and vasovagal events in the elderly. It is further postulated that adenosine stimulates production of NO, which is also recently a focus for exacerbating vasodilatation and thus a fall in blood pressure. In a 1995 study by Li et al., the addition of theophylline antagonized the production by arterial, but not by venous, endothelial cells.

TABLE 20-3 Drug Treatment of Recurrent Vasovagal Syncope

Current therapies
Low-dose β blockers
Fludrocortisone
Disopyramide
Theophylline
Verapamil
Fluoxetine
Alpha agonists
Future possibilities
Inhibitors of NO synthesis/blockade of action
Inhibitors of acetylcholine production
Modulation of theophylline treatment regime (i.e., in elderly)

These new foci provide exciting future possibilities for treatment that may include targeting decreased production of NO, either by inhibition of synthesis or by blockade of its action.

Despite the fact that there is uneasiness regarding medical therapy of vasovagal syncope, many new strategies have become feasible recently. There are many who firmly believe that when this type of syncope is associated with bradycardia or asystole, drug therapy is very effective. Emphasis must, however, continue to be placed on the inclusion of non-pharmacologic measures into treatment plans as research on the newest pharmacologic therapy continues.

SUGGESTED READINGS

Frishman WH, Shevell T: Drug treatment of orthostatic hypotension and vasovagal syncope, in Frishman WH, Sonnenblick EH (eds): *Cardiovascular Pharmacotheraputics*. New York, McGraw-Hill, 1997, pp 1231–1246.

Low PA, Gilden JL, Freeman R, et al., for the Midodrine Study Group: Efficacy of midodrine versus placebo in neurogenic orthostatic hypotension: A randomized, double-blind multicenter study. *JAMA* 277:1046, 1997.

Robertson D: Treatment of cardiovascular disorders: Orthostatic hypotension, in Melmon KL, Morelli HF, Hoffman BB, et al (eds): *Clinical Pharmacology, Basic Principles of Therapeutics*, 3d ed. New York, Macmillan, 1992, pp 84–103.

Robertson D: Therapy of orthostatic hypotension, in Singh BN, Dzau V, Vanhoutte PM, Woosley RL (eds): *Cardiovascular Pharmacology and Therapeutics*. New York, Churchill-Livingstone, 1994, pp 1015–1023.

Sra JS, Jazayeri MR, Avitall B: Comparison of cardiac pacing with drug therapy in the treatment of neurocardiogenic (vasovagal) syncope with bradycardia or asystole. *N Engl J Med* 328:1085, 1993.

Chapter 21 Drug Treatment of Infective Endocarditis

Mark H. Goldberger, Gary E. Kalkut, Joseph N. Cosico, and William H. Frishman

Infective endocarditis (IE) is a disease with protean manifestations resulting from endovascular infection within the heart. The location of infection is usually the heart valves; however, the chordae tendinae, mural endocardium, or septal defects may be involved. The initial event in the pathogenesis of IE is endothelial damage at a site of turbulent blood flow. Fibrin, leukocytes, and platelets are deposited on the abnormal endothelial surface, forming a sterile vegetation referred to as *nonbacterial thrombotic endocarditis*. Pathogenic organisms gaining access to the bloodstream may become incorporated in the fibrin-platelet network, resulting in infected vegetation, the pathologic hallmark of IE. Continued deposition of fibrin and platelets protects microorganisms from cellular defense mechanisms and perhaps from contact with antimicrobials and allows the density of organisms to reach high levels. Virulent bacteria such as *Staphylococcus aureus* or *Streptococcus pneumoniae* with the capacity to adhere to less severely damaged endothelium may cause infection on apparently normal heart valves.

Embolization, one of the dread complications of the disease, occurs when portions of friable vegetation are lost in the circulation. Vegetation on the left side of the heart gives rise to systemic emboli leading to organ and limb infarction, including stroke or coronary artery occlusion. Right heart vegetation embolizes to the lungs. Rarely, in the setting of a septal defect or elevated right atrial pressures with a patent foramen ovale, paradoxical emboli to the systemic circulation occur with right-sided valvular lesions. Emboli from either side of the heart may be septic or bland.

From the vegetation, infection may spread locally to damage the valve itself or its supporting structures. The valvular incompetence that ensues can result in hemodynamic compromise and congestive heart failure. Invasion of the myocardium, through direct spread or embolization, may cause abscesses that can lead to myocardial dysfunction, continued sepsis, and conduction abnormalities, including complete heart block. In the absence of effective therapy, the vegetation is a source of continuous bacteremia, leading to peripheral foci of infection and eventually death. Some of the more subtle manifestations of the disorder are caused by the immunologic response to the persistent bacteremia, including glomerulonephritis, arthritis, Osler nodes, Janeway lesions, and Roth spots.

THERAPY

In the absence of antibacterial chemotherapy, bacterial endocarditis is a uniformly fatal disease; host defense mechanisms alone are inadequate.

Furthermore, therapy of bacterial endocarditis requires the use of bactericidal agents. The goals of therapy are the eradication of all organisms within the vegetation and the prevention of embolic and immunologic phenomena and valve destruction. Several factors make this vegetation particularly difficult to treat. Because it is endovascular, white blood cells alone are ineffective in eliminating the infection. Antibiotic therapy is problematic because (1) the inner layers of the vegetation may be exposed to very low concentrations of antibiotic because of poor penetrability, (2) those antibacterial agents which require active growth for killing (most cell wall active agents) are relatively ineffective against the slow-growing organisms found deep within the vegetation, and (3) high density of bacteria in vegetation may produce exceedingly high local levels of antibiotic modifying enzymes.

For these reasons, the therapy of IE customarily has required high doses of bactericidal agents for prolonged periods of time. A controversial issue has been the usefulness of serum inhibitory and bactericidal levels in monitoring therapy of endocarditis. As initially reported by Schlichter, the trough serum inhibitory concentration (SIC) is determined by serially diluting the patient's serum obtained just prior to the next dose of antibiotic and testing the ability of these dilutions to inhibit the growth of a standard inoculum of the patient's bacterial isolate. The highest serum dilution to inhibit growth is the SIC. The serum bactericidal concentration (SBC) is determined by subculturing those tubes with inhibited growth onto fresh agar and demonstrating killing of the initial inoculum. The highest serum dilution to accomplish this degree of killing is the SBC. The same determinations can be made for peak inhibitory and bactericidal levels by drawing serum shortly after administration of an antibiotic dose.

Although previously the American Heart Association (AHA) recommended that the peak SBC be maintained at 1:8 or higher in the treatment of *S. viridans* endocarditis, clinical experience has not supported an association between these levels and clinical outcome. Current AHA guidelines do not recommend the use of serum bactericidal titers in most cases of IE. These levels may be helpful in circumstances where response to antimicrobial therapy is poor, in disease due to unusual organisms, and in therapy with unconventional agents.

The first sign of successful therapy often is the patient's increased sense of well-being. In uncomplicated IE, fever generally resolves over days to a week or more, and the patient remains afebrile. Immune-complex nephritis and arthritis generally parallel the course of the infection, although some patients may be left with residual impairment of renal function. In IE caused by *S. aureus*, blood cultures may remain positive beyond 1 week. Some of these patients are cured with medical therapy. Persistently positive cultures, however, usually imply failure to eradicate the initial focus of infection, spread of infection to the myocardium, or metastasis to a distant focus. Persistent fever may be caused by one of these factors, superinfection, or drug fever. It often is difficult in any one patient to identify with certainty the etiology of persistent or recurrent fever. Repeated examination of the patient, preferably by the same observer, is of paramount importance. The development of a new murmur, a pericardial friction rub, heart failure, or embolic phenomena in such a patient suggests continued active endocarditis. Complaints of bone or joint pain, abdominal pain, or persistent bacteriuria should direct attention to a new focus.

The importance of obtaining a microbiologic isolate cannot be overemphasized. Although the initial selection of antibiotics can be made empirically, an optimal regimen can be prescribed only when an isolate is available for susceptibility testing. The timing of initial therapy depends on the patient's presentation. In a patient with subacute illness, antibiotic therapy should be withheld until the diagnosis is made securely. In the patient with suspected acute IE, blood cultures should be obtained and empiric antibiotic therapy begun immediately.

Patients with an acute presentation of IE (often injection drug users) require empiric therapy prior to culture results. Staphylococci and streptococci (including enterococci) are the most common pathogens with occasional cases due to gram-negative bacilli. The combination of penicillin, a penicillinase-resistant penicillin, and an aminoglycoside will provide effective empiric coverage for the majority of cases. In many places, community-acquired methicillin-resistant *S. aureus* (MRSA) IE occurs in at least 10 to 15% of cases, so that vancomycin should be substituted for the penicillin and the penicillinase-resistant penicillin.

Once the infecting organism is isolated and antimicrobial susceptibility determined, the antibiotic regimen should be adjusted accordingly (Table 21-1).

Discussion of therapeutic approaches to the treatment of the more common bacterial isolates follows.

Nonenterococcal Streptococcal Endocarditis

Approximately 30 to 55% of all cases of IE are caused by penicillin-susceptible streptococci. *S. viridans*, a heterogeneous group of organisms, accounts for the majority, with the remainder caused by group G, nonenterococcal group D, and other streptococci. For these patients, there are several recommended regimens (see Table 21-1). For most patients with highly sensitive streptococci (minimal inhibitory concentration [MIC] for penicillin, <0.1 μg/mL), single-drug therapy for 4 weeks or a combination of penicillin and gentamicin for 2 weeks has replaced 4 weeks of penicillin given with streptomycin for 2 weeks as conventional therapy. Regimens containing β-lactam antibiotics achieve cure in at least 98% of cases. Vancomycin appears to be as effective as penicillin when given for 4 weeks in viridans streptococcal IE.

TABLE 21-1 Treatment Regimens for Infective Endocarditis

Organism	Regimen	Duration, weeks	Comments
Penicillin-susceptible *Streptococcus veridans* and *Streptococcus bovis* (Minimum inhibitory concentration ≤ 0.1 μg/mL)[a]	Aqueous crystalline penicillin G sodium 12–18 million U/24 h IV either continuously or in six equally divided doses	4	Preferred in most patients older than 65 yr and in those with impairment of the eighth nerve or renal function
	Ceftriaxone sodium 2 g once-daily IV or IM (Patients should be informed that IM injection of ceftriaxone is painful)	4	
	Aqueous crystalline penicillin G sodium 12–18 million U/24 h IV either continuously or in six equally divided doses	2	When obtained 1 h after a 20–30 min IV infusion or IM injection, serum concentration of gentamicin of approximately 3 μg/mL desirable; trough concentration should be <1 μg/mL
	With gentamicin sulfate 1 mg/kg IM every 8 h[b]	2	
	Vancomycin hydrochloride 30 mg/kg per 24 h IV in two equally divided doses, not to exceed 2 g/24 h unless serum levels are monitored[c]	4	Vancomycin therapy recommended for patients allergic to β-lactams; peak serum concentrations of vancomycin should be obtained 1 h after completion of the infusion and should be in the range of 30–45 μg/mL for twice-daily dosing
Streptococcus viridans and *Streptococcus bovi* relatively resistant to penicillin G (minimum inhibitory concentration ≤0.1 μg/mL)[a]	Aqueous crystalline penicillin G sodium 18 million U/24 h IV either continuously or in six equally divided doses	4	Cefazolin or other first-generation cephalosporin may be substituted for penicillin in patients whose penicillin hypersensitivity is not the immediate type
	With gentamicin sulfate 1 mg/kg IM or IV every 8 h[b]	2	

	Vancomycin hydrochloride 30 mg/kg 24 h IV in two equally divided doses, not to exceed 2 g/24 h unless serum levels are monitored[c]	4	Vancomycin therapy recommended for patients allergic to β-lactams
Enterococci[d]	Aqueous crystalline penicillin G sodium 18–30 million U/24 h IV either continuously or in six equally divided doses	4–6	4-wk therapy recommended for patients with symptoms <3 mo in duration, 6-wk therapy recommended for patients with symptoms >3 mo duration
	With gentamicin sulfate 1 mg/kg IM or IV every 8 h[b]	4–6	
	Ampicillin sodium 12 g/24 h IV either continuously or in six equally divided doses	4–6	Same as above
	With gentamicin sulfate 1 mg/kg IM or IV every 8 h[b]		
	Vancomycin hydrochloride 30 mg/kg per 24 h IV in two equally divided doses, not to exceed 2 g/24 h unless serum levels are monitored[c]	4–6	Vancomycin therapy recommended for patients allergic to β-lactams; cephalosporins not acceptable alternatives for patients allergic to penicillin
	With gentamicin sulfate 1 mg/kg IM or IV every 8 h[b]		
Straphylococcus in the absence of prosthetic material[e] (methicillin-susceptible staphylococci)	Regimens for non-β-lactam allergic patients:		
	Nafcillin sodium or oxacillin sodium 2 g IV every 4 h	4–6	Benefit of additional aminoglycosides not established
	With optional addition of gentamicin sulfate 1 mg/kg IM or IV every 8 h[b]	3–5 days	

(continued)

TABLE 21-1 Treatment Regimens for Infective Endocarditis *(continued)*

Organism	Regimen	Duration, weeks	Comments
	Regimens for β-lactam allergic patients:		
	Cefazolin (or other first-generation cephalosporins in equivalent dosages) 2 g IV every 8 h	4–6	Cephalosporin should be avoided in patients with immediate-type hypersensitivity to penicillin
	With optional addition of gentamicin sulfate 1 mg/kg every 8 h[b]	3–5 days	
	Vancomycin hydrochloride 30 mg/kg per 24 h IV in two equally divided doses, not to exceed 2 g/24 h unless serum levels are monitored[b]	4–6	Recommended for patients allergic to penicillin
(Methicillin-resistant) staphylococci)	Vancomycin hydrochloride 30 mg/kg per 24 h in two equally divided doses, not to exceed 2 g/24 h unless serum levels are monitored[c]	4–6	
Staphylococcus in the presence of a prosthetic valve or other prosthetic material[a] (methicillin-susceptible staphylococci)	Nafcillin sodium or oxacillin sodium 2 g IV every 4 h	≥6	First-generation cephalosporins or vancomycin should be used in patients allergic to β-lactam
	With rifampin 300 mg orally every 8 h[f]	≥6	
	And with gentamicin sulfate 1 mg/kg IM or IV every 8 h[b,g]	2	Cephalosporin should be avoided in patients immediate-type hypersensitivity to penicillin or with methicillin-resistant staphylococci
(Methicillin-resistant staphylococci)	Vancomycin hydrochloride 30 mg/kg per 24 h IV in 2 or 4 equally divided doses, not to exceed 2 g/24 h unless serum levels are monitored[c]	≥6	

	With rifampin 300 mg orally every 8 h[f]	≥6	Rifampin increases the amount of warfarin sodium required for antithrombotic therapy
	And with gentamicin sulfate 1 mg/kg IM or IV every 8 h[b,g]	2	
HACEK Microorganisms[a] (*Haemophilus parainfluenzae*, *Haemophilus aphrophilus*, *Actinobacillus actinomycetemcomitans*, *Cardiobacterium hominis*, *Eikenella corrodens*, and *Kingella kingae*)	Ceftriaxone sodium 2 g once-daily IV or IM	4	Cefotaxime sodium or other third-generation cephalosporin may be substituted
	Ampicillin sodium 12 g/24 h IV either continuously or in 6 equally divided doses[i]	4	
	With gentamicin sulfate 1 mg/kg IM or IV every 8 h[b]	4	
In the presence of prosthetic valve:			
Diptheroids	Aqueous penicillin G 20 million U/24 h plus Gentamicin sulfate 1 mg/kg IV every 8 h, or Vancomycin 0.5 g IV every 6 h	6	Vancomycin for penicillin-allergic patients
Fungi	Amphotericin B up to 1 mg/kg per 24 h IV plus Flucytosin 35 mg/kg orally every 6 h	6	Surgical consultation advised
Empirical regimen, bacteria not identified	Vancomycin 0.5 g IV every 6 h plus Gentamicin sulfate 1 mg/kg IV every 8 h		

(continued)

TABLE 21-1 Treatment Regimens for Infective Endocarditis *(concluded)*

[a]Dosages recommended are for patients with normal renal function. IV = intravenous; IM = intramuscular.

[b]Dosing of gentamicin on a milligram per kilogram basis will produce a higher serum concentration in obese patients than in lean patients. Therefore, in obese patients, dosing should be ideal body weight (for men, 50 kg + 2.3 kg per inch over 5 ft; for women, 45 kg + 2.3 kg per inch over 5 ft). Relative contraindications of the use of gentamicin are age >65 y, renal impairment, or impairment of the eighth nerve. Other nephrotoxic agents such as nonsteroidal anti-inflammatory drugs should be used cautiously in patients receiving gentamicin.

[c]Vancomycin dosage should be reduced in patients with impaired renal function. Vancomycin given on a milligram per kilogram basis will produce higher serum concentration in obese patients; dosing should be based on ideal body weight (see above). Each dose of vancomycin should be infused over at least 1 h to reduce the risk of the histamine release "red man" syndrome.

[d]All enterococci causing endocarditis must be tested for antimicrobial susceptibility to select optimal therapy. This is for endocarditis due to gentamicin- or vancomycin-susceptible enterococci, *streptococcus viridans* with minimum inhibitory concentration of >0.5 μg/mL, nutritionally variant *streptococcus viridans*, or prosthetic valve endocarditis caused by viridans streptococci or *Streptococcus bovis*. Dosages are for patients with normal renal function.

[e]For treatment of endocarditis due to penicillin-susceptible staphylococci (minimum inhibitory concentration ≤0.1 μg/mL), aqueous crystalline penicillin G can be used for 4–6 wk instead of nafcillin or oxacillin. Shorter antibiotic courses have been effective in some drug addicts with right-sided endocarditis due to *Staphylococcus aureus*.

[f]Rifampin plays a unique role in the eradication of staphylococcal infection involving prosthetic material; combination therapy is essential to prevent emergence of rifampin resistance.

[g]Use during initial 2 wk.

[i]Ampicillin should not be used if laboratory tests show β-lactamase production.

Source: Adapted from Wilson WR, Karchmer AW, Dajani AS, et al: Antibiotic treatment of adults with infective endocarditis due to streptococci, enterococci, staphylococci, HACEK microorganisms. *JAMA* 274:1706–1713, 1995, and Douglas JL, Cobbs CG: Prosthetic valve endocarditis, in Kaye D (ed): *Infective Endocarditis,* 2d ed. New York, Raven Press, 1992, pp 375–396.

Gentamicin is now preferred to streptomycin in combined regimens because of its broad clinical use, approved intravenous or intramuscular route of administration, and widespread availability of serum drug levels. In vitro and clinical data demonstrate the efficacy of gentamicin combined with penicillin in streptococcal IE. Some authorities continue to recommend penicillin for 4 weeks with gentamicin for the initial 2 weeks for sensitive *S. viridans* IE if the course is complicated or the duration of disease is longer than 3 months. Consideration of a patient's age, renal status, eighth cranial nerve function, and drug allergy guide the choice of therapy. Outpatient treatment, for all or part of therapy, has become feasible with current regimens. The largest experience with outpatient therapy is with ceftriaxone for sensitive *S. viridans* endocarditis; however, staphylococcal, enterococcal, and some gram-negative disease may be suitable for outpatient therapy with a variety of antibiotics. Therapy with ceftriaxone and netilmicin is synergistic against susceptible *S. viridans* and more effective than either agent alone in an animal model of IE, raising the possibility of 2-week once-daily therapy of IE. Durack predicts that outpatient therapy will be used in the treatment of at least 50% of all IE patients in the future.

From 15 to 20% of *S. viridans* require more than 0.1 μg/mL of penicillin for inhibition. Endocarditis caused by these organisms should be treated with penicillin for 4 weeks, combined with gentamicin for the first 2 weeks, although data are limited and clinical trials showing superior efficacy of the combined regimen over a single agent are lacking. Endocarditis due to penicillin-resistant streptococci (MIC $>$ 0.5 μg/mL) and nutritionally variant streptococci (*Streptococcus adjacens*, *Streptococcus defectivus*) should be treated with the antibiotic combinations recommended for enterococcal IE.

The significance of antibiotic tolerance for treating *S. viridans* IE is controversial. Most streptococci are inhibited and killed by low concentrations of penicillin. Tolerant strains, however, require a much higher concentration ($>$32 times) to kill the organism than is required for inhibition of growth. Although in animal models tolerant strains are killed more slowly than nontolerant ones, differences in treatment outcomes for human IE have not been demonstrated. Therefore, penicillin-tolerant *S. viridans* is treated according to the recommendations mentioned earlier based on the determination of penicillin MIC; measurement of the minimum bactericidal concentration (MBC) is usually not necessary.

Enterococcal Endocarditis

Enterococci may cause either subacute or acute IE. This occurs most commonly in women of childbearing age after obstetric procedures and in older men. This group of organisms was formerly classified as group

D streptococci but is now considered a separate genus *Enterococcus*. Enterococci account for 5 to 20% of isolates from patients with IE. Enterococcal isolates from patients with bacterial IE include *Enterococcus faecium*, *Enterococcus faecalis*, and *Enterococcus durans*. *Streptococcus bovis* and *Streptococcus equinus* are group D streptococci that may be confused with enterococci, but these streptococci usually are highly sensitive to penicillin and should be treated the same way as infections caused by *S. viridans*.

Enterococci are usually relatively resistant and highly tolerant to penicillin, exhibiting MICs of 1 to 4 μg/mL and MBCs of equal to or greater than 100 μg/ mL. Similar tolerance has been demonstrated for vancomycin. The cephalosporins are not clinically useful for treating these infections, although some strains of *E. faecalis* are susceptible to imipenem-cilastatin. The MIC for penicillin, ampicillin, and vancomycin should be determined for enterococci causing IE. β-lactamase-producing strains of enterococci have been reported over the past decade. Therapy for infections with these organisms would include vancomycin or ampicillin-sulbactam in combination with gentamicin.

Synergistic killing has been demonstrated in vitro for most enterococci with the combination of penicillin or vancomycin and streptomycin or gentamicin. However, enterococcal isolates with high-level (MIC $\geq$ 500 to 2000 μg/mL) resistance to these aminoglycosides are now isolated with increasing frequency. Bactericidal synergy between a cell wall active antibiotic and aminoglycosides is lost in the presence of high-level resistance. Testing for high-level resistance to streptomycin and gentamicin is currently recommended for enterococcal IE; the other available aminoglycosides are not useful if high-level resistance to gentamicin is demonstrated. Treatment for IE due to strains with high-level aminoglycoside resistance is controversial. Standard recommendations include high-dose ampicillin or vancomycin for 8 to 12 weeks with a strong consideration for valve replacement for patients failing therapy.

Enterococci resistant to vancomycin are an increasing problem in the United States. Infection with these organisms, which are also often resistant to penicillins, has been associated with nosocomial acquisition, severe underlying disease, and previous use of antibiotics. There is no consensus about treatment of IE with multiresistant enterococci. Combinations of drugs have been used with some success in animal models of IE, but there are no clinical data to guide therapy. Infectious disease consultation is recommended for patients with resistant enterococcal IE.

When penicillin or vancomycin can be combined with gentamicin or streptomycin, 4 weeks of therapy appears adequate for most patients. Six weeks is recommended if symptoms have been present for more than 3 months or infection is on a prosthetic valve.

Endocarditis Caused by *Staphylococcus aureus*

S. aureus generally causes acute bacterial IE in patients with no prior history of valvular disease. It is the infecting agent in 25 to 45% of IE cases and may be more common at community hospitals than in university referral centers. Among intravenous drug users with IE, staphylococci account for 65 to 82% of cases. Standard therapy is a penicillinase-resistant penicillin such as nafcillin or oxacillin or a first-generation cephalosporin. The penicillins are favored because in vitro cephalosporins appear more sensitive to β-lactamases at the high organism densities (inoculum effect) expected in a valvular vegetation. It is not clear that this inoculum effect is important clinically.

Vancomycin is recommended for patients with severe allergy to β-lactams. For methicillin-sensitive *S. aureus* (MSSA) IE, there is evidence that vancomycin is not as rapidly bactericidal as nafcillin and may have higher failure rates in IE. Karchmer cautions against using vancomycin because of dosing convenience, and allergy testing and penicillin desensitization in appropriate patients should be attempted. Vancomycin is the drug of choice for IE due to MRSA, which continues to increase in the United States. The response of patients with MRSA IE appears to be slower than that of patients treated with β-lactams with MSSA disease.

Methicillin-sensitive *S. aureus* is killed more rapidly in vitro and in animal models of IE with the combination of a penicillinase-resistant penicillin and gentamicin. In a large clinical trial, the combination of nafcillin and gentamicin for 2 weeks was associated with a more rapid clearing of bacteremia in staphylococcal IE compared with nafcillin alone, but without improved survival and with more renal toxicity. Gentamicin is currently recommended as an optional addition to a β-lactam agent for the initial 3 to 5 days of treatment. A short course of gentamicin also can be added to vancomycin for MSSA or MRSA IE, although nephrotoxic effects of this combination may be more common.

Staphylococcal IE in intravenous drug users usually involves the tricuspid valve and has a significantly better prognosis than left-sided disease from *S. aureus*, with a mortality of under 5%. Two-week antibiotic regimens combining nafcillin and an aminoglycoside have been used successfully in selected stable patients with tricuspid valve IE. There are few clinical data on the efficacy of cephalosporins or vancomycin in 2-week regimens, and these drugs are not recommended.

Rifampin is an extremely potent antistaphylococcal drug that achieves excellent tissue and intracellular concentrations. Resistance emerges rapidly when used as a single agent but usually not when combined with other effective drugs. In vitro, the effect of rifampin in combination with β-lactams or vancomycin is variable depending on experimental conditions. There was no advantage to vancomycin and rifampin compared with vancomycin alone in a clinical study of MRSA IE. Rifampin is not recommended for native valve staphylococcal endocarditis, although it does have a role in the treatment of prosthetic valve infections.

Indication for Surgery

Valvular surgery can be lifesaving for certain groups of patients with endocarditis. Indications for surgery include congestive heart failure (CHF), persistent bacteremia, fungal endocarditis, and unstable prosthesis. A detailed discussion of indications for surgery in infective endocarditis is beyond the scope of this chapter.

Anticoagulation and Infective Endocarditis

Vegetation is a complex mass of fibrin, platelets, leukocytes, and organisms in which the more deeply situated colonies metabolize slowly. These slow-growing organisms are relatively resistant to antibiotics. Further, impaired diffusion of antibiotics to deeper colonies effectively lowers the concentration of drug for which these organisms are exposed. It is therefore reasonable to attempt to limit the size of the vegetation to enhance the antibiotic efficacy.

There is experience with such therapy, both in the laboratory and in vivo. In a rabbit model of endocarditis in which sterile vegetation (nonbacterial thrombotic endocarditis) was induced by placing a catheter across the aortic valve and subsequently infecting it by the intravenous administration of bacteria, pretreatment with warfarin prevented the initial formation of vegetation but not the development of endocarditis. Large instances of vegetation were seen only in nonanticoagulated animals, and the duration of penicillin therapy needed to sterilize the smaller instances of vegetation seen in the anticoagulated animals was halved. In another study, warfarin increased the bacterial inoculum needed to cause endocarditis in this model. Once induced, the warfarin-treated vegetation had fewer colony-forming units and was more prone to spontaneously become sterile than vegetation in the nonanticoagulated animals. Despite such improvement, the warfarin-treated animals had significantly shortened survival in both of these studies.

The use of anticoagulant in patients with infective endocarditis was initially introduced in the beginning of the antibiotic era to improve the penetration of antibiotic into the infected vegetation. Several groups suggested that therapy with a combination of antibiotic and anticoagulant could be more effective in treating endocarditis than antibiotic alone. In these studies, a high incidence of cerebral hemorrhage was seen in these patients. Several authors advocated that anticoagulation be contraindicated in the treatment of endocarditis. Echocardiography, in particular transesophageal echo-cardiography (TEE), has added additional information that enables the clinician to assess the patient at risk for embolization. There is no suggestion that anticoagulation alone reduces the incidence of embolic events in infective endocarditis. One study showed that in patients with infective endocarditis the rate of cerebral embolic events was promptly reduced after antibiotic therapy was begun, but there was no change in the incidence of emboli with or without anticoagulant therapy.

Prosthetic valve endocarditis and anticoagulation deserve attention. With the exception of bioprosthetic valves and normal sinus rhythm, patients with prosthetic heart valves are anticoagulated. Some physicians also anticoagulate bioprosthetic valves for the first 3 months after implantation. The risk-benefit ratio of continuing anticoagulation must be assessed carefully in each patient. In a study from the Mayo Clinic, 3 of 38 patients (8%) with adequate anticoagulation had cerebrovascular events, whereas 10 of 14 patients (71%) who were either not anticoagulated or were subtherapeutically anticoagulated had events. Other groups showed different results. A retrospective study from the Massachussetts General Hospital showed that 23% of hemorrhagic CNS events occured in the endocarditis patients receiving anticoagulants, who represented 3% of the sample. Other studies confirmed that antibiotic therapy is more important than anticoagulation in preventing neurologic complications. Should a cerebral event occur in a patient with endocarditis, immediate CT of the head is essential to rule out cerebral hemorrhage, which would necessitate discontinuation of anticoagulation. The Cerebral Embolism Study Group published its recommendation based on patients who did not have endocarditis. The group recommended that nonhypertensive patients with no evidence of hemorrhage on CT 24 to 48 h after a stroke should be started on anticoagulation, although a delay of 7 days is warranted in patients with large cerebral infarctions.

The decision to continue anticoagulation in the setting of endocarditis is often a difficult one to make. Recently, the Fourth ACCP Consensus Conference on Antithrombotic Therapy published its recommendation on anticoagulation in infective endocarditis.

1. It is strongly recommended that anticoagulant therapy not be given to patients in normal sinus rhythm with uncomplicated infective endocarditis involving a native valve or a bioprosthetic valve. This grade C* recommendation is based on the increased incidence of hemorrhage in these patients and the lack of demonstrated efficacy of anticoagulant therapy in this setting.
2. It is recommended that long-term warfarin therapy be continued when endocarditis occurs in patients with a mechanical prosthetic valve unless there are specific contraindications. This grade C* recommendation is based on the frequency of systemic thromboembolism in these patients. However, it is to be noted that the risk of intracranial hemorrhage is substantial.

*Grade C = results come from nonrandomized cohort studies or case series.

3. The indications for anticoagulant therapy when systemic embolism occurs during the course of infective endocarditis involving a native or bioprosthetic heart valve are uncertain. The therapeutic decision should consider comorbid factors, including atrial fibrillation (AF), evidence of left atrial thrombus, evidence and size of valvular vegetations, and particularly the success of antibiotic therapy in controlling the infective endocarditis.

Prophylaxis for Endocarditis

The bloodstream is invaded daily by bacteria introduced by activities of normal living, invasive medical procedures, and disease. Yet endocarditis is a comparatively rare disease. When it occurs, there are often predisposing factors. Animal models have helped to identify these factors.

Durack and Beeson, using a modification of the Garrison and Freedman model, demonstrated that the intravenous injection of a large bacterial inoculum into rabbits would cause only a transient bacteremia; normal valvular endothelium was not infected. Endocarditis would not result unless a substrate of nonbacterial thrombotic endocarditis had been induced by damaging the valvular endothelium with a catheter prior to inoculation. In humans, such damage can be the result of several factors. Turbulent blood flow (through a damaged prosthetic or regurgitant valve, a septal defect, or even idiopathic hypertrophic subaortic stenosis) creates jets whose impact can destroy the integrity of the endothelium, expose collagen, and result in platelet activation and adhesion. Such jets create low-pressure "sinks" distal to the origin of the jet into which bacteria are deposited.

The concept of endocarditis prophylaxis is based on identifying situations in which patients have predisposing factors for the development of endocarditis. Approximately 75% of patients with endocarditis have preexisting cardiac abnormalities. Although precise figures are lacking, the ranking of risk can be based on the frequency of each preexisting cardiac disorder in large series of patients with endocarditis who are compared with the general population.

Before recommending prophylactic antibiotics for any given patient, several factors must be recognized: (1) only a small proportion of all cases of infective endocarditis can be attributed to bacteremia caused by medical, surgical, or dental procedures; (2) antibiotic recommendations derive from in vitro susceptibility data and animal models; efficacy in patients has not been determined for any regimen in any situation; and (3) occasionally a patient will have a serious allergy to the antibiotic.

The cardiac conditions and other indications for which the AHA recommends antibiotic prophylaxis are in Table 21-2. Mitral valve prolapse (MVP) deserves special comment. In a case-control study, Clemens et al. calculated an eightfold increase in endocarditis risk.

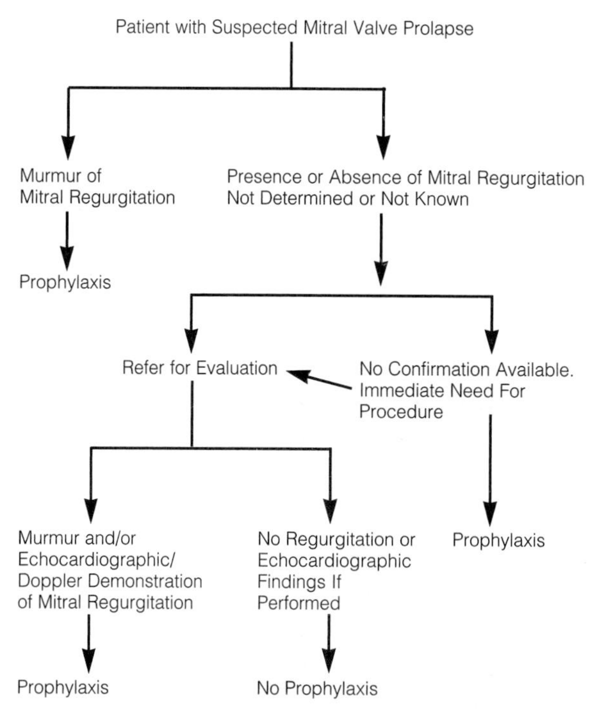

FIG. 21-1 Clinical Approach to Determination of the Need for prophylaxis in patients with suspected mitral valve prolapse. For more details on the role of echocardiography in the diagnosis of mitral valve prolapse, see the text and the 1997 AHA Recommendations.

Hickey et al. calculated a fivefold increase in the risk. However, the incidence of endocarditis remains low. According to AHA guidelines, patients with MVP and valvular regurgitation should receive antibiotic prophylaxis before selected procedures and interventions. (see Table 21-2). The latest AHA guidelines are summarized in Fig. 21-1.

The current AHA recommended prophylaxis regimens are found in Table 21-3.

The efficacy of prophylaxis is debated. Van der Meer et al., in a case-controlled study, estimated a 49% efficacy for prophylaxis. Imperiale et al. estimated a 91% protective efficacy for prophylaxis. The study involved a small number of patients. A retrospective study of 533 patients with valvular prostheses who underwent dental or surgical procedures

TABLE 21-2 Recommendations for Prophylaxis of Endocarditis[a]

Cardiac Conditions

Endocarditis prophylaxis recommended
- *High-risk category*
  - Prosthetic cardiac valves, including bioprosthetic and homograft valves
  - Previous bacterial endocarditis
  - Complex cyanotic congenital heart disease (single-ventricle states, transposition of the great arteries, tetralogy of Fallot)
  - Surgically constructed systemic pulmonary shunts or conduits
- *Moderate-risk category*
  - Most congenital cardiac malformations (other than above and below)
  - Acquired valvar dysfunction (rheumatic heart disease)
  - Hypertrophic cardiomyopathy
  - Mitral valve prolapse with valvar regurgitation and/or thickened leaflets[b]

Endocarditis prophylaxis not recommended
- *Negligible-risk category* (no greater risk than the general population)
  - Isolated secundum atrial septal defect
  - Surgical repair of atrial septal defect, ventricular septal defect, or patent ductus arterious (without residual beyond 6 months)
  - Previous coronary artery bypass graft surgery
  - Mitral valve prolapse without valvar regurgitation
  - Physiologic, functional, or innocent heart murmurs
  - Previous Kawasaki disease without valvular dysfunction
  - Previous rheumatic fever without valvular dysfunction
  - Cardiac pacemakers (intravascular and epicardial) and implanted defibrillators

Dental Procedures

Endocarditis prophylaxis recommended[c]
- Dental extractions
- Peridontal procedures, including surgery, scaling and root planing, probing, and recall maintenance
- Dental implant placement and reimplantation of avulsed teeth
- Endodontic (root canal) instrumentation or surgery beyond the apex
- Subgingival placement of antibiotic fibers or strips
- Initial placement of orthodontic bands but not brackets
- Intraligamentary local anesthetic injections
- Prophylactic cleaning of teeth or implants where bleeding is anticipated

Endocarditis prophylaxis not recommended
- Restorative dentistry[d] (operative and prosthodontic) with or without retraction cord[e]
- Local anesthetic injections (nonintraligamentary)
- Intracanal endodontic treatment; post placement and buildup
- Placement of rubber dams
- Postoperative suture removal
- Placement of removable prosthodontic or orthodontic appliances
- Taking of oral impressions
- Fluoride treatments

TABLE 21-2 *(continued)*

- Taking of oral radiographs
- Orthodontic appliance adjustment
- Shedding of primary teeth

Other Procedures

Endocarditis prophylaxis recommended
- Respiratory tract
  - Tonsillectomy and/or adenoidectomy
  - Surgical operations that involve respiratory mucosa
  - Bronchoscopy with rigid bronchoscope[f]
- Gastrointestinal tract[g]
  - Sclerotherapy for esophageal varices
  - Esophageal stricture dilation
  - Endoscopic retrograde cholangiography with biliary obstruction
  - Biliary tract surgery
  - Surgical operations that involve intestinal mucosa
- Genitourinary tract
  - Prostatic surgery
  - Cystoscopy
  - Urethral dilation

Endocarditis prophylaxis not recommended
- Respiratory tract
  - Endotracheal intubation
  - Bronchoscopy with a flexible bronchoscope, with or without biopsy
  - Tympanostomy tube insertion
- Gastrointestinal tract
  - Transesophageal echocardiography[h]
  - Endoscopy with or without gastrointestinal biopsy
- Genitourinary tract
  - Vaginal hysterectomy[i]
  - Vaginal delivery
  - Cesarean section
  - In uninfected tissue:
    - Urethral catheterization
    - Uterine dilatation and curettage
    - Therapeutic abortion
    - Sterilization procedures
    - Insertion or removal of intrauterine devices

Other
- Cardiac catheterization, including balloon angioplasty
- Implanted cardiac pacemakers, implanted defibrillators and coronary stents
- Incision or biopsy of surgically scrubbed skin
- Circumcision

[a]This table lists selected conditions and procedures but is not meant to be all-inclusive.
[b]Generally, patients with mitral valve prolapse without regurgitation are at low risk and the risk-benefit of chemoprophylaxis is not known.
[c]Prophylaxis is recommended for patients with high- and moderate-risk cardiac conditions.

TABLE 21-2 *(concluded)*

[d]This includes restoration of decayed teeth (filling cavities and replacement of missing teeth.
[e]Clinical judgment may indicate antibiotic use in selected circumstances that may create significant bleeding.
[f]In patients who have prosthetic heart valves, a previous history of endocarditis, or surgically constructed systemic-pulmonary shunts or conduits, physicians may choose to administer prophylactic antibiotics even for low-risk procedures that might involve the respiratory, genitourinary, and/or gastrointestinal tracts.
[g]Prophylaxis is recommended for high-risk patients; it is optional for medium-risk patients.
[h]Prophylaxis is recommended for high-risk patients; it is optional for medium-risk patients.
[i]Prophylaxis is optional for high-risk patients.
Source: Adapted from AHA recommendations, *JAMA* 264:2919, 1990.

TABLE 21-3 Recommended Regimens for Chemophylaxis

Situation	Agent	Regimen*
Dental–Respiratory Tract Procedures		
Standard regimen	Amoxicillin	Adults 2.0 g; children 50 mg/kg orally 1 h before procedure
Unable to take oral medications	Ampicillin	Adult 2.0 g IM or IV; children 50 mg/kg IM or IV within 30 min before procedure
Allergic to penicillin	Clindamycin or	Adults 600 mg; children 20 mg/kg orally 1 h before procedure
	Cephalexin or cefadroxil[†]	Adults 2.0 g; children 50 mg/kg orally 1 h before procedure
	Azithromycin or clarithromycin	Adults 500 mg; children 15 mg/kg orally 1 h before procedure
Allergic to penicillin and unable to take oral medications	Clindamycin or	Adults 600 mg; children 20 mg/kg IV with 30 min before procedure
	Cefazolin[†]	Adults 1.0 g; children 25 mg/kg IM or IV within 30 min before procedure
Gastrointestinal-Genitourinary Procedures		
High-risk patients	Ampicillin + gentamicin	Adults: Ampicillin 2.0 g IM or IV + gentamicin 1.5 mg/kg (not to exceed 120 mg) within 30 min or starting procedure; 6 h later ampicillin 1 mg IM or IV or amoxicillin 1 mg orally.

TABLE 21-3 *(continued)*

Situation	Agent	Regimen*
		Children: Ampicillin 50 mg/kg IM or IV (not to exceed 2.0 g) + gentamicin 1.5 mg/kg within 30 min or starting procedure; 6 h later ampicillin 25 mg/kg IM or IV or amoxicillin 25 mg/kg orally.
High-risk patient allergic to ampicillin/amoxicillin	Vancomycin + gentamicin	Adult: Vancomycin 1.0 g IV or 1–2 h + gentamicin 1.5 mg/kg IV or IM (not to exceed 120 mg); complete injection/infusion within 30 min of starting procedure Children: Vancomycin 20 mg/kg IV or 1–2 h + gentamicin 1.5 mg/kg IV or IM; complete injection/infusion within 30 min of starting procedure
Moderate-risk patients	Amoxicillin or ampicillin	Adults: Amoxicillin 2.0 g orally 1 h before procedure or ampicillin 2.0 g IM or IV within 30 min of starting procedure Children: Amoxicillin 50 mg/kg orally 1 h before procedure or ampicillin 50 mg/kg IM or IV within 30 min of starting procedure.
Moderate-risk patients allergic to ampicillin/amoxicillin	Vancomycin	Adults: Vancomycin 1.0 g IV or 1–2 h; complete infusion within 30 min of starting procedure Children: Vancomycin 20 mg/kg over 1–2 h; complete infusion within 30 min of starting procedure

*Total children's dose should not exceed adult dose; no second dose of vancomycin or gentamicin is recommended.

†Cephalosporins should not be used in individuals with immediate-type hypersensitivity reaction (uticaria, angioedema, and anaphylaxis) to penicillins.

Source: Adapted from Dajani AS, Tubert KA, Wilson W, et al: Prevention of endocarditis and recommendation of the American Heart Association. *JAMA* 277:1798, 1997.

was done. Six cases of endocarditis occurred in 229 patients with no prophylaxis as compared with no episodes of endocarditis in 304 patients who received antibiotic prophylaxis.

There are cases of apparent failure of antibiotic prophylaxis. Durack summarized the cases submitted to the National AHA Registry. MVP was the most common underlying cardiac lesion. Two-thirds of the bacteria causing endocarditis were sensitive to the antibiotics that have been given prophylactically.

There are also case reports of patients diagnosed with endocarditis temporally related to endoscopic procedures. Schlaeffer et al. reported on 16 patients with bacteremia that developed after endoscopy. Twelve presented with endocarditis. A case of *Streptococcus sangus* endocarditis temporally related to transesophageal echocardiography has been reported in a patient with MVP and a flail posterior leaflet.

A controversial area is the need for prophylaxis in patients who have had permanent pacemaker implants. Pacemakers, Swan-Ganz catheters, and central venous catheters rarely have been associated with endocarditis. Animal studies have demonstrated that the longer a catheter remains in situ, the lower is the risk of endocarditis. This is probably the result of the restoration of endothelial integrity. Pacemaker electrodes are not considered an indication for prophylaxis by the AHA. A recent article on pacemaker endocarditis also concluded that regular antibiotic prophylaxis is not indicated in pacemaker patients having minor invasive procedures.

Rheumatic Fever

The Jones criteria for the diagnosis of rheumatic fever were updated in 1992. The guidelines include both major and minor manifestations, as well as the need for supporting evidence of antecedent group A streptococcal infection. These are summarized in Table 21-4.

Prevention of recurrent rheumatic fever depends on continuous prophylaxis with appropriate antibiotics. The risk of recurrence decreases with time after the previous episode. The risk increases if there are two or more previous attacks of rheumatic fever. The risk also increases in the presence of rheumatic heart disease. Parents of young children, teachers, physicians, nurses, allied medical personnel, military personnel, and other individuals living in crowded conditions have an increased risk of exposure to recurrent streptococcal infection.

The recommendations for treatment of acute streptococcal pharyngitis and prevention of rheumatic fever have been updated recently. They are summarized in Table 21-5.

Prosthetic Valve Endocarditis

Infection of a prosthetic valve is an especially serious problem. Classically, such prosthetic valve infections have been divided into two

TABLE 21-4 Guidelines for the Diagnosis of Initial Attack of Rheumatic Fever (Jones Criteria, Updated 1992)*

Major manifestations	Minor manifestations	Supporting evidence of antecedent group A streptococcal infection
Carditis	Clinical findings	Positive throat culture or rapid streptococcal antigen test
Polyarthritis	Arthralgia	
Chorea	Fever	
Erythema marginatum	Laboratory findings	
Subcutaneous nodules	Elevated acute phase reactants:	Elevated or rising streptococcal antibody titer
	Erythrocyte sedimentation rate	
	C-reactive protein	
	Prolonged PR interval	

*If supported by evidence of preceding group A streptococcal infection, the presence of two major manifestations or of one major and two minor manifestations indicates a high probability of acute rheumatic fever.
Source: Adapted from AHA Writing Group: Guidelines for the diagnosis of rheumatic fever: Jones Criteria Update1992. *Circulation* 87:302, 1992.

groups: early and late. In early prosthetic valve endocarditis (PVE), the infection becomes manifest within 2 months of insertion of the prosthesis. In general, early PVE is caused by organisms introduced during the surgical procedure or, if the implant replaced an infected valve, residual infection. In contrast, late PVE usually is caused by the introduction of pathogens into the circulation after the time of surgery. Consequently, early PVE more commonly is caused by staphylococcal species (largely *Staphylococcus epidermidis*), gram-negative organisms, and diphtheroids, whereas late disease is similar in microbial spectrum to native valve endocarditis. *S. epidermidis* is the most common causative organism in PVE.

The pathology of infection is dependent on the class of valve used. Of 22 patients with infected mechanical valves studied at necropsy by Arnett and Roberts, all had valve ring abscesses. Dehiscence, causing severe valvular regurgitation, occurred in 14 of the 22 patients, and prosthetic valve obstruction by vegetative material occurred in 6. Conversely, in porcine heterografts, the infection frequently developed in the fibrin layer that covers the cusps and can spread to involve the subadjacent collagen; valve ring abscess is infrequent. Regurgitation with porcine valves occurs most often because the valve leaflets are destroyed rather than resulting from suture line dehiscence. There are also reported cases in which fibrinous membranes developed on the atrial surface of a prosthetic mitral valve, leading to fatal obstruction of left ventricular inflow.

TABLE 21-5 Treatment of Acute Streptococcal Pharyngitis and Prevention of Rheumatic Fever

Clinical presentation of streptococcal tonsillopharyngitis

Common finding	Findings not suggesting Group A β-Hemolytic streptococcal infection
Symptoms	
Sudden onset sore throat	Coryza
Pain on swallowing	Hoarseness
Fever	Cough
Headache	Diarrhea
Abdominal pain	
Nausea and vomiting	
Signs	
Tonsillopharyngeal erythema/exudate	Conjunctivitis
Soft palate petechiae ("doughnut" lesions)	Anterior stomatitis
	Discrete ulcerative lesions

Treatment of streptococcal tonsillopharyngitis†

Agent	Dose	Mode	Duration
Benzathine Penicillin G	600,000 U for patients ≤27 kg (60 lb) 1,200,000 U >27 kg (60 lb) or	IM	Once
Penicillin V (phenoxymethyl penicillin)	Children: 250 mg 2–3 times daily Adolescents and adults: 500 mg 2–3 times daily	Oral	10 days
For individuals allergic to penicillin			
Erythromycin			
Estolate	20–40 mg/kg/per day 2–4 times daily (maximum 1g/day) or	Oral	10 days
Ethylsuccinate	40 mg/kg/per day 2–4 times daily (maximum 1 g/day)	Oral	10 days

Duration of secondary rheumatic fever prophylaxis

Category	Duration
Rheumatic fever with carditis and residual heart disease (persistent valvular disease)*	At least 10 y since last episode and at least until age 40 y, sometimes life-long prohylaxis
Rheumatic fever with carditis but no residual heart disease (no valvular disease)*	10 y or well into adulthood, whichever is longer
Rheumatic fever without carditis	5 y or until age 21 y, whichever is longer

TABLE 21-5 *(continued)*

Secondary prevention of rheumatic fever (prevention of recurrent attacks)		
Agent	Dose	Mode
Benzathine penicillin G	1,200,000 U every 4 weeks‡	IM
	or	
Penicillin V	250 mg twice daily	Oral
	or	
Sulfadiazine	0.5 g once daily for patients ≤27 kg (60 lb) 1.0g once daily for patients >27 kg (60 lb)	Oral
For individuals allergic to penicillin and sulfadiazine		
Erythromycin	250 mg twice daily	Oral

*These findings are noted primarily in children older than 3 years of age and adults. Symptoms and signs in younger children can be different and less specific.

†The following are not acceptable: sulfonamides, trimethoprim, tetracyclines, and chloramphenicol.

‡Clinical or echocardiographic evidence. In high-risk situations, administrations every 3 weeks is justified and recommended.

Source: Adapted from Dajani A, Taubert K, Ferrieri P, et al: Treatment of acute streptococcal pharyngitis and prevention of rheumatic fever: A statement for health professionals. *Pediatrics* 96:758, 1995.

The diagnosis of PVE can be elusive, especially when fever and bacteremia complicate the early postoperative period. Even when an extracardiac source can be identified, the possibility of valve seeding cannot be ignored because virtually any organism can establish a focus of infection on a newly implanted prosthetic valve. However, in a study of 32 patients who developed bacteremia postoperatively, only 2 (6.3%) were thought to have PVE. Bacteremia in a patient with a recently implanted prosthetic valve is an ominous sign. A recent review of six studies revealed an approximately 50% overall mortality.

Echocardiography, in particular TEE, has become an essential test in the diagnostic workup and evaluation of prosthetic valve endocarditis. Peterson et al. showed that TEE was more sensitive than transthoracic echocardiography (TTE) in diagnosing vegetation or abscesses. Daniel et al. studied 120 patients with 148 prosthetic valves. Thirty-three were found to have endocarditis at surgery or autopsy. TTE identified vegetation in 36% of the infected valves. TEE diagnosed 27 of 33, or 82%. Daniel and associates also showed the superiority of TEE in diagnosing abscesses associated with endocarditis.

In a large review, mortality for medically treated patients was 61.4%, whereas for those who also received surgery it was 38.5%. These data were obtained from studies without controls; thus selection bias clearly played some role in determining these figures.

For bacterial PVE, the susceptibility of the etiologic agent to antimicrobial agents is an especially important factor for outcome. Organisms resistant to conventional therapy, such as methicillin-resistant staphylococci or gram-negative bacilli, are more likely to require surgery. It also is important to note that many survivors of complicated *S. epidermidis* PVE required valve replacement within the ensuing 6 months of bacteriologic cure. In contrast, the somewhat less aggressive endocarditis caused by penicillin-susceptible streptococcal infection is more often cured medically.

A relatively unique situation in PVE is the development of infection caused by methicillin-resistant *S. epidermidis*. It has been demonstrated conclusively that these patients were more likely to survive if their antibiotic regimen included vancomycin, and furthermore, the addition of rifampin and gentamicin increased survival.

Sett and colleagues reviewed prosthetic valve endocarditis in porcine bioprostheses. In this series, all patients with early PVE died. Ninety-one percent with late PVE survived with a combined medical and surgical approach. The authors recommended a combined medical and surgical approach in PVE with *S. aureus*, *Candida albicans*, or gram-negative organisms.

Fungal PVE, like its counterpart on native valves, is notoriously unresponsive to medical therapy, and therefore, early surgery should be performed once the diagnosis is made. Even when surgically treated, however, there is a high incidence of recurrent endocarditis (Table 21-6).

Valvular dysfunction caused by incompetence, stenosis of the outflow track, or perivalvular leak is unlikely to respond to medical management and should be treated with prompt surgery prior to hemodynamic compromise. The development of conduction abnormalities suggests an annular abscess. In some studies, 69% of patients with conduction abnormalities and infection of a prosthetic aortic valve have annular abscesses. Many of these patients do not survive despite therapy. It is therefore prudent to follow all patients carefully and to use the earliest sign of valvular destruction, dysfunction, myocardial invasion, or failure of bacteriologic cure as an indication for urgent surgery. The treatment of PVE requires close consultation with a cardiac surgeon and infectious disease specialist. According to Thielkeid and Cobbs, several general observations can be made regarding the role of surgery in the management of PVE. First, the mortality of surgery is no greater (and may be less) than the mortality of medical therapy (see Table 21-6). The risk of recurrent PVE after surgery is usually acceptable. Baumgartner and associates reported a reinfection rate following valve replacement for PVE of 15% over an average follow-up of 3.6 years. This reflects a linear rate of 4.1% per patient per year. Finally, when prosthetic valve replacement is clinically indicated, surgery should be performed without delay.

TABLE 21-6 An Estimate of Microbiologic Cure Rates for Various Forms of Endocarditis*

	Antimicrobial therapy alone, %		Antimicrobial therapy plus surgery, %	
Native-Valve Endocarditis (NVE)				
Streptococcus spp: *viridans* group, group A, *S. bovis*, and *S. pneumoniae*; *Neisseria gonorrhoeae*	>95		>95	
Enterococcus faecalis	90		>90	
Staphylococcus aureus (in young drug addicts)	90		>90	
Staphylococcus aureus (in older patients)	50		70	
Gram-negative aerobic bacilli†	40		65	
Fungi	<5		50	
	Early PVE	Late PVE	Early PVE	Late PVE
Prosthetic-Valve Endocarditis (PVE)				
Streptococcus spp: *viridans*, group A, *S. bovis*, and *S. pneumoniae*	‡	80	‡	90
Neisseria gonorrhoeae				
Enterococcus faecalis	‡	60	‡	75
Staphylococcus aureus	25	40	50	60
Staphylococcus epidermidis	20	40	60	70
Gram-negative aerobic bacilli	<10	20	40	50
Fungi	<1	<1	30	40

*Morbidity and mortality for bacteriologic cure are significantly greater than these figures indicate.

†Excluding *Haemophilus* spp

‡Insufficient data to estimate rate.

Source: Adapted from Durack DT: Infective and noninfective endocarditis, in Schlant RC, Alexander RW, O'Rourke RA, et al (eds): *Hurst's The Heart*, 8th ed. New York, McGraw-Hill, 1994, pp 1681–1709.

SUGGESTED READINGS

AHA Writing Group: Guidelines for the diagnosis of rheumatic fever: Jones criteria update 1992. *Circulation* 87:302, 1992.

American Heart Association Recommendations. *JAMA* 264:2919, 1990.

American Heart Association Guidelines. *JAMA* 277:1798, 1997.

Bansal RC: Infective endocarditis. *Med Clin North Am* 79:1205, 1995.

Bayer AS, Ward JI, Gintzon LE, et al: Evaluation of new clinical criteria for the diagnosis of infective endocarditis. *Am J Med* 96:211, 1994.

Child JS (ed): Diagnosis and management of infective endocarditis cardiology clinic. 14(3):327–470, 1996.

Dajani A, Taubert K, Ferrieri P, et al: Treatment of acute streptococcal pharyngitis and prevention of rheumatic fever: A statement for health professionals. *Pediatrics* 96(4 part 1):758, 1995.

Douglas JL, Cobbs CG: Prosthetic valve endocarditis, in Kaye D (ed): *Infective Endocarditis*, 2nd ed. New York, Raven Press, 1992, pp 375–396.

Durack DT: Infective and noninfective endocarditis, in Schlant RC, Alexander RW, O'Rourke RA, et al. (eds): *Hurst's The Heart*, 8th ed. New York: McGraw-Hill, 1994, p 1681.

Durack DT: Infective endocarditis, in Hoeprich PD, Jordan MC, Ronald AR (eds): *Infectious Diseases*, 5th ed. Philadelphia, JB Lippincott, 1994, pp 1233–1248.

Durack DT: Prevention of infective endocarditis. *N Engl J Med* 332:38, 1995.

Goldberger, MH, Kalkut GE, Frishman WH: Infective endocarditis, in Frishman WH, Sonnenblick EH (eds): *Cardiovascular Pharmacotherapeutics*. New York: McGraw-Hill, 1997, pp 1247–1266.

Prevention of recurrent attacks of rheumatic fever (secondary prevention), in *AMA Drug Evaluation Annual 1995*. Chicago, American Medical Association, 1995, Chap 61, pp 1357–1358.

Scheld WM, Sande MA: Endocarditis and intravascular infections, in Mandell GL, Douglas RG Jr, Bennett JE, Dolin R (eds): *Principles and Practice of Infectious Diseases*, 4th ed. New York, Churchill-Livingstone, 1995, pp 740–783.

Wilson WR, Karchmer AW, Dajani AS, et al: Antibiotic treatment for infective endocarditis due to streptococci, enterococci, staphylococci, and HACEK organisms. *JAMA* 274:1706, 1995.

Chapter 22 Cardiovascular Drug Interactions

Lionel H. Opie

Cardiovascular drug interactions are numerous, sometimes unpredictable, and potentially serious to patient and physician. Fortunately, serious interactions are relatively uncommon and often avoidable by simple clinical precautions based on a prior knowledge of the properties of the drugs in question. There are two types of drug interactions: pharmacokinetic and pharmacodynamic. *Pharmacokinetic interactions* concern all interactions at any stage of the pharmacokinetic steps that most drugs go through, that is, absorption, distribution in the blood and binding to plasma proteins, metabolism (often in the liver), and excretion (often in the urine). Active metabolites may have additional interactions. *Pharmacodynamic interactions*, on the other hand, result from additive cardiovascular hemodynamic or electrophysiologic effects. An example is added atrioventricular nodal block from the combination verapamil-digoxin. Although such an interaction could be predicted, its clinical relevance depends on specific unpredictable physiologic or pathologic variations found in the AV node of that particular individual.

This chapter analyzes cardiovascular drug interactions in two ways. First, the *major organ sites* of such interactions are considered, starting with the heart itself and specifically considering the sinoatrial (SA) and atrioventricular (AV) nodes, the intraventricular conduction system, the myocardial contractile mechanism, and proarrhythmic drug interactions. Thereafter follows an evaluation of vascular smooth muscle as a site for drug interactions, after which come hepatic and renal interactions. There are only a few interactions at the level of plasma proteins. Second, the *major classes of cardiovascular drugs* are sequentially considered in order, namely: (1) β-adrenergic blockers, (2) antianginal vasodilators including the calcium channel antagonists (CCAs), (3) diuretics, (4) angiotensin converting enzyme (ACE) inhibitors, (5) digitalis and other positive inotropic drugs, (6) antiarrhythmic drugs, (7) antithrombotic drugs, and (8) lipid-lowering agents.

THE HEART AS A SITE FOR DRUG INTERACTIONS

Sinoatrial and Atrioventricular Nodes

The SA node responds to at least three pacemaker currents, including I_f, $I_{Ca(L)}$, and I_k. The definition of two of these currents is as follows: I_f is the inward "funny" sodium current initially described in Purkinje fibers, and I_k is the delayed rectifier outward potassium current. Of these pacemaker currents, two are susceptible to β-adrenergic blockers and one to CCAs. The reason the combination of a β blocker with a CCA does not arrest the heart is severalfold. First, one of the pacemaker currents, I_k, is affected by neither. Second, the CCA effect is on the long-acting calcium current $I_{Ca(L)}$. The transient calcium current $I_{Ca(T)}$, which probably accounts for the initial phases of depolarization in the SA and AV nodes, is not affected by CCAs. Third, it is only the CCAs of the verapamil and diltiazem type that are effective on the SA node. Dihydropyridines (DHPs, i.e., nifedipinelike compounds) have a much less marked effect on these nodes. In contrast, sinoatrial arrest has been reported when an intravenous bolus of verapamil or diltiazem is given to predisposed patients already receiving a beta blocker.

Thus adverse drug interactions at the level of the SA node causing excess bradycardia, excess tachycardia, or AV block often involve beta blockers, CCAs, or digitalis.

Intraventricular Conduction System

There are a number of antiarrhythmics (class Ia and Ic sodium channel blockers) that inhibit the intraventricular (His-Purkinje) conduction system. These drugs (quinidine, flecainide, propafenone) should not be given together because they may produce serious additive intraventricular conduction defects.

Proarrhythmic Drug Interactions

There are three basic proarrhythmic mechanisms. First, prolongation of the QT interval may occur, especially in the presence of hypokalemia and/or bradycardia. The type of arrhythmia produced by QT prolongation is highly specific, namely, torsades de pointes.

Second, agents increasing myocardial levels of cyclic adenosine monophosphate (cyclic AMP) or cytosolic calcium levels cause arrhythmias through a different mechanism, namely, the precipitation of afterpotentials with triggered activity and risk of ventricular tachycardia and/or fibrillation (Table 22-1). All agents decreasing plasma potassium levels, such as β-adrenergic stimulants or excess diuretic usage, promote afterdepolarizations and arrhythmias.

Myocardial Contractile Mechanism

There are a number of drugs with negative inotropic effects, including β blockers, CCAs, and certain antiarrhythmic agents. Often a relatively well-functioning left ventricle is able to withstand cotherapy with these drugs, but when the left ventricle (LV) is diseased, then even one of these drugs may precipitate adverse heart failure.

VASCULAR SMOOTH MUSCLE AS A SITE FOR DRUG INTERACTIONS

In vascular smooth muscle, there can be interactions to cause excess vasoconstriction, for example, the combination of a drug inhibiting the reuptake of norepinephrine from the nerve terminals (such as cocaine)

TABLE 22-1 Potentially Proarrhythmic Drug Interactions: Agents Increasing Myocardial Cyclic AMP or Cell Calcium Levels or Decreasing Plasma Potassium Levels*

Cardiac drug	Interacting drug	Mechanism	Consequence	Prophylaxis
PDE III inhibitors Amrinone Milrinone Enoximone	All proarrhythmic drugs, particularly β-adrenergic stimulants	Increase of myocardial cyclic AMP especially in presence of ischemia	Risk of VT/VF	Caution in presence of acute myocardial ischemia; avoid chronic use in LV failure; monitor. Avoid cotherapy with proarrhythmic drugs.
β-adrenergic stimulants Dopamine Dobutamine Norepinephrine Epinephrine	All proarrhythmic drugs	Increase of myocardial cyclic AMP; decrease of plasma potassium	Risk of VT/VF	As above. Check plasma potassium.
Bronchodilators Theophylline Aminophylline	All proarrhythmic drugs	Inhibition of PDE; increase of cyclic AMP; decrease of plasma potassium	Risk of VT/VF (not common)	Caution in asthmatics with cardiac arrhythmia problems or heart failure. Avoid bronchodilators for asthma if proarrhythmic drugs are being given.
Digitalis Digoxin	All proarrhythmic drugs, particuarly β-adrenergic stimulants or PDE inhibitors	Inhibition of sodium pump with increase of cytosolic calcium and calcium-induced afterdepolarizations	VT associated with AV nodal block	Caution in hypokalemia or cotherapy with proarrhythmic drugs.
Diuretics Thiazides Loop diuretics	Digoxin; other proarrhythmic drugs, including those prolonging action potential duration	Decreased plasma K^+ with increased afterdepolarizations; sensitization to digoxin arrhythmias	VT/VF; torsades de pointes	Check plasma potassium; use K^+-retaining diuretic such as triamterene or amiloride.

*AMP = adenosine monophosphate; AV = atrioventricular; LV = left ventricle; PDE = phosphodiesterase; VT = ventricular tachycardia; VF = ventricular fibrillation.

Source: For references, see Opie LH: Interactions with cardiovascular drugs. *Curr Prob Cardiol* 18:529, 1993.

together with therapeutic administration of monoamine oxidase (MAO) inhibitors, which also inhibit the reuptake of norepinephrine in the nerve terminals. The combination of cocaine with these inhibitors, for example, could theoretically promote a powerful coronary vasoconstriction. When dopamine is infused into a patient receiving monoamine oxidase inhibitors, there is risk of severe hypertension from excess sensitivity to dopamine.

Conversely, there may be a number of drug interactions causing excess vasodilation and hypotension, for example, the combination of the α_1 blocker prazosin with the powerful CCA vasodilator nifedipine.

Vascular smooth muscle also can be the site of drug interactions that lessen the effects of antihypertensive or antifailure therapy, such as the nonsteroidal anti-inflammatories (NSAIDs).

HEPATIC INTERACTIONS OF DRUGS

Pharmacokinetic Interactions

Many cardiovascular drugs are metabolized in the liver, generally via the cytochrome oxidase system. Although cytochrome P450 is the collective name for the system, there are many isoenzymes of which P450 IID6 is the relevant one in humans. This system can be induced by drugs such as phenytoin, barbiturates, and rifampin. Accordingly, such drugs accelerate the breakdown of cardiovascular drugs that are metabolized in the liver, reducing the blood level and the therapeutic efficacy (Table 22-2). On the other hand, cimetidine, which inhibits the oxidase system, permits excess circulating levels to build up with a greater therapeutic effect. Thus cimetidine can increase blood levels of a host of drugs, including the antiarrhythmics quinidine, lidocaine, and procainamide; the CCAs nifedipine and verapamil; and the β blocker propranolol (see Table 22-2). Cimetidine, therefore, probably increases the blood levels of all cardiovascular drugs metabolized in the liver. A similar danger may theoretically occur during the use of other cytochrome inhibitory drugs, such as quinidine or propafenone. Ranitidine seems free of this adverse side effect, at least as far as nifedipine is concerned. Cardiovascular drugs that are metabolized by the liver, such as verapamil, propranolol, or metoprolol, also can interact with each other (with risk of increased nodal inhibition and negative inotropic effect) or verapamil and prazosin with an increased hypotensive effect.

Pharmacodynamic Interactions

These occur whenever altered hepatic blood flow changes rates of first-pass liver metabolism. For example, when a β blocker and lidocaine are given together, as may occur during acute myocardial infarction, the β blocker reduces both the hepatic blood flow to the liver and the rate of hepatic metabolism of lidocaine. The consequence is an increased

TABLE 22-2 Cardiovascular Drug Pharmacokinetic Interactions by Hepatic Mechanisms*

Cardiac drug	Interacting drug	Mechanism	Consequence	Prophylaxis
Lipid-soluble β blockers Propranolol Metoprolol Labetalol Timolol Acebutolol	Cytochrome oxidase inducers (rifampin, barbiturates, phenytoin); opposite effects with cimetidine	Induction of hepatic cytochrome oxidase enhances hepatic metabolism of β blocker to reduce blood level; opposite effects with cimetidine	Decreased therapeutic effect of β blocker with inducers; increased effect with cimetidine	*Inducers*: Avoid cotherapy or increase β-blocker dose *Cimetidine*: Reduce dose of both drugs
Calcium antagonists				
Verapamil	Metoprolol	V decreases M metabolism presumably by inhibition of oxidase	Excess M effects such as bradycardia and negative inotropism	Reduce M dose
Verapamil	Cimetidine	C inhibits cytochrome oxidase system	Blood level of V rises	Reduce V dose
Nifedipine	Cimetidine	As above	Blood level of N rises	Reduce N dose
Nifedipine	Diltiazem	D decreases N metabolism	Blood level of N rises	Reduce N dose
Antiarrhythmics				
Quinidine	Cimetidine	C inhibits cytochrome oxidase system	Blood level of Q rises	Reduce Q dose
Procainamide	Cimetidine	C inhibits cytochrome oxidase system	Increased blood level of P	Reduce P dose
Lidocaine	Cimetidine	C inhibits cytochrome oxidase system	Blood level of L rises	Reduce L dose

*C = cimetidine; L = lidocaine; M = metoprolol; P = procainamide; Q = quinidine.
Source: For references, see Opie LH: Interactions with cardiovascular drugs. *Curr Prob Cardiol* 18:529, 1993.

blood lidocaine level with the risk of lidocaine toxicity. Conversely, by increasing hepatic blood flow, nifedipine has the opposite effect, so the breakdown of propranolol is increased, resulting in lower blood levels of propranolol. The combination nifedipine-atenolol, the latter agent not being metabolized in the liver at all, therefore, seems theoretically better than nifedipine-propranolol.

RENAL INTERACTIONS OF DRUGS

A number of drugs interact with each other by competing for renal clearance mechanisms or altering the rate of renal clearance of the other drug. For example, the renal clearance of digoxin is decreased by quinidine, leading to an elevation of digoxin levels. This renal interaction drew the attention of cardiologists because it showed that apparently established properties of a drug could perhaps be explained more simply by drug interactions. For example, "quinidine syncope" could be caused by digitalis-induced arrhythmias, precipitated by cotherapy with quinidine. Other antiarrhythmics inhibiting the renal excretion of digoxin include verapamil, amiodarone, and propafenone.

PLASMA PROTEIN BINDING AS A SITE FOR DRUG INTERACTIONS

Sulfinpyrazone powerfully displaces warfarin, so the dose of warfarin required may be dramatically less. In dogs, prazosin displaces digoxin from plasma and other binding sites.

EFFECTS OF AGING

Few studies give details of drug interactions in the elderly. By extrapolation from known changes with age in pharmacokinetics, certain projections can be made. In general, disease of the SA and AV nodes is more common, myocardial contractile activity more likely to be depressed, and renal function more probably impaired. Nonrenal clearance of drugs such as flecainide may be impaired. The major way of avoiding adverse interactions is by ruthlessly cutting out redundant drugs and reducing excess doses of the remaining drugs so as to reduce the risk of interactions. Nonetheless, a classic error is to presume that all elderly patients have impaired renal function and therefore need a lower than standard digoxin dose. In fact, the standard dose of 0.25 mg digoxin daily remains correct for elderly patients, provided that the creatinine clearance is 90 mL/min or more.

INTERACTIONS OF β-ADRENERGIC BLOCKING DRUGS

A number of pharmacodynamic and pharmacokinetic interactions are possible (Table 22-3). For example, β blockers may have adverse pharmacodynamic interactions with CCAs to cause excess hypotension,

TABLE 22-3 Drug Interactions of β-Adrenergic Blocking Agents*

Cardiac drug	Interacting drugs	Mechanism	Consequence	Prophylaxis
Hemodynamic Interactions				
All β blockers	Calcium antagonists, especially IR nifedipine	Added hypotension	Risk of myocardial ischemia	Blood pressure control, adjust dose
	Verapamil or diltiazem	Added negative inotropic effect	Risk of myocardial ischemia	Check for CHF, adjust doses
	Flecainide	Added negative inotropic effect	Hypotension	Check LV function, flecainide levels
Electrophysiologic Interactions				
All β blockers	Verapamil	Added inhibition of SA, AV nodes	Bradycardia, asystole, complete heart block	Exclude "sick sinus" syndrome, AV nodal disease, adjust dose
	Diltiazem	Added negative inotropic effect	Excess hypotension	Exclude predrug LV failure
Hepatic Interactions				
Propranolol (P)	Cimetidine (C)	C decreases P metabolism	Excess propranolol effects	Reduce both drug doses
	Lidocaine (L)	Low hepatic blood flow	Excess lidocaine effects	Reduce lidocaine dose
Metoprolol (M)	Verapamil (V)	V decreases M metabolism	Excess M effects	Reduce M dose
	Cimetidine (C)	C decreases M metabolism	Excess M effects	Reduce both drug doses
Labetalol (L)	Cimetidine (C)	C decreases L metabolism	Excess L effects	Reduce both drug doses
Antihypertensive Interactions				
β blockers	Indomethacin (I), NSAIDs	I inhibits vasodilatory prostaglandins	Decreased antihypertensive effect	Omit indomethacin; use alternative drugs

*AV = atrioventricular; CHF = congestive heart failure; IR = instant release; LV = left ventricular.

Source: Adapted from Opie LH: Adverse cardiovascular drug interactions, in Schlant RC, Alexander RW (eds): *The Heart*, 8th ed. New York, McGraw-Hill, 1994, pp 1971–1985, with permission.

undue bradycardia, or AV nodal block. Now that β blockers are used with increasing frequency in the acute phase of myocardial infarction and often given intravenously, they may depress hepatic blood flow, thereby decreasing hepatic inactivation of lidocaine. Examples of pharmacokinetic interactions are those of cimetidine with drugs such as propranolol, metoprolol, and labetalol, which are metabolized by the cytochrome oxidase system in the liver (see Table 22-3).

INTERACTIONS OF ANTIANGINAL VASODILATORS INCLUDING CALCIUM CHANNEL ANTAGONISTS

The chief drug interactions of nitrates are pharmacodynamic (Table 22-4). During triple therapy of angina pectoris by nitrates, β blockers, and CCAs, the efficacy of the combination may be less than expected, probably because each of the drugs can predispose to excess hypotension. Unexpectedly, high doses of intravenous nitroglycerin may induce heparin resistance by altering the activity of antithrombin III. Nitroglycerin also potentially interferes with the clotting mechanism in another way, through lessening the therapeutic potency of the tissue plasminogen activator alteplase.

Many of the interactions of CCAs are *pharmacodynamic*, such as added effects on the nodes (verapamil or diltiazem plus β blockers or excess digitalis) or on the systemic vascular resistance, with the risk of excess hypotension in predisposed subjects. There may be two important properties of CCAs that distinguish the specific compounds from each other. First, accumulating evidence suggests that short-acting compounds with acute vasodilatory effects induce acute hypotension and repetitive neurohumoral activation and tachycardia. Thus the long-acting second-generation CCAs, such as amlodipine and nifedipine gastrointestinal therapeutic system (GITS), are less likely to cause acute vasodilatory drug interactions than shorter-acting compounds. Second, the DHPs, such as nifedipine, amlodipine, and others, need to be distinguished from the non-DHPs, such as verapamil and diltiazem. The DHPs have rather specific vascular dilatory effects, whereas the non-DHPs also inhibit the SA and AV nodes and are more negatively inotropic. Thus the DHPs have potentially fewer cardiac pharmacodynamic interactions, whereas the non-DHPs also interact with other nodal-inhibitory drugs such as β blockers and digoxin.

In addition, there can be *pharmacokinetic* interactions. Hepatic metabolic interactions are numerous. Drugs metabolized by the cytochrome oxidase system, such as nifedipine and verapamil, have their breakdown inhibited by cimetidine but not by ranitidine. Verapamil and diltiazem, both metabolized by the cytochrome oxidase system in the liver, can inhibit the hepatic oxidation of some other drugs whose blood levels therefore increase (see Table 22-2). For example, the blood level of cyclosporine may increase during diltiazem therapy, and during verapamil therapy, the blood levels of prazosin, theophylline, and quinidine may all increase. Diltiazem also can interfere with hepatic nifedipine metabolism, potentiating dihydropyridine side effects when the drugs are used together.

Although NSAIDs reduce the therapeutic efficacy of many antihypertensives, an important exception is that nifedipine retains its potency.

Another pharmacokinetic interaction, in this case at the level of the kidney, is that occurring between verapamil and digoxin, whereby digoxin clearance is decreased with consequent risk of digoxin toxicity. In the case of nifedipine and diltiazem, such interactions with digoxin appear to be much less. Nonetheless, it is impossible to generalize without prior knowledge. Whereas nicardipine causes only a modest rise of digoxin levels, nitrendipine has an effect almost as severe as that of verapamil in that digoxin levels approximately double. Amlodipine has virtually no pharmacokinetic interaction with digoxin.

Of still unknown clinical importance is an experimental interaction between diltiazem and r-tPA (recombinant tissue-type plasminogen activator) that leads to excess bleeding. Whether this is a drug-specific or a class effect remains to be established.

INTERACTIONS OF DIURETICS

Loop Diuretics

Hypokalemia, as may occur when loop diuretics are given acutely and intravenously, may precipitate digitalis toxicity. An interesting and complex set of interactions between furosemide and captopril has emerged. On the one hand, captopril decreases the renal excretion of furosemide that is required for the diuretic effect of the latter (Table 22-5); this may explain why captopril reduces furosemide-induced natriuresis to less than half. This effect of captopril in altering furosemide excretion seems not to be shared by other ACE inhibitors. There is an important pharmacodynamic interaction between captopril and furosemide. Both these agents are able to dilate the postglomerular efferent arterioles. When captopril is given in a standard dose of 25 mg, furosemide has little or no diuretic effect. On the other hand, only minute doses of captopril, such as 1 mg, enhance the diuretic effect of furosemide. The proposed mechanism is that the very low dose of captopril still allows sufficient circulating angiotensin II to maintain efferent arteriolar tone and thereby to keep the glomerular filtration rate sufficiently high for the furosemide to act. Both these pharmacokinetic and pharmacodynamic interactions therefore argue for a low-dose captopril combination with furosemide. On the other hand, in patients with a low serum sodium, which is an indirect indicator of a high renin state, it is the high aldosterone levels that retain sodium and stimulate vasopressin secretion, the latter causing the hyponatremia. Therapy of such

TABLE 22-4 Drug Interactions of Antianginal Vasodilators Including Calcium Antagonists*

Cardiac drug	Interacting drugs	Mechanism	Consequence	Prophylaxis
Nitrates				
All nitrates	Calcium antagonists	Excess vasodilation	Syncope, dizziness	Monitor BP
	Prazosin (PZ)	Excess vasodilation	Syncope, dizziness	Monitor BP and start with low PZ dose
Calcium Antagonists				
Verapamil (V)	β blockers	SA and AV nodal inhibition	Added nodal and negative inotropic effects	Care during cotherapy
		Myocardial failure		Check ECG, BP, heart size
	Cimetidine	Hepatic metabolic interaction	Blood V rises	Adjust dose
	Digitalis poisoning	Added SA and AV nodal inhibition	Asystole; complete heart block after IV verapamil	Avoid IV verapamil in digitalis poisoning
	Digoxin (D)	Decreased digoxin clearance	Risk of D toxicity	Halve D dose; blood D level
	Disopyramide	Pharmacodynamic	Hypotension, constipation	Check BP, LV and gut
	Flecainide (F)	Added negative inotropism	Hypotension	Check LV, F levels
	Prazosin (PZ)	Hepatic interaction	Excess hypotension	Check BP during cotherapy
	Quinidine (Q)	Added α receptor inhibition; V decreases Q clearance	Hypotension	Check Q levels and BP
	Theophylline (T)	Inhibition of hepatic metabolism	Increased blood T levels	Reduce T, check levels

Nifedipine (N) and other DHPs	β blockers	Added negative inotropism	Excess hypotension	Check BP, use test dose of N
	Cimetidine	Hepatic metabolic interaction	Increased blood N levels	Decreased N dosage by 40%
	Digoxin (D)	Minor/modest changes in digoxin	Increased digoxin levels	Check D levels
	Prazosin (PZ)	PZ blocks α reflex to N	Postural hypotension	Test dose of N or PZ
	Propranolol (P)	N and P have opposite effects on blood liver	N decreases P levels; increases N levels	Readjust P and N doses if needed
	Quinidine (Q)	N improves poor LV function; Q clearance faster	Decreased Q effect	Check Q levels
Diltiazem (D)	β blockers	Added SA nodal inhibition Negative inotropism	Bradycardia, hypotension	Check ECG and LV function
	Cimetidine	Hepatic metabolic interactions	Increased D levels	Reduce D dose by one-third
	Cyclosporine (C)	Hepatic metabolism of C inhibited	Increased blood C levels	Decrease C dose
	Digoxin (D)	Some fall in D clearance	Only in renal failure	Check D levels
	Flecainide (F)	Added negative inotropism	Hypotension	Check LV; F levels
Nicardipine (see also nifedipine)	Cyclosporine (C)	Hepatic metabolism of C inhibited	Increased blood C levels	Decrease C dose
	Digoxin (D)	Decreased D clearance	Blood D doubles	Decrease D, D levels

*AV = atrioventricular; SA = sinoatrial node; LV = left ventricle; BP = blood pressure; ECG = electrocardiogram.
Source: Adapted from Opie LH: Adverse cardiovascular drug interactions, in Schlant RC, Alexander RW (eds): *The Heart*, 8th ed. New York, McGraw-Hill, 1994, pp 1971–1985, with permission.

TABLE 22-5 Drug Interactions of Diuretics*

Cardiac drug	Interacting drugs	Mechanism	Consequence	Prophylaxis
Loop and thiazide diuretics	Indomethacin and other NSAIDs	Pharmacodynamic	Decreased anti-hypertensive effect	Adjust diuretic dose or add another agent
	Probenecid	Decreased tubular excretion of diuretic	Decreased diuretic effect	Increase diuretic dose
	ACE inhibitors	Excess diuretics, high renins	Excess hypotension; prerenal uremia	Low diuretic dose; test dose ACE inhibitor
Furosemide (F)	Captopril	Decreased tubular excretion of F; added efferent arteriolar vaso-dilation	Decreased diuretic effect; decreased glomerular flow; diuretic effect of F less	Increase furosemide dose? Ultra low-dose captopril? Avoid captopril?
K^+-retaining diuretics	ACE inhibitors	Added K^+ retention	Hyperkalemia	Check K^+ levels

*ACE = angiotensin converting enzyme; NSAIDs = nonsteroidal anti-inflammatory drugs.
Source: Adapted from Opie LH: Adverse cardiovascular drug interactions, in Schlant RC, Alexander RW (eds): *The Heart*, 8th ed. New York, McGraw-Hill, 1994, pp 1971–1985, with permission.

patients by furosemide alone is ineffective and the addition of captopril in a standard dose may achieve improvement.

Quite apart from the preceding complex interactions, it is generally regarded as a wise precaution to reduce the diuretic dose of patients with congestive heart failure before adding an ACE inhibitor. The aim of this procedure is to lessen excessive first-dose hypotension. Overdiuresis tends to result in activation of the renin-angiotensin system and greater sensitivity to ACE inhibition.

Thiazide Diuretics

Indomethacin and other nonsteroidal anti-inflammatory drugs decrease the antihypertensive effect of thiazides. Probenecid decreases the urinary excretion of thiazide and loop diuretics so that the diuretic efficacy is reduced. Although thiazide diuretics and the nifedipine-like CCAs should have added hypotensive effects, they often do not. The proposed mechanism for this lack of an additive pharmacodynamic effect is that the dihydropyridine CCAs such as nifedipine have a significant diuretic effect on their own.

Potassium-Retaining Diuretics

These may interact with ACE inhibitors to cause added potassium retention and hyperkalemia, especially in the presence of renal failure.

INTERACTIONS OF ANGIOTENSIN CONVERTING ENZYME INHIBITORS

In general, these agents have few drug interactions (Table 22-6). In patients with congestive heart failure, excessive first-dose hypotension should be avoided to lessen the risk of renal impairment, which may lead to accumulation and interaction of renal-excreted drugs.

Because of potential hyperkalemia with potassium-sparing diuretics, the ideal combination with an ACE inhibitor is a thiazide diuretic or furosemide but without a potassium-retaining component. In patients receiving NSAIDs, which tend to decrease renal plasma flow in their own right, addition of an ACE inhibitor can further decrease the glomerular filtration rate, with added risk of hyperkalemia. Captopril may interact with probenecid, which inhibits its tubular excretion, and as mentioned earlier, there is a serious interaction with the loop diuretic furosemide.

In patients with severe congestive heart failure, the acute combination of aspirin and an ACE inhibitor decreases the peripheral vasodilation. Lower aspirin doses seem to have little or no hemodynamic interference, but there are no true dose-response or chronic studies. It is best to keep the dose of aspirin as low as possible when combined with ACE inhibitors.

TABLE 22-6 Drug Interactions of Angiotensin Converting Enzyme (ACE) Inhibitors and Vasodilators*

Cardiac drug	Interacting drugs	Mechanism	Consequence	Prophylaxis
ACE Inhibitors				
All (or probably all)	Diuretics	High renin levels in overdiuresed patients	First-dose hypotension, risk of renal failure	Low test dose; first dose effect may be less with perindopril
All	K^+-sparing diuretics	Added K^+ retention	Hyperkalemia	Avoid combination
	Aspirin (acute) NSAIDs	Less PG vasodilation	Less fall in SVR	Decrease dose of aspirin; avoid NSAIDs
Captopril (C)	Immunosuppressive drugs, procainamide, hydralazine	Added immune effects	Increased risk of neutropenia	Avoid combination; check neutrophils
	Probenecid (P)	P inhibits excretion of C	Small rise in C levels	Decrease dose of C
	Loop diuretics	C inhibits renal excretion of furosemide (F)	Decrease F efficacy	Change from C; or minimize C dose; or increase F dose
	Digoxin (D)	Decreased renal clearance	Small rise in D levels	Sometimes decrease dose of D

Vasodilators.				
Hydralazine/NP	Digoxin	Increased renal D excretion	Decreased D levels	Check D levels
Prazosin (P), doxazosin, terazosin	Nifedipine	Pharmacodynamic	Excess hypotension	Test dose of nifedipine
	Nitrates	Pharmacodynamic	Syncope, hypotension	Decrease PZ dose
	Verapamil	Hepatic metabolism	Synergistic anti-hypertensive effect	Adjust doses
Hydralazine (H)	NSAIDs	Diminished vaso-dilator effect of H	Less therapeutic effect	Avoid cotherapy; increase dose of H

*C = captopril; F = furosemide; D = digoxin; NP = nitroprusside; NSAIDs = nonsteroidal anti-inflammatory drugs; P = probenecid; PG = prostaglandins; PZ = prazosin; SVR = systemic vascular resistance.

Source: Adapted from Opie LH: Adverse cardiovascular drug interactions, in Schlant RC, Alexander RW (eds): *The Heart*, 8th ed. New York, McGraw-Hill, 1994, pp 1971–1985, with permission.

INTERACTIONS OF OTHER VASODILATORS

Hydralazine or nitroprusside can increase renal clearance of digoxin with the possible result of increased tubular excretion. Theoretically, blood digoxin levels should be checked during the use of hydralazine as a nonspecific vasodilator for heart failure. In practice, however, the addition of an unloading agent should improve congestive heart failure, enhance renal plasma flow, and therefore exaggerate the renal clearance of digoxin. For these reasons, digoxin levels should be checked during cotherapy with hydralazine.

Hydralazine, like other vasodilators, including ACE inhibitors, has its antihypertensive efficacy lessened by NSAIDs.

In the case of prazosin, the α_1 antagonist, there may be an interaction with the CCAs verapamil and nifedipine resulting in excess hypotension with the first dose of prazosin. Prazosin given to dogs displaces digoxin from plasma and other binding sites to increase blood levels by about 25%. In the case of the synergistic hypotensive effects of verapamil and prazosin, part may be explained by a pharmacokinetic-hepatic interaction, which, therefore, is less acute.

INTERACTIONS OF DIGOXIN AND POSITIVE INOTROPIC AGENTS

The kidney is the most common site at which the pharmacokinetics of digoxin can be altered by other cardiovascular drugs.

Potentially interacting drugs including quinidine, verapamil, nitrendipine, propafenone, and amiodarone all increase blood digoxin levels, and their common mechanism of action is decreased renal clearance of digoxin (Table 22-7). If the digoxin is being given for therapy of congestive heart failure, there is a risk that, in addition, poor renal function may be present. In the presence of renal failure, drugs ordinarily causing a modest or minimal rise in blood digoxin levels, such as diltiazem or nifedipine, sometimes can precipitate digoxin toxicity. It needs reemphasis, however, that the majority of CCAs, with the exception of amlodipine and possibly felodipine, should not be given to patients with heart failure.

If the digoxin is being given to inhibit the AV node, as in the therapy of refractory paroxysmal supraventricular nodal tachycardia, then the most likely interaction is with verapamil. Since patients with this condition often have normal myocardial function, an increase in blood digoxin is normally not serious although as a precaution the blood level of digoxin should be checked during such cotherapy.

When cotherapy elevates digoxin levels, the features of *digitalis toxicity* may depend on the agent added as well as on the underlying condition of the heart. With quinidine, tachyarrhythmias become more likely; amiodarone and verapamil seem to repress the ventricular arrhythmias of digitalis toxicity so that bradycardia and AV block are

TABLE 22-7 Drug Interactions of Digitalis and Other Positive Inotropic Agents

Cardiac drug	Interacting drugs	Mechanism	Consequence	Prophylaxis
Positive Inotropic Agents				
Digitoxin	Verapamil	Nonrenal clearance of digitoxin falls	Digitoxin levels up by one-third	Check digitoxin level
	Other drugs interacting with digoxin	? Altered digitoxin clearance	? Digitoxin levels increase	Check digitoxin level
Digoxin (D)	Amiodarone	Reduce renal clearance of D	D level may double	Check D level; halve dose
	Captopril	Reduced D clearance	Blood D increases	Check D dose
	Diltiazem	Variable decrease of D clearance	Variable blood D increases	Check D level
	Diuretics; potassium-sparing amiloride/triamterene	Reduced extrarenal D clearance	D levels up by 20%	Check D level
	spironolactone (S)	S reduces renal D clearance		Complex effects; check D level
	Nifedipine	Variable fall of D clearance	Variable blood D rises	Check D level
	Nitrendipine	Reduced D clearance	Blood D doubles	Check D level; halve dose
	Prazosin (PZ)	PZ displaces D from binding sites	Blood D rises	(Needs confirmation in humans)
	Propafenone	Not defined	D level increases	Check D level
	Quinidine, quinine	Reduced D clearance	Blood D doubles	Check D level, halve dose
	Verapamil	Reduced D clearance	Blood D doubles or more	Check D level, halve dose
Sympathomimetic Inotropes				
Dobutamine Amrinone Milrinone	Thiazide diuretics	Additive hypokalemic effects	Arrhythmias	Check blood potassium

Source: Adapted from Opie LH: Adverse cardiovascular drug interactions, in Schlant RC, Alexander RW (eds): *The Heart*, 8th ed. New York, McGraw-Hill, 1994, pp 1971–1985, with permission.

more likely. Because of numerous interactions of digoxin with antiarrhythmic drugs (see Table 22-7), it is of some comfort that there are several such drugs that have little or no pharmacokinetic interactions with digoxin, including procainamide, disopyramide, lidocaine, phenytoin, mexiletine, encainide, and sotalol. During cotherapy of digoxin with sotalol, recently released in the United States, it should be noted that hypokalemia not only exaggerates the arrhythmogenic effects of digoxin but also those of sotalol and must therefore be rigorously avoided. Even normal blood levels of digoxin, not usually causing toxicity, can become toxic when the blood potassium falls, as occurs during cotherapy with potassium-losing diuretics.

Diuretics also may directly precipitate digitalis toxicity. Hypokalemia, when really severe (plasma potassium below 2 to 3 mEq/L), may actually inhibit the tubular secretion of digoxin.

Potassium-sparing diuretics (amiloride, triamterene, and spironolactone) as well as captopril decreased digoxin clearance by about 20 to 30%. Since such combinations with digoxin are frequently used in the therapy of congestive heart failure, the blood digoxin level must frequently be monitored. Blood digoxin levels respond to inducers or inhibitors of the hepatic cytochrome P450 oxidase system.

Digoxin absorption may be interfered with by co-therapy with cholestyramine, probably because digoxin binds to the resin. Digoxin should therefore be given several hours before the resin, or digoxin capsules may be used. Furthermore, such capsules also lead to less interaction with kaolin pectate, which can also reduce digoxin absorption, and with erythromycin and tetracycline which increase blood digoxin levels by inhibiting gastrointestinal flora that inactivate digoxin

INTERACTIONS OF ANTIARRHYTHMIC DRUGS

These agents have truly numerous and sometimes serious interactions (Table 22-8). Some of the most frequent are with (1) digoxin, (2) diuretics, and (3) hepatic enzyme inducers. The last can alter the metabolism of agents such as quinidine and other antiarrhythmics that are metabolized in the liver. Cimetidine decreases the hepatic metabolism of these agents, whereas phenytoin, barbiturates, and rifampin have opposite effects (Table 22-8). To some extent the kinetic and other interactions of antiarrhythmics have been reduced recently because of the tendency to use cotherapy at lower doses, thereby avoiding dose-related side effects as in the case of quinidine and mexiletine. Also, the indiscriminate use of antiarrhythmic agents has lessened since recent studies have stressed potential proarrhythmic effects.

Adenosine

Of particular interest are the antiarrhythmic effects of the new agent adenosine, that is used to inhibit certain supraventricular tachycardias.

It has an indirect effect, similar to that of the CCA verapamil, by enhancing the flow of the current $I_{k(ACh)}$. Aminophylline or theophylline, by competing with adenosine for the receptor sites, completely inhibits the adenosine-induced effect on AV conduction. Dipyridamole, on the other hand, inhibits the breakdown of adenosine and/or its uptake into the tissues, so that the amount of adenosine available for the antiarrhythmic effect is enhanced. Effective doses of adenosine on patients receiving sustained dipyridamole therapy may only be one quarter to one eighth of the normal doses.

INTERACTIONS OF ANTIHYPERTENSIVE DRUGS

Interactions for diuretics, β-adrenergic blockers, CCAs, angiotensin converting enzyme inhibitors, and α-adrenergic blockers have already been considered. In general, NSAIDs interfere severely with antihypertensive efficacy of all antihypertensives. An important exception is nifedipine (and, presumably, other dihydropyridines). Unlike other NSAIDs, aspirin and sulindac may be less prone to this potentially negative interaction. When CCAs are used as antihypertensives, part of their effect is by natriuresis, so adding a diuretic is often relatively ineffective, especially in the case of nifedipine.

INTERACTIONS OF ANTITHROMBOTIC DRUGS

Aspirin

Blood levels of uric acid may be increased by both aspirin and thiazide diuretics, so special care is required when cotherapy is given to patients with gout or a family history thereof. Conversely, aspirin may decrease the uricosuric effects of sulfinpyrazone and probenecid. Aspirin has some effects similar to those of the NSAIDs, also inhibiting the function of vasodilatory prostaglandin. Thus it may reduce the natriuretic effect of spironolactone and some of the benefits of ACE inhibitors in severe congestive heart failure (see Table 22-6), according to acute studies. Aspirin-induced gastrointestinal bleeding may be a greater hazard in patients receiving corticosteroid therapy or NSAIDs. Aspirin breakdown is increased by agents inducing the hepatic cytochrome oxidase system such as barbiturates, phenytoin, and rifampin. High-dose aspirin may evoke a bleeding tendency and exaggerate anticoagulant-induced bleeding. Thus aspirin plus warfarin causes more bleeding than dipyridamole plus warfarin in patients who have undergone bypass surgery. The current trend toward low-dose aspirin should decrease the significance of all these drug interactions.

Warfarin (Coumadin)

Warfarin is suspected in a large number of drug interactions, possibly as many as 80. It follows that drug interactions must be suspected

TABLE 22-8 Drug Interactions of Antiarrhythmic Drugs*

Cardiac drug	Interacting drugs	Mechanism	Consequence	Prophylaxis
Class IA				
Quinidine (Q)	Amiodarone	Added QT effects; blood Q rises	Torsades de pointes	Check QT, potassium
	Antibiotics (some)	Quinidine inhibits muscarinic receptors	Increased antibiotic-induced muscular weakness	Clinical care, drug levels
	Anticholinesterases	Quinidine inhibits muscarinic receptors	Decreased ACh efficacy in myasthenia gravis	Avoid Q if possible blood
	Antihypertensive agents	Added hypotensive and added SA nodal effects	Hypotension, excess bradycardia	Regulate BP
	β Blockers			Check BP, ECG
	Cimetidine (C)	C inhibits oxidative metabolism of Q	Increased Q levels, risk of toxicity	Q levels, consider ranitidine
	Digoxin (D)	Decreased D clearance	Risk of D toxicity	Check D dose levels
	Diltiazem	Added inhibition of SA node	Excess bradycardia	Check ECG, heart rate
	Disopyramide	Added QT prolongation	Torsades de pointes	Check QT, potassium
	Diuretic, potassium-losing	Hypokalemia and QT prolongation	Torsades de pointes	Check QT, potassium
	Hepatic enzyme inducers (phenytoin, barbiturates, rifampin)	Increased Q hepatic metabolism	Decreased Q levels	Q levels, doses

	Nifedipine	Increased Q clearance	Decreased Q levels	Q levels, doses
	Sotalol	Added QT prolongation,	Torsades de pointes	Check QT, potassium
	Verapamil	Decreased Q clearance	Excess bradycardia	Check ECG, Q levels
	Warfarin	Hepatic interaction with Q	Bleeding	Check prothrombin time
Procainamide (P)	Captopril	Combined immune effects	Theoretical risk of neutropenia	Cotherapy with care
	Cimetidine	Decreased renal P clearance	Prolonged P half-life, excess P effect	Reduce P dose; consider ranitidine
Disopyramide (D)	Agents prolonging APD* (quinidine, amiodarone, sotalol)	Added QT prolongation, especially if hypokalemic	Torsades de pointes	Check QT, potassium
	β Blockers	Combined negative inotropism	Hypotension	Low doses
	Cimetidine	Hepatic D metabolism falls	Increased blood D levels	
	Digitalis toxicity	Added SA, AV nodal depression	SA, AV block	Avoid D in digitalis toxicity
	Hepatic enzyme inducers (phenytoin, rifampin, barbiturates)	Enhanced D hepatic metabolism	Blood D levels fall; readjust D dose	Readjust D dose

(*continued*)

TABLE 22-8 Drug Interactions of Antiarrhythmic Drugs* (*concluded*)

Cardiac drug	Interacting drugs	Mechanism	Consequence	Prophylaxis
	Drugs inhibiting SA or AV nodes/conduction system (quinidine, β blockers, methyldopa, digoxin)	Pharmacodynamic additive effects	SA, AV block; conduction block	Check ECG; decrease doses
	Pyridostigmine	Inhibition of cholinesterase activity	Beneficial effect of P on D; harmful effect of D on P	In myasthenia gravis, avoid D
Class IB				
Lidocaine (lignocaine)	Verapamil	Combined negative inotropism	Hypotension	Avoid IV D or V cotherapy
	Cimetidine	Decreased hepatic metabolism	Increased L levels	Decrease L infusion rate
	Halothane	Decreased hepatic blood flow	Increased L levels	Decrease L infusion rate
	Propranolol	Decreased hepatic blood flow	Increased L levels	Decrease L infusion rate
	Other β blockers	Decreased hepatic blood flow	Increased L levels	Decrease L infusion rate
Mexiletine	Hepatic enzyme inducers (phenytoin, barbiturates, rifampin)	Increased hepatic metabolism	Decreased plasma M levels	Increase M dose
Class IC				
Flecainide (F)	Amiodarone	Unknown	Blood F rises; added effects on nodes, myocardium	Decrease F dose

	Digoxin (D)	Decreased D clearance	Blood D rises slightly	Check D level
	Drugs inhibiting SA or AV nodes, IV conduction, or myocardial function	Pharmacodynamic, additive	SA, AV block; conduction block; negative inotropism	Decrease D dose
	Cimetidine	Decreased hepatic F loss	Blood F rises	Check F dose
Propafenone	Digoxin	Pharmacokinetic	Increased D level	Decrease D dose
Class III				
Amiodarone (A)	Drugs prolonging QT interval (quinidine, disopyramide, phenothiazines, tricyclic antidepressants, thiazide diuretics, sotalol)	Pharmacodynamic additive effects	Torsades de pointes	Avoid low K^+; avoid combinations
	Quinidine (Q)	Pharmacokinetic	Blood Q rises	Check Q levels
	Procainamide (P)	Pharmacokinetic	Blood P rises	Check P dose
Sotalol	Diuretic, K^+-losing	Hypokalemia plus class III action	Torsades de pointes	Exclude low K^+; use K^+-retaining diuretic

*APD = action potential duration; IV = intravenous; ACh = acetylcholine.

Source: Adapted from Opie LH: Adverse cardiovascular drug interactions, in Schlant RC, Alexander RW (eds): *The Heart*, 8th ed. New York, McGraw-Hill, 1994, pp 1971–1985, with permission.

whenever there is cotherapy with another agent. The safest rule is to tell patients having oral anticoagulation not to use any new or over-the-counter drugs without consultation and for the physician to carefully check any added compounds (Table 22-9). More frequent measurements of the prothrombin time [now replaced by international normalized ratio (INR)] are required when potentially interfering drugs are added.

Interfering drugs include those which reduce absorption of vitamin K or warfarin such as cholestyramine. Sulfinpyrazone increases warfarin levels by displacing it from plasma proteins. Other interfering drugs are those which induce hepatic enzymes (barbiturates, phenytoin, rifampin) to increase the rate of warfarin metabolism in the liver.

Yet other drugs decrease the hepatic degradation of warfarin to increase the anticoagulant effect, including antibiotics such as metronidazole and cotrimoxazole. Cimetidine likewise inhibits hepatic degradation; on first principles, ranitidine should not. Other potentiating cardiovascular agents are allopurinol, clofibrate, quinidine, and amiodarone. Amiodarone is especially dangerous because its very long half-life means a very long potentiation of warfarin. Heparin or aspirin may potentiate bleeding, though there are large interindividual variations. Very high doses of aspirin impair synthesis of clotting factors.

It must be reemphasized that sulfinpyrazone has a powerful effect in displacing warfarin from blood proteins, so that the dose of warfarin required may be reduced to only 1 mg.

Heparin

The physical properties of heparin are such that it is incompatible in a water solution with certain substances, including antibiotics, antihistamines, phenothiazides, and hydrocortisone. Direct pharmacokinetic or pharmacodynamic drug interactions, however, have not been described, apart from the resistance to heparin induced by high doses of intravenous nitroglycerin.

INTERACTIONS OF LIPID-LOWERING AGENTS

These increasingly popular drugs seem to have some serious interactions (Table 22-10). Warfarin may interact with some lipid-lowering agents either by decreased absorption (cholestyramine) or by hepatic interference (bezafibrate, gemfibrozil). Clofibrate (no longer used) and gemfibrozil increase the effects of warfarin. Probucol potentially prolongs the QT interval, particularly in the presence of additional agents such as thiazide diuretics or group IA or III antiarrhythmics; the risk is that torsades de pointes may be precipitated. The new hydroxymethylglutaryl coenzyme A (HMG-CoA) reductase inhibitors such as lovastatin, simvastatin, and pravastatin should not be combined with

TABLE 22-9 Drug Interactions of Antithrombotic Agents*

Cardiac drug	Interacting drugs	Mechanism	Consequence	Prophylaxis
Aspirin (A)	Hepatic enzyme inducers (barbiturates, phenytoin, rifampin)	Increased A metabolism	Decreased A effect	Adjust A dose; check A side effects
	Sulfinpyrazone (S) probenecid (P)	A decreases urate excretion	Decreased uricosuric effect of S or P	Increase dose of S or P
	Thiazide diuretics	A decreases urate excretion	Hyperuricemia	Low diuretic dose
	Warfarin (W)	A is antithrombotic	Excess bleeding	Check INR
	ACE inhibitors	? via PGs	Decreased ACEI effect	Decrease A dose[†]
Sulfinpyrazone (S)	Warfarin	S displaces W from plasma proteins	Excess bleeding	Check INR
Warfarin (W)	*Potentiating drugs*			
	Allopurinol	Mechanism unknown	Excess bleeding	Check INR
	Amiodarone	Mechanism unknown	Sensitizes to W for 1–2 months	Avoid combination
	Aspirin	Added bleeding tendency	Excess bleeding	Check INR
	Cimetidine	Decreased W degradation	Increased blood W	Check INR
	Quinidine	Hepatic interaction	Excess bleeding	Check INR
	Sulfinpyrazone	Displaces W from plasma proteins	Excess bleeding	Check INR
	Inhibitory drugs			
	Cholestyramine Colestipol	Decreased absorption of W	Decreased W effect	Check INR

*ACEI = angiotensin converting enzyme inhibitor; INR = international normalization ratio.
[†]See Table 22-5.

Source: Adapted from Opie LH: Adverse cardiovascular drug interactions, in Schlant RC, Alexander RW (eds): *The Heart*, 8th ed. New York, McGraw-Hill, 1994, pp 1971–1985, with permission.

TABLE 22-10 Drug Interactions of Lipid-Lowering Agents*

Cardiac drug	Interacting drugs	Mechanism	Consequence	Prophylaxis
Probucol	Thiazides, groups IA and III	Probucol-induced diarrhea with potassium loss?	QT prolongation	Check potassium; avoid combinations
Fibric acids (gemfibrozil, bezafibrate fenofibrate)	Warfarin	Hepatic interference	Risk of bleeding	Check INR
Bile acid sequestrants (cholestyramine, colestipol)	Warfarin (W)	Decreased absorption	Decreased W effect	Check INR
HMG-CoA reductase inhibitors (lovastatin, pravastatin, simvastatin)	Fibrates cyclosporine, erythromycin, nicotinic acid	Added risk of myositis	Rhabdomyolysis and risk of renal failure	Check creatine phosphokinase levels

*INR = international normalized ratio.

Source: Adapted from Opie LH: Adverse cardiovascular drug interactions, in Schlant RC, Alexander RW (eds): *The Heart*, 8th ed. New York, McGraw-Hill, 1994, pp 1971–1985, with permission.

fibrates because of the increased danger of myositis with rhabdomyolysis and the risk of renal failure, as explained in the product package inserts. Concurrent therapy with nicotinic acid or cyclosporine or erythromycin also increases the risk of rhabdomyolysis. As a precaution, serum creatine kinase levels should be checked at the commencement of cotherapy and whenever doses are increased. Nonetheless, according to the product package inserts on lovastatin and simvastatin, there is no assurance that such monitoring will prevent the occurrence of severe myopathy.

SUGGESTED READINGS

Opie LH: Interactions with cardiovascular drugs. *Curr Prob Cardiol* 18:529, 1993.

Opie LH: Adverse cardiovascular drug interactions, in Schlant RC, Alexander RW (eds): *The Heart*, 8th ed. New York, McGraw-Hill, 1994, pp 1971–1985.

Opie LH, Frishman WH, Thadani U: Calcium channel antagonists (calcium entry blockers), in Opie LH (ed): *Drugs for the Heart*, 4th ed. Philadelphia, WB Saunders, 1995, pp 50–82.

Opie LH: Cardiovascular drug interactions, in Frishman WH, Sonnenblick EH (eds): *Cardiovascular Pharmacotherapeutics.* New York, McGraw-Hill, 1997, pp 1383–1400.

Appendix 1 Pharmacokinetic Properties of Approved Cardiovascular Drugs

Sylvia Thomas, Angela Cheng and William H. Frishman

APPENDIX 1 Pharmacokinetics

Generic name	Bioavailability (%)	Protein binding (%)	Volume of distribution (liters/kg)	Half-life (hours)	Urinary excretion (% unchanged)	Clearance ($mL \cdot min^{-1} \cdot kg^{-1}$)	Therapeutic range	References
Abciximab	NA	—	—	0.5	—	—	—	Faulds D, Sorkin EM: Abciximab (c7E Fab): A review of its pharmacology and therapeutic potential in ischemic heart disease. *Drugs* 48:583–598, 1994.
Acebutolol	37 ± 12	26 ± 3	1.2 ± 0.3	2.7 ± 0.4	40 ± 11	6.8 ± 0.8	—	Singh BN, Thoden WR, Wahl J: Acebutolol: A review of its pharmacology, pharmacokinetics, clinical uses, and adverse effects. *Pharmacotherapy* 6:45–63, 1986.
Adenosine	—	—	0.11–0.19	<10 sec.	—	59–152	—	Blardi P, Laghi-Pasini F, Urso R, et al: Pharmacokinetics of exogenous adenosine in man after infusion. *Eur J Clin Pharmacol* 44:505–507, 1993.

Key: ↑ = increased; ↓ = decreased; **CAD** = coronary artery disease; **CHF** = congestive heart failure; **Cl** = clearance; **eld** = elderly; **F** = bioavailability; **HI** = hepatic impairment; **ID** = insufficient data; **MI** = myocardial infarction; **NA** = not applicable; **neo** = neonate; **RI** = renal impairment; **SL** = sublingual; $t_{1/2}$ = half-life; **TOP** = topical; ***Vd*** = volume of distribution.

APPENDIX 1 *(continued)*

Generic name	Bioavailability (%)	Protein binding (%)	Volume of distribution (liters/kg)	Half-life (hours)	Urinary excretion (% unchanged)	Clearance (mL · min^{-1} · kg^{-1})	Therapeutic range	References
Alteplase	—	—	0.10–0.17	3–5 min $t_{1/2}$ is ↑ in HI	—	9.8–10.4 Cl is ↓ in HI	0.45 μg/mL	Seifried E, Tanswell P, Rijken DC, et al: Pharmacokinetics of antigen and activity of recombinent tissue-type plasminogen activator after infusion in healthy volunteers. *Arzneimittelforschung* 38: 418–422, 1988.
Amiloride	15–25	23	17 ± 4	6–9 $t_{1/2}$ is ↑ in RF	49 ± 10 Cl is ↓ in eld and RI	9.7 ± 1.9	38–48 ng/mL	Vidt DG: Mechanism of action, pharmacokinetics, adverse effects, and therapeutic uses of amiloride hydrochloride, a new potassium-sparing diuretic. *Pharmacotherapy* 1:179–187, 1981.
Amiodarone	46 ± 22	99.98 ± 0.01	66 ± 44	25 ± 12 days	0	1.9 ± 0.4	1.0–2.5 μg/mL	Freeman MD, Somberg JC: Pharmacology and pharmacokinetics of amiodarone. *J Clin Pharmacol* 31:1061–1069, 1991.
Amlodipine	74 ± 17	93 ± 1	16 ± 4	39 ± 8 $t_{1/2}$ is ↑ in eld and HI	10	5.9 ± 1.5 Cl is ↓ in eld and HI	—	Abernethy DR: The pharmacokinetic profile of amlodipine. *Am Heart J* 118:1100–1103, 1989.

Amrinone	93 ± 12	35–49	1.3 ± 0.3	4.4 ± 1.4[1] 2.0 ± 0.6[2] $t_{1/2}$ is ↑ in CHF and neo	25 ± 10	4.0 ± 1.6[1] 8.9 ± 2.7[2] Cl is ↓ in CHF and neo	3.7 µg/mL	Steinberg C, Notterman DA: Pharmacokinetics of cardiovascular drugs in children; inotropes and vasopressors. *Clin Pharmacokinet* 27:345-367, 1994. [1]Slow acetylators [2]Fast acetylators
Anagrelide	—	—	12	1.3 h[1] 3 days[2]	<1	2.1	—	Spencer, CM, Brogden RN: Anagrelide: A review of its pharmacodynamic and pharmacokinetic properties, and therapeutic potential in the treatment of thrombocythaemia. *Drugs* 47:809–822, 1994. [1]Plasma half-life [2]Terminal elimination half-life
Anisindione	Variable	97–99	—	3–5 days	—	—	—	
Anistreplase	—	—	0.084 ± 0.027	1.2 ± 0.4	—	0.92 ± 0.36 Cl is ↓ in HI	—	Gemmill JD, Hogg KJ, Burns JMA, et al:. A comparison of the pharmacokinetic properties of streptokinase and anistreplase in acute myocardial infarction. *Br J Clin Pharmacol* 31:143–147, 1991.

Key: ↑ = increased; ↓ = decreased; **CAD** = coronary artery disease; **CHF** = congestive heart failure; **Cl** = clearance; **eld** = elderly; **F** = bioavailability; **HI** = hepatic impairment; **ID** = insufficient data; **MI** = myocardial infarction; **NA** = not applicable; **neo** = neonate; **RI** = renal impairment; **SL** = sublingual; $t_{1/2}$ = half-life; **TOP** = topical; ***Vd*** = volume of distribution.

APPENDIX 1 (*continued*)

Generic name	Bioavailability (%)	Protein binding (%)	Volume of distribution (liters/kg)	Half-life (hours)	Urinary excretion (% unchanged)	Clearance ($mL \cdot min^{-1} \cdot kg^{-1}$)	Therapeutic range	References
Ardeparin	90[1]	—	0.19[1]	3[1] (2.5–3.3) ↑ in RI	—	0.65–0.98[1] ↓ in RI	0.1–0.2 units/mL[2]	Troy S, Fruncillo R, Ozawa T, et al: The dose proportionality of the pharmacokinetics of ardeparin, a low molecular weight heparin, in healthy volunteers. *J Clin Pharmacol* 35:1194–1199. 1995. [1]Based on plasma antifactor Xa activity [2]Plasma antifactor Xa level at 6 or 12 hours postdose
Aspirin	50–100[1]	76–90	0.15–0.2	2.4–19[2] $t_{1/2}$ is ↑ in HI	2–30[3]	0.18–0.88 Cl is ↓ in HI and neo	150–300 μg/mL	Furst DE, Tozer TN, Melmon KL: Salicylate clearance, the resultant of protein binding and metabolism. *Clin Pharmacol Ther* 26: 380–389, 1979. [1]Dependent on formulation [2]Dependent on dose [3]Dependent on urinary pH
Atenolol	50–60	5–15	0.95 ± 0.15	6.1 ± 2.0 $t_{1/2}$ is ↑ in RI and eld	94 ± 8	2.0 ± 0.2 Cl is ↓ in eld and RI	0.1–1 μg/mL	Wadworth AN, Murdoch D, Brogden RN: Atenolol: A reappraisal of its pharmacological properties and therapeutic use in cardiovascular disorders. *Drugs* 42:468–510, 1991.

Atorvastatin	12	≥ 98	8	14 (11–24) ↑ in elderly	<2	—	—	Lea AP, McTavish D: Atorvastatin: A review of its pharmacology and therapeutic potential in the management of hyperlipidaemias. *Drugs* 53:828–847, 1997.
Atropine	50	14–22	2.0 ± 1.1 V_d is ↑ in child	3.5 ± 1.5 $t_{1/2}$ is ↑ in eld and child	57 ± 8	8 ± 4 Cl is ↓ in eld	—	Kentala E, Kaila T, Iisalo E, et al: Intramuscular atropine in healthy volunteers: A pharmacokinetic and pharmacodynamic study. *Int J Clin Pharmacol Ther Toxicol* 28:399–404, 1990.
Benazepril	37	95–97	0.12	0.6 10–11[1]	<1 18[1]	0.3–0.4	—	Kaiser G, Ackermann R, Brechbukler S, et al: Pharmacokinetics of the angiotensin converting enzyme inhibitor benazepril HCl (CGS 14 824 A) in healthy volunteers after single and repeated administration. *Biopharm Drug Dispos* 10:365–376, 1989. [1]Active metabolite
Bendroflu-methiazide	100	94	1.48	3–3.9	30	5.3 ± 1.4	—	Beermann B, Groschinsky-Grind M, Lindstrom B: Pharmacokinetics of bendroflumethiazide. *Clin Pharmacol Ther* 22:385–388, 1977.

Key: ↑ = increased; ↓ = decreased; **CAD** = coronary artery disease; **CHF** = congestive heart failure; **Cl** = clearance; **eld** = elderly; **F** = bioavailability; **HI** = hepatic impairment; **ID** = insufficient data; **MI** = myocardial infarction; **NA** = not applicable; **neo** = neonate; **RI** = renal impairment; **SL** = sublingual; $t_{1/2}$ = half-life; **TOP** = topical; ***Vd*** = volume of distribution.

APPENDIX 1 (*continued*)

Generic name	Bioavailability (%)	Protein binding (%)	Volume of distribution (liters/kg)	Half-life (hours)	Urinary excretion (% unchanged)	Clearance $(mL \cdot min^{-1} \cdot kg^{-1})$	Therapeutic range	References
Bepridil	60	>99	8 ± 5	12–24	<1	5.3 ± 2.5	—	Benet LZ: Pharmacokinetics and metabolism of bepridil. *Am J Cardiol* 55: 8C–13C, 1985.
Betaxolol	76–89	50–55	4.9–9.8	14–22 $t_{1/2}$ is ↑ in eld	15	4.7 Cl is ↓ in eld	20–50 ng/mL	Frishman WH, Tepper D, Lazar EJ, et al: Betaxolol: A new long-acting $beta_1$-selective adrenergic blocker; *J Clin Pharmacol* 30:686–692, 1990.
Bisoprolol	85–91	30–35	3.2 ± 0.5	8.2–12 $t_{1/2}$ is ↑ in RI	50–60	3.7 ± 0.7 Cl is ↓ in RI	—	Lancaster SG, Sorkin EM: Bisoprolol: A preliminary review of its pharmacodynamic and pharmacokinetic properties, and therapeutic efficacy in hypertension and angina pectoris. *Drugs* 36: 256–285, 1988.
Bretylium	23 ± 9	0–8	5.9 ± 0.8	5–10 $t_{1/2}$ is ↑ in RI	70–80	10.2 ± 1.9 Cl is ↓ in RI	—	Rapaport WG: Clinical pharmacokinetics of bretylium. *Clin Pharmacokinet* 10:248–256, 1985.
Bumetanide	55–89	99 ± 0.3	0.13 ± 0.03 V_d is ↑ in RI and HI	0.3–1.5 $t_{1/2}$ is ↑ in RI, HI, and CHF	62 ± 20	2.6 ± 0.5 Cl is ↓ in RI, HI, and CHF	—	Cook JA, Smith DE, Cornish LA, et al: Kinetics, dynamics, and bioavailability of bumetanide in healthy subjects and patients with congestive heart failure.

								Clin Pharmacol Ther 44:487–500, 1988.
Captopril	65–75	30 ± 6	0.81 ± 0.18	2.2 ± 0.5 $t_{1/2}$ is ↑ in RI and CHF	40–50	12.0 ± 1.4 Cl is ↓ in RI	0.05–0.5 μg/mL	Duchin KL, McKinstry DN, Cohen AI, et al: Pharmacokinetics of captopril in healthy subjects and in patients with cardiovascular diseases. *Clin Pharmacokinet* 14:241–259, 1988.
Carteolol	85	23–30	—	5–7 $t_{1/2}$ is ↑ in RI	50–70	—	—	Chrisp P, Sorkin EM: Ocular carteolol: A review of its pharmacological properties, and therapeutic use in glaucoma and ocular hypertension. *Drugs Aging* 2:58–77, 1992.
Carvedilol	25	95	1.5 ± 0.3	7–10[1] $t_{1/2}$ is ↑ in HI	<2	8.7 ± 1.7 Cl is ↓ in HI	—	Dunn CJ, Lea AP, Wagstaff AJ: Carvedilol: A reappraisal of its pharmacological properties and therapeutic use in cardiovascular disorders. *Drugs* 54:161–185, 1997. [1]Apparent mean terminal elimination half-life

Key: ↑ = increased; ↓ = decreased; **CAD** = coronary artery disease; **CHF** = congestive heart failure; **Cl** = clearance; **eld** = elderly; **F** = bioavailability; **HI** = hepatic impairment; **ID** = insufficient data; **MI** = myocardial infarction; **NA** = not applicable; **neo** = neonate; **RI** = renal impairment; **SL** = sublingual; $t_{1/2}$ = half-life; **TOP** = topical; ***Vd*** = volume of distribution.

APPENDIX 1 (*continued*)

Generic name	Bioavailability (%)	Protein binding (%)	Volume of distribution (liters/kg)	Half-life (hours)	Urinary excretion (% unchanged)	Clearance (mL · min^{-1} · kg^{-1})	Therapeutic range	References
Cerivastatin	60 (39–100)	>99	0.3	2–3	<2	2.9–3.1[1]	—	Bayer: Baycol package insert, West Haven, CT; 1997. [1]Plasma clearance
Chlorothiazide	10–21	20–80	0.20 ± 0.08	1.5 ± 0.2 $t_{1/2}$ is ↑ in RI and CHF	92 ± 5	4.5 ± 1.7 Cl is ↓ in RI	—	Osmon MA, Patel RB, Irwin DS, et al: Bioavailability of chlorothiazide from 50, 100, and 250 mg solution doses. *Biopharm Drug Dispos* 3:89–94, 1982.
Chlorthalidone	64 ± 10	75 ± 1	0.10 ± 0.04	47 ± 22 $t_{1/2}$ is ↑ in eld	65 ± 9	0.04 ± 0.01 Cl is ↓ in eld	—	Williams RL, Blume CD, Lin ET, et al: Relative bioavailability of chlorthalidone in humans: Adverse influence of polyethylene glycol. *J Pharm Sci* 71:533–535, 1982.
Clofibrate	95 ± 10	95–98	0.11 ± 0.02	12–22 $t_{1/2}$ is ↑ in RI	5.7 ± 2.1	0.12 ± 0.01 Cl is ↓ in RI	162–200 μg/mL	Gugler R, Kurten JW, Jensen CJ, et al: Clofibrate disposition in renal failure and acute and chronic liver disease. *Eur J Clin Pharmacol* 15:341–347, 1979.
Clonidine	95	20	2.1 ± 0.4	12–16 $t_{1/2}$ is ↑ in RI	40–60	3.1 ± 1.2 Cl is ↓ in RI	0.2–2 ng/mL	Lowenthal DT, Matzek KM, McGregor TR: Clinical pharmacokinetics of clonidine. *Clin Pharmacokinet* 14:287–310, 1988.

Clopidogrel	—	98	—	8[1]	50	—	—	Sanofi: Plavix package insert, New York, NY; 1997. [1]Half life of primary metabolite (inactive carboxylic-acid derivative)
Dalteparin	87	—	0.04–0.06	3–5 $t_{1/2}$ is ↓ in RI	—	0.27–0.41	0.1–0.6 anti-Xa units/mL	Simonean G, et al: Pharmacokinetics of a low molecular weight heparin (Fragmin®) in young and elderly subjects. *Thromb Res* 66:603–607, 1992.
Danaparoid	100[1]	—	0.11–0.13[1]	24[1] ↑ in RI	—	0.086–0.190[2]	0.15–0.40 units/mL[3]	Skoutakis VA: Danaparoid in the prevention of thromboembolic complications. *Ann Pharmacother* 31:876–887, 1997. [1]Based on plasma antifactor Xa activity [2]Total plasma clearance of plasma antifactor Xa activity [3]Plasma antifactor Xa level at 6 hours postdose; further studies are needed to determine if a therapeutic window exists for danaparoid.

Key: ↑ = increased; ↓ = decreased; **CAD** = coronary artery disease; **CHF** = congestive heart failure; **Cl** = clearance; **eld** = elderly; **F** = bioavailability; **HI** = hepatic impairment; **ID** = insufficient data; **MI** = myocardial infarction; **NA** = not applicable; **neo** = neonate; **RI** = renal impairment; **SL** = sublingual; $t_{1/2}$ = half-life; **TOP** = topical; ***Vd*** = volume of distribution.

APPENDIX 1 (*continued*)

Generic name	Bioavailability (%)	Protein binding (%)	Volume of distribution (liters/kg)	Half-life (hours)	Urinary excretion (% unchanged)	Clearance (mL · min^{-1} · kg^{-1})	Therapeutic range	References
Dexfenfluramine	69	36	10.5–14	13–24	7–19	8.6–11.5	15–92 ng/mL	Cheymol G, et al: The pharmacokinetics of dexfenfluramine in obese and non-obese subjects. *Br J Clin Pharmacol* 39:684–687, 1995.
Dicoumarol	Variable	99	—	1–2 days	—	—	—	
Digitoxin	>90	97 ± 0.5	0.54 ± 0.14 V_d is ↑ in child	6.7 ± 1.7 days	32 ± 15	0.055 ± 0.018 Cl is ↑ in child	14–26 ng/mL	Mooradian AD: Digitalis: An update of clinical pharmacokinetics, therapeutic monitoring techniques and treatment recommendations. *Clin Pharmacokinet* 15:165–179, 1988.
Digoxin	70 ± 1.3	20–25	—	39 ± 13 $t_{1/2}$ ↑ in RI, CHF, eld	60 ± 11	[(0.8 mL/min/kg) (wt in kg) + Cl_{cr}][1]; ↑ in neo, child	0.5–2 ng/mL	Mooradian AD: Digitalis: An update of clinical pharmacokinetics, therapeutic monitoring techniques and treatment recommendations. *Clin Pharmacokinet* 15:165–179, 1988. [1]Total digoxin clearance in patients without CHF (mL/min)
Diltiazem	40–67	70–80	3.1 ± 1.2 V_d ↓ in RI	3.7–6	2–4	12 ± 4 Cl is ↓ in RI	50–200 ng/mL	Echizen H, Eichelbaum M: Clinical pharmacokinetics of verapamil, nifedipine and diltiazem. *Clin Pharmacokinet* 11:425–449, 1986.

Dipyridamole	37–66	91–99	—	10–12	<5	—	—	Gregov D, Jenkins A, Duncan E, et al: Dipyridamole: Pharmacokinetics and effects on aspects of platelet function in man. *Br J Clin Pharmacol* 24:425–434, 1987.
Disopyramide	83 ± 11	68–89	0.59 ± 0.15	4–10 $t_{1/2}$ ↑ in RI, CHF	55 ± 6	1.2 ± 0.4 Cl ↓ in MI, CHF, RI, HI	2–4 μg/mL	Siddoway LA, Woosley RL: Clinical pharmacokinetics of disopyramide. *Clin Pharmacokinet* 11: 214–222, 1986.
Dobutamine	NA	ID	0.20 ± 0.08	2.4 ± 0.7 min	0	59 ± 22 Cl ↑ in child	40–190 ng/mL	Steinberg C, Notterman DA: Pharmacokinetics of cardiovascular drugs in children: Inotropes and vasopressors. *Clin Pharmacokinet* 27:345–367, 1994.
Dopamine	NA	0	—	2 min	<5	—	—	Kulka PJ, Tryba M: Inotropic support of the critically ill patient. *Drugs* 45: 654–667, 1993.
Doxazosin	63 ± 14	98.9 ± 0.5	1.5 ± 0.3	19–22	—	1.7 ± 0.4	—	Donelly R, Meredith PA, Elliott HL: Pharmacokinetic-pharmacodynamic relationships of α-adrenoceptor antagonists. *Clin Pharmacokinet* 17:264–274, 1989.

Key: ↑ = increased; ↓ = decreased; **CAD** = coronary artery disease; **CHF** = congestive heart failure; **Cl** = clearance; **eld** = elderly; **F** = bioavailability; **HI** = hepatic impairment; **ID** = insufficient data; **MI** = myocardial infarction; **NA** = not applicable; **neo** = neonate; **RI** = renal impairment; **SL** = sublingual; $t_{1/2}$ = half-life; **TOP** = topical; ***Vd*** = volume of distribution.

APPENDIX 1 (*continued*)

Generic name	Bioavailability (%)	Protein binding (%)	Volume of distribution (liters/kg)	Half-life (hours)	Urinary excretion (% unchanged)	Clearance (mL · min^{-1} · kg^{-1})	Therapeutic range	References
Enalapril	41 ± 15	< 50	1.7 ± 0.7	1.3 11[1] $t_{1/2}$ is ↑ in RI and HI	54 40[1]	4.9 ± 1.5 Cl is ↓ in RI, eld, CHF, neo and ↑ in child	5–20 ng/mL	Louis WJ, Conway EL, Krum H, et al: Comparison of the pharmacokinetics and pharmacodynamics of perindopril, cilazapril and enalapril. *Clin Exp Pharmacol Physiol* 19 (Suppl 19):55–60, 1992. [1]Enalaprilat
Encainide	25–90[1]	75–85	3.6–3.9	1–2[2] 6–11[3]	5[2] 40–45[3]	30[2] 2.5[3]	250 ng/mL	Brogden RN, Todd PA: Encainide: A review of its pharmacological properties and therapeutic efficacy. *Drugs* 34: 519–538, 1987. [1]Depends on metabolic phenotype [2]Fast oxidizer [3]Slow oxidizer
Enoxaparin	92	—	0.08	4.5 $t_{1/2}$ is ↑ in RI	8–20	0.3 ± 0.1 Cl is ↓ in RI	—	Bendetowicz AV, Beguin S, Caplain H, et al: Pharmacokinetics and pharmacodynamics of a low molecular weight heparin (enoxaparin) after subcutaneous injection, comparison with

								unfractionated heparin—a three-way crossover study in healthy volunteers. *Thromb Haemost* 71:305–313, 1994.
Esmolol	NA	55	1.9 ± 1.3	0.13 ± 0.07 $t_{1/2}$ is ↓ in child	<1	170 ± 70 Cl is ↓ in CAD and ↑ in child	—	Weist D: Esmolol: A review of its therapeutic efficacy and pharmacokinetic characteristics. *Clin Pharmacokinet* 28: 190–202, 1995.
Ethacrynic acid	100	90	—	0.5–1	65	—	—	
Felodipine	20	99.6 ± 0.2	10 ± 3	10–17 $t_{1/2}$ is ↑ in eld, CHF	<1	12 ± 5 Cl is ↓ in eld, HI, CHF	—	Edgar B, Lundborg P, Regardh CG: Clinical pharmacokinetics of felodipine: A summary. *Drugs* 34(Suppl 3):16–27, 1987.
Fenoldopam	5.7	88	0.23–0.66	0.16	1	24.8–38.2	3.5–14.25 μg/L	Brogden RN and Markham A: Fenoldopam: A review of its pharmacodynamic and pharmacokinetic properties and intravenous clinical potential in the management of hypertensive urgencies and emergencies. *Drugs* 54(4):634–650, 1997.

Key: ↑ = increased; ↓ = decreased; **CAD** = coronary artery disease; **CHF** = congestive heart failure; **Cl** = clearance; **eld** = elderly; **F** = bioavailability; **HI** = hepatic impairment; **ID** = insufficient data; **MI** = myocardial infarction; **NA** = not applicable; **neo** = neonate; **RI** = renal impairment; **SL** = sublingual; $t_{1/2}$ = half-life; **TOP** = topical; ***Vd*** = volume of distribution.

APPENDIX 1 (*continued*)

Generic name	Bioavailability (%)	Protein binding (%)	Volume of distribution (liters/kg)	Half-life (hours)	Urinary excretion (% unchanged)	Clearance (mL · min^{-1} · kg^{-1})	Therapeutic range	References
Flecainide	85–90	40–50	4.9 ± 0.4	12–30 $t_{1/2}$ is ↑ in RI, HI, CHF and ↓ in child	10–50	5.6 ± 1.3 Cl is ↓ in RI, HI, CHF	0.4–0.8 μg/mL	Funck-Bretano C, Becquemont L, Kroemer HK, et al: Variable disposition kinetics and electrocardiographic effects of flecainide during repeated dosing in humans: Contribution of genetic factors, dose-dependent clearance and interaction with amiodarone. *Clin Pharmacol Ther* 55: 256–269, 1994.
Fluvastatin	9–50	98	—	1.2 $t_{1/2}$ is ↑ in HI	<5	—	—	Tse FLS, Jaffe JM, Troendle A: Pharmacokinetics of fluvastatin after single and multiple doses in normal volunteers. *J Clin Pharmacol* 32:630-638, 1992.
Fosinopril	36 ± 7	≥ 95	0.13 ± 0.03	11.3 ± 0.7[1] $t_{1/2}$ is ↑ in RI	<2	0.51 ± 0.10 Cl is ↓ in HI, RI	—	Hui KK, Duchin KL, Kripalani KJ, et al: Pharmacokinetics of fosinopril in patients with various degrees of renal function. *Clin Pharmacol Ther* 49: 457–467, 1991.

[1]Fosinoprilat

Furosemide	61 ± 17	98.8 ± 0.2	0.11 ± 0.02	0.5–1.0 $t_{1/2}$ ↑ in RI, CHF, neo, HI, eld	66 ± 7	2.0 ± 0.4 Cl is ↓ in RI, CHF, neo, eld	ID	Hammarlund-Udenaes M, Benet LZ: Furosemide pharmacokinetics and pharmacodynamics in health and disease—an update. *J Pharmacokinet Biopharm* 17:1–46, 1989.
Gemfibrozil	98 ± 1	> 97	0.14 ± 0.03	1.1 ± 0.2	<1	1.7 ± 0.4	—	Todd PA, Ward A: Gemfibrozil, a review of its pharmacodynamic and pharmacokinetic properties and therapeutic use in dyslipidaemia. *Drugs* 36:314–339, 1988.
Guanabenz	ID	95	93–147	4–14	<1	—	—	Holmes B, Brogden RN, Heel RC, et al: Guanabenz: A review of its pharmacodynamic properties and therapeutic efficacy in hypertension. *Drugs* 26: 212–229, 1983.
Guanadrel	85	<20	—	10–12 $t_{1/2}$ ↑ in RI	40	—	—	Finnerty FA Jr, Brogden RN: Guanadrel: A review of its pharmacodynamic and pharmacokinetic properties and therapeutic use in hypertension. *Drugs* 30:22–31, 1985.

Key: ↑ = increased; ↓ = decreased; **CAD** = coronary artery disease; **CHF** = congestive heart failure; **Cl** = clearance; **eld** = elderly; **F** = bioavailability; **HI** = hepatic impairment; **ID** = insufficient data; **MI** = myocardial infarction; **NA** = not applicable; **neo** = neonate; **RI** = renal impairment; **SL** = sublingual; $t_{1/2}$ = half-life; **TOP** = topical; ***Vd*** = volume of distribution.

APPENDIX 1 (*continued*)

Generic name	Bioavailability (%)	Protein binding (%)	Volume of distribution (liters/kg)	Half-life (hours)	Urinary excretion (% unchanged)	Clearance ($mL \cdot min^{-1} \cdot kg^{-1}$)	Therapeutic range	References
Guanethidine	3–30	—	—	4–8 days	50	0.8	8–17 ng/mL	Woosley RL, Nies AS: Guanethidine. *N Engl J Med* 295:1053–1057, 1976.
Guanfacine	80	70	6.3	10–30	40–75	—	5–10 ng/mL	Sorkin EM, Heel RC: Guanfacine: A review of its pharmacodynamic and pharmacokinetic properties and therapeutic efficacy in the treatment of hypertension. *Drugs* 31:301–336, 1986.
Heparin	NA	—	0.058 ± 0.01	1–2[1]	≤50	0.5–0.6[2]	—	Estes JW: Clinical pharmacokinetics of heparin. *Clin Pharmacokinet* 5:204–220, 1980. [1]Increases with dose [2]Plasma clearance
Hydralazine	16 ± 15[1] 35 ± 4[2]	87	1.5 ± 1.0	2–4 $t_{1/2}$ is ↑ in CHF	1–15	56 ± 13 Cl is ↓ in CHF	—	Mulrow JP, Crawford MH: Clinical pharmacokinetics and therapeutic use of hydralazine in congestive heart failure *Clin Pharmacokinet* 16:86–89, 1989. [1]Rapid acetylator [2]Slow acetylator

Hydrochlo-rothiazide	65–75	58 ± 17	0.83 ± 0.31	2–15 $t_{1/2}$ is ↑ in RI, CHF and eld	>95	4.9 ± 1.1 Cl is ↓ in RI, CHF and eld	—	Beerman B, Groschinsky-Grind M: Pharmacokinetics of hydrochlorothiazide in man. *Eur J Clin Pharmacol* 12: 297–303, 1977.
Hydroflu-methiazide	50	74	—	12–27	40–80	—	—	Brors O, Jacobsen S: Pharmacokinetics of hydroflumethiazide during repeated oral administration to healthy subjects. *Eur J Pharmacol* 15:281–286, 1979.
Ibutilide	—	40	11	6 ± 4	7	29	—	Jungbluth GL, et al: Evaluation of the pharmacokinetics and pharmacodynamics of ibutilide fumarate and its enantiomers in healthy male volunteers (Abstract). *Pharm Res* 8:S249, 1991.
Indapamide	93	71–79	0.86–1.57	14–18	7	—	—	Caruso FS, Szabadi RR, Vukovich RA: Pharmacokinetics and clinical pharmacology of indapamide. *Am Heart J* 106: 212–220, 1983.

Key: ↑ = increased; ↓ = decreased; **CAD** = coronary artery disease; **CHF** = congestive heart failure; **Cl** = clearance; **eld** = elderly; **F** = bioavailability; **HI** = hepatic impairment; **ID** = insufficient data; **MI** = myocardial infarction; **NA** = not applicable; **neo** = neonate; **RI** = renal impairment; **SL** = sublingual; $t_{1/2}$ = half-life; **TOP** = topical; ***Vd*** = volume of distribution.

APPENDIX 1 (*continued*)

Generic name	Bioavailability (%)	Protein binding (%)	Volume of distribution (liters/kg)	Half-life (hours)	Urinary excretion (% unchanged)	Clearance ($mL \cdot min^{-1} \cdot kg^{-1}$)	Therapeutic range	References
Irbesartan	60–80	~90	0.76–1.33	11–15	1	2.3–2.6	—	Gillis JC and Markham A: Irbesartan: A review of its pharmacodynamic and pharmacokinetic properties and therapeutic use in the management of hypertension. *Drugs* 54(6): 885–902, 1997.
Isosorbide dinitrate	22 ± 14[1] 45 ± 16[2]	28 ± 12	3.9 ± 1.5	1.0 ± 0.5	<1	45 ± 20 Cl is ↓ in HI	—	Fung HL: Pharmacokinetics and pharmacodynamics of organic nitrates. *Am J Cardiol* 60:4H–9H, 1987. [1]Oral [2]Sublingual
Isosorbide mononitrate	93 ± 13	<4	0.73 ± 0.09	4.9 ± 0.8	<5	1.80 ± 0.24	100 ng/mL	Abshagen UWP: Pharmacokinetics of isosorbide mononitrate. *Am J Cardiol* 70:61G–66G, 1992.
Isoxsuprine	100	ID	—	1.25	—	—	—	
Isradipine	15–24 F is ↑ in eld and HI	97	4.0 ± 1.9	8 ± 5	0	10 ± 1	—	Fitton A, Benfield P: Isradipine: A review of its pharmacodynamic and pharmacokinetic properties and therapeutic use in cardiovascular disease. *Drugs* 40:31–74, 1990.

Labetalol	18 ± 5 F ↑ in eld, HI	50	9.4 ± 3.4	4.9 ± 2.0 $t_{1/2}$ ↑ in eld	<5	25 ± 10 Cl ↓ in eld	—	Donnelly R, Macphee GJA: Clinical pharmacokinetics and kinetic-dynamic relationships of dilevalol and labetalol. *Clin Pharmacokinet* 21:95–109, 1991.
Lidocaine	NA	50–70	1.1 ± 0.4	1.8 ± 0.4 $t_{1/2}$ is ↑ in HI, neo	<10	9.2 ± 2.4 Cl is ↓ in CHF, HI	1.5–6 μg/mL	Thompson PD, Melmon KL, Richardson JA, et al: Lidocaine pharmacokinetics in advanced heart failure, liver disease and renal disease in humans. *Ann Intern Med* 78:499–508, 1973.
Lisinopril	25 ± 20 F ↓ in CHF	0	2.4 ± 1.4	12 $t_{1/2}$ is ↑ in eld RI	88–100	4.2 ± 2.2 Cl is ↓ in CHF, RI, eld	—	Sica DA, Cutler RE, Parmer RJ, et al: Comparison of the steady-state pharmacokinetics of fosinopril, lisinopril and enalapril in patients with chronic renal insufficiency. *Clin Pharmacokinet* 20:420–427, 1991.

Key: ↑ = increased; ↓ = decreased; **CAD** = coronary artery disease; **CHF** = congestive heart failure; **Cl** = clearance; **eld** = elderly; **F** = bioavailability; **HI** = hepatic impairment; **ID** = insufficient data; **MI** = myocardial infarction; **NA** = not applicable; **neo** = neonate; **RI** = renal impairment; **SL** = sublingual; $t_{1/2}$ = half-life; **TOP** = topical; ***Vd*** = volume of distribution.

APPENDIX 1 (*continued*)

Generic name	Bioavailability (%)	Protein binding (%)	Volume of distribution (liters/kg)	Half-life (hours)	Urinary excretion (% unchanged)	Clearance (mL · min^{-1} · kg^{-1})	Therapeutic range	References
Losartan	33 F is ↑ in HI	98	0.49	1.5–2.5 6–9[1]	4	8.6 Cl is ↓ in HI	—	Ohtawa M, Takayama F, Saitoh K, et al: Pharmacokinetics and biochemical efficacy after single and multiple oral administration of losartan, an orally active non-peptide angiotensin II receptor antagonist, in humans. *Br J Clin Pharmacol* 35:290–297, 1993. [1]Active metabolite
Lovastatin	<5	>95	—	3–4	<5	4–18 Cl is ↓ in RI	—	McKenney JM: Lovastatin: A new cholesterol-lowering agent. *Clin Pharmacol* 7:21–36, 1988.
Mecamylamine	ID	—	—	ID	50[1]	—	—	[1]Depends on urinary pH
Methyldopa	42 ± 16	1–16	0.46 ± 0.15	1.8 ± 0.6 $t_{1/2}$ is ↑ in RI, neo	40 ± 13	3.7 ± 1.0 Cl is ↓ in RI	—	Skerjanee A, Campbell NRC, Robertson S, et al: Pharmacokinetics and presystemic gut metabolism of methyldopa in healthy human subjects. *J Clin Pharmacol* 35:275–280, 1995.

Metolazone	40–65	95[1]	1.6	14	70–95	—	—	Tilstone WJ, Dargie H, Dargie EN, et al: Pharmacokinetics of metolazone in normal subjects and in patients with cardiac or renal failure. *Clin Pharmacol Ther* 16:322–329, 1974. [1]50–78% is bound to erythrocytes
Metoprolol	38 ± 14 F is ↑ in HI	11 ± 1	4.2 ± 0.7	3–4 $t_{1/2}$ is ↑ in HI, neo	10 ± 3	15 ± 3	50–100 ng/mL	Dayer P, Leemann T, Marmy A, et al: Interindividual variation of beta-adrenoceptor blocking drugs, plasma concentration and effect: Influence of genetic status on behaviour of atenolol, bopindolol and metoprolol. *Eur J Clin Pharmacol* 28:149–153, 1985.
Mexiletine	87 ± 13	50–60	4.9 ± 0.5	9.2 ± 2.1 $t_{1/2}$ ↑ in MI, CHF, RI, and HI	10	6.3 ± 2.7 Cl is ↓ in MI, RI (Cl_{cr} <10 mL/min), HI	0.5–2.0 μg/mL	Monk JP, Brogden RN: Mexiletine: a review of its pharmacodynamic and pharmacokinetic properties, and therapeutic use in the treatment of arrhythmias. *Drugs* 40:374–411, 1990.

Key: ↑ = increased; ↓ = decreased; **CAD** = coronary artery disease; **CHF** = congestive heart failure; **Cl** = clearance; **eld** = elderly; **F** = bioavailability; **HI** = hepatic impairment; **ID** = insufficient data; **MI** = myocardial infarction; **NA** = not applicable; **neo** = neonate; **RI** = renal impairment; **SL** = sublingual; $t_{1/2}$ = half-life; **TOP** = topical; ***Vd*** = volume of distribution.

APPENDIX 1 (*continued*)

Generic name	Bioavailability (%)	Protein binding (%)	Volume of distribution (liters/kg)	Half-life (hours)	Urinary excretion (% unchanged)	Clearance (mL · min^{-1} · kg^{-1})	Therapeutic range	References
Mibefradil	>90	>99	2.8	17–25	<1	—	—	Reid JL, Petrie JR, Glen SK, Meredith PA, Elliott HL: Clinical pharmacology of the novel calcium antagonist mibefradil. *J Cardiovasc Pharmacol* 27(Suppl A):S22–S26, 1996.
Midodrine	90–93[1]	—	4–4.6[1]	0.5 3[1]	2–4	19.7–24.3[2]	—	McTavish D, Goa KL: Midodrine: A review of its pharmacological properties and therapeutic use in orthostatic hypotension and secondary hypotensive disorders. *Drugs* 38:757–777, 1989. [1]Based on desglymidodrine, active metabolite of midodrine. [2]Total body plasma clearance of desglymidodrine
Milrinone	≥80	70	0.32 ± 0.08	0.80 ± 0.22 $t_{1/2}$ is ↑ in CHF, RI	85 ± 10	6.1 ± 1.3 Cl is ↓ in CHF, RI	150–250 ng/mL	Young RA, Ward A: Milrinone: A preliminary review of its pharmacological properties and therapeutic use. *Drugs* 36:158–192, 1988.
Minoxidil	ID	0	2.7 ± 0.7	3.1 ± 0.6[1]	20 ± 6	24 ± 6	—	Fleishaker JC, Andreadis NA, Welshman IR, et al: The pharmacokinetics of 2.5 to 10 mg oral doses of minoxidil in healthy

								volunteers. *J Clin Pharmacol* 29: 162–167, 1989. [1]Hypertensives
Moexipril	13	90	—	1.3 2–9[1]	<10	—	—	Van Hecken A, et al: Moexipril does not alter the pharmacokinetics or pharmacodynamics of warfarin. *Eur J Clin Pharmacol* 45:291–293, 1993. [1]Moexiprilat
Moricizine	38	95	4.4	1.5–3.5 $t_{1/2}$ is ↑ in HI	<1	—	—	Fitton A, Buckley MM: Moricizine: A review of its pharmacological properties, and therapeutic efficacy in cardiac arrhythmias. *Drugs* 40:138–167, 1990.
Nadolol	34 ± 5	20 ± 4	1.9 ± 0.2	16 ± 2 $t_{1/2}$ is ↑ in RI and child	73 ± 4	2.9 ± 0.6 Cl is ↓ in RI	—	Morrison RA, Singhvi SM, Creasey WA, et al: Dose proportionality of nadolol pharmacokinetics after intravenous administration to healthy subjects. *Eur J Clin Pharmacol* 33:625–628, 1988.
Nicardipine	18 ± 11	98–99.5	1.1 ± 0.3	2–4 $t_{1/2}$ is ↑ in HI	<1	10.4 ± 3.1 Cl is ↓ in HI	0.1 μg/mL	Singh BN, Josephson MA: Clinical pharmacology, pharmacokinetics and hemodynamic effects of nicardipine. *Am Heart J* 119:427–434, 1990.

Key: ↑ = increased; ↓ = decreased; **CAD** = coronary artery disease; **CHF** = congestive heart failure; **Cl** = clearance; **eld** = elderly; **F** = bioavailability; **HI** = hepatic impairment; **ID** = insufficient data; **MI** = myocardial infarction; **NA** = not applicable; **neo** = neonate; **RI** = renal impairment; **SL** = sublingual; $t_{1/2}$ = half-life; **TOP** = topical; ***Vd*** = volume of distribution.

APPENDIX 1 (*continued*)

Generic name	Bioavailability (%)	Protein binding (%)	Volume of distribution (liters/kg)	Half-life (hours)	Urinary excretion (% unchanged)	Clearance (mL · min^{-1} · kg^{-1})	Therapeutic range	References
Nicotinic acid	88	<20	—	0.75–1	[1]	—	—	[1]Increases with ↑ dose
Nifedipine	50 ± 13	96 ± 1	0.78 ± 0.22	2.5 ± 1.3	<1	7.0 ± 1.8	47 ± 20 ng/mL	Soons PA, Schoemaker HC, Cohen AF, et al: Intraindividual variability in nifedipine pharmacokinetics and effects in healthy subjects. *J Clin Pharmacol* 32:324–331, 1992.
Nimodipine	10 ± 4 F is ↑ in HI	98	1.7 ± 0.6	1.1 ± 0.3 $t_{1/2}$ is ↑ in HI and RI	<1	19 ± 6 Cl is ↓ in HI and RI	—	Langley MS, Sorkin EM: Nimodipine: A review of its pharmacodynamic and pharmacokinetic properties, and therapeutic potential in cerebrovascular disease. *Drugs* 37:669–699, 1989.
Nisoldipine	3.7 F is ↑ in HI	99	4–5	8–9 $t_{1/2}$ is ↑ in HI	—	—	—	Baksi AK, Edwards JS, Ahr G: A comparison of the pharmacokinetics of nisoldipine in elderly and young subjects. *Br J Clin Pharmacol* 31:367–370, 1991.
Nitroglycerin	Oral:<1 SL: 38 ± 26 TOP: 72 ± 20	60	2.9	1–4 min	—	—	—	Thadani U, Whitsett T: Relationship of pharmacokinetic and pharmacodynamic properties of the organic nitrates. *Clin Pharmacokinet* 15:32–43, 1988.

Penbutolol	100	80–98	—	5 $t_{1/2}$ is ↑ in RI	<10	—	—	Brockmeier D, Hajdu P, Henke W, et al: Penbutolol: Pharmacokinetics, effect on exercise tachycardia, and in vitro inhibition of radioligand binding. *Eur J Clin Pharmacol* 35:613–623, 1988.
Pentoxi-fylline	33 ± 13 F is ↑ in HI	0	4.2 ± 0.9	0.9 ± 0.3 $t_{1/2}$ is ↑ in eld and HI	0	60 ± 13 Cl is ↓ in eld and HI	—	Ward A, Clissold SP: Pentoxifylline: A review of its pharmacodynamic and pharmacokinetic properties, and its therapeutic efficacy. *Drugs* 34:50–97, 1987.
Pindolol	75 ± 9 F is ↓ in RI	40–60	2.3 ± 0.9	3.6 ± 0.6 $t_{1/2}$ is ↑ in RI and HI	35–50	8.3 ± 1.8 Cl is ↓ in RI and HI	—	Guerret M, Cheymol G, Aubry JP, et al: Estimation of the absolute oral bioavailability of pindolol by two analytical methods. *Eur J Clin Pharmacol* 25:357–359, 1983.
Polythiazide	ID	84	—	25.7	25	—	—	
Pravastatin	18 ± 8	43–48	0.46 ± 0.04	1.8 ± 0.8	20	13.5[1] Cl is ↓ in HI	—	Quion JAV, Jones PH: Clinical pharmacokinetics of pravastatin. *Clin Pharmacokinet* 27:94–103, 1994. [1]Clearance after intravenous dose

Key: ↑ = increased; ↓ = decreased; **CAD** = coronary artery disease; **CHF** = congestive heart failure; **Cl** = clearance; **eld** = elderly; **F** = bioavailability; **HI** = hepatic impairment; **ID** = insufficient data; **MI** = myocardial infarction; **NA** = not applicable; **neo** = neonate; **RI** = renal impairment; **SL** = sublingual; $t_{1/2}$ = half-life; **TOP** = topical; ***Vd*** = volume of distribution.

APPENDIX 1 (*continued*)

Generic name	Bioavailability (%)	Protein binding (%)	Volume of distribution (liters/kg)	Half-life (hours)	Urinary excretion (% unchanged)	Clearance (mL · min^{-1} · kg^{-1})	Therapeutic range	References
Prazosin	48–68	95 ± 1	0.60 ± 0.13	2.9 ± 0.8 $t_{1/2}$ is ↑ in CHF, eld	<1	3.0 ± 0.3 Cl is ↓ in CHF	—	Vincent J, Meredith PA, Reid JL, et al: Clinical pharmacokinetics of prazosin—1985. *Clin Pharmacokinet* 10:144–154, 1985.
Probucol	2–8	95	—	12–500	0	—	23.6 ± 17.2 μg/mL	
Procainamide	83 ± 16	16 ± 5	1.9 ± 0.3	3.0 ± 0.6 $t_{1/2}$ is ↑ in RI and MI, and ↓ in child and neo	67 ± 8	3.2[1] & 1.1[2] Cl is ↑ in child and ↓ in MI	3–10 μg/mL	Karlson E: Clinical pharmacokinetics of procainamide. *Clin Pharmacokinet* 3:97–107, 1978. [1]Fast acetylator [2]Slow acetylator
Propafenone	5–50[1]	85–95	3.6 ± 2.1	2–10[2] 10–32[3]	<1	17 ± 8 Cl is ↓ in HI	0.2–1.5 μg/mL	Bryson HM, Palmer KJ, Langtry HD, et al: Propafenone: A reappraisal of its pharmacology, pharmacokinetics and therapeutic use in cardiac arrhythmias. *Drugs* 45:85–130, 1993. [1]Dose dependent [2]Fast metabolizers [3]Slow metabolizers

Propranolol	26 ± 10	87 ± 6	4.3 ± 0.6	3–5 $t_{1/2}$ is ↑ in HI	<0.5	11.4–17.1 Cl is ↓ in HI	20 ng/mL	McDevitt DG: Comparison of pharmacokinetic properties of beta-adrenoceptor blocking drugs. *Eur Heart J* 8(Suppl M): 9–14, 1987.
Quinapril	60	97	0.4	2.2 ± 0.2[1] $t_{1/2}$ is ↑ in eld and RI	Trace	2.0 ± 0.6 Cl is ↓ in eld and RI	—	Wadworth AN, Brogden RN: Quinapril: A review of its pharmacological properties and therapeutic efficacy in cardiovascular disorders. *Drugs* 41:378-399, 1991. [1]Quinaprilat
Quinidine	70–80 71 ± 17	87 ± 3	2.7 ± 1.2	6.2 ± 1.8 $t_{1/2}$ is ↑ in RI and eld	18 ± 5	4.7 ± 1.8 Cl is ↓ in RI, eld and severe CHF	2–6 μg/mL	Verme CN, Ludden TM, Clementi WA, et al: Pharmacokinetics of quinidine in male patients: A population analysis. *Clin Pharmacokinet* 22:468–480, 1992.
Ramipril	50–60	56	—	14 ± 7[1] $t_{1/2}$ is ↑ in RI	<2%	1.1 ± 0.4 Cl is ↓ in RI	—	Meisel S, Shamiss A, Rosenthal T: Clinical pharmacokinetics of ramipril. *Clin Pharmacokinet* 26:7–15, 1994. [1]Ramiprilat

Key: ↑ = increased; ↓ = decreased; **CAD** = coronary artery disease; **CHF** = congestive heart failure; **Cl** = clearance; **eld** = elderly; **F** = bioavailability; **HI** = hepatic impairment; **ID** = insufficient data; **MI** = myocardial infarction; **NA** = not applicable; **neo** = neonate; **RI** = renal impairment; **SL** = sublingual; $t_{1/2}$ = half-life; **TOP** = topical; ***Vd*** = volume of distribution.

APPENDIX 1 (*continued*)

Generic name	Bioavailability (%)	Protein binding (%)	Volume of distribution (liters/kg)	Half-life (hours)	Urinary excretion (% unchanged)	Clearance ($mL \cdot min^{-1} \cdot kg^{-1}$)	Therapeutic range	References
Reserpine	50	—	—	33	<1	—	—	
Reteplase	—	—	0.086[1]	13–16 min[2]	—	3.6–6.4[3]	2000 IU/mL (activity) 4200 μg/L (antigen)	Noble S, McTavish D: Reteplase: A review of its pharmacological properties and clinical efficacy in the management of acute myocardial infarction. *Drugs* 52: 589–605, 1996. [1]Apparent volume of distribution during the terminal elimination phase [2]Effective half-life [3]Plasma clearance
Simvastatin	<5	94	—	1.9	<0.5	7.6	—	Mauro VF, MacDonald JL: Simvastatin: A review of its pharmacology and clinical use. *DICP Ann Pharmacother* 25:257–264, 1991.
Sodium nitroprusside	NA	ID	—	3–4 min 3–4 days[1] $t_{1/2}$ ↑ in RI	—	—	—	Schulz V: Clinical pharmacokinetics of nitroprusside, cyanide, thiosulphate and thiocyanate. *Clin Pharmacokinet* 9: 239–251, 1984. [1]Thiocyanate

Sotalol	90–100	0	2.0 ± 0.4	7–15 $t_{1/2}$ is ↑ in RI and eld	80.1	2.6 ± 0.5 Cl is ↓ in RI and eld	—	Antonaccio MJ, Gomoll A: Pharmacology, pharmacodynamics and pharmacokinetics of sotalol. *Am J Cardiol* 65: 12A–21A, 1990.
Spironolactone	60–70	>90	—	1.3–1.4 13–24[1] $t_{1/2}$ is ↑ in eld	<1	— Cl is ↓ in eld	—	Overdick HW, Merkus FW: The metabolism and biopharmaceutics of spironolactone in man. *Rev Drug Metab Drug Interact* 5:273–302, 1987. [1]Half-life of canrenone
Streptokinase	NA	—	0.08 ± 0.04	0.61 ± 0.04	0	1.7 ± 0.7	—	Gemmill JD, Hogg KJ, Burns JMA, et al: A comparison of the pharmacokinetic properties of streptokinase and anistreplase in acute myocardial infarction. *Br J Clin Pharmacol* 31:143–147, 1991.
Terazosin	90	90–94	0.80 ± 0.18	9–12	12 ± 3	1.1 ± 0.2	—	Titmarsh S, Monk JP: Terazosin: A review of its pharmacodynamic and pharmacokinetic properties and therapeutic efficacy in essential hypertension. *Drugs* 33:461–477, 1987.

Key: ↑ = increased; ↓ = decreased; **CAD** = coronary artery disease; **CHF** = congestive heart failure; **Cl** = clearance; **eld** = elderly; **F** = bioavailability; **HI** = hepatic impairment; **ID** = insufficient data; **MI** = myocardial infarction; **NA** = not applicable; **neo** = neonate; **RI** = renal impairment; **SL** = sublingual; $t_{1/2}$ = half-life; **TOP** = topical; ***Vd*** = volume of distribution.

APPENDIX 1 (*continued*)

Generic name	Bioavailability (%)	Protein binding (%)	Volume of distribution (liters/kg)	Half-life (hours)	Urinary excretion (% unchanged)	Clearance ($mL \cdot min^{-1} \cdot kg^{-1}$)	Therapeutic range	References
Ticlopidine	80–90	98	—	4–5 days $t_{1/2}$ is ↑ in RI	trace	8–21 Cl is ↓ in RI	1–2 μg/mL	Saltiel E, Ward A: Ticlopidine: A review of its pharmacodynamic and pharmacokinetic properties and therapeutic efficacy in platelet-dependent disease states. *Drug* 34:222–262, 1987.
Timolol	50	<10[1] 60[2]	2.1 ± 0.8	3–5	15	7.3 ± 3.3	—	McGourty JC, Silas JH, Fleming JJ, et al: Pharmacokinetics and beta-blocking effects of timolol in poor and extensive metabolizers of debrisoquin. *Clin Pharmacol Ther* 38:409–413, 1985. [1]By equilibrium dialysis. [2]By ultrafiltration
Tocainide	89 ± 5	10–15	3.0 ± 0.2	13.5 ± 2.3 $t_{1/2}$ is ↑ in RI	38 ± 7	2.6 ± 0.5 Cl is ↓ in CHF and RI	3–9 μg/mL	Roden DM, Woosley RL: Drug therapy: Tocainide. *N Engl J Med* 315:41–45, 1986.
Tolazoline	NA	—	1.61 ± 0.21	3–10[1]	—	—	—	Ward RM, Daniel CH, Kendig JW, et al: Oliguria and tolazoline pharmacokinetics in the newborn. *Pediatrics* 77: 307–315, 1986. [1]In neonates

Torsemide	80–90	97–99	0.16	3–4	27	—	—	Knauf H, Spahn H, Mutschler E: The loop diuretic torsemide in chronic renal failure: Pharmacokinetic and pharmacodynamics. *Drugs* 41(Suppl 3):23–34, 1991.
Trandolapril	40–60[1]	80	—	0.7–1.3 16–24[1] $t_{1/2}$ is ↑ in RI	—	—	—	Wiseman LR, McTavish D: Trandolapril: A review of its pharmacodynamic and pharmacokinetic properties, and therapeutic use in essential hypertension. *Drugs* 48:71–90, 1994. [1]Trandolaprilat
Triamterene	54 ± 12	61 ± 2	13.4 ± 4.9	4.2 ± 0.7 $t_{1/2}$ is ↑ in RI and eld	21	63 ± 20 Cl is ↓ in HI, RI, and eld	—	Gilfrich HJ, Kremer G, Möhrke W, et al: Pharmacokinetics of triamterene after IV administration to man: Determination of bioavailability. *Eur J Clin Pharmacol* 25:237–241, 1983.
Trichlormethiazide	ID	—	—	2.3–7.3	ID	—	—	Sketris IS, Skoutakis VA, Acchiardo SR, et al: The pharmacokinetics of trichlormethiazide in hypertensive patients with normal and compromised renal function. *Eur J Clin Pharmacol* 20:453–457, 1981.

Key: ↑ = increased; ↓ = decreased; **CAD** = coronary artery disease; **CHF** = congestive heart failure; **Cl** = clearance; **eld** = elderly; **F** = bioavailability; **HI** = hepatic impairment; **ID** = insufficient data; **MI** = myocardial infarction; **NA** = not applicable; **neo** = neonate; **RI** = renal impairment; **SL** = sublingual; $t_{1/2}$ = half-life; **TOP** = topical; ***Vd*** = volume of distribution.

APPENDIX 1 (*continued*)

Generic name	Bioavailability (%)	Protein binding (%)	Volume of distribution (liters/kg)	Half-life (hours)	Urinary excretion (% unchanged)	Clearance $(mL \cdot min^{-1} \cdot kg^{-1})$	Therapeutic range	References
Urokinase	NA	—	—	10–20 min $t_{1/2}$ ↑ in HI	—	—	—	Maizel AS, Bookstein JJ: Streptokinase, urokinase, and tissue plasminogen activator: Pharmacokinetics, relative advantages, and methods for maximizing rates and consistency of lysis. *Cardiovasc Intervent Radiol* 9:236–244, 1986.
Valsartan	25 (10–35)	95 (94–97)	0.24	6	<13	0.48	—	Criscione L, et al: Valsartan: Preclinical and clinical profile of an antihypertensive angiotensin-II antagonist. *Cardiovasc Drug Rev* 13:230–250, 1995.
Verapamil	22 ± 8	90 ± 2	5.0 ± 2.1	4.0 ± 1.5 $t_{1/2}$ is ↑ in HI and eld	<3	15 ± 6 Cl is ↓ in HI and eld	80–300 ng/mL	McTavish D, Sorkin EM: Verapamil: An updated review of its pharmacodynamic and pharmacokinetic properties and therapeutic use in hypertension. *Drugs* 38:19–76, 1989.

Warfarin	93 ± 8	99 ± 1	0.14 ± 0.06	37 ± 15	<2	0.045 ± 0.024	2.2 ± 0.4 µg/mL	Chan E, McLachlan AJ, Pegg M, et al: Disposition of warfarin enantiomers and metabolites in patients during multiple dosing with *rac*-warfarin. *Br J Clin Pharmacol* 37:563–569, 1994.

Key: ↑ = increased; ↓ = decreased; **CAD** = coronary artery disease; **CHF** = congestive heart failure; **Cl** = clearance; **eld** = elderly; **F** = bioavailability; **HI** = hepatic impairment; **ID** = insufficient data; **MI** = myocardial infarction; **NA** = not applicable; **neo** = neonate; **RI** = renal impairment; **SL** = sublingual; $t_{1/2}$ = half-life; **TOP** = topical; ***Vd*** = volume of distribution.

Appendix 2 Therapeutic Use of Available Cardiovascular Drugs

William H. Frishman, Adam J. Spiegel, Angela Cheng, and Sylvia Thomas

ALPHA-ADRENERGIC BLOCKERS

1. Doxazosin (Cardura)

Indication

Hypertension
Benign prostatic hyperplasia

Dosage

Adults: As an antihypertensive, initiate at 1mg/d. Increase gradually to individual requirements, depending on periodic blood pressure. May increase every 1–2 wk to 2, 4, 8, and 16 mg/d as needed.

Elderly: Use lowest possible dose to initiate therapy.

Children: Safety and effectiveness not established.

Preparation

Cardura (Roerig): 1, 2, 4, and 8 mg tablets

2. Prazosin (Prazosin, Minipress)

Indication

Hypertension

Dosage

Adults: As an antihypertensive, initiate in 1 mg capsules two to three times daily. Maintain at individual requirements, most commonly 6–15 mg a day in two to three divided doses. Limit: Doses above 20 mg usually do not have increased effect. Some patients respond to up to 40 mg/d.

Elderly: Use lowest possible dose because of risk for postural hypotension.

Children: Under 7 y of age, initiate at 250 μg (0.25 mg) two to three times daily, adjusted to response. In children 7–12 y of age, initiate at 500 μg (0.5 mg) two to three times daily, adjusted to response.

Preparation

Prazosin (generic); Minipress (Pfizer Labs): 1, 2, 5 mg capsules

3. Terazosin (Hytrin)

Indication

Hypertension
Benign prostatic hyperplasia

Dosage

Adults: As an antihypertensive, initiate therapy with 1-mg tablets taken at bedtime. There seems to be little benefit in exceeding a dose of 20 mg/d. Usual maintenance is 1–5 mg/d.

Elderly: Because of sensitivity, the lowest dose should be used to initiate therapy.

Children: Safety and effectiveness not established

Preparation

Hytrin (Abbott Laboratories): 1, 2, 5, 10 mg tablets and capsules

ANGIOTENSIN CONVERTING ENZYME INHIBITORS

1. Benazepril (Lotensin)

Indication

Hypertension

Dosage

Adults: Initial dose is 10 mg/d, increased to the usual effective dose of 20–40 mg/d. The maximum dose is 80 mg/d. In renovascular hypertension, renal failure, or in patients in whom diuretics have not been discontinued, the starting dose should be 5 mg.

Elderly: Usually respond well; dose reduction generally not required.

Children: Safety and effectiveness not established.

Preparation

Lotensin (CibaGeneva Pharmaceuticals): 5, 10, 20, 40 mg tablets

2. Captopril (Captopril, Capoten)

Indication

Hypertension
Neonatal hypertension
Congestive heart failure
Left ventricular dysfunction after myocardial infarction
Diabetic nephropathy

Dosage

Hypertension

Adults: Initially 12.5 mg, usually as two divided doses, increased if necessary to 75–300 mg/d depending on severity of hypertension and clinical response. Some may require dosage three times daily. In renovascular hypertension, when diuretics have not been discontinued or in renal impairment, initial dose should be 6.25 mg, titrated cautiously according to response.

Congestive Heart Failure

Adults: Initially, 6.25 mg, increased according to clinical response. The usual daily dose is 50–150 mg/d in two or three divided doses.

Elderly: Initiate with the lowest dose possible and titrate according to clinical response.

Children: Initially 0.3 mg/kg body weight increased to maximum of 6 mg/kg body weight given in divided doses. (*Note*: Safety and effectiveness not firmly established.)

Preparation

Captopril (generic); Capoten (Bristol-Myers-Squibb): 12.5, 25, 50, 100 mg tablets

3. Enalapril (Vasotec) and Enalaprilat (Vasotec I.V.)

Indication

Hypertension
Congestive heart failure
Left ventricular dysfunction—asymptomatic

Dosage

Hypertension

Adults: Initial oral dose is 5 mg/d, increased to the usual effective maintenance dose of 10–20 mg/d (maximum, 40 mg once daily can be given in two divided doses). In renovascular hypertension or in patients in whom diuretics were not discontinued 2–3 d previously, the starting dose should be 2.5 mg.

Intravenously: An initial dose of 0.625 mg should be used in patients who are sodium- and water-depleted or who have renal failure. Patients should be observed 1 h after dose to watch for hypotension. If response is inadequate after 1 h, 0.625 mg dose can be repeated and therapy continued at a dose of 1.25 mg every 6 h.

Elderly: Initially 2.5 mg orally, titrated according to clinical response.

Children: Safety and effectiveness not established.

Congestive Heart Failure

Adults: Initially 2.5 mg once or twice daily, titrated according to clinical response. The usual maintenance dose is 5–20 mg/d given in two divided doses.

Preparation

Vasotec (Merck & Co.): 2.5, 5, 10, 20 mg tablets
Vasotec I.V. (Merck & Co.): 1.25 mg/mL intravenous solution

4. Fosinopril (Monopril)

Indication

Hypertension
Congestive heart failure

Dosage

Hypertension

Adults: Initial dose is 10 mg/d, increased to the usual effective dose of 20–40 mg/d. In renovascular hypertension or in patients in whom diuretics have not been discontinued, the starting dose should be 5 mg.

Elderly: Usually respond well; dose reduction generally not required.

Children: Safety and effectiveness not established.

Congestive Heart Failure

Adults: Initial dose is 10 mg/d, increased to the usual effective dose of 20–40 mg/d. A 5 mg initial dose may need to be used in patients with renal failure.

Preparation

Monopril (Bristol-Myers-Squibb): 10, 20 mg tablets

5. Lisinopril (Prinivil, Zestril)

Indication

Hypertension
Congestive heart failure
Improves survival after acute myocardial infarction

Dosage

Hypertension

Adults: Initial dose 10 mg/d, adjusted to usual effective dose range of 10–40 mg/d according to response (maximum daily dose, 40 mg).

Elderly: Initial dose 2.5 mg/d, adjusted according to response and in line with age-related decline in renal function.

Children: Safety and effectiveness not established.

Congestive Heart Failure

Adults: Initial dose 5 mg/d, administered under medical observation especially in patients with low blood pressure. Usual effective dosage range is 5–20 mg/d, single daily dose.

Myocardial Infarction

Within 24 h of MI, initiate treatment with 5 mg/d, followed by 5 mg after 24 h, 10 mg after 48 h, and then 10 mg/d for 6 weeks. Patients with low systolic blood pressure should receive an initial dose of 2.5–5 mg.

Preparation

Prinivil (Merck & Co.): 2.5, 5, 10, 20, 40 mg tablets
Zestril (Zeneca): 2.5, 5, 10, 20, 40 mg tablets

6. Moexipril Hydrochloride (Univasc)

Indication

Hypertension

Dosage

Adults: Initial dose is 7.5 mg once daily for adults not receiving diuretics. It should be given 1 h before meals. The usual effective dose range is 7.5 to 30 mg daily, in one or two divided doses.

Elderly: No adjustment is needed.

Children: Safety and effectiveness not established.

Note: In patients with renal impairment or in patients in whom diuretics have not been discontinued, initiate with 3.75 mg once daily with careful clinical monitoring.

Preparation

Univasc (Schwarz Pharma): 7.5, 15 mg tablets

7. Quinapril (Accupril)

Indication

Hypertension
Congestive heart failure

Dosage

Hypertension

Adults: Initial dose is 10 mg, increased (at 2-wk intervals) to a maximum of 80 mg/d according to response, given as a single dose or two divided doses. In renovascular hypertension or in patients in whom diuretics have not been discontinued, the starting dose should be 2.5–5 mg.

Elderly: Initially, 2.5 mg; titrated according to response.

Children: Safety and effectiveness not established.

Congestive Heart Failure

Adults: Initial dose is 5 mg twice daily titrated to clinical response. The usual maintenance dose is 20–40 mg/d in 2 divided doses.

Preparation

Accupril (Parke-Davis): 5, 10, 20, 40 mg tablets

8. Ramipril (Altace)

Indication

Hypertension
Congestive heart failure immediately following myocardial infarction

Dosage

Hypertension

Adults: Initial dose is 2.5 mg/d, increased if necessary by 2.5–5 mg/d, up to 20 mg/d. In renovascular hypertension or in patients in whom diuretics have not been discontinued, the starting dose should be 1.25 mg/d.

Elderly: The starting dose should be low, 1.25 mg/d, and adjusted according to response.

Children: Safety and effectiveness not established.

Congestive Heart Failure

For the treatment of post-infarction patients, the recommended starting dose is 2.5 mg twice daily and then increased if tolerated to 5 mg twice daily. If hypotension develops, use 1.25 mg twice daily.

Preparation

Altace (Hoechst-Roussel): 1.25, 2.5, 5, 10 mg capsules

9. Trandolapril (Mavik)

Indication

Hypertension
Heart failure post MI
Left ventricular dysfunction post MI

Dosage

Adults: Initial dose is 1 mg once daily for adults not receiving diuretics in non-African American patients and 2 mg in African American patients. Dose may be adjusted after 1 week according to patient response. Patients receiving concurrent diuretics should start with 0.5 mg daily. The usual effective dose is 0.5 mg to 4 mg daily. For heart failure post myocardial infarction or left ventricular dysfunction post myocardial infarction, the recommended starting dose is 1 mg once daily. Following the intitial dose, all patients should be titrated as tolerated toward a target dose of 4 mg daily. If a 4 mg dose is not tolerated, patient can continue with the greatest tolerated dose.

Elderly: If renal and hepatic function are normal, no dosage adjustment is necessary. In patients with renal insufficiency (creatine clearance $\leq$ 30 mL/min/1.73 m^2) or in patients with hepatic cirrhosis, the initial dose should be 0.5 mg daily.

Children: Safety and effectiveness not established.

Preparation

Mavik (Knoll): 1, 2, 4 mg tablets

ANGIOTENSIN II RECEPTOR BLOCKERS

1. Irbesartan (Avapro)

Indication

Hypertension

Dosage

Adults: Initial dose is 150 mg once daily; may be increased to 300 mg once daily. No additional benefit conferred by daily dosage of greater than 300 mg or twice-daily dosing.

Elderly: No dosage adjustment is necessary.

Children: Safety and efficacy not established.

Preparation

Avapro (Bristol-Myers Squibb/Sanofi): 75, 150, 300 mg tablets

2. Losartan (Cozaar)

Indication

Hypertension

Dosage

Adults: Oral, 50 mg once a day.

Note: In patients with possible volume depletion and those with a history of hepatic function impairment, an initial dose of 25 mg once a day is recommended.

For maintenance, an oral dosage of 25–100 mg may be given once a day or divided into two doses.

Note: If adequate blood pressure control is not achieved by losartan alone, a low dose of a diuretic may be added for an additive effect.

Elderly: Use of losartan in a limited number of patients 65 years of age and older has not demonstrated geriatric-specific problems that would limit the usefulness of losartan in the elderly.

Children: Safety and efficacy not established.

Preparation

Cozaar (Merck & Co.): 25, 50 mg tablets

3. Valsartan (Diovan)

Indication

Hypertension

Dosage

Adults: Oral 80 mg once daily; may be increased to 320 mg once daily in patients using valsartan as monotherapy who are not volume depleted. No additional benefit conferred by dividing doses.

Elderly: No geriatric-specific problems that would limit the usefulness of valsartan in the elderly.

Children: Safety and effectiveness not established.

Preparation

Diovan (CibaGeneva): 80, 160 mg tablets

ANTIARRHYTHMIC AGENTS

1. Disopyramide (Disopyramide Phosphate, Norpace, Norpace CR)

Indication

Life-threatening ventricular arrhythmias
Supraventricular tachycardia

Dosage

Adults: *Capsules*: As an antiarrhythmic, the usual adult dosage is 600 mg/d divided into 150 mg every 6 h for immediate release capsules. The range of adult dosage is 400–800 mg/d.

Extended release capsules: As an antiarrhythmic, 300 mg (base) q 12 h (200 mg q 12 h for body weight <50 kg). When transferring from regular oral dose, first dose of extended-release capsules should be given 6 h after last regular dose. Limit to 800 mg (base) daily.

Note: Extended-release capsules not for initial dosage; maintenance dosages only. Doses up to 1.6 g (base) have been used (regular and extended) in severe refractory ventricular tachycardia, but such high doses are restricted to the hospitalized patient.

Elderly: May be more sensitive to adult dose. Dose reduction required.

Children: Dosing is age-specific. Equally divided, administered q 6 h (or other individually appropriate intervals). Extended-release capsules not recommended.

Up to 1 y, 10–30 mg (base)/kg body weight daily
1–4y, 10–20 mg (base)/kg body weight daily
4–12y, 10–15 mg (base)/kg body weight daily
12–18y, 6–15 mg (base)/kg body weight daily

Note: Children should be hospitalized during initial period of therapy to allow close monitoring until maintenance dose is established.

Preparation

Disopyramide phosphate (generic); Norpace (Searle & Co.): 100, 150 mg capsules
Disopyramide phosphate extended release (generic); Norpace CR (Searle & Co.): 100, 150 mg extended-release capsules

2. Flecainide (Tambocor)

Indication

Supraventricular arrhythmias
Ventricular arrhythmias
Life-threatening ventricular tachycardia

Dosage

Adults: For sustained ventricular tachycardia, initiate at 100 mg every 12 h, increase in increments of 50 mg twice daily every 4 d as needed. Maintenance dose, 150 mg every 12 h; limit to 400 mg/d. For patients with paroxysmal supraventricular tachycardia and patients with paroxysmal atrial fibrillation, initiate at 50 mg every 12 h; increase in increments of 50 mg twice daily every 4 d as needed; limit to 300 mg/d in patients with paroxysmal supraventricular tachycardia.

Elderly: May be more sensitive to adult dose. Half-life may be increased; therefore, reduced dose and wider intervals should be used.

Children: Safety and effectiveness not established in individuals under 18.

Preparation

Tambocor (3M Pharmaceuticals): 50, 100, 150 mg tablets

3. Ibutilide (Corvert)

Indication

Rapid conversion of atrial fibrillation and/or flutter

Dosage

Adults: For adults $\geq$ 60 kg, use 1 mg undiluted or in 50 mL 0.9% NaCl or D_5W. Dose may be repeated after 10 min if needed. For adults <60 kg, 0.01 mg/kg is given. When arrhythmia is controlled, the infusion should be stopped. No dosage adjustment is needed in renal or hepatic insufficiency.

Elderly: No geriatric specific problems.

Children: Safety and efficacy have not been established.

Preparation

Corvert (Pharmacia and Upjohn): 10 mL vial, 0.1 mg/mL

4. Lidocaine (Lidocaine Hydrochloride, Xylocaine)

Indication

Ventricular arrhythmias
Ventricular arrhythmias associated with acute myocardial infarction
Ventricular arrhythmias resulting from digitalis toxicity
Ventricular arrhythmias caused by cardiac surgery or catheterization

Dosage

Elderly: May be more susceptible to dehydration, and renal function may be reduced; reduce dose and then increase slowly.

Children: Not recommended in children under 2 y of age.

Direct Intravenous Injection

Adults: As an antiarrhythmic, loading dose of 1 mg/kg body weight (usually 50–100 mg) at a rate of 25–50 mg/min, repeated after 5 min if necessary; usually followed by continuous intravenous infusion. Limit to 300 mg (4.5 mg/kg body weight) in 1 h period.

Children: Loading dose, 1 mg/kg body weight at a rate of 25–50 mg/min, repeated after 5 min if necessary, and not exceeding a total of 3 mg/kg; usually followed by continuous intravenous infusion.

Continuous Intravenous Infusion

Adults: As an antiarrhythmic (usually following a loading dose), 20–50 μg (0.02–0.05 mg)/kg body weight per minute at a rate of 1–4 mg/min. Limit to 300 mg (about 4.5 mg/kg body weight) in a 1-h period.

Children: As an antiarrhythmic (usually following a loading dose), 30 μg (0.03 mg) (range, 20–50 μg; 0.02–0.05 mg)/kg body weight/min.

Intramuscular

Adults: As an antiarrhythmic, 3–4 mg/kg body weight (approximately 300 mg for a 70 kg adult), repeated after 60–90 min if necessary. Limit to 300 mg in a 1-h period. Single dose of 300 mg may be administered by a patient using the self-injection dose form.

Children: Dosage not established (self-injection form not recommended in children <50 kg).

Note: Use intramuscular form only when electrocardiographic equipment is available. Administration into deltoid muscle is preferred. Intravenous route preferred due to local discomfort.

Sterile Lidocaine Hydrochloride USP

Adults: As an antiarrhythmic, continuous intravenous infusion (usually following loading dose), 20–50 μg (0.02–0.05 mg)/kg body weight per minute at rate of 1–4 mg/min. Limit to 300 mg (about 4.5 mg/kg body weight) in a 1 h period.

Children: As an antiarrhythmic (usually following a loading dose), 30 μg (0.03 mg) (range, 20–50 μg; 0.02–0.05 mg)/kg body weight/min.

Lidocaine Hydrochloride and Dextrose Injection USP

Adults: As an antiarrhythmic, continuous intravenous infusion (usually following loading dose), 20–50 μg (0.02–0.05 mg)/kg body weight at a rate of 1–4 mg/min. Limit to 300 mg (about 4.5 mg/kg body weight) in a 1 h period.

Children: As an antiarrhythmic (usually following a loading dose), 30 μg (0.03 mg) (range 20–50 μg; 0.02–0.05 mg)/kg body weight/min.

Preparation

Lidocaine for IV admixtures (generic): 40, 100, 200 mg/mL
Xylocaine (Astra): 40, 200 mg/mL for IV admixtures
Lidocaine direct intravenous injection (generic); Xylocaine (Astra): 10, 20 mg/mL
Lidocaine intramuscular injection (generic); Xylocaine (Astra), LidoPen Auto-Injector (Survival Technology): 100 mg/mL (3 mL for self-injection)
Sterile lidocaine hydrochloride (generic): 1, 2 g
Lidocaine hydrochloride and dextrose injection (generic): 1, 2, 4, 8 mg/mL

4. Mexiletine (Mexitil)

Indication

Life-threatening ventricular tachycardia
Recurrent ventricular arrhythmias

Dosage

Adults: Initiate in capsule form at 200 mg every 8 h, increase or decrease in increments or decrements of 50–100 mg/dose every 2–3 d as needed. For rapid control of ventricular arrhythmias, loading dose of 400 mg may be administered followed by 200 mg dose 8 h later. Limit to 1200 mg/d when given every 8 h (i.e., 400 mg/ dose) or 900 mg/d when given every 12 h (i.e., 450 mg/ dose).

Note: Dosage adjustments no more frequently than every 2–3 d. Some patients may tolerate twice-daily dosing. For patients adequately maintained on dose of 300 mg or less every 8 h, total daily dose may be given, divided every 12 h. Patients not adequately controlled by dosing every 8 h may respond to dosing every 6 h.

Elderly: Use normal adult dose. There may be little need to reduce dose except in severe renal impairment.

Children: Safety and effectiveness not established.

Preparation

Mexitil (Boehringer Ingelheim): 150, 200, 250 mg capsules

5. Moricizine (Ethmozine)

Indication

Life-threatening ventricular arrhythmias

Dosage

Adults: In tablet form, give 600–900 mg/d in three divided doses (every 8 h); increase, if necessary, in increments of 150 mg/d at 3 day intervals. Limit to 900 mg/d.

Note: In patients with hepatic function impairment or significant renal function impairment, an initial dose of 600 mg/d or less is recommended. In patients whose arrhythmias are well controlled, dosing every 12 h may be used to aid compliance.

Elderly: May be more susceptible to proarrhythmic effects. Lower doses recommended due to age-related decline in clearance.

Children: Safety and effectiveness not established in individuals under 18 y of age.

Preparation

Ethmozine (Roberts): 200, 250, 300 mg tablets

6. Procainamide (Procainamide Hydrochloride, Pronestyl, Pronestyl SR, Procanbid)

Indication

Life-threatening ventricular tachycardia
Life-threatening ventricular arrhythmia
Supraventricular arrhythmias

Dosage

Capsules and Tablets

Adults: For ventricular arrhythmias, 1 g initially, then 50 mg/kg body weight per day in eight divided doses (every 3 h); adjust to response and tolerability. Maintenance dose, up to 6 g/d. Sustained-release preparations are given every 6 h, or twice daily depending on formulation.

Elderly: Use lower dose and increase slowly (hypotension may result)

Parenteral

Adults: Intravenous injection of 100 mg diluted to allow slow intravenous injection at a rate not exceeding 50 mg/min and repeated at 5 min intervals until arrhythmia is controlled or a maximum dose of 1 g is achieved. Intravenous injection of 500–600 mg diluted appropriately and administered at a constant rate over 25–30 min (may be maintained at a dose rate of 2–6 mg/min).

Intramuscular injection of 50 mg/kg of body weight per day in divided doses given every 3–6 h.

Note: Continuous monitoring of blood pressure with patient in supine position is highly recommended. Phenylephrine and norepinephrine injections should be available to counteract severe hypotension.

Children: Intramuscular dosing not recommended.

Preparation

Pronestyl (Princeton Pharm): 250, 375, 500 mg tablets
Procainamide hydrochloride tablets (generic): 375, 500 mg tablets
Procanbid (Parke-Davis): 500, 1000 mg extended-release tablets
Procainamide hydrochloride extended-release tablets (generic): 250, 500, 750 mg tablets
Procainamide hydrochloride capsules (generic); Pronestyl (Princeton Pharm): 250, 375, 500 mg capsules
Procainamide hydrochloride injection (generic): 100, 500 mg/mL

7. Propafenone (Rythmol)

Indication

Life-threatening ventricular arrhythmias
Supraventricular arrhythmias

Dosage

Adults: As an antiarrhythmic use tablets; initiate at 150 mg every 8 h; increase after 3–4 d, if necessary, to 225 mg every 8 h; may be further increased after an additional 3–4 d, to 300 mg every 8 h.

Elderly: Lower doses required.

Children: Safety and effectiveness not established.

Preparation

Rythmol (Knoll): 150, 225, 300 mg tablets

8. Quinidine (Quinidine Gluconate, Quinidine Sulfate, Quinaglute Dura-tabs, Quinidine Polygalacturonate, Quinidex, Cardioquin)

Indication

Maintenance of sinus rhythm after cardioversion of atrial fibrillation/flutter
Conversion of atrial fibrillation/flutter

Atrial flutter
Life threatening ventricular arrhythmias

Dosage

Adults: *Quinidine polygalacturonate tablets*: Initiate in 275–825 mg dose every 3–4 h for three to four doses; dose can be increased by 137.5–275 mg every third or fourth dose until rhythm is restored or toxic effect occurs. Maintenance dose, 275 mg two to three times daily. *Quinidine sulfate capsules and tablets:* As an anti-arrhythmic, initiate at 200–300 mg three to four times daily. With paroxysmal supraventricular tachycardia, administer 400–600 mg every 2–3 h until paroxysm is terminated. In atrial flutter, administer by individual titration following digitalization. With conversion of atrial fibrillation, administer 200 mg every 2–3 h for five to eight doses, with subsequent daily increases as needed. Maintenance dose, 200–300 mg three to four times daily (do not exceed 3–4 g daily). *Quinidine gluconate extended-release tablets:* Maintenance dose of 324–648 mg every 8–12 h. *Quinidine sulfate extended-release tablets USP:* 300–600 mg every 8–12 h. *Quinidine gluconate injection USP:* Initiate 600 mg intramuscularly, then up to 400 mg every 2 h if necessary; adjust each dose by the effect of the previous dose. Intravenously, administer 800 mg (500 mg quinidine) in 50 mL of 5% dextrose at a rate of 1 mL/min with electrocardiographic and blood pressure monitoring.

Elderly: Dose reduction required in renal and hepatic impairment.

Children: Safety and effectiveness not established.

Preparation

Quinidine gluconate extended-release tablets (generic); Quinaglute Dura-Tabs (Berlex): 324 mg extended-release tablets
Cardioquin (Purdue Frederick): 275 mg polygalacturonate tablets
Quinidine sulfate extended-release tablets (generic); Quinidex Extentabs (A.H. Robins): 300 mg extended-release tablets
Cin-Quin (Solvay): 100, 200, 300 mg tablets
Quinidine sulfate tablets USP (generic): 200, 300 mg tablets
Cin-Quin (Solvay): 200, 300 mg capsules
Quinidine sulfate capsules USP (generic): 300 mg capsules
Quinidine gluconate injection (Lilly): 80 mg/mL (50 mg/mL quinidine)

9. Tocainide (Tonocard)

Indication

Life-threatening ventricular arrhythmias

Dosage

Adults: Initiate at 400 mg every 8 h; adjust as needed. Maintenance dose, 1200–1800 mg/d in three divided doses (some patients may tolerate twice-daily dosings).

Elderly: May be more susceptible to hypotension. Reduce dose because of age-related decline in clearance.

Children: Safety and effectiveness not established.

Preparation

Tonocard (Astra Merck): 400, 600 mg tablets

10. Amiodarone (Cordarone, Cordarone IV)

Indication

Life-threatening ventricular arrhythmias

Dosage

Adults: Loading dose in tablets is 800 mg to 1.6 g/d for 1–3 wk or longer until initial therapeutic response or side effects occur; may be given in divided doses with meals for doses >1 g daily or if adverse gastrointestinal side effects occur. When adequate control or excessive side effects occur, reduce dose to 600–800 mg/d for 3 wk. Maintenance dose, 200–400 mg/d. Lower-dosing regimens (oral maintenance of 100–200 mg/d) are under investigation for use in patients with pronounced cardiac dysfunction or in patients with propensity for cardiac arrhythmias, such as atrial fibrillation. For intravenous infusion, the recommended total dose for the first 24 h is about 1000 mg. Initiate intravenous infusion at 150 mg over the first 10 min (15 mg/min), then 360 mg over the next 6 h (1 mg/min), then 540 mg over the remaining 18 h (0.5 mg/min). After the first 24 h, the maintenance infusion rate is 0.5 mg/min (720 mg/24 h). Intravenous amiodarone concentrations should not exceed 2 mg/mL unless a central venous catheter is used.

Elderly: Dose reduction may be required.

Children: Safety and effectiveness not established. However, amiodarone has been given to children. Loading dose in tablets is 10 mg/kg of body weight per day for 10 d or until an initial therapeutic response or side effects occur. When adequate control or excessive side effects occur, the dose is reduced to 5 mg/kg of body weight per day for several weeks and then decreased gradually to the lowest effective maintenance dose. Usual maintenance dose is 2.5 mg/kg of body weight per day or 200 mg/ 1.72 m^2 of body surface per day.

Preparation

Cordarone (Wyeth-Ayerst Labs): 200 mg tablets
Cordarone IV (Wyeth-Ayerst): 3 mL ampul, 50 mg/mL

11. Bretylium (Bretylium Tosylate)

Indication

Ventricular fibrillation
Life-threatening ventricular arrhythmias
Ventricular tachycardias refractory to first-line treatment

Dosage

Adults: With bretylium tosylate injection, for ventricular fibrillation, existing and life-threatening, initiate over 1 min a 5 mg/kg body weight undiluted intravenous infusion, followed by 10 mg/kg body weight infusions every 15–30 min if necessary, to a total of 30 mg/kg body weight daily. Maintenance infusion (intermittent) should be diluted and administered in a dose of 5–10 mg/kg body weight over a 10–30 min period, repeated every 6 h. For other ventricular arrhythmias, administer diluted intravenous infusion (intermittent) in a dose of 5–10 mg/kg body weight over a 10–30 min period, repeated every 1–2 h if necessary. Maintenance infusion every 6–8 h as above, or constant infusion, diluted and administered at a rate of 1–2 mg/min.

With intramuscular administration, 5–10 mg/kg body weight administered undiluted and repeated every 1–2 h as necessary. Maintenance dose, 5–10 mg/kg body weight, undiluted, every 6–8 h.

Adults and Adolescents: Bretylium tosylate in 5% dextrose injection. For ventricular tachycardia, unstable ventricular arrhythmias, maintenance dose by intravenous infusion (intermittent) 5–10 mg/kg body weight over a 10–30 min period, repeated every 6–8 h, or constant infusion 1– 2 mg/min.

Elderly: Dose reduction may be required in renal impairment.

Children: Safety and effectiveness not established.

Preparation

Bretylium tosylate injection (generic): 50, 100 mg/mL
Bretylium tosylate in 5% dextrose injection (generic): 1, 2, 4 mg/mL

12. Adenosine (Adenocard)

Indication

Supraventricular tachycardia
AV reciprocating tachycardia
Wolff-Parkinson-White syndrome

Dosage

Adults: Administer as rapid bolus by peripheral intravenous route. Initial dose, 3–6 mg over 2 s. Second dose (if first dose does not eliminate supraventricular tachycardia within 1–2 min): 6–12 mg over 2 s. Third dose (if second dose does not eliminate supraventricular tachycardia within 1–2 min): 12 mg over 2 s. Additional or higher doses not recommended.

Elderly: No dose adjustment usually necessary.

Children: Some studies suggest a regimen of 37.5–50 μg/kg initially. Studies performed to date on adenosine's use as an antiarrhythmic have not demonstrated pediatric-specific problems that would limit the usefulness of this medication in the pediatric population.

Preparation

Adenocard (Fujisawa USA): vials of 6 mg in 2 mL. NaCl solution Injection of 6, 12 mg prefilled disposable syringes.

13. Atropine (Atropine Sulfate)

Indication

Sinus bradycardia
Ventricular irritability (associated with fall in heart rate)
Sinus node suppression or dysfunction
Acute atrioventricular node block

Dosage

Adults: Usual dose, 0.4–2 mg as one or two bolus injections or as intravenous infusion over 30 min.

Elderly: Use with caution because of susceptibility to adverse effects.

Children: Usual initial dose, 0.01 mg/kg; maximum, 0.4 mg. If necessary, repeat every 4–6 h.

Preparation

Atropine sulfate injection (generic): 0.05, 0.1, 0.3, 0.4, 0.5, 0.8, 1 mg/mL

ANTIOBESITY DRUGS

1. Dexfenfluramine (Redux)

Indication

Management of obesity in patients on a reduced calorie diet with a body mass ≥30 kg/m^2 with no risk factors or ≥27 kg/m^2 with risk factors (hypertension, diabetes, hyperlipidemia)

Dosage

15 mg twice daily with meals

Preparation

Redux (Wyeth-Ayerst) 15-mg capsules

ANTITHROMBOTIC THERAPY: ANTICOAGULANTS

1. Anisindione (Miradon)

Indication

Deep vein thrombosis
Pulmonary thromboembolism (treatment or prophylaxis)
Anticoagulation
Myocardial infarction
Adjunctive management of coronary occlusion
Cardioversion of chronic atrial fibrillation
Prosthetic heart values
Cerebral thromboembolism

Dosage

Adults: Initial dose should be 300 mg/d, reducing on successive days to 200 and 100 mg/d. Maintenance should be adjusted according to prothrombin time. The usual maintenance dose lies in the range of 25–250 mg/d.

Elderly: This group is more sensitive to the action of anisindione. Half the usual adult dose should be used initially, with adjustment in line with prothrombin time.

Children: Not recommended; no adequate clinical experience

Preparation

Miradon (Schering): 50 mg tablets

2. Dicumarol (Dicumarol)

Indication

Deep vein thrombosis (treatment or prophylaxis)

Pulmonary thromboembolism (treatment or prophylaxis)
Anticoagulation
Myocardial infarction
Embolism due to atrial fibrillation (treatment or prophylaxis)
Peripheral arterial embolism (treatment or prophylaxis)

Dosage

Adults: Initial dose 200–300 mg/d on the first day. Subsequent dosage based on prothrombin time. Maintenance dose 25–200 mg/d as indicated by prothrombin-time determinations.

Elderly: This group is more sensitive to the action of dicoumarol. Half the usual dose should be used initially, with adjustment in line with prothrombin time.

Children: Not recommended; no adequate clinical experience.

Preparation

Dicumarol (Abbott): 25-mg tablets

3. Heparin (Heparin)

Indication

Embolism due to atrial fibrillation (treatment or prophylaxis)
Venous thrombosis (treatment or prophylaxis)
Pulmonary embolism (treatment or prophylaxis)
Peripheral arterial embolism
Disseminated intravascular coagulation
Catheter occlusion
Cardiac surgery (to prevent clotting) during extracorporeal circulation
Cyanotic congenital heart disease
Hemodialysis
Peritoneal dialysis
Cerebral thrombus (stroke in evolution)
Blood clotting during extracorporeal circulation
Prophylaxis of recurrent cerebral thromboembolism
Prophylaxis after thrombolytic therapy
Relief of unstable angina

Dosage

Heparin Calcium or Heparin Sodium Injection

Note: All of the following doses must be adjusted in the individual patient as determined by coagulation test results.

Adults: *Full-dose regimen:* Subcutaneous, deep (intrafat) 10,000–20,000 USP units, then 8000–10,000 USP units every 8 h or 15,000–20,000 units every 12 h. This schedule may be preceded by a loading dose of 5000 USP units of intravenous injection. *Intravenous:* Initiate 10,000 USP units, then 5000–10,000 USP units every 4–6 h, or 100 USP units/kg body weight every 4 h. The dose may be administered undiluted or diluted with 50–100 mL of 0.9% sodium chloride injection. *Intravenous infusion:* 20,000–40,000 USP units in 1000 mL of 0.9% sodium chloride over 24 h. This schedule is usually preceded by a loading dose of 35–70 USP units/kg body weight or 5000 USP units. It is then usually administered at a rate of 1000 USP units/h. *Heart–blood vessel surgery:* Intravenous initially not less than 150 USP units/kg body weight. Doses often used are 300 USP units/kg body weight for procedures <60 min, and 400 mg/kg body weight for procedures >60 min. Subsequent doses should be based on coagulation test results. *Disseminated intravascular coagulation:* Intravenous 50–100 USP units/kg body weight every 4 h, administered by continuous infusion or as a single injection. Discontinue if no improvement within 4–8 h. *Adjusted-dose regimen:* Subcutaneous, deep (intrafat), established dose to be injected every 12 h. The required dose is determined by adjusting heparin dose until the mid-interval (6 h after injection) activated partial thromboplastin time (APTT) is maintained at 1.5 times the control value. Low-dose (prophylactic) regimen—subcutaneous, deep (intrafat), 5000 USP units 2 h before surgery and every 8–12 h thereafter for 7 d or until patient is fully ambulatory, whichever is longer.

Children: *Intravenous:* Initially 50 USP units/kg body weight, then 50–100 USP units/kg body weight every 4 h or as determined by coagulation test results. *Intravenous infusion:* Loading dose of 50 USP units/kg body weight then 100 USP units/kg body weight added and absorbed every 4 h or 20,000 USP units/m^2 body surface every 24 h, as determined by coagulation test results. *Heart–blood vessel surgery:* Intravenous, initially not less than 150 USP units/kg body weight. Doses of 300 USP units are often used for procedures lasting <60 min. Subsequent doses should be based on coagulation test results.

Heparin Solution in Sodium Chloride Injection

Adults: Intravenous infusion, 20,000–40,000 USP units over 24 h. This schedule is usually preceded by a loading dose of 35–70 USP units/kg body weight or 5000 USP units administered by intravenous injection. The infusion is often administered at a rate of 1000 USP units/h; however, dosage must be adjusted as determined by coagulation test results.

Elderly: The elderly, especially women, may be more susceptible to hemorrhage during treatment; risk also increases when age-related renal impairment is significant.

Children: *Intravenous infusion:* Initially 50 USP units/kg body weight as loading dose, then 100 USP units/kg body weight added and absorbed every 4 h or 20,000 USP units/m^2 body surface over 24 h, or as determined by coagulation test results. *Disseminated intravascular coagulation*: 25–50 USP units/kg of body weight every 4 h, administered as a single injection or by continuous infusion. The medication should be discontinued if no improvement occurs within 4–8 h.

Note: At one time, 1 mg of heparin sodium was equivalent to 100 USP units. However, this is no longer the case because of increased purification. Other medications should not be added to infusion solutions containing heparin. Full-dose heparin therapy is contraindicated whenever suitable blood coagulation tests cannot be performed at regular intervals.

Preparation

Heparin calcium injection USP from porcine intestinal mucosa: 25,000 USP units/mL (in single unit dose containers providing 5000 USP units/0.2 mL; 12,500 USP units/0.5 mL; and 20,000 USP units/0.8 mL). *Heparin sodium injection USP from beef lung:* 1000, 5000, 10,000, 20,000 USP units/mL (with preservative); 1000, 5000 USP units/mL (without preservative). *From porcine intestinal mucosa:* 100, 2500, 5000, 7500, 20,000, 25,000, 40,000 USP units/mL (with preservative; benzyl alcohol); 1000, 5000 USP units/mL (without preservative).

Note: Single-unit dose containers may also provide the quantities of heparin sodium listed above in volumes other than 1 mL.

Heparin sodium in sodium chloride injection (from porcine intestinal mucosa:—with 0.9% sodium chloride, 2 USP units/mL (1000 USP units/500 mL; 2000 USP units/1000 mL). With 0.45% sodium chloride, 50 USP units/mL (12,500 USP units/250 mL; 25,000 USP units/500 mL); 100 USP units/mL (25,000 USP units/250 mL).

Heparin: Special Formulation

3a. Low-Molecular Weight Heparin, Ardeparin Sodium (Normiflo)

Indication

Prevention of deep-vein thrombosis (DVT) following knee replacement surgery

Dosage

Adults: 50 anti-Xa units/kg of body weight subcutaneously every 12 h. Begin treatment at the evening of the day of surgery or the following morning. Continue treatment for up to 14 d or until the patient is fully ambulatory, whichever is shorter.

Children: Safety and effectiveness have not been established.

Preparation

Normiflo (Wyeth-Ayerst Laboratories): 5000 anti-Xa units/0.5 mL, 10,000 anti-Xa units/0.5 mL, in packages of 10 tubex sterile cartridge-needle units.

3b. Low-Molecular-Weight Heparin, Dalteparin (Fragmin)

Indication

Prevention of DVT in patients undergoing abdominal surgery

Dosage

2500 to 5000 IU daily by subcutaneous injection. In patients undergoing abdominal surgery with a risk of thromboembolic complications, administer 2500 IU subcutaneously starting 1–2 h prior to surgery and repeated once daily for 5–10 d postoperatively. In patients at high risk for thromboembolic complications (e.g., malignancy), administer 5000 IU subcutaneously the evening before surgery and repeat once daily for 5–10 d postoperatively. Alternatively, in patients with malignancy, the first 5000-IU dose can be administered as 2500 IU subcutaneously 1–2 h prior to surgery, with an additional 2500-IU subcutaneous dose 12 h later and then 5000 IU once daily for 5–10 d.

Preparation

Fragmin (Pharmacia and Upjohn): 2500 IU in 0.2 mL single use syringe, 5000 IU in 0.2 mL single use syringe

3c. Danaparoid Sodium (Orgaran)

Indication

Prophylaxis of postoperative DVT in patients undergoing elective hip replacement surgery

Dosage

Adults: In patients undergoing hip replacement surgery, the dose is 750 anti-Xa units twice daily administered by subcutaneous injections. Begin first dose 1–4 h preoperatively and second dose not sooner than 2 h after surgery. Usual duration of treatment is 7–10 d but can be given up to 14 d. Patients with serum creatinine $\geq$ 2.0 mg/dL should be monitored carefully.

Elderly: No dosage adjustment is necessary.

Children: Safety and effectiveness have not been established.

Preparation

Orgaran (Organon): 0.6 mL (750 anti-Xa units) of danaparoid sodium in one ampule, boxes of 10 ampules; 0.6 mL (750 anti-Xa units) of danaparoid sodium in one disposable prefilled syringe (each prefilled syringe is affixed with a 25 gauge $\times$ 5/8 inch needle), boxes of 10 syringes.

3d. Low-Molecular-Weight Heparin, Enoxaparin (Lovenox)

Indication

Prophylaxis of DVT (following hip or knee replacement and abdominal surgery)

Dosage

For patients undergoing hip or knee replacement surgery, the dose is 30 mg twice daily by subcutaneous injection for 7–10 d. Provided that hemostasis has been established, the initial dose should be given 12–24 h postoperatively. Up to 14 d of therapy has been well tolerated. In patients undergoing abdominal surgery who are at risk for thromboembolic complications, the dose is 40 mg once daily by subcutaneous injection for 7–10 d. Initial dose should be given 2 h prior to surgery. Up to 12 d administration has been well tolerated.

Preparation

Lovenox (Rhone-Poulenc Rorer): 30 mg per 0.3 mL single-dose syringes, 40 mg per 0.4 mL single-dose syringes.

4. Warfarin (Coumadin)

Indication

Pulmonary embolism (prophylaxis or treatment)
Thromboembolic complications associated with prosthetic cardiac valve replacement
Venous thrombosis (prophylaxis or treatment)
Transient ischemic attacks

Dosage

Adults: Initial oral dose 2–5 mg/d; adjust to maintenance dose of 2–10 mg/d as indicated by PT or INR determination. The intravenous dosages would be the same as those which would be used orally if the patient could take the drug by the oral route. Administer as a slow bolus injection over 1–2 min into a peripheral vein. Each 5-mg vial should be reconstituted with 2.7 mL of sterile water for injection to yield 2 mg/mL. IM administration is not recommended.

Elderly: Half the usual dose initially, with adjustment as indicated by PT or INR determination.

Children: Start treatment with lower dose and adjust as indicated by PT or INR determination. Safety and effectiveness in children below the age of 18 have not been established.

Preparation

Coumadin (Dupont Pharmaceuticals): 1, 2, 2.5, 3, 4, 5, 6, 7.5, 10 mg tablets
Powder for injection, lyophilized: 5-mg vials

ANTITHROMBOTIC THERAPY: ANTIPLATELET AGENTS

1. Abciximab (ReoPro)

Indication

Adjunctive therapy to prevent cardiac ischemic complications in patients undergoing percutaneous coronary intervention (PCI) and in patients with unstable angina not responding to conventional medical therapy when a PCI is planned within 24 hours.

Dosage

Adults: For prophylaxis of PCI-related thrombosis, use intravenous bolus dose of 250 μg (0.25 mg)/kg of body weight administered 10 to 60 min prior to the start of PCI, followed by a 12-hour continuous infusion of 0.125 μg/kg/min (to a maximum of 10 μg/min). For the specific indication in patients with unstable angina, use intravenous bolus dose of 0.25 mg/kg, followed by an 18- to 24-hour infusion of 10 μg/min concluding 1 hour after the procedure.

Note: The safety and efficacy of abciximab have been only studied with concomitant administration of heparin and aspirin. The continuous infusion of abciximab should be stopped in cases of failed PCI, since there is no evidence for the efficacy of abciximab in that setting.

Elderly: There may be an increased risk of major bleeding in patients over 65 years of age. Caution is recommended.

Children: Safety and efficacy have not been established.

Preparation

ReoPro (Lilly): 2 mg/mL (5 mL single-use vial)

2. Anagrelide (Agrylin)

Indication

Treatment of essential thrombocythemia to reduce the elevated platelet count and the risk of thrombosis

Dosage

Initiate treatment with anagrelide under close medical supervision. Initial dose is 0.5 mg four times daily or 1 mg twice daily, which should be maintained for at least 1 week. Dosage should then be adjusted to the lowest effective dosage required to reduce and maintain platelet count below 600,000/μL and ideally to the normal range. Dosage should be increased by not more than 0.5 mg/d in any one week. Maximum dose is 10 mg/d or 2.5 mg in a single dose. Most patients will experience an adequate response at a dose of 1.5 to 3.0 mg/d. Monitor patients with known or suspected heart disease, renal insufficiency, or hepatic dysfunction closely.

Note: To monitor the effect of anagrelide and prevent the occurrence of thrombocytopenia, platelet counts should be performed every 2 d during the first week of treatment and at least weekly thereafter until the maintenance dosage is reached.

Children: Safety and effectiveness not established in patients under 16 y of age. However, anagrelide has been used successfully in eight pediatric patients (age range 8 to 17 y), including three patients with essential thrombocythemia, who were treated at a dose of 1 to 4 mg/d.

Preparation

Agrylin (Roberts): 0.5, 1-mg capsules

3. Aspirin

Indication

Transient cerebral ischemic attacks

Cerebral thromboembolism (prophylaxis)
Recurrent cerebral thromboembolism (prophylaxis)
Myocardial infarction (prophylaxis) in patients with unstable angina pectoris
Myocardial reinfarction (prophylaxis)
Thromboembolism (prophylaxis) following orthopedic surgery and insertion of arteriovenous shunt
Alone or in combination with dipyridamole to reduce thromboembolic complications in patients with prosthetic heart valves
Alone or in combination with dipyridamole to reduce the risk for thrombosis and/or reocclusion of saphenous vein aortocoronary bypass grafts
Alone or in combination with dipyridamole for maintaining patency following coronary or peripheral vascular angioplasty and for treating patients with peripheral vascular insufficiency caused by arteriosclerosis
Kawasaki disease to reduce occurrence of cardiovascular complications preventing embolic events in patients with atrial fibrillation

Dosage

Adults: *Tablets:* As platelet aggregation inhibitor, 80–325 mg/d with the following exceptions: TIAs in males; TIAs associated with mitral valve prolapse (325 mg–1 g/d); thromboembolism (cerebral, recurrent, 1 g/d reduced to 325 mg/d if higher dose not tolerable); prevention of thrombosis or occlusion of coronary bypass graft (325 mg 7 h postoperatively via nasogastric tube, then 325 mg three times daily concurrently with 75 mg of dipyridamole. Dipyridamole may be discontinued 1 wk postoperatively, but aspirin should be continued indefinitely.)

Chewable tablets: As platelet aggregation inhibitor, 80–160 mg/d, usually in combination with dipyridamole.

Delayed-release tablets, aspirin and caffeine tablets; aspirin, alumina, and magnesia tablets, buffered aspirin tablets: As platelet aggregation inhibitor, 80–325 mg/d with the following exceptions: TIAs in males; TIAs associated with mitral valve prolapse (325–1300 mg daily); thromboembolism (cerebral, recurrent, 1 g/d reduced to 325 mg/d if higher dose not tolerable); prevention of thrombosis or occlusion or coronary bypass graft (325 mg 7 h postoperatively via nasogastric tube, then 325 mg 3 times daily concurrently with 75 mg of dipyridamole. Dipyridamole may be discontinued 1 wk postoperatively, but aspirin should be continued indefinitely).

Note: Although the doses recommended above for the use of aspirin as a platelet inhibitor have been found effective in clinical studies, optimum dosage has not been established. For indications other than prevention of TIA or recurrent cerebral thromboembolism, lower doses are often used. A few studies have shown that 160 mg of aspirin every 24 h or 325 mg every 48 h may effectively inhibit platelet aggregation while minimizing the risk for aspirin-induced side effects.

Aspirin, alumina, and magnesium oxide tablets: For TIAs in males only, 1 g/d or reduced to 325 mg/d.

Elderly: May be more susceptible to toxic effects of aspirin.

Children: Not recommended in those under 12 y of age; risk for Reye's syndrome.

Preparation

Available in a wide range of preparations

3a. Clopidogrel (Plavix)

Indication

Reduction of atherosclerotic events in patients with atherosclerosis documented by recent stroke, recent MI or established peripheral arterial disease.

Dosage

Adults: 75 mg once daily.

Elderly: No dosage adjustment necessary.

Children: Safety and efficacy have not been established.

Preparation

Plavix (Sanofi): 75 mg tablets

4. Dipyridamole (Dipyridamole, Persantine)

Indication

Cardiac valve or mitral valve replacement
Prosthetic valve replacement
Thallium myocardial perfusion imaging
Thromboembolism (prophylaxis, adjunct)
Platelet aggregation (prophylaxis)

Dosage

Adults: Orally, as a platelet aggregation inhibitor, administer 75–100 mg 4 times daily in combination with a coumarin anticoagulant. Limit to 400 mg/d. (Diagnostic adjunct, orally, 300–400 mg as a single dose administered prophylactically 45 min prior to the injection of the radiopharmaceutical agent, or as an intravenous infusion, 0.57 mg/kg of body weight, administered at a rate of 0.142 mg/kg of body weight per minute for 4 min (not to exceed 60 mg over 4 min). The radiopharmaceutical is injected within 3–5 min after completion of the dipyridamole infusion.

Elderly: No dose adjustment necessary.

Children: Dose based on body weight; no specific information available for this group.

Preparation

Dipyridamole (generic); Persantine (Boehringer Ingelheim): 25, 50, 75 mg tablets; Persantine (Boehringer Ingelheim): 5 mg/mL (10 mg/2 mL ampule)

5. Ticlopidine (Ticlid)

Indication

Stroke, thromboembolic, initial or recurrent (prophylactic agent in patients with transient cerebral ischemic attacks)

Dosage

Adults: 250 mg orally twice daily with food.

Elderly: No dosage reduction required.

Children: Not recommended; no adequate experience.

Preparation

Ticlid (Roche): 250 mg tablets

ANTITHROMBOTIC THERAPY: THROMBOLYTIC AGENTS

1. Alteplase (Activase)

Indication

Pulmonary thromboembolism, acute (treatment)
Coronary arterial thrombosis, acute (treatment)
Myocardial infarction
Acute ischemic stroke within 3 h of symptoms if patient does not show evidence of intracranial bleeding on CT scan.

Dosage

Adults: Parenterally (3 h infusion), for lysis of coronary artery thrombi associated with myocardial infarction, 100 mg adminis-

tered as 60 mg (34.8 million IU) in the first hour, (of which 6–10 mg is administered as a bolus over the first 1–2 min), 20 mg (11.6 million IU) over the second hour, and 20 mg (11.6 million IU over the third hour. For smaller patients, (<65 kg), a dose of 1.25 mg/kg administered over 3 h, as described above, may be used. As a general guideline, no other medication should be added to tPA-containing solutions. If the clinical situation warrants, research has shown that lidocaine hydrochloride, propranolol hydrochloride, and metoprolol tartrate are acceptable for simultaneous administration (piggybacking) through the same tubing. Several drugs have exhibited incompatibility with tPA solutions. Heparin sodium has been shown to lower alteplase activity as a result of a physical incompatibility. Morphine sulfate activity is reduced by tPA. Dopamine hydrochloride has been shown to reduce alteplase activity and results in particulate formation. Dobutamine can result in precipitate formation and is not compatible with tPA. One study on alteplase has shown a significantly greater incidence of intracranial hemorrhage with total doses of 150 mg than with total doses of 100 mg. Therefore, the 150 mg dose is not recommended. For pulmonary embolism, administer 100 mg over a 2 h period. *Accelerated infusion*: The recommended dose administered is 100 mg as a 15 mg IV bolus, followed by a 50 mg infusion over the next 30 minutes and then 35 mg infused over the next 60 minutes. For patients weighing ≤67 kg, the recommended dose is administered as a 15 mg IV bolus, followed by 0.75 mg/kg infused over the next 30 minutes (not to exceed 50 mg), and then 0.50 mg/kg over the next 60 minutes (not to exceed 35 mg). The safety and efficacy of this accelerated infusion of alteplase regimen have only been investigated with concomitant administration of heparin and aspirin.
In acute ischemic stroke, the recommended dose is 0.9 mg/kg (maximum 90 mg) infused over 60 minutes, with 10% of the total dose administered as an IV bolus over 1 minute. The safety and efficacy of this regimen with concomitant administration of heparin and aspirin during the first 24 h of symptoms has not been investigated.

Note: It is recommended that heparin be used in conjunction with alteplase for the treatment of acute pulmonary embolism. Heparin administration may be initiated, provided that the patient's activated partial thromboplastin or thrombin time value is no higher than twice the control value, near the end of or immediately following the alteplase infusion.

Elderly: Generally, the adult dose can be used, but body weight should be considered. Patients over 75 y of age, especially those with suspected arterial degeneration are at an increased risk for unwanted bleeding; monitor closely. Patients weighing less than 65 kg may require a lower weight-adjusted dose.

Children: Safety and effectiveness not established.

Preparation

Activase (Genentech): 50 mg (29 million IU), 100 mg (58 million IU) vials for reconstitution and injection

2. Anistreplase (Eminase)

Indication

Acute myocardial infarction
Coronary arterial thrombosis

Dosage

Adults: Parenterally, 30 U intravenously over 2–5 min within 6 h of infarction if possible.

Note: Slowly add 5 mL of sterile water for injection into the vial containing anistreplase, directing the stream of water against the side of the vial. Gently roll (do not shake) the vial to mix the powder with the liquid. Other measures to minimize foaming should also be used. The reconstituted solution should not be further diluted before administration or added to infusion solutions. No other medications should be added to the vial containing anistreplase.

Elderly: Generally, the same dose should be used; however, those over 75 y of age, especially those with suspected arterial degeneration, may be at risk for unwanted bleeding; close monitoring is required.

Children: Safety and effectiveness not established.

Preparation

Eminase (Roberts): 30 units per single-dose vial

3. Reteplase (Retavase)

Indication

Acute myocardial infarction
Coronary arterial thrombosis

Dosage

Adults: Reteplase should be administered as two 10-unit bolus injections each administered over 2 min, the second dose given

30 min after the initiation of the first injection. Injections should be given through an intravenous line in which no other medications (e.g., heparin) are being injected or infused. If reteplase is to be administered through an intravenous line containing heparin, the line should be flushed before and after reteplase administration with either 0.9% sodium chloride or 5% dextrose solution. Reteplase should be reconstituted with 10 mL of sterile water for injection (without preservatives) to yield a solution of 1 unit/mL. The vial should be gently swirled to dissolve the drug, taking precaution to avoid shaking. Once dissolved, 10 mL should be withdrawn from the vial into a syringe for administration to the patient. Approximately 0.7 mL will remain in the vial due to overfill. When reteplase is reconstituted as directed, the solution may be used within 4 h when stored at 2–30°C (36–86°F). Prior to administration, the product should be inspected for particulate matter and discoloration.

Children: Safety and effectiveness not established.

Preparation

Retavase (Boehringer Mannheim): 10.8 units (18.8 mg) per single use vial.

4. Streptokinase (Streptase, Kabikinase)

Indication

Pulmonary thromboembolism, acute (treatment
Coronary arterial thrombosis, acute (treatment)
Deep venous thrombosis
Cannula, arteriovenous clearance
Catheter, intravenous clearance

Dosage

Adults: *Acute myocardial infarction:* A single intravenous dose of 1.5×10^6 units should be infused over 1 h. *Thrombosis/embolism:* 250,000 IU over 30 min. Maintenance dose is 100,000 IU/h for 24–72 h. *Deep vein thrombosis:* 250,000 IU over 30 min. Maintenance dose is 100,000 IU/h for 72 h. *Pulmonary embolism:* 250,000 IU over 30 min. Maintenance dose is 100,000 IU/h for 24–72 h. *Intracoronary:* After placing catheter in the appropriate position in the affected vessel, initial bolus averages 15,000– 20,000 IU with maintenance dose of 2000–4000 IU/min for 60 min. *Intraarterial peripheral artery occlusion:* 5000 IU/h. *Arteriovenous cannula, occlusion:* 250,000 IU in 2 mL intravenous solution instilled into the occluded limb(s) of the catheter slowly. Each cannula limb is then clamped off for 2 h, and the patient is observed for any adverse effects. The contents of the cannula limb(s) are aspirated and flushed with saline, and the cannula is reconnected.

Elderly: Those over 75 y of age may be more susceptible to unwanted bleeding events.

Children: Recommended maintenance dose is 20 IU/mL blood volume. Dosage in children has not been established.

Preparation

Kabikinase (Kabi Pharmaceuticals); Streptase (Behringwerke/Astra): 250,000, 750,000, 1,500,000 IU/vial

4. Urokinase (Abbokinase)

Indication

Pulmonary thromboembolism, acute (treatment)
Catheter, intravenous clearance
Cannula, arteriovenous clearance
Coronary arterial thrombosis

Dosage

Adults: Parenterally, for acute pulmonary embolism, intravenously, initiate at 4400 IU/kg body weight over a 10 min period, then 4400 IU/kg body weight per hour for 12 h.

Note: Consult manufacturer's production information for recommendations concerning rate of infusion, based on recommended dilution volume of the product.

For coronary artery thrombosis: Intraarterially 6000 IU/min for up to 2 h.

Note: Prior to intracoronary arterial administration of urokinase, it is recommended that 2500–10,000 USP heparin units be administered via direct intravenous injection. Prior heparin administration should be considered when calculating the dose. The average total dose of urokinase required for lysis of coronary artery thrombi is 500,000 IU. Urokinase administration should be continued until the artery is maximally opened, usually 15–30 min after its initial opening. The medication has been administered for periods of up to 2 h.

For intravenous catheter clearance: After disconnecting the intravenous tubing, fill catheter with solution containing 5000 IU/mL of urokinase.

Elderly: Generally, the adult dose can be used. However, those older than 75 y of age, especially those with suspicion of arterial degeneration, may be at increased risk for unwanted bleeding.

Children: Dosage not established.

Note: Because urokinase contains no preservatives, it should not be reconstituted until immediately prior to use. Also, any unused solution must be discarded. Filaments may form in the solution during reconstitution, especially if the vial is shaken. Avoid shaking the vial. If necessary, the solution may be filtered through a 0.45-μm or smaller cellulose membrane filter.

Preparation

Abbokinase Open-Cath: (Abbott): 5000, 9000 IU per mL vial (urokinase for catheter clearance)
Abbokinase (Abbott): 250,000 IU per 5-mL vial (urokinase for injection)

β-ADRENERGIC BLOCKERS

NONSELECTIVE β BLOCKERS WITHOUT ISA

1. Nadolol (Corgard, Nadolol)

Indication

Angina pectoris
Hypertension

Dosage

Adults: *Hypertension:* Initially, 40 mg/d, orally increased gradually in increments of 40–80 mg. Limit to 320 mg/d if necessary. *Angina:* Initially, 40 mg/d, orally, increased by 40–80 mg at 3–7 d intervals. Limit 160–240 mg/d.

Elderly: Low initial dose should be used to assess senstivity to side effects.

Note: Because of long half-life, once-a-day dosage is sufficient to provide stable plasma concentrations; however, this level may not be achieved for up to 5 d after initiation or change of therapy.

Children: Safety and efficacy not established.

Preparation

Corgard (Bristol-Myers Squibb): 20, 40, 80, 120, 160 mg tablets

2. Propranolol (Propranolol, Inderal, Inderal LA)

Indication

Hypertension
Angina pectoris
Myocardial infarction
Arrhythmias (supraventricular postoperative, ventricular)
Hypertrophic subaortic stenosis
Essential tremors
Hypertrophic cardiomyopathy
Migraine headache prophylaxis
Pheochromocytoma

Dosage

Extended Release Capsules

Adults: As an antihypertensive: 80 mg once daily; increase gradually up to 160 mg once daily as needed. Doses up to 640 mg/d have been used in some patients. As an antianginal agent: 80 mg once daily; increase dosage gradually every 3–7 d as needed up to 320 mg/d. Vascular headache prophylaxis: 80 mg once daily; increase dosage gradually as needed up to 240 mg once daily.

Elderly: Have increased or decreased sensitivity to adult dose

Children: Dosage not established.

Oral Solution and Tablets

Adults: As an antianginal agent: 10–20 mg 3–4/d; increase gradually every 3–7 d. Limit to 320 mg/d if necessary. *As an antiarrhythmic:* 10–30 mg 3–4/d; adjusted as needed and tolerated. *As an anithypertensive:* 40 mg twice daily; increase gradually up to 320 mg if necessary (up to 1 g has been used by some clinicians). *As a hypertrophic cardiomyopathy adjunct:* 20–40 mg 3–4/d; adjust as needed. *As a prophylactic for myocardial infarction:* 180–240 mg/d in divided doses. *As a pheochromocytoma therapy adjunct:* 20 mg three times daily to 40 mg three or four times daily (as necessary to achieve sufficient blockade) for 3 d prior to surgery, concomitantly with alpha-adrenergic blocking medication (should never be started until latter is partially established). Doses of 30–160 mg/d in divided doses have been used for inoperable tumors. As a vascular headache prophylactic, 20 mg four times daily; increase gradually to 240 mg/d (given in divided doses) if necessary. As an antitremor agent, 40 mg twice daily; adjust as needed and tolerated to a maximum dose of 320 mg daily.

Children: As an antiarrhythmic or antihypertensive, give initially 500 μg (0.5 mg) to 1 mg/kg body weight per day in two to four divided doses; adjust as necessary to treat hypertension and prevent supraventricular tachycardia.

Note: Prepare solution by mixing with liquid such as water, juice, or soda. After first glass is finished, rinse with more liquid and drink to make certain all medication is ingested. Propranolol oral solution may also be mixed with semisolid food (e.g., applesauce, pudding).

Parenteral

Adults: As an antiarrhythmic, administer intravenously 1–3 mg at a rate not to exceed 1 mg/min, repeated after 2 min, and again after 4 h if necessary.

Note: A dose of one-tenth the oral dose may be used during surgery to temporarily replace oral dosing.

Elderly: May have increased or decreased sensitivity to adult dose.

Children: As an antiarrhythmic, administer as slow intravenous infusion, 10–100 μg (0.01– 0.1 mg)/kg body weight, to a maximum of 1 mg per dose, every 6–8 h if necessary.

Preparation

Inderal (Wyeth-Ayerst), propranolol (generic): 10, 20, 40, 60, 80 mg tablets
Propranolol extended-release capsules (generic); Inderal LA (Wyeth-Ayerst): 60, 80, 120, 160 mg extended-release capsules
Propranolol injection (generic); Inderal injection (Wyeth-Ayerst): 1 mg/mL

3. Sotalol (Betapace)

Indication

Ventricular arrhythmias
Refractory ventricular arrhythmias

Dosage

Adults: Usual initial oral dose is 80 mg twice daily. Dosage may be increased gradually every 2–3 d to 240 or 320 mg/d if necessary (daily dose is usually given in 2 divided doses).

Elderly: Dose should be adjusted in those with poor renal function or poor left ventricular function.

Children: Safety and effectiveness not established.

Preparation

Betapace (Berlex): 80, 160, 240 mg tablets

4. Timolol (Timolol, Blocadren, Timoptic XE)

Indication

Hypertension
Myocardial infarction
Open angle glaucoma
Headache, vascular (prophylaxis)

Dosage

Adults: *For hypertension:* Initially give 10 mg twice daily in tablet form; increase at 1 wk intervals. Maintenance dose, 20–40 mg/d in 2–4 divided doses; increase to 30 mg twice daily if necessary. *For myocardial reinfarction:* 10 mg twice daily in clinically stable patients. Treatment is initiated 4 wk after initial infarct. Maintenance dose, 20 mg/d (may be given as single daily dose). Limit to 30 mg/d (10 mg in morning, 20 mg in evening).

Elderly: May have increased or decreased sensitivity. Reduced metabolic and excretory capabilities may lead to increased myocardial depression; age-related peripheral vascular disease and beta-blocker–induced hypothermia are increased risks.

Children: Safety and efficacy not established.

Preparation

Timolol (generic); Blocadren (Merck & Co): 5, 10, 20 mg tablets
Timolol (generic): 0.25 and 0.50% ophthalmic solution
Timoptic (Merck & Co.): 0.25 and 0.5% ophthalmic solution
Timoptic XE (Merck & Co.): 0.25 and 0.5% ophthalmic gel

β_1-SELECTIVE ADRENERGIC BLOCKERS WITHOUT ISA

1. Atenolol (Atenolol, Tenormin)

Indication

Hypertension
Angina pectoris
Myocardial infarction

Dosage

Adults: *Tablets*: *As an antianginal agent:* Initially use 50 mg/d; increase gradually to 100 mg after 1 wk if necessary. Some patients may require up to 200 mg/d. *As an antihypertensive:* Initially use 25–50 mg/d; increase to 50–100 mg/d after 2 wk if necessary. *As prophylaxis for myocardial infarction:* In patients who tolerated the full intravenous dose (5 mg over 5 min), initially give 50 mg 10 min after the last intravenous dose, followed by another 50 mg 12 h later. A dose of 100 mg/d or 50 mg twice daily may then be given for 6–9 d or until discharge from the hospital. *In renal impairment:* Adjust dose according to creatinine clearance (mL/min/1.73 m^2): <15, administer 50 mg every other day; 15–35, 50 mg/d; >35, 100 mg/d. *Parenteral:* For myocardial infarction prophylaxis, initially give 5 mg over 5 min; may be repeated 10 min later.

Elderly: May have increased or decreased sensitivity.

Children: Safety and effectiveness not established.

Preparation

Atenolol (generic); Tenormin (Zeneca): 25, 50, 100 mg tablets
Tenormin injection (Zeneca): 0.5 mg/mL, 10 mL ampule

2. Betaxolol (Kerlone)

Indication

Hypertension

Dosage

Adults: As an antihypertensive, initially give 10 mg/d in tablets; double after 7–14 d if necessary. May be combined with other anti-hypertensive agents such as diuretics for additive effect.

Elderly: May have increased or decreased sensitivity; initial dose of 5 mg should be considered. *Renal function impairment (undergoing hemodialysis):* Initially give 5 mg/d, with increments of 5 mg/d every 14 d, to a maximum daily dose of 20 mg as necessary.

Children: Safety and effectiveness not established.

Preparation

Kerlone (Searle): 10, 20 mg tablets

3. Bisoprolol Fumarate (Zebeta)

Indication

Mild to moderate hypertension

Dosage

Adults: The usual starting dose is 5 mg once daily. If the antihypertensive effect of 5 mg is inadequate, the dose may be increased to 10 mg and then, if necessary, to 20 mg once daily.

Elderly: Elderly patients are more likely to have age-related peripheral vascular disease, which may require caution in patients receiving beta-adrenergic blocking agents. In addition, the risk of beta-blocker–induced hypothermia may be increased in elderly patients.

Children: Use of beta-adrenergic blocking agents in a limited number of neonates, infants, and children has not demonstrated pediatric-specific problems that would limit the usefulness of these medications in children.

Preparation

Zebeta (Lederle): 5, 10 mg tablets

4. Esmolol (Brevibloc)

Indication

Arrhythmias
Control of ventricular rate in patients with atrial fibrillation, atrial flutter preoperatively and postoperatively, and other emergency situations

Dosage

The 250 mg/mL strength of esmolol hydrochloride injection must be diluted before administration by intravenous infusion. Concentrations of more than 10 mg/mL may produce irritation. The 10 mg/mL strength may be given by direct infusion. If a reaction occurs at the infusion site, the infusion should be stopped and resumed at another site. Use of butterfly needles for administration is not recommended.

Adults: Parenterally, for supraventricular tachycardia (dosage established by means of a series of loading and maintenance doses), administer a loading intravenous infusion of 500 μg (0.5 mg)/kg body weight per minute for 1 min followed by a maintenance intravenous infusion of 50 μg (0.05 mg)/kg body weight per minute for 4 min. If adequate response is not observed at end of 5 min, repeat sequence with loading intravenous infusion (as above) followed by an increased maintenance infusion rate of 100 μg/kg per minute (0.1 mg/kg/min). The sequence is repeated until an adequate response is obtrained, with an increment of 50 μg (0.05 mg)/kg of body weight per minute in the maintenance dose at each step. As desired end point (defined as desired heart rate/undesirable decrease in blood pressure) is approached, loading dose may be omitted and increments in maintenance dose reduced to 25 μg (0.025 mg) or less. If desired, interval between titration steps may be increased from 5 to 10 min. Established maintenance dose usually does not exceed 200 μg (0.2 mg)/kg body weight per minute (owing to risk for hypotension) and can be given for up to 48 h. Maintenance doses as low as 25 μg/kg per minute and as high as 300 μg/kg per minute have been found to be adequate. *Intraoperative and postoperative tachycardia and/or hypertension*: In the intraoperative and postoperative settings it is not always advisable to slowly titrate the dose of esmolol hydrochloride to a therapeutic effect. Therefore, two dosing options are presented: immediate control dosing and a gradual control dosing when the physician has time to titrate. *Immediate control*: For intraoperative treatment of tachycardia and/or hypertension, give an 80-mg (approximately 1 mg/kg) bolus dose over 30 s followed by a 150 μg/kg per minute infusion, if necessary. Adjust the infusion rate as required up to 300 μg/kg per minute to maintain desired heart rate and/or blood pressure. *Gradual control*: For postoperative tachycardia and hypertension, the dosing schedule is the same as that used in supraventricular tachycardia (see above).

Elderly: Reduced metabolic and excretory capabilities may lead to increased myocardial depression; age-related peripheral vascular disease and beta-blocker–induced hypothermia are increased risks.

Children: Safety and effectiveness not established.

Preparation

Brevibloc (Ohmeda): injection: 10 mg/mL (*Note:* This strength is prediluted and may be used for loading dose.), 100 mg/10 mL vial; 250 mg/mL (25% alcohol; *Note:* Must be diluted before use.), 2.5 g/10 mL ampule

5. Metoprolol (Metoprolol tartrate, Lopressor)

Indication

Hypertension

Angina
Myocardial infarction

Dosage

Adults: *Tablets:* As an antianginal or antihypertensive, initially give 100 mg/d in single or divided doses; increase at 1 wk intervals as needed. Limit to 450 mg/d.

Note: To maintain satisfactory blood pressure control, some patients may require division of total daily dose into three separate doses.

For myocardial infarction prophylaxis (early treatment), give 50 mg every 6 h starting 15 min after the last intravenous dose or as soon as clinical condition allows for patients who tolerate full intravenous dose (dose of 25–50 mg may be used for patients who do not). Continue for 48 h followed by (late treatment) 100 mg twice daily for at least 3 mo and possibly as long as 1–3 y. *Injection:* For myocardial infarction prophylaxis (early treatment), give rapid intravenous injection, 5 mg every 2 min for three doses.

Elderly: For all indications, may have increased or decreased sensitivity.

Children: Safety and effectiveness not established.

Preparation

Metoprolol tartrate (generic); Lopressor (Geigy): 50, 100 mg tablets
Metoprolol tartrate injection (generic); Lopressor injection (Geigy): 1 mg per mL (5 mL ampules)

5a. Metoprolol succinate (Toprol XL)

Dosage

Hypertension: Initial dosage, 50–100 mg in a single dose. Titrate weekly; maximal daily dose, 400 mg. *Angina*: Initial dose, 100 mg in a single dose. Titrate every 1–2 wk; maximal daily dose, 400 mg.

Preparation

Toprol XL (Astra USA): 50, 100, 200 mg extended-release tablets

β BLOCKERS WITH ISA

1. Acebutolol (Acebutolol, Sectral)

Indication

Hypertension
Ventricular arrhythmias

Dosage

Adults: *For hypertension:* Initially give 400 mg daily as single dose or two divided doses; adjust to response. *As an antiarrhythmic:* Initially give 400 mg/d in two divided doses; adjust to response. Maintenance dose up to 1200 mg/d. As an antianginal, initially give 400 mg/d at breakfast or 200 mg twice daily. In some severe forms, up to 300 mg three times daily may be required; up to 1200 mg/d has been used.

Note: Reduce dose in renal function impairment as follows:

Creatine clearance, mL/min/1.73 m²	Normal dose to be given, %
<50	50
<25	25

Elderly: Daily doses should not exceed a total of 800 mg. May have increased or decreased sensitivity.

Children: Safety and efficacy not established.

Preparation

Acebutolol (generic); Sectral (Wyeth-Ayerst): 200, 400 mg capsules

2. Carteolol (Cartrol)

Indication

Hypertension
Glaucoma

Dosage

Adults: For hypertension, initially give 2.5 mg/d in tablet form; adjust to response. Limit to 10 mg/d.

Note: Recommend dosage interval be increased as follows in renal function impairment:

Creatine clearance, mL/min/1.73 m²	Dosage interval, h
>60	24
20–60	48
<20	72

Elderly: May have increased or decreased sensitivity.

Children: Safety and efficacy not established.

Preparation

Cartrol (Abbott): 2.5, 5 mg tablets

3. Penbutolol (Levatol)

Indication

Hypertension

Dosage

Adults: For hypertension, give 20 mg/d in tablet form (2 wk of therapy is required to see full effect).

Elderly: Reduced metabolic and excretory capabilities may lead to increased myocardial depression; age-related peripheral vascular disease and beta-blocker-induced hypothermia are increased risks.

Children: Safety and effectiveness not established.

Preparation

Levatol (Schwartz Pharma): 20 mg tablets

4. Pindolol (Pindolol, Visken)

Indication

Hypertension

Dosage

Adults: For hypertension, initially give 5 mg in tablet form twice daily; increase in increments of 10 mg/d at 2–3 wk intervals as tolerated. Limit to 60 mg/d. Once the optimal daily dose has been reached, once-daily dosing may be used.

Note: Many hypertensive patients require a maintenance dose of 5 mg twice daily to provide an adequate reduction in blood pressure.

Elderly: May have increased or decreased sensitivity.

Children: Safety and efficacy not established.

Preparation

Pindolol (generic); Visken (Sandoz): 5, 10, mg tablets

DUAL-ACTING β BLOCKERS

1. Carvedilol (Coreg)

Indication

Congestive heart failure (NYHA class II or III)
Hypertension

Dosage

Adults: For congestive heart failure, dosage of carvedilol must be individualized and closely monitored during the up-titration. Dosing of digitalis, diuretics and ACE inhibitors (if used) must be stabilized prior to initiation of carvedilol. Initiate carvedilol with 3.125 mg twice daily for 2 wk. If this dose is tolerated, it can then be increased to 6.25 mg twice daily. Dosing should then be doubled every 2 wks to the highest level tolerated by the patient. The maximum recommended dose is 25 mg twice daily in patients weighing less than 85 kg and 50 mg twice daily in patients weighing more than 85 kg. If bradycardia occurs (pulse rate <55 beats/min), the dose of carvedilol should be reduced.

For hypertension, initiate dose at 6.25 mg twice daily. After 7–14 d, the dose may be increased to 12.5 mg twice daily if tolerated and needed. After an additional 7–14 d, 25 mg twice daily may be given if tolerated and needed. Total daily dose should not exceed 50 mg.

Note: Carvedilol should be taken with food to slow the rate of absorption and reduce the incidence of orthostatic hypotension. Since carvedilol is metabolized primarily by the liver, it should not be given to patients with severe hepatic impairment.

Elderly: Although plasma levels of carvedilol average about 50% higher in the elderly compared with young subjects, adjustment of dosage has not been recommended by the manufacturer.

Children: Safety and effectiveness are not established.

Preparation

Coreg (SmithKline Beecham): 3.125, 6.25, 12.5, 25 mg tablets

2. Labetalol (Normodyne, Trandate)

Indication

Hypertension
Severe hypertension (parenteral)

Dosage

Adults: *Tablets*: As an antihypertensive, initially give 100 mg twice daily, adjust in 100 mg increments two times daily every 2–3 d until desired response is reached. Maintenance dose, 200–400 mg twice daily. For severe hypertension, doses of 1.2–2.4 g daily in two to three divided doses may be needed.

Note: May be administered in three divided doses if necessary because of side effects.

Parenteral: As an antihypertensive, inject 20 mg intravenously (0.25 mg/kg body weight for an 80 kg patient) slowly over 2 min; additional injections of 40 and 80 mg may be given at 10 min intervals until desired blood pressure is reached or total of 300 mg has been given, or administer intravenous infusion at a rate of 2 mg/min; adjust to response. Total dose may range from 50–300 mg.

Elderly: May have increased or decreased sensitivity to both oral and intravenous forms.

Children: Safety and effectiveness not established.

Preparation

Normodyne (Schering Co.): 100, 200, 300 mg tablets; 5 mg/mL injection (4, 8 mL disposable syringes; 20, 40 mL vials)
Trandate (Glaxo Wellcome): 100, 200, 300 mg tablets; 5 mg/mL injection (20, 40 mL vials)

CALCIUM ANTAGONISTS

1. Amlodipine (Norvasc)

Indication

Hypertension
Angina

Dosage

Adults: Initially, give 5 mg once daily. May be increased to a maximum dose of 10 mg, depending on individual response. The dose does not need adjusting with concurrent therapy with thiazides, beta blockers, or ACE inhibitors.

Elderly: Normal dosage recommended.

Children: Safety and effectiveness not established.

Preparation

Norvasc (Pfizer Labs): 2.5, 5, 10 mg tablets

2. Bepridil (Vascor)

Indication

Angina

Dosage

Adults: Individualize therapy according to each patient's response and clinical judgment. Usual initial dose is 200 mg in tablet form once daily. Upward adjustment may be made after 10 d depending on patient's response. Usual maintenance dose is 300 mg once daily. Maximum daily dose is 400 mg.

Elderly: Same initial dose as above. However, careful monitoring must be done after therapeutic response is demonstrated.

Note: If nausea occurs, administer the drug with meals or at bedtime.

Children: Safety and effectiveness not established.

Preparation

Vascor (McNeil Pharmaceutical): 200, 300, 400 mg tablets

3. Diltiazem (Diltiazem, Cardizem, Cardizem SR, Cardizem CD, Dilacor XR, Tiazac)

Indication

Angina (Cardizem Tabs, Cardizem CD)
Hypertension (Cardizem SR, Dilacor XR, Tiazac, Cardizem CD)
Arrhythmias
Paroxysmal supraventricular tachycardia (Cardizem injectable)
Atrial fibrillation or flutter (Cardizem injectable)

Dosage

Adults and Adolescents: *Tablets*: As an antianginal agent, usual initial dose is 30 mg four times daily (before meals and at bedtime). Dosage should be increased gradually at 1–2 d intervals; maximum daily dose, 360 mg.

Elderly: Half-life may be increased; also, more likely to have age-related renal impairment.

Children: Safety and effectiveness not established.

Preparation

Cardizem (Hoechst Marion Roussel): 30, 60, 90, 120 mg tablets
Diltiazem (generic): 30, 60, 90, 120 mg tablets

Diltiazem: Special Formulations

3a. Sustained-Release (Cardizem CD)

Dosage

As monotherapy for hypertension, initially, 180–240 mg once daily. The usual dose range in clinical trials was 240–360 mg/d.

Individual patients may respond to higher doses of up to 480 mg once daily. For angina, start with 120 or 180 mg once daily. Dose may be titrated upward every 7–14 d up to a maximum of 480 mg once daily if necessary.

Preparation

Cardizem CD (Hoechst Marion Roussel): 120, 180, 240, 300 mg capsules

3b. Sustained-Release (Extended-release Diltiazem, Cardizem SR)

Dosage

As monotherapy for hypertension, start with 60–120 mg twice daily, although some patients may respond well to lower doses. Usual dose range is 240–360 mg/d.

Preparation

Extended-release Diltiazem capsules (generic); Cardizem SR (Hoechst Marion Roussel): 60, 90, 120 mg capsules

3c. Sustained-Release (Dilacor XR)

Dosage

For hypertension, start with 180–240 mg once daily. Adjust dose as needed depending on antihypertensive response. In clinical trials, the therapeutic dose range is 180–540 mg once daily. For angina, start with 120 mg once daily. Dose may be titrated upward every 7–14 d up to a maximum of 480 mg once daily if necessary.

Preparation

Dilacor XR (Rhone-Poulenc Rorer): 120, 180, 240 mg capsules

3d. Extended-Release (Tiazac)

Dosage

Usual starting dose is 120–240 mg once daily. Maximum effect is observed after 14 d. In clinical trials doses up to 540 mg daily were effective.

Preparation

Tiazac (Forest): 120, 180, 240, 300, 360 mg extended-release capsules

3e. Intravenous

Dosage

Direct intravenous single injections (bolus): Initial 0.25 mg/kg body weight administered as a bolus over 2 min (20 mg is reasonable dose for average patient). If response inadequate, a second dose may be administered after 15 min (25 mg is a reasonable dose of 0.35 mg/kg body weight). Intravenous infusion: An IV infusion may be administered for continued reduction of the heart rate (up to 24 h) in patients with atrial fibrillation or atrial flutter. Start an infusion at a rate of 10 mg/h immediately after bolus administration of 0.25 or 0.35 mg/kg. Some patients may maintain response to an initial rate of 5 mg/h. The infusion rate may be increased in 5 mg/h increments up to 15 mg/h as needed. Infusion duration longer than 24 h and infusion rates $>$ 15 mg/h are not recommended (refer to package insert for proper dilution of diltiazem for continuous infusion).

Preparation

Cardizem Injectable (Hoechst Marion Roussel): 5 and 10 mL vials (5 mg/mL)

4. Felodipine (Plendil)

Indication

Hypertension

Dosage

Adults: 5 mg once daily (range, 2.5–10 mg as a single daily dose).

Elderly: Treatment should be initiated at 2.5 mg once daily because of possible accumulation. Maximum dose, 10 mg once daily. Closely monitor blood pressure.

Children: Safety and effectiveness not established.

Preparation

Plendil (Astra Merck): 2.5, 5, 10 mg extended-release tablets

5. Isradipine (DynaCirc, Dynacirc)

Indication

Hypertension

Dosage

Adults: Initially, give 2.5 mg orally twice daily alone or in combination with a thiazide diuretic. If necessay, adjust in increments of 5 mg/d at 2–4 wk intervals. Limit to 20 mg/d.

Elderly: 1.25 mg twice daily should be used to initiate therapy.

Note: In renal and hepatic impairment, initiate therapy at 1.25 mg twice daily.

Children: Safety and effectiveness not established.

Preparation

DynaCirc (Sandoz): 2.5, 5 mg capsules

Isradipine: Special Formulations

5a. Controlled-Release Isradipine (DynaCirc CR)

Dosage

Initially give 5 mg once daily; if necessary, the dose may be adjusted in increments of 5 mg at 2–4 week intervals, up to a maximum of 20 mg/d.

Preparation

DynaCirc CR (Sandoz): 5, 10 mg gastrointestinal therapeutic system (GITS) controlled-release tablets

6. Mibefradil (Posicor)

Indication

Hypertension
Chronic stable angina pectoris

Dosage

Adults: For hypertension and angina, the initial dose is 50 mg once a day. The dose can be increased to 100 mg once daily in both hypertension and angina if necessary.

Elderly: No dosage adjustment is necessary.

Children: Safety and effectiveness are not established.

Preparation

Posicor (Roche) 50 and 100 mg tablets

7. Nicardipine (Cardene, Cardene IV, Cardene SR)

Indication

Hypertension (Cardene, Cardene SR)
Short-term treatment of hypertension when oral therapy cannot be given (Cardene IV)
Angina (Cardene)

Dosage

Adults: As an antianginal or antihypertensive agent, administer 20 mg in capsules three times daily; increase to 90–120 mg/d to obtain optimal clinical response. Beta blocker may be added with beneficial results in angina.

Elderly: Initial dose, 20 mg three times daily, followed by careful titration to avoid excessive lowering of systolic blood pressure.

Note: In renal impairment, initiate at 20 mg three times daily and titrate carefully. Dosage must be individualized for patients.

Children: Safety and effectiveness not established.

Preparation

Cardene (Roche): 20, 30 mg capsules

Nicardipine: Special Formulations

7a. Sustained-Release Nicardipine (Cardene SR)

Dosage

Initiate treatment with 30 mg twice daily. The effective dose ranges from 30–60 mg twice daily.

Preparation

Cardene SR (Syntex): 30, 45, 60 mg sustained-release capsules

7b. Intravenous Nicardipine (Cardene IV)

Dosage

Intravenously administered nicardipine injection must be diluted before infusion. Administer (concentration of 0.1 mg/mL) by slow, continuous infusion. Blood pressure lowering effect is seen within minutes. For gradual blood pressure lowering, initiate at 50 mL/h (5 mg/h). Infusion rate may be increased by 25 mL/h (2.5 mg/h) every 15 min to a maximum of 150 mL/h (15 mg/h). For rapid blood pressure reduction, initiate at 50 mL/h. Increase infusion rate by 25 mL/h every 5 min to a maximum of 150 mL/h until desirable blood pressure lowering is achieved. Infusion rate must be decreased to 30 mL/h (3 mg/h) when desirable blood pressure is reached. Conditions requiring infusion adjustment include hypotension and tachycardia. The intravenous infusion rate required to produce an average plasma concentration equivalent to a given oral dose at steady state is shown below:

Oral dose	Equivalent intravenous infusion rate
20 mg every 8 h	0.5 mg/h
30 mg every 8 h	1.2 mg/h
40 mg every 8 h	2.2 mg/h

Preparation

Cardene IV (Wyeth-Ayerst): 2.5 mg/mL in 10 mL ampules

8. Nifedipine (Nifedipine, Adalat, Adalat CC, Procardia, Procardia XL)

Indication

Vasospastic angina (Nifedipine, Adalat, Procardia, Procardia XL)
Chronic stable angina (Nifedipine, Adalat, Procardia, Procardia XL)
Hypertension (Adalat CC, Procardia XL)

Dosage (Nifedipine, Procardia, Adalat)

Adults and Adolesents: As an antianginal, initiate capsules at 10 mg three times daily, gradually increasing over 7–14 d as needed. Capsules may be bitten or punctured and administered bucally or sublingually in patients unable to swallow medication; peak plasma concentrations may be achieved slightly earlier.

Note: For hospitalized patients under close supervision, dosage may be increased by 10 mg increments over 4–6 h periods until symptoms are controlled.

Elderly: Initiate treatment at 10 mg twice daily. *Hepatic impairment:* Initiate treatment at 10 mg twice daily, with careful monitoring.

Children: Safety and effectiveness not established.

Note: New labeling states that immediate-release product should not be used for hypertension, hypertensive crisis, acute MI and some forms of unstable angina and chronic stable angina.

Preparation

Nifedipine (generic); Adalat (Bayer Pharmaceutical); Procardia (Pfizer Pharmaceuticals): 10, 20 mg capsules

Nifedipine: Special Formulations

8a. Sustained-Release

Dosage

Sustained-release tablets: give 30–60 mg once daily, adjust over 7–14 d period as needed [limit, 90 mg (antianginal), 120 mg (antihypertensive)]. Titration to doses above 90 mg daily is not recommended by the manufacturer.

Note: Swallow extended-release tablets whole, without breaking, crushing, or chewing.

Preparation

Adalat CC (Bayer): 30, 60, 90 mg tablets

8b. Extended-Release

Dosage

For hypertension and angina it is recommended that the drug be administered orally once daily on an empty stomach. Titration should proceed over a 7–14 d period starting with 30 mg/d. The usual maintenance dosage is 30–60 mg/d. Titration to doses above 120 mg/d is not recommended.

Preparation

Procardia XL (Pfizer): 30, 60, 90 mg tablets

9. Nimodipine (Nimotop)

Indication

Subarachnoid hemorrhage
Associated neurologic deficits

Dosage

Adults: 60 mg in capsules every 4 h, beginning within 96 h of subarachnoid hemorrhage and continuing for 21 d.

Elderly: Decrease dose; elderly may be more sensitive to drug's effects.

Children: Safety and effectiveness not established.

Preparation

Nimotop (Bayer Pharmaceutical): 30 mg capsules

10. Verapamil (Verapamil, Extended-Release Verapamil, Calan, Calan SR, Isoptin, Isoptin SR, Verelan, Covera HS)

Indication

Hypertension (all of the above)
Angina (Verapamil, Covera HS)
Tachyarrhythmias (Verapamil)
Arrhythmias (Verapamil)

Dosage

Tablets

Adults and Adolescents: As an antianginal, antiarrhythmic, and antihypertensive, initiate at 80–120 mg three times daily, increase at daily or weekly intervals as needed. Limit to 480 mg/d in divided doses.

Note: An initial dose of 40 mg three times daily is recommended in those who may have an increased response to verapamil. Total daily dose range is 240–480 mg.

Elderly: Initiate at 40 mg three times daily; adjust as needed.

Children: For infants less than 1 y of age and children between the ages of 1 and 15 y, give 4–8 mg/kg body weight daily in divided doses.

Extended-Release Capsules (Verelan)

Adults and Adolescents: As an antihypertensive, initiate at 240 mg once daily; increase in increments of 120 mg/d at daily or weekly intervals as needed and tolerated.

Note: Initiate dose at 120 mg/d for patients who may have an increased response to verapamil. Total daily dose range, 240–480 mg.

Children: Not established.

Extended-Release Tablets

Adults and Adolescents: As an antihypertensive, initiate at 120–240 mg once daily with food; increase in increments of 40–120 mg/d at daily or weekly intervals as needed. Total daily dose range, 240–480 mg.

Children: Not established.

Extended-Release Tablets (controlled onset)

Adults and Adolescents: Initiate with 180 mg dose at bedtime for both hypertension and angina; if an inadequate response, the dose may be titrated upward to 540 mg/d given at bedtime.

Children: Not established.

Parenteral

Adults: Initiate as 5–10 mg [or 75–150 μg/kg body weight (0.075–0.15 mg/kg)] slowly over at least 2 min with continuous electrocardiographic and blood pressure monitoring. If response is inadequate, 10 mg [or 150 μg/kg body weight (0.15 mg/kg)] may be administered 30 min after completion of initial dose.

Elderly: Administer intravenous dose slowly over 3 min to minimize undesired effects

Children: In infants up to 1 y of age, initiate at 100–200 μg/kg body weight (0.1–0.2 mg/kg as an IV bolus over at least 2 min). Usual range, 0.75–2 mg. In children 1–15 y, initiate at 100–300 μg/kg body weight (0.1– 0.3 mg/kg) as an IV bolus over at least 2 min. Usual range, 2–5 mg (not to exceed 5 mg). Repeat above dose 30 min after the first dose if the initial response is not adequate. Do not exceed 10 mg as a single dose.

Note: Parenteral verapamil is indicated for cardiac arrhythmias; close monitoring, emergency equipment, and medications should be available for parenteral dosing. Verapamil hydrochloride injection is physically and chemically compatible with a Ringer's 5% dextrose, or 0.9% sodium chloride injection. Verapamil hydrochloride is physically incompatible with albumin, amphotercin B injection, hydralazine hydrochloride injection, aminophylline, and sulfamethoxazole and trimethoprim injection. Precipitation of verapamil hydrochloride will occur in any solution with a pH higher than 6.0.

Preparation

Verapamil (generic) 40, 80, 120 mg tablets; Calan (Searle); Isoptin (Knoll): 40, 80, 120 mg tablets
Verapamil extended-release (generic) 120, 180, 240 mg; Calan SR (Searle); Isoptin SR (Knoll): 120, 180, 240 mg extended-release oral caplets
Verelan (Wyeth-Ayerst, Lederle): 120, 180, 240, 360 mg extended-release capsules
Covera HS (Searle): 180, 240, 360 mg extended-release controlled-onset tablets
Verapamil injection (generic); Isoptin injection (Knoll): 2.5 mg/mL (5 mg/2 mL)

CENTRALLY ACTING ANTIHYPERTENSIVE AGENTS

1. Clonidine (Clonidine, Catapres)

Indication

Hypertension

Dosage

Adults: Initially, give 0.1 mg orally two times daily; can be increased at intervals of 0.1 mg/d and can be done weekly. Maintenance dose is 0.2–0.6 mg/d in divided doses. Maximum dose is 2.4 mg/d. In severe hypertension, in the urgent situation, the total dosage used is 0.5–0.7 mg. Control blood pressure on maintenance doses.

Elderly: Treatment should be individualized to ensure minimum dosage. Dose reduction may be required in line with age-related reduction in renal function.

Children: Safety and effectiveness not established.

Preparation

Clonidine (generic); Catapres (Boehringer Ingelheim): 0.1, 0.2, 0.3 mg tablets

Clonidine: Special Formulation

1a. Catapres-TTS

Dosage

Initiate with one TTS-1 (2.5 mg) patch; increase to next largest dose every 1–2 wk for additional control or use a combination of patches. The maximum dosage is two TTS-3 patches.

Preparation

Catapres-TTS-1 (Boehringer Ingelheim): 2.5 mg (delivering 0.1 mg/d)
Catapres-TTS-2 (Boehringer Ingelheim): 5.0 mg (delivering 0.2 mg/d)
Catapres-TTS-3 (Boehringer Ingelheim): 7.5 mg (delivering 0.3 mg/d)

1b. Clonidine Hydrochloride (Duraclon)

Indication

Treatment of severe pain in cancer patients who are not adequately relieved by opioid analgesics alone.

Dosage

Adults: Initial dose of clonidine for continuous epidural infusion is 30 μg/h. Dosage may be titrated up or down depending on pain relief and occurrence of adverse events. Experience with dosage rate > 40 μg/h is limited.

Children: Initiate dose with 0.5 μg/kg per hour and cautiously adjust based on the clinical response.

Note: Clonidine must not be used with a preservative.

Preparation

Duraclon (Fujisawa): 100 μg/mL in 10-mL vials (preservative-free)

2. Guanabenz (Guanabenz, Wytensin)

Indication

Hypertension

Dosage

Adults: Usual starting dose is 4 mg in tablet form twice daily; dose may be adjusted every 1–2 wk in increments of 4–8 mg/d until maximal dose of 32 mg/d (given twice daily) is achieved.

Elderly: Initiate therapy at lower dose and titrate more slowly.

Children: Safety and effectiveness not established.

Preparation

Wytensin (Wyeth-Ayerst): 4, 8 mg tablets
Guanabenz (generic): 4, 8 mg tablets

3. Guanfacine (Guanfacine, Tenex)

Indication

Hypertension (in patients already taking thiazide diruetics)

Dosage

Adults: Starting dose, 1 mg at bedtime in patients already taking a thiazide diuretic; increase dose at 3–4 wk if necessary to 2 mg/d. Dose can be increased after an additional 3–4 wk to 3 mg.

Elderly: Dose reduction needed in patients with impaired renal function.

Children: Safety and effectiveness not established.

Preparation

Guanfacine (generic); Tenex (A.H. Robins): 1, 2 mg tablets

4. Methyldopa (Methyldopa, Aldomet)

Indication

Hypertension

Dosage

Oral

Adults: Initially, give 250 mg 2–3 per day for 2 d; adjust at intervals of not less than 2 d according to response to a maximum of 3 g/d on a twice-per-day regimen. In patients who have received previous antihypertensive therapy, limit dosage initially to 500 mg/d.

Children: Dose should be based on body weight: initially, 10 mg/kg body weight per day given in two to four oral doses. Dosage should be adjusted in daily increments of 10 mg/kg (according to response) to a maximum of 65 mg/kg or 3 g per day, whichever is less.

Elderly: Individualize treatment to ensure minimum dosage. Initially, the dose should not exceed 125 mg twice daily and it should be increased slowly. Do not exceed a daily dose of 2 g.

Intravenous

Adults: Add the dose, 250–500 mg, to 100 mL of 5% dextrose or give in 5% dextrose in water in a concentration of 10 mg/mL. Administer intravenously over 30–60 min every 6 h if necessary (maximum 1 g every 6 h).

Children: Dose should be based on body weight: 20–40 mg/kg per day in divided doses every 6 h. It should not exceed 65 mg/kg or 3 g per day, whichever is the smaller amount.

Preparation

Methyldopa (generic); Aldomet (Merck & Co.): 125, 250, 500 mg tablets
Methyldopa injection (generic); Aldomet injection (Merck & Co.): 50 mg per mL, 250 mg/5 mL
Aldomet Oral Suspension (Merck & Co.): 250 mg/5 mL

DIURETICS

LOOP DIURETICS

1. Bumetanide (Bumetanide, Bumex)

Indication

Edema associated with CHF

Dosage

Adults: As a diuretic, give 500 μg (0.5 mg) to 2 mg/d as a single daily dose. May be increased by the addition of a second or third daily dose with intervals of 4–5 h between doses. An intermittent dose schedule (administration on alternate days for 3–4 d, with 1–2 d in between) may also be used. *Parenteral:* As a diuretic, give 500 μg (0.5 mg) to 1 mg intravenously or intramuscularly; repeat at intervals of 2–3 h if necessary.

Note: Intravenous administration preferred; slow, controlled rate over 2 min.

Elderly: May be sensitive to adult dose; use lower dose.

Children: 0.015 mg/kg orally every other day to 0.1 mg/kg daily.

Preparation

Bumetanide (generic); Bumex (Roche): 0.5, 1, 2 mg tablets
Bumex injection (Roche): 0.25 mg/mL (benzyl alcohol, 1%)

2. Ethacrynic Acid (Edecrin)

Indication

Edema (CHF, cirrhosis, renal disease)
Ascites caused by malignancy, idiopathic edema, or lymphedema

Dosage

Oral

Adults: As a diuretic, initiate at 50–100 mg/d in single or divided doses, with increments of 25–50 mg/d as needed. Maintenance dose is usually 50–200 mg/d; limit to 400 mg/d.

Elderly: May be sensitive to adult dose; reduce dose.

Children: Initiate at 25 mg (taken immediately after breakfast). If necessary, this should be increased every 2–3 d by 25 mg/d until effective dosage is achieved. Not recommended in infants. Dose should not exceed 2–3 mg/kg/d orally.

Parenteral

Adults: As a diuretic, give 50 mg (base) or 500 μg (0.5 mg) to 1 mg/kg body weight intravenously over several minutes. Repeat in 2–4 h if necessary, then every 4–6 h if patient is responsive. In some emergencies, injection may be repeated every hour. Maximum single dose in adults should not exceed 100 mg.

Elderly: May be sensitive to adult dose; reduce dose.

Children: Give 1 mg (base)/kg body weight intravenously over 20–30 min. Not recommended in infants.

Note: Intramuscular or subcutaneous administration is not recommended. If a second injection is required, use of a different site is recommended to prevent thrombophlebitis.

Preparation

Edecrin (Merck & Co.): 25, 50 mg tablets
Edecrin intravenous (Merck & Co.): 50 mg (base)

3. Furosemide (Furosemide, Lasix)

Indication

Hypertension
Edema (CHF, cirrhosis, renal disease)

Dosage

Oral (Liquid or Tablets)

Adults: As a diuretic, initiate at 20–80 mg as a single dose, increasing by 20–40 mg at 6–8 h intervals until desired response is reached. Maintain by titration and as a single daily dose, divided daily dose, dose given once a day every other day, or dose given once a day for 2–4 consecutive days of the week. Limit to 600 mg/d. As an antihypertensive, initiate at 40 mg twice daily; adjust to response.

Elderly: May be sensitive to adult dose.

Children: As a diuretic, initiate at 2 mg/kg body weight as a single dose; increase by 1–2 mg/kg body weight at 6–8 h intervals, until desired response is achieved.

Note: In chronic renal failure, doses up to 4 g/d have been used. Doses as large as 5 mg/kg body weight may be required in children with nephrotic syndrome. Doses of more than 6 mg/kg body weight are not recommended. Extend dosing interval in neonates.

Parenteral

Adults: As a diuretic, intramuscularly or intravenously, initiate at 20–40 mg as a single dose; increase by 20 mg at 2 h intervals until desired response is reached. Maintain by titration; give once or twice daily. This dose should be administered over several minutes. For a hypertensive crisis (accompanied by pulmonary edema or acute renal failure) initiate intravenously at 100–200 mg. As antihypertensive, give intravenously at 40–80 mg.

Elderly: May be sensitive to adult dose.

Children: As a diuretic, intramuscularly or intravenously, initiate at 1 mg/kg body weight as a single dose; increase by 1 mg/kg body weight at 2 h intervals until desired response is reached.

Note: In acute pulmonary edema (not accompanied by hypertensive crisis), usual dose is 40 mg given intravenously repeated as 80 mg in 1 h, if satisfactory response not obtained. Intravenous administration is preferred over intramuscular administration. Intravenous administration should be at a slow, controlled rate not exceeding 4 mg/min. Doses of more than 6 mg/kg body weight are not recommended. Extend dosing interval in neonates.

Preparation

Furosemide (generic); Lasix (Hoechst Marion Roussel): 20, 40, 80 mg tablets
Furosemide oral solution (generic); Lasix oral solution (Hoechst Marion Roussel): 10 mg/mL (alcohol, 11.5%)
Furosemide injection (generic); Lasix injection and prefilled syringe (Hoechst Marion Roussel): 10 mg/mL (2, 4, and 10 mL)

4. Torsemide (Demadex, Demadex IV)

Indication

Hypertension
Edema associated with hepatic and renal disease
Edema associated with CHF and cirrhosis

Dosage

Oral (Tablets)

Adults: Oral and intravenous doses are therapeutically equivalent. *For edema:* A result of congestive heart failure, 10–20 mg once daily; titrate by doubling dose to a maximum of 200 mg/d. A result of renal disease, 20 mg once daily; titrate as above. A result of hepatic disease, 5–10 mg once daily; titrate to maximum of 40 mg/d. *For hypertension:* 5 mg once daily; double dose in 4–6 wk if needed; maximum dose 10 mg/d.

Children: No information available.

Elderly: Risk for postural hypotension, circulatory collapse, thromboembolic event, renal function impairment.

Preparation

Demadex (Boehringer Mannheim): 5, 10, 20, 100 mg tablets
Demadex IV (Boehringer Mannheim): 10 mg/mL (in 2 mL and 5 mL ampules)

THIAZIDE-TYPE DIURETICS

1. Bendroflumethiazide (Naturetin)

Indication

Hypertension
Edema
Adjunct for mild CHF

Dosage

Adults: As a diuretic, initially give 2.5–10 mg once or twice daily, once every other day, or once a day for 3–5 d/wk. Maintain a 2.5–5 mg/d, every other day, or once a day for 3–5 d. As an antihypertensive, give 2.5–20 mg/d as single dose or two divided doses; adjust to response.

Elderly: May be more sensitive to adult dose.

Children: As a diuretic, initially give up to 400 μg (0.4 mg)/kg body weight or 12 mg/m^2 body surface daily, as single dose or two divided doses; adjust to response. As an antihypertensive, 50–400 μg (0.05–0.4 mg)/kg body weight or 1.5–12 mg/m^2 body surface area daily, as a single dose or two divided doses; adjust to response.

Preparation

Naturetin (Apothecon): 5, 10 mg tablets

2. Benzthiazide (Exna)

Indication

Hypertension
Edema
Adjunct for CHF

Dosage

Adults: *As an antihypertensive*: Initiate at 25–50 mg/d as a single daily dose. Maintenance dose should be given according to individual; maximum, 200 mg/d. *As a diuretic*: Initiate at 50–

200 mg/d. If dosage exceeds 100 mg/d, administer in two doses, after the morning and evening meal. Maintenance dose should be 50–150 mg/d in two divided doses.

Elderly: May be more sensitive to adult dose; adjust accordingly.

Children: Initiate at 1–4 mg/kg body weight or 30–120 mg/m^2 body surface area daily, in single or divided doses. Adjust to response.

Preparation

Exna (Robins Company): 50 mg tablets (scored)

3. Chlorothiazide (Chlorothiazide, Diuril)

Indication

Hypertension
Adjunct for CHF
Edema

Dosage

Oral

Adults: Use suspension or tablets as a diuretic or antihypertensive, 125 mg to 1 g/d as a single dose or as divided doses; adjust to response.

Elderly: May be more sensitive to adult dose.

Children: Up to 6 mo of age, give 10–30 mg/kg body weight daily as two divided doses; adjust to response. For children older than 6 mo, give 10–20 mg/kg body weight daily as two divided doses; adjust to response.

Parenteral

Adults: As a diuretic or antihypertensive, give 500 mg to 1 g intravenously daily in single or two divided doses.

Elderly: May be more sensitive to adult dose.

Children: Not recommended.

Note: Solutions of chlorothiazide are incompatible with whole blood or its derivatives. Chlorothiazide should not be administered intramuscularly or subcutaneously. Care must be taken to avoid extravasation during intravenous administration. Reconstituted solution may be stored at room temperature for 24 h, after which it must be discarded.

Preparation

Chlorothiazide (generic); Diuril (Merck & Co.): 250, 500 mg tablets (scored)
Diuril oral suspension (Merck & Co.): 50 mg/mL
Diuril injection (Merck & Co.): 500 mg (base)

4. Chlorthalidone (Chlorthalidone, Hygroton, Thalitone)

Indication

Hypertension
Edema
Adjunct for CHF

Dosage

Adults: As a diuretic, give 25–50 mg/d or 50–100 mg once every other day, or once a day for 3 d/wk. As an antihypertensive, give 12.5–25 mg/d; adjust to response. Use lower doses if possible. Consider adding potassium-sparing diuretic to regimen.

Elderly: May be more sensitive to adult dose.

Children: Give 1–2 mg/kg body weight or 60 mg/m^2 body surface area once daily, 3 d/wk; adjust to response.

Preparation

Chlorthalidone (generic); Hygroton (Rhone-Poulenc Rorer): 25, 50, 100 mg tablets
Thalitone (Horus Therapeutics): 15, 25 mg tablets

5. Hydrochlorothiazide (Hydrochlorothiazide, Hydrodiuril, Esidrex, Oretic)

Indication

Hypertension
Edema
Adjunct for CHF

Dosage

Adults: As an antihypertensive, initiate at 12.5–25 mg as a single or divided dose. Maintenance dose should be 25 mg. For CHF, initiate at 25–100 mg/d for several days. Maintenance dose should be 25–50 mg/d. Use lower doses if possible. Consider adding potassium-sparing diuretic to regimen at these doses. For edema, intermittent therapy (every other day or 3–5 d/wk) may be useful and associated with fewer side effects.

Children: For those 6 mo to 2 y of age, give 12.5–37.5 mg/d in two doses. For those ages 2 to 12 y, give 37.5–100 mg/d in two doses.

Elderly: Because of sensitivity to electrolyte disturbance, start with low dose (12.5–25 mg); increase according to response and renal function.

Preparation

Hydrochlorothiazide (generic); Esidrex (Ciba); HydroDIURIL (Merck & Co.): 25, 50, 100 mg tablets
Oretic (Abbott Labs): 25, 50 mg tablets
Hydrochlorothiazide oral solution (generic): 10 mg/mL

6. Hydroflumethiazide (Hydroflumethiazide, Diucardin, Saluron)

Indication

Hypertension
Edema
Adjunct for CHF

Dosage

Adults: As a diuretic, initiate at 25–100 mg 1 to 2 times daily, once every other day, or once a day for 3–5 d/wk. As an antihypertensive, give 50–100 mg/d as single dose or as two divided doses; adjust to response. May require 200 mg/d in divided doses.

Elderly: May be sensitive to adult dose.

Children: Initiate at 1 mg/kg body weight or 30 mg/m^2 body surface area once daily; adjust to response.

Preparation

Hydroflumethiazide (generic); Diucardin (Wyeth-Ayerst): Saluron (Roberts): 50 mg tablets

7. Indapamide (Indapamide, Lozol)

Indication

Hypertension
Edema related to CHF

Dosage

Adults: Give 1.25–2.5 mg/d in the morning; adjust to response after 1 wk (for edema) or after 4 wk (for hypertension). Limit to 5 mg/d as a single dose.

Elderly: May be more sensitive; reduce dose.

Note: The lowest effective dose should be used to minimize potential electrolyte imbalance. Intermittent dosage schedules may reduce this possibility.

Children: Safety and effectiveness not established.

Preparation

Indapamide (generic); Lozol (Rhone-Poulenc Rorer): 1.25, 2.5 mg tablets

8. Methyclothiazide (Methyclothiazide, Enduron)

Indication

Hypertension
Edema
Adjunct to CHF

Dosage

Adults: As a diuretic, give 2.5–10 mg/d; adjust to response. Maximum effective single dose is 10 mg. As an antihypertensive, give 2.5–5 mg/d; adjust to response.

Children: Give 50–200 μg/kg body weight or 1.5–6 mg/m^2 body surface area daily; adjust to response.

Elderly: May be sensitive to adult dose; lower dose required.

Preparation

Methyclothiazide (generic); Enduron (Abbott): 2.5, 5 mg tablets

9. Metolazone (Zaroxolyn, Mykrox)

Indication

Hypertension
Edema
Adjunct for CHF

Dosage

Adults: Extended-release: As a diuretic, give 5–20 mg/d. As an antihypertensive, give 2.5 mg/d; adjust to response. *Prompt tablets*: As an antihypertensive, initiate at 500 μg (0.5 mg)/d; adjust to response. Maintenance dose should be 500 μg (0.5 mg) to 1 mg/d. Limit to 1 mg/d.

Elderly: May be sensitive to adult dose.

Note: Extended-release and prompt tablets are not bioequivalent.

Children: (1.5–14 y of age) Edema (furosemide resistant) 0.2–0.4 mg/kg/d (extended release form) in one or two divided doses. May be given with furosemide 2–4 mg/kg/d. For infants, dosage is as follows:

Weight, kg	Dose, mg
<7	0.3
7–14	0.65

Preparation

Zaroxolyn (Medeva Pharmaceuticals): 2.5, 5, 10 mg extended tablets
Mykrox (Medeva Pharmaceuticals): 500 μg (0.5 mg) prompt tablets

10. Polythiazide (Renese)

Indication

Hypertension
Edema
Adjunct for CHF

Dosage

Adults: As a diuretic, give 1–4 mg/d, once every other day, or once a day for 3–5 d/wk. As an antihypertensive, give 2–4 mg/d; adjust to response.

Elderly: May be sensitive to dose; use lower dose.

Children: Give 20–80 μg (0.02–0.08 mg)/kg body weight or 500 μg (0.5 mg) to 2.5 mg/m^2 body surface area once daily; adjust to response.

Preparation

Renese (Pfizer): 1, 2, 4 mg tablets

11. Quinethazone (Hydromox)

Indication

Hypertension
Edema
Adjunct for CHF

Dosage

Adults: Give 25–100 mg/d orally as a single dose or in two divided doses; adjust to response. Doses of 150–200 mg/d may be needed.

Elderly: May be sensitive to hypotensive and electrolytic effects; may have age-related renal function impairment.

Children: Dosage not yet established.

Preparation

Hydromox (Lederle): 50 mg tablets

12. Trichlormethiazide (Trichlormethiazide, Metahydrin, Naqua)

Indication

Hypertension
Edema
Adjunct for CHF

Dosage

Adults: As a diuretic or antihypertensive, initiate at 1–4 mg/d; adjust to response.

Elderly: May be sensitive to adult dose; use lower dose.

Children: For those older than 6 mo of age; initiate at 70 μg (0.07 mg)/kg body weight or 2 mg/m^2 body surface area daily as single dose or two divided doses; adjust to response.

Preparation

Metahydrin (Hoechst Marion Roussel); Naqua (Schering): 2, 4 mg tablets
Trichlormethiazide (generic): 4 mg tablets

POTASSIUM-SPARING DIURETICS

1. Amiloride (Amiloride, Midamor)

Indication

Hypertension (adjunct treatment)
Edema (adjunct treatment)
Hypokalemia

Dosage

Adults: As a diuretic or antihypertensive, give 5 mg/d as a single dose. Increase by 5 mg/d increments to maximum dose of 20 mg/d.

Elderly: Dose should be reduced according to renal function and electrolyte balance.

Children: *For diuretic use*: 0.625 mg/kg/24 h for patients weighing 6–20 kg. *For adolescents*: 5–20 mg/24 h to maximum of 40 mg/24 h.

Preparation

Amiloride (generic); Midamor (Merck & Co.): 5 mg tablets

2. Spironolactone (Spironolactone, Aldactone)

Indication

Edema associated with CHF
Nephrotic syndrome
Primary hyperaldosteronism
Cirrhosis
Hypertension
Hypokalemia

Dosage

Adults: As a diuretic, initiate at 25–200 mg/d in two to four divided doses for at least 5 d. Maintenance dose should be 75–400 mg/d in two to four divided doses. As an antihypertensive, initiate at 50–100 mg/d as a single dose or two divided doses for at least 2 wk, then gradually adjust every 2 wk as necessary, up to 200 mg/d. Limit: May be increased to up to three times initial dose or to a maximum of 400 mg/d.

Elderly: Start with lowest dose and adjust upward according to response.

Children: As a diuretic or antihypertensive, initiate at 1–3 mg/kg body weight or 30–90 mg/m^2 body surface area daily as a single dose or two to four divided doses; adjust after 5 d. Limit: May be increased to up to three times the initial dose. Maximum dose is 200 mg/d. Maintenance dose should eventually be reduced to 1–2 mg/kg/d.

Neonates: 0.5 mg/kg orally every 8 h.

Preparation

Aldactone (Searle): 25, 50, 100 mg tablets
Spironolactone (generic): 25 mg tablets

3. Triamterene (Dyrenium)

Indication

Cirrhosis
Edema (CHF, cirrhosis, nephrotic syndrome, steroid-induced edema, hyperaldosteronism)
Potassium conservation

Dosage

Adults: As a diuretic, initiate capsules at 50–100 mg/d; adjust to response. Limit to 300 mg/d.

Elderly: May be sensitive to adult dose; dose reduction required.

Children: As a diuretic, initiate at 2–4 mg/kg body weight or 120 mg/m^2 body surface area daily or on alternate days in divided doses. Maintenance dose is up to 6 mg/kg body weight daily; limit to 300 mg/d in divided doses.

Preparation

Dyrenium (SmithKline Beecham): 50, 100 mg capsules

INOTROPIC AGENTS

PHOSPHODIESTERASE INHIBITORS

1. Amrinone (Inocor)

Indication

CHF (short-term)

Dosage

Adults: Amrinone lactate injection (with sodium metabisulfite, 0.25 mg/mL)—initial dose should be 0.75 mg/kg body weight given by slow intravenous injection over 2–3 min. Repeat after 30 min if necessary. For longer-term therapy, use 0.005–0.01 mg/kg body weight per minute up to a total daily dose of 10 mg/kg. For infusion, the drug may be given diluted with sodium chloride (0.45 or 0.9%) to produce a solution of 1–3 mg/mL.

Note: Diluted solutions should be used within 24 h. Amrinone should not be diluted with solutions containing dextrose (slow-developing chemical interaction occurs over 24 h). However, amrinone injection may be injected into running dextrose infusions through a Y connector or directly into tubing where preferable.

Elderly: Precise dosage not known; initial dose and maintenance dose may require a reduction in line with age-related renal impairment.

Children: Safety and effectiveness not established.

Preparation

Inocor lactate injection (Sanofi Winthrop Pharmaceuticals): 5 mg/mL (with sodium metabisulfite, 0.25 mg/mL)

2. Milrinone (Primacor)

Indication

Congestive heart failure (short term)

Dosage

Adults: For parenteral administration, the initial dose should be 0.05 mg/kg body weight given by slow intravenous infusion over 10 min, followed by an intravenous infusion at a rate of 0.0005 mg/kg/min; adjust according to response (range 0.000375–0.00075 mg/kg/min). The total daily dose should not exceed 1.13 mg/kg. For infusion, the drug may be diluted with dextrose or saline solution.

Elderly: No specific experience; dose should be reduced in line with age-related renal impairment.

Children: Safety and effectiveness not established.

Preparation

Primacor injection (Sanofi Winthrop Pharmaceuticals): 1 mg/mL (10 and 20 mL; single-dose containers and 5 mL sterile cartridge needle unit)

BETA AND DOPAMINE-RECEPTOR AGONISTS

1. Dobutamine (Dobutamine, Dobutrex)

Indication

Cardiogenic shock
Heart failure

Dosage

Adults: *Injection*: Rates of infusion for concentrations of 250, 500, and 1000 μg/mL are as follow:

Drug delivery rate, μg/kg/min	Infusion delivery rate, 250 μg/mL* (mL/kg/min)	Infusion delivery rate, 500 μg/mL† (mL/kg/min)	Infusion delivery rate, 1000 μg/mL‡ (mL/kg/min)
2.5	0.01	0.005	0.0025
5.0	0.02	0.01	0.005
7.5	0.03	0.015	0.0075
10.0	0.04	0.02	0.01
12.5	0.05	0.025	0.0125
15.0	0.06	0.03	0.015

*250 mg/L of dilutent.
†500 mg/L or 250 mg/500 mL of dilutent.
‡1000 mg/L or 250 mg/250 mL of dilutent.

Solution must be further diluted to at least 50 mL before administration in a compatible intravenous solution, that is, 5–10% dextrose, 0.45–0.9% sodium chloride, or lactated Ringer's. Dobutamine is incompatible with alkaline solutions and should not be mixed with solutions such as 5% sodium bicarbonate injection. Dobutamine injection should not be used in conjunction with other agents or dilutents containing both sodium bisulfite and ethanol. Mixture or administration of dobutamine through the same intravenous line as heparin, hydrocortisone sodium succinate, cefazolin, cefamandole, neutral cephalothin, penicillin, or sodium ethacrynate is not recommended.

Preparation

Dobutrex injection (Lilly): 12.5 mg (base)/mL
Dobutamine injection (generic): 12.5 mg/mL (125, 250, 500 mg)

2. Dopamine (Dopamine)

Indication

Hypotension
Cardiogenic shock
Congestive heart failure

Dosage

Adults: Initially give dopamine intravenously at an infusion rate of 0.001–0.005 mg/kg per minute. Increase by increments of

0.001–0.004 mg/kg per minute at intervals of 10–30 min according to response. Lower initial doses are applicable for chronic heart failure (initially, 0.0005–0.002 mg/kg per minute, increased according to response). Most patients respond to a dose <0.020 mg/ kg per minute. The lower starting dose should be used in patients with occlusive vascular disease (0.001 mg/kg per minute). Severely ill patients should be given a high initial dose (0.005 mg/ kg per minute), increased gradually by increments of 0.005–0.01 mg/kg per minute to a maximum of 0.020–0.050 mg/kg per minute, according to response.

Note: Dopamine must be diluted before use; if not prediluted.

Elderly: Recommend lower dose than in adults if occlusive vascular disease suspected.

Preparation

Dopamine hydrochloride injection USP (generic);
Dopamine hydrochloride and dextrose injection USP (generic): 800 μg (0.8 mg) 1.6 mg, and 3.2 mg of dopamine hydrochloride per milliliter in 5% dextrose.

3. Norepinephrine (Norepinephrine, Levophed)

Indication

Hypotensive, acute
Adjunct therapy in cardiac arrest

Dosage

Adults: Norepinephrine bitartrate injection contains 50% norepinephrine. Administer in intravenous infusion, at rate of 8–12 μg (0.008–0.012 mg) (base)/min; adjust to establish and maintain desired blood pressure. Administer maintenance dose at rate of 2–4 μg (0.002–0.004 mg) (base)/min.

Note: Norepinephrine bitartrate injection is a concentrated, potent drug that must be diluted in dextrose-containing solutions prior to infusion. Dosage should be titrated according to patient response. Occasionally, hypotensive patients have required much higher doses [as high as 68 mg (base) daily]; however, in patients requiring very large doses, occult blood volume depletion should always be suspected and corrected if present. Central venous pressure monitoring may be helpful in detecting and treating this situation.

Children: For acute hypotension, administer intravenous infusion initially at rate of 2 μg (0.002 mg) (base)/min, or 2 μg

(0.002 mg)/m^2 per minute; adjust to maintain desired blood pressure. For severe hypotension (in cardiac arrest), administer intravenous infusion, initially at rate of 0.1 μg (0.0001 mg) (base)/kg per minute; adjust to establish and maintain desired blood pressure.

Preparation

Norepinephrine (generic); Levophed injection (Sanofi Winthrop Pharmaceuticals): 1 mg (base)/mL (2 mg norepinephrine bitartrate contains 1 mg norepinephrine)

4. Midodrine (ProAmantine)

Indication

Orthostatic hypotension

Dosage

Adults: Begin with 2.5 mg at breakfast and lunch and increase in 2.5 mg increments as needed until a maximum dose of 10 mg 3 times daily has been reached. Dosing should take place during the daytime hours when the patient is upright, pursuing daily activities. Do not give midodrine after the evening meal or < 4 h before bedtime due to the risk of supine hypertension.

Preparation

ProAmantine (Roberts): 2.5 and 5 mg tablets

DIGITALIS

1. Digitoxin (Digitoxin, Crystodigin)

Indication

Supraventricular arrhythmias
Congestive heart failure

Dosage

Adults and Children > 12 y: *Rapid*: Initially give 600 μg (0.6 mg) dose, then 400 μg (0.4 mg) after 4–6 h and 200 μg (0.2 mg) after another 4–6 h. Follow with daily maintenance dose as needed. *Slow*: Give 200 μg (0.2 mg) twice daily for 4 d. Follow with daily maintenance dose as needed. Limit to 1.6 mg over 1–2 d. Maintenance dose is in range of 0.05–0.3 mg once daily. The therapeutic blood level to aim for is 13–25 ng/mL.

Elderly: Initiate and maintain with half the adult dose; adjust according to response.

Preparation

Crystodigin (Lilly): 50 μg (0.05 mg), 100 μg (0.1 mg) tablets
Digitoxin (generic): 100 μg (0.1 mg), 200 μg (0.2 mg) tablets

2. Digoxin (Digoxin, Lanoxin, Lanoxicaps)

Indication

Congestive heart failure
Supraventricular arrhythmias

Dosage

Adults: *Rapid capsules*: Initally, give 400–600 μg (0.4–0.6 mg) with additional doses of 100–300 μg (0.1–0.3 mg) every 6–8 h as needed and tolerated until desired effect is clinically evident. *Slow capsules:* Give total of 50–350 μg (0.05–0.35 mg) divided and administered in two doses daily, repeated for 7–22 d as needed to reach steady-state serum concentrations. Maintenance dose should be 50–350 μg (0.05–0.35 mg) administered as one or two doses daily as needed and tolerated. *Rapid elixir:* Give total of 0.75– 1.25 mg divided into two or more doses, each then being administered every 6–8 h. *Slow elixir:* Give 125–500 μg (0.125–0.5 mg) once daily for 7 d. Maintenance dose 125–500 μg (0.125–0.5 mg) once daily. *Injection:* Initially, give 400–600 μg (0.4–0.6 mg) intravenously with additional doses of 100–300 μg (0.1–0.3 mg) every 4–8 h as needed and tolerated until desired effect is clinically evident. Intravenous maintenance dose should be 125–500 μg (0.125–0.5 mg) per day in divided doses or as single dose.

Note: May be administered undiluted or may be diluted with a fourfold or greater volume (to reduce risk of precipitation) of sterile water for injection, 0.9% sodium chloride injection, or 5% dextrose injection for intravenous administration.

Rapid tablets: Give total of 0.75–1.25 mg divided into two or more doses, each then being administered every 6–8 h. *Slow tablets:* Give 125–500 μg (0.125–0.5 mg) once daily for 7 d. Maintenance dose should be 125–500 μg (0.125–0.5 mg) given once daily.

Children: For all dosage forms, doses are per kilogram of body weight. In small children (especially premature and immature infants), careful titration of dose is required, along with close monitoring of serum concentrations and electrocardiogram.

Preparation

Lanoxin (Glaxo Wellcome): 0.125, 0.25, 0.5 mg tablets
Digoxin (generic): 0.125, 0.25 mg tablets
Lanoxicaps (Glaxo Wellcome): 0.05, 0.1, 0.2 mg capsules
Digoxin elixir (generic); Lanoxin (Glaxo Wellcome): 50 μg (0.05 mg)/mL
Lanoxin injection (Glaxo Wellcome): 100 μg (0.1 mg), 250 μg (0.25 mg)/mL
Digoxin injection (generic): 250 μg (0.25 mg)/mL

Usual Digitalizing Dosages with Normal Renal Function Based on Lean Body Weight

Age	Capsules*	Elixir†
Premature neonates	15–25 μg/kg	20–35 μg/kg
Full-term neonates	20–30 μg/kg	20–35 μg/kg
1 mo–2 y	30–50 μg/kg	35–60 μg/kg
2–5 y	25–35 μg/kg	30–40 μg/kg
5–10 y	15–30 μg/kg	20–35 μg/kg
≥10 y	8–12 μg/kg	Rapid: 0.75–1.25 mg; slow‡: 125–500 μg
Age	**Injection***	**Tablets†**
Premature neonates	15–25 μg/kg	20–35μg/kg
Full-term neonates	20–30 μg/kg	20–35 μg/kg
1 mo–2 y	30–50 μg/kg	35–60 μg/kg
2–5 y	25–35 μg/kg	30–40 μg/kg
5–10 y	15–30 μg/kg	20–35 μg/kg
≥10 y	8–12 μg/kg	Rapid: 0.75–1.25 mg; slow‡: 125–500 μg

*Administer each of the following total amounts in three or more divided doses, with the initial portion representing approximately one-half the total, doses then being given every 4–8 h.
†Administer each of the following total amounts in two or more divided doses at 6–8 h intervals.
‡Dose is given once daily for 7 d.

2a. Digoxin Immune Fab(Ovine) (Digibind)

Indication

Potentially life threatening digoxin and digitoxin intoxication

Dosage

Adults and Adolescents: As an antidote to digitalis glycoside toxicity, intravenous, in an amount equimolar to the amount of digoxin or digitoxin in the patient's body [total body load (TBL)].

A dose of 38 mg of digoxin immune fab(ovine) binds approximately 0.5 mg of digoxin or digitoxin.
Approximate dose of digoxin immune fab(ovine) when amount of digoxin ingested is known:

No. of digoxin tablets or capsules ingested*	Dose of digoxin immune fab(ovine)	
	mg	No. of 38 mg vials
25	380	10
50	760	20
75	1140	30
100	1520	40
150	2280	60
200	3040	80

*0.25 mg tablets with 80% bioavailability, or 0.2 mg capsules.

Elderly: More likely to have age-related renal function impairment, which may require caution in patients receiving this medication.

Children: In small children, monitoring for volume overload is important.

Preparation

Digibind (Glaxo Wellcome): *Injection*: 38 mg/vial (with 75 mg sorbitol)

LIPID-LOWERING DRUGS

BILE-ACID SEQUESTRANTS

1. Cholestyramine (Questran)

Indication

Hypercholesterolemia (type IIa hyperlipoproteinemia)
Pruritus associated with partial biliary obstruction

Dosage

Adults and Adolescents: *Oral suspension*: Initially give 4 g (anhydrous cholestyramine resin) 1–2 times daily at mealtime. Maintenance dose is up to 4 g (anhydrous cholestyramine resin) 6 times daily at mealtime and at bedtime. Maximum recommended daily dose is 24 g (anhydrous cholestyramine resin).

Note: The administration time for cholestyramine may be modified to avoid interference with absorption of other medications. Oral suspension should be mixed with fluids before taking.

Children: Not established.

Elderly: No precautions necessary.

Preparation

Questran light (Bristol-Myers Squibb Co.): 60 single-dose 5 g packets, 42 dose cans at 210 g per can
Questran powder (Bristol-Myers Squibb Co.): 60 single-dose 9 g packets, 42 dose cans at 378 g per can

2. Colestipol (Colestid)

Indication

Hypercholesterolemia (type IIa hyperlipoproteinemia)

Dosage

Adults: *Granules:* Usual daily dose is 5–30 g, taken in divided doses one to two times daily; daily dose should not exceed 30 g. Initial dose should be 5–10 g/d; increase by 5 g at 1–2 mo intervals. *Tablets*: Usual daily dose is 2–16 g, taken in divided doses. Initial dose is 2 g once or twice a day; increase by 2 g once or twice daily at 1–2 mo intervals.

Elderly: No dosage adjustment necessary.

Children: Safety and effectiveness not established.

Preparation

Colestid (Pharmacia & Upjohn): 1 g tablets
Colestid unflavored granules (Pharmacia & Upjohn Co.): 5 g single-dose packet, 300 and 500 g (5 g per level scoop)
Colestid flavored granules (orange flavor with aspartame, Upjohn): 7.5 g single dose packets, 450 g (7.5 g per level scoop)

FIBRIC-ACID DERIVATIVES

1. Clofibrate (Clofibrate, Atromid-S)

Indication

Hyperlipidemia

Dosage

Adults: 1.5–2 g/d in capsular form in two to four divided doses. Limit to 2 g/d.

Elderly: No dose reduction required, but treatment should be individualized to ensure lowest dose is used.

Children: Safety and effectiveness not established.

Preparation

Clofibrate (generic); Atromid-S (Wyeth-Ayerst): 500 mg capsules

2. Gemfibrozil (Gemfibrozil, Lopid)

Indication

Hyperlipidemia (hypertriglyceridemia, type IIb hyperlipoproteinemia)

Dosage

Adults: Usual dose is 1200 mg/d in two divided doses, 30 min before the morning and evening meals. In patients with type V hyperlipidemia, dosage may be increased to 1500 mg/d.

Elderly: No dosage adjustment required, but treatment should be individualized to ensure minimum dosage is used.

Children: Safety and effectiveness not established.

Preparation

Gemfibrozil (generic); Lopid (Parke-Davis): 600 mg tablets

NICOTINIC ACID

1. Nicotinic Acid (Niacin) (Nicotinic acid, Niacor, Nicobid, Nicolar, Slo-Niacin, Nicotinex Elixir)

Indication

Hypercholesterolemia
Hypertriglyceridemia
Types IIa, IV, and V hyperlipoproteinemia

Dosage

Adults: Using conventional and extended-release tablets, normal dose is 1–2 g three times daily with meals. Maximum dose is 6–8 g daily.

Note: Because of the possible increased hepatotoxicity observed with sustained-release niacin, it is recommended that the daily dosage of this preparation not exceed 2 g.

Elderly: Start with lower dose (100 mg three times daily) and increase according to response and tolerability.

Children: Safety and effectiveness not established.

Preparation

Niacin tablets (generic): 25, 50, 100, 125, 250, 400, 500 mg tablets
Nicolar (Rhone-Poulenc Rorer); Niacor (Upsher-Smith): 500 mg tablets
Slo-Niacin (Upsher-Smith): 250, 500, 750 mg extended-release tablets
Niacin extended-release tablets (generic): 125, 250, 400, 500, 750, 1000 mg tablets
Nicobid (Rhone-Poulenc Rorer): 125, 250, 300, 400, 500 mg extended-release capsules
Nicotinic acid extended-release capsules (generic): 125, 250, 400, 500 mg capsules
Nicotinex elixir (Fleming): 50 mg/5 mL (14% alcohol)

LIPID-LOWERING AGENTS: HMG-COA REDUCTASE INHIBITORS

1. Atorvastatin (Lipitor)

Indication

Hypercholesterolemia (types IIa and IIb)
Homozygous familial hypercholesterolemia

Dosage

Adults: Initiate with 10 mg once a day; maintenance dose is 10–80 mg daily. Atorvastatin can be administered as a single dose at any time of the day, with or without food. Adjust dose to results of lipid levels at intervals of 2–4 wk as needed.

Elderly: No dosage adjustment is necessary.

Children: For homozygous familial hypercholesterolemia, dosage of 10–80 mg daily has been used.

Preparation

Lipitor (Parke-Davis): 10, 20, 40 mg tablets.

2. Cerivastatin (Baycol)

Indication

Primary hypercholesterolemia (types IIa and IIb)
Mixed dyslipidemia

Dosage

Adults: Initial dose is 0.3 mg once daily in the evening, with or without food. For patients with $Cl_{Cr} \leq 60$ ml/min/1.73 m^2, the initial dose is 0.2 mg once daily in the evening.

Elderly: No dosage adjustment is necessary.

Children: Safety and effectiveness have not been established.

Preparation

Baycol (Bayer): 0.2, 0.3 mg tablets

3. Fluvastatin (Lescol)

Indication

Hypercholesterolemia (types IIa and IIb)
To slow the progression of atherosclerosis in patients with coronary artery disease.

Dosage

Adults: The recommended starting dose for the majority of patients is 20 mg once daily at bedtime. The recommended dosing range is 20–80 mg/d (divide 80 mg dose for twice daily administration). Increase at 4 wk intervals according to response.

Elderly: No dose adjustment appears necessary.

Children: Safety and effectiveness not established.

Preparation

Lescol (Sandoz): 20, 40 mg (base) capsules

4. Lovastatin (Mevacor)

Indication

Hypercholesterolemia (types IIa and IIb)
To slow the progression of atherosclerosis in patients with coronary heart disease

Dosage

Adults and Adolescents: Initially, give 20 mg/d in tablet form with evening meal; adjust at 4 wk intervals. Maintenance dose should be 10–80 mg/d as single or divided doses, with meals. Limit to 80 mg/d.

Elderly: Dose reduction may not be needed; preliminary studies show good response.

Children: Safety and effectiveness not established.

Preparation

Mevacor (Merck & Co.): 10, 20, 40 mg tablets

5. Pravastatin (Pravachol)

Indication

Hypercholesterolemia (types IIa and IIb)
Prevention of first heart attack and reduction of death from cardiovascular disease in patients at risk of first heart attack
In patients with CAD including prior MI to slow up the progression of coronary atherosclerosis and to reduce the risk of acute coronary events.

Dosage

Adults: Administer 10–40 mg/d in tablet form at bedtime. Adjust to response at 4 wk intervals.

Elderly: Give 20 mg or less per day.

Children: Safety and effectiveness not established.

Preparation

Pravachol (Bristol-Myers Squibb Co.): 10, 20, 40 mg tablets

6. Simvastatin (Zocor)

Indication

Hypercholesterolemia (types IIa and IIb)
Hypertriglyceridemia
In patients with CAD, reduces risk of death from heart disease
Reduces risk of nonfatal myocardial infarction
Reduces risk of undergoing myocardial revascularization procedures

Dosage

Adults: Initial dose, 5–10 mg in tablet form at night; increase at 4 wk intervals according to response. Maintenance dose, 5–40 mg/d, taken as single dose before retiring to bed.

Elderly: Initial dose, 5 mg/d.

Children: Safety and effectiveness not established.

Preparation

Zocor (Merck & Co.): 5, 10, 20, 40 mg tablets

NEURONAL AND GANGLIONIC BLOCKERS

1. Guanadrel (Hylorel)

Indication

Hypertension

Dosage

Adults: Initially, give 5 mg twice daily. Adjust dosage weekly or monthly until blood pressure is controlled—using standing blood pressure measurements as basis. Maintenance dose is usually 20–75 mg/d in two to four divided doses. Maximum dose, usually 100 mg/d.

Elderly: Lower dosage recommended; elderly are more susceptible to hypotensive effects of drug.

Children: Safety and effectiveness not established.

Preparation

Hylorel (Medeva Pharmaceuticals): 10, 25 mg tablets

2. Guanethidine (Guanethidine, Ismelin)

Indication

Hypertension
Hypertensive crisis
Renal hypertension

Dosage

Adults: Initially, give 10 or 12.5 mg/d orally; increased gradually according to response (10 or 12.5 mg increments at weekly intervals). Maintenance dose is 25–50 mg/d. Dosage may be increased more rapidly and to higher levels under careful hospital supervision.

Elderly: Use lower dose.

Children: 0.2 mg/kg body weight. Daily dose can be increased by 0.2 mg/kg body weight at 7–10 d intervals, if necessary, to control blood pressure.

Preparation

Guanethidine (generic); Ismelin (CibaGeneva): 10, 25 mg tablets

3. Mecamylamine (Inversine)

Indication

Hypertension
Malignant hypertension, uncomplicated
Hyperreflexia
Smoking cessation

Dosage

Adults: Initially, give 2.5 mg twice daily; increase in increments of 2.5 mg every 2 d according to response. Smallest dose should be taken in the mornings to limit the orthostatic adverse effects of the drug. The average maintenance dose is 25 mg/d in three divided doses.

Elderly: Lower dose recommended.

Note: Recommend that mecamylamine be administered at consistent times in relationship to meals. Administration after meals may cause a more gradual absorption and smoother control of blood pressure; therefore, administration after meals may be preferable to administration on an empty stomach.

Children: Safety and effectiveness not established.

Preparation

Inversine (Merck & Co.): 2.5 mg tablets

4. Reserpine (Reserpine)

Indication

Hypertension

Dosage

Adults: 0.1–0.25 mg/d, taken at meals to avoid gastric irritation.

Children: 0.005–0.02 mg/kg (5–20 μg/kg) or 0.15–0.60 mg/m^2 (150–600 μg) body surface area in one or two divided daily doses. Dose $>$ 0.25 mg daily is generally not recommended due to increased possibility of mental depression and other side effects.

Elderly: More sensitive to the hypotensive and CNS effects.

Preparation

Reserpine (generic) 0.1, 0.25 mg tablets

VASODILATORS

1. Cyclandelate (Cyclandelate, Cyclospasmol)

Indication

Adjunctive therapy for intermittent claudication
Arteriosclerosis obliterans
Thrombophlebitis (to control associated vasospasm and muscular ischemia)
Nocturnal leg cramps
Raynaud's phenomenon
Ischemic cerebrovascular disease (selected cases)

Note: The FDA has classified cyclandelate as being ineffective for its labeled indications.

Dosage

Adults: Give 1.2–1.6 g/d orally before meals and at bedtime. Dosage should be reduced by decrements of 200 mg until a maintenance dose of 400–800 mg/d in two to four divided doses is reached.

Elderly: Treatment similar to that for younger people.

Children: Safety and effectiveness not established.

Preparation

Cyclandelate (generic); Cyclospasmol (Wyeth-Ayerst): 200, 400 mg capsules

2. Diazoxide (Diazoxide, Hyperstat IV, Proglycem)

Indication

Hypertensive emergencies (intravenous)
Hypoglycemia (oral)

Dosage

Hypertension

Adults: Intravenously, give 150–300 mg or 1–3 mg/kg body weight every 5–15 min if necessary to obtain desired response. Further doses may be administered every 4–24 h as needed to maintain desired blood pressure until oral antihypertensive medication is effective, usually within 4–5 d. Limit to 1.2 g/d.

Note: Treatment is most effective if intravenous administration is completed within 10–30 s. Patient should remain recumbent during and for 15–30 min after administration.

Children: Intravenous 1–3 mg/kg body weight or 30–90 mg/m^2 body surface area, every 5–15 min as necessary to obtain desired response. Further doses may be given every 4–24 h, as needed to maintain desired blood pressure until oral antihypertensive medication is effective. In hypertensive emergencies, usual initial dose is 150 mg (in 20 mL solution) intravenously. Injection should be rapid and not exceed 30 s.

Elderly: May require reduction in dose or lengthening of dosage interval.

Oral

Adults and Adolescents: Oral, initially 1 mg/kg of body weight every 8 h, adjusted according to clinical response. For maintenance, 3 to 8 mg/kg of body weight a day, divided into two or three equal doses every 12 or 8 h, respectively.

Neonates and Infants: Oral, 3.3 mg/kg body weight every 8 h, adjusted according to clinical response. For maintenance, 8 to 15 mg/kg of body weight a day divided into two or three equal doses every 12 or 8 h.

Elderly: More likely to have age-related renal function impairment, which may require a reduction in dosage and/or longer dosing interval.

Preparation

Hyperstat IV (Schering): 15 mg/mL, or 20 mL ampules containing diazoxide, 300 mg
Proglycem (Baker Norton): 50 mg capsules
Proglycem oral suspension (Baker Norton): 50 mg/mL

3. Fenoldopam (Corlopam)

Indication

Short term management of severe hypertension
Malignant hypertension

Dosage

Adults: The initial dose of fenoldopam is chosen according to the desired magnitude and rate of blood pressure reduction in a given clinical situation. In general, there is a greater and more rapid blood pressure reduction as the initial dose is increased. Lower initial doses (0.03–0.1 μg/kg/min) titrated slowly have been associated with less reflex tachycardia than have higher initial doses (≥ 0.3 μg/kg/min). The recommended increments for titration are 0.05–0.1 μg/kg/min at intervals of ≥ 15 minutes.

Doses below 0.1 μg/kg/min have very modest effects and appear only marginally useful in patients with severe hypertension. Fenoldopam infusion can be abruptly discontinued or gradually tapered prior to discontinuation. Oral antihypertensive agents can be added during fenoldopam infusion or following its discontinuation. Patients in clinical trials have received intravenous fenoldopam for a maximum of 48 hours.

Note: Fenoldopam should be administered by continuous intravenous infusion only. A bolus dose should not be used. The fenoldopam injection ampule concentrate must be diluted with the appropriate amount of 0.9% sodium chloride or 5% dextrose before infusion. Please see package insert for details of proper dilution.

Elderly: Age does not influence the pharmacokinetics of fenoldopam. Dosage is the same as in younger adults.

Children: Safety and effectiveness not established.

Preparation

Corlopam (Neurex): 10 mg/mL in single-dose ampules of 5 mL.

4. Hydralazine (Hydralazine, Apresoline)

Indication

Cardiac failure
Systemic hypertension
Hypertensive emergencies
Severe aortic regurgitation

Dosage

Oral

Adults: For hypertension, give 40 mg/d for the first 2–4 d, 100 mg/d for the balance of wk 1, and 200 mg/d for wk 2 and subsequent weeks in four divided daily doses. Maintain dose at lowest effective level. Limit to 300 mg/d. Higher doses have been used in the treatment of congestive heart failure.

Children: For hypertension, give 750 μg (0.75 mg)/kg body weight or 25 mg/m^2 body surface area per day divided into four doses; increase gradually over 3–4 wk as needed. Limit to 7.5 mg/kg body weight or 200 mg/d.

Elderly: May be more sensitive to adult dose.

Parenteral

Adults: For hypertension, give 10–40 mg intravenously or intramuscularly; repeat as needed.

Children: For hypertension, give 1.7–3.5 mg/kg body weight intravenously or intramuscularly; or 50–100 mg/m^2 body surface area per day; divide into 4–6 daily doses.

Preparation

Hydralazine (generic); Apresoline (CibaGeneva): 10, 25, 50, 100 mg tablets
Hydralazine hydrochloride injection (generic); Apresoline (Ciba-Geneva): 20 mg/mL in 1 mL ampules

5. Isoxsuprine (Vasodilan)

Indication

Cerebrovascular insufficiency (possibly effective)
Peripheral vascular disease (possibly effective)
Raynaud's phenomenon (possibly effective)

Dosage

Adults: Give 10–20 mg orally three to four times daily with meals, milk, or antacid to reduce gastrointestinal irritation.

Children: Not recommended.

Elderly: Same dosage as for adults.

Preparation

Isoxsuprine (generic); Vasodilan (Apothecon): 10, 20 mg tablets

6. Minoxidil (Minoxidil, Loniten, Rogaine)

Indication

Resistant or refractory hypertension
Severe hypertension
Topical use for male-pattern baldness of the vertex of the scalp

Dosage

Adults: Usual initial dose is 5 mg/d orally as a single or divided dose; may be increased by 10 mg every 3 d (seldom necessary to exceed 50 mg/d). Maintenance dose should be at 10–40 mg/d. Limit to 100 mg/d. *Topical* (for male-pattern baldness): Apply 1 mL to affected areas of scalp twice daily (morning and night). Wash hands after applying.

Elderly: May require reduced dosage (see above).

Children: For children under 12 y, the usual dose should be 0.2 mg/kg daily in single or divided doses, initially to a maximum of 1.0 mg/kg per day. Maximum daily dose, 50 mg.

Note: Allow interval of at least 3 d between each dosage for full effect; 3–7 d of treatment are needed for maximum blood pressure response.

Preparation

Minoxidil (generic); Loniten (Upjohn): 2.5, 10 mg tablets
Rogaine topical solution (Pharmacia & Upjohn): 2% per 60 mL (20 mg/mL)

7. Pentoxifylline (Trental)

Indication

Intermittent claudication

Dosage

Adults: Usual initial dose is 400 mg three times daily with meals, reduced to 400 mg twice daily if gastrointestinal or central nervous system side effects occur.

Elderly: May be more sensitive to effects of usual adult dose; dosage reduction may be required.

Children: Not recommended.

Preparation

Trental (Hoechst Marion Roussel): 400 mg tablets

8. Phenoxybenzamine (Dibenzyline)

Indication

Hypertension (in pheochromocytoma)

Dosage

Adults: Give 20 mg/d in two divided doses; increase by 10 mg every second day until response occurs. Maintenance dose, 20–40 mg two to three times daily.

Children: Give 0.2 mg/kg or 6 mg/m^2/d (to 10 mg maximum dose). Increase dosage every 4 d until response occurs. Maintenance dose, 0.4–1.2 mg/kg or 12–36 mg/m^2/d in three to four divided doses.

Elderly: May be more sensitive to effects of adult dosage.

Preparation

Dibenzyline (SmithKline Beecham): 10 mg capsules

9. Phentolamine (Regitine)

Indication

Pheochromocytoma
Dermal necrosis from extravasation of norepinephrine

Dosage

Adults: *Preoperative:* 5 mg intravenously 1–2 h before surgery; repeat if necessary. *During surgery:* 5 mg intravenously or 0.5–1 mg/min intravenous infusion; adjust to response. *Hypertensive crisis:* 5–20 mg. *Clonidine withdrawal:* 5–10 mg intravenously at 5 min intervals, up to 20–30 mg. *Following extravasation of norepinephrine:* infiltrate 5–10 mg in 10 mL of sodium chloride injection; effective if given within 12 h of extravasation.

Children: *Preoperative:* 1 mg intramuscularly or intravenously; 100 μg (0.1 mg)/kg or 3 mg/m^2 1–2 h prior to surgery; repeat if necessary. *During surgery:* 1 mg intravenously; 100 μg (0.1 mg)/kg; or 3 mg/m^2 intravenously. *For blood pressure reduction:* 0.1– 0.2 mg/kg, up to a maximum of 10 mg.

Elderly: May be more sensitive to adult dose.

Note: Reconstituted solution should be used when prepared. Do not store remainder.

Preparation

Regitine (Ciba-Geneva): 5 mg IV solution in 1 mL vials

10. Tolazoline (Priscoline)

Indication

Pulmonary hypertension (in the newborn)

Dosage

Newborns: For pulmonary hypertension, the recommended dose is 1–2 mg/kg body weight via scalp vein over a 5–10 min period. Maintenance is best with 1–2 mg/kg body weight/h, increased if necessary (in increments of 1–2 mg/kg/h) up to 6–8 mg/kg/h. May be withdrawn gradually when arterial blood gases remain stable. If necessary, the initial bolus dose may be repeated during the maintenance infusion.

Elderly: Not applicable.

Preparation:

Priscoline (CibaGeneva): 25 mg/mL in 4 mL ampules

VASODILATORS: NITRATES AND NITRITES

1. Erythrityl Tetranitrate (Cardilate)

Indication

Angina pectoris

Dosage

Adults: Initiate at 5–10 mg three to four times daily—administer orally, sublingually, or bucally. Adjust as needed and tolerated. Limit to 100 mg/d.

Children: Dosage not established.

Elderly: May be more sensitive to adult dose. Lower if necessary.

Note: Regular tablet currently marketed may be used for oral, sublingual, or buccal dosage; however, sublingual form is not useful for the treatment of acute angina attacks.

Preparation

Cardilate (Burroughs Wellcome): 10 mg tablets

2. Isosorbide Dinitrate (Isosorbide dinitrate, Isordil, Dilatrate SR, Sorbitrate)

Indication

Hypertensive emergencies
Angina (treatment and prophylaxis)

Dosage

Adult: As an antianginal agent, give 5–20 mg in tablet form 3 times daily; adjust as needed and tolerated. Dose range, 5–40 mg 3 times daily. Usual range, 10–40 mg 3 times daily. Elderly may be more sensitive to hypotensive effect. Use with caution in those with impaired renal function; may require reduction in dose.

Note: A daily nitrate-free interval of at least 14 h is advisable to minimize tolerance. The optimal interval will vary with the individual patient, dose, and regimen.

Children: Safety and effectiveness not established.

Preparation

Isosorbide dinitrate capsules (generic); Dilatrate SR (Schwarz): 40 mg extended-release capsules
Isordil (Wyeth-Ayerst); Sorbitrate (Zeneca): 5, 10, 20, 30, 40 mg tablets

Isosorbide dinitrate (generic): 2.5, 5, 10, 20, 30 mg tablets
Sorbitrate (Zeneca): 5, 10 mg chewable tablets
Isosorbide dinitrate extended-release tablets (generic); Isordil (Wyeth-Ayerst); Sorbitrate SA (Zeneca): 40 mg extended-release tablets
Isosorbide dinitrate sublingual (generic); Isordil (Wyeth-Ayerst); Sorbitrate (Zeneca): 2.5, 5, 10 mg sublingual tablets

3. Isosorbide Mononitrate (Ismo, Monoket, Imdur)

Indication

Angina (treatment and prophylaxis)

Dosage

Adults: For angina prophylaxis, tablets should be swallowed whole. Give 20 mg (Ismo, Monoket) twice daily with doses given 7 h apart. An initial dose of 5 mg twice daily may be appropriate for persons of small stature. Imdur may be initiated at 30 or 60 mg once daily. Dosage of Imdur may be increased to 120 mg once daily after several days if necessary.

Elderly: May be more sensitive to hypotensive effects. Use caution in those with impaired renal function; may require reduction in dosage.

Children: Safety and effectiveness not established.

Preparation

Ismo (Wyeth-Ayerst): 20 mg tablets
Monoket (Schwarz): 10, 20 mg tablets
Imdur (Key Pharmaceuticals): 60 mg extended-release tablets

4. Nitroglycerin (Nitroglycerin, Nitrogard, Nitrolingual, Nitro-bid, Nitrostat, Transderm-Nitro, Nitroglyn, Minitran, Deponit, Nitrodisc)

Indication

Hypertension (intravenous)
Controlled hypotension (intravenous)
Angina (therapy and prophylaxis)
Congestive heart failure
Intubation
Acute myocardial infarction

Dosage

Adults: For angina, give 150–600 μg (0.15–0.6 mg) sublingual tablets; repeat every 5 min as needed to relieve angina attacks. Place tablet(s) under tongue and allow to dissolve. If no relief is achieved after three tablets in 15 min, contact physician and go to hospital.

Elderly: May be more sensitive to hypotensive effects or have age-related renal function impairment; lower dosage may be required.

Children: Has been used.

Preparation

Nitrostat (Parke-Davis): 0.15, 0.3, 0.4, 0.6 mg sublingual tablets

Nitroglycerin: Special Formulations

4a. Lingual Aerosol

Dosage

For angina, spray on or under the tongue one or two metered doses (400 or 800 μg, 0.4 or 0.8 mg) repeating every 5 min as needed for relief of angina attacks. Limit to 1.2 mg/d. If no relief is achieved after three doses in 15 min, call physician and go to hospital. Do not shake before use. Do not inhale.

Preparation

Nitrolingual spray (Rhone-Poulenc Rorer): 400 μg (0.4 mg) per metered dose

4b. Parenteral, Adult

Dosage

For angina, hypertension, or cardiac load reduction, give as intravenous infusion initially at 5 μg/ min (0.005 mg); increase by increments of 5 μg/ min at 3–5 min intervals until desired effect is obtained or to 20 μg/min. Dosage may be increased beyond 20 μg/min by 10 μg/min increments at 3–5 min intervals, then by 20 μg/min increments until desired effect is reached. Slow dosage increments and frequency as partial effect are noted.

Note: Intravenous infusion is not direct, but must be given through a special nonpolyvinylchloride (non-PVC) intravenous infusion set or infusion pump. Dilute as instructed by manufacturer. Do not administer with other medications.

Preparation

Nitrostat injection (Parke-Davis): 0.8, 5, 10 mg/ mL
Nitro-Bid IV (Hoechst Marion Roussel): 5, 10 mg/mL
Nitroglycerin injection (generic): 0.5, 0.8, 1, 5, 10 mg/mL

4c. Oral, Adult, Extended-Release Buccal Tablets

Dosage

For angina, initially give 1 mg dissolved in place on the oral mucosa every 5 h during waking hours. Increase dosage in strength and/or frequency as needed. Do not chew or swallow tablet. Available in 1, 2, and 3 mg tablets.

Preparation

Nitrogard (Forest Pharmaceuticals): 1, 2, 3 mg tablets

4d. Extended-Release Capsules

Dosage

For angina, give 2.5, 6.5, or 9 mg every 12 h; increase to every 8 h if needed and tolerated. Swallow capsules whole with a glass of water.

Note: Tolerance may develop when nitroglycerin is administered without a nitrate-free interval. Consider administering on a reduced schedule (once or twice daily).

Preparation

Nitroglycerin extended-release capsules (generic); Nitroglyn (Kenwood): 2.5, 6.5, 9 mg capsules

4e. Extended-Release Tablets

Dosage

For angina, 1.3, 2.6, or 6.5 mg every 12 h; increase to every 8 h if needed and tolerated. Swallow tablet whole with glass of water.

Note: Tolerance may develop when nitroglycerin is administered without a nitrate-free interval. Consider administering on a reduced schedule (once or twice daily).

Preparation

Generic: 2.6, 6.5, 9 mg tablets

4f. Topical Ointment

Dosage

For angina, initiate at 15–30 mg (1–2 in) every 8 h, increasing by one-half inch per application every 6 h to a maximum of 75 mg (5 in) per application every 4 h.

Note: Any regimen of nitroglycerin ointment administration should include a daily nitrate-free interval of about 10–12 h to avoid tolerance. To apply the ointment using the dose-measuring paper applicator, place the applicator on a flat surface, printed side down. Squeeze the necessary amount of ointment from the tube onto the applicator, place the applicator (ointment side down) on the desired area of skin (usually on nonhairy skin of chest or back), and tape the applicator into place. Do not rub in.

Preparation

Generic; Nitro-Bid (Hoechst Marion Roussel): 2%

4g. Transdermal Patch

Dosage

For angina, apply one patch to skin every 24 h, with the smallest patch in place for 12–14 h, removing 10–12 h before applying new patch. Apply patch to clean, dry, hairless skin of chest, inner upper arm, or shoulder. Avoid placing below knee or elbow. Vary site of placement to avoid skin irritation. Apply a new patch if first patch loosens or falls off. Patches are available for delivering 0.1, 0.2, 0.3, 0.4, 0.6 and 0.8 mg/h of nitroglycerin.

Preparation

Generic 0.1, 0.2, 0.4, 0.6 mg/h; Transderm-Nitro (Summit): 0.1, 0.2, 0.4, 0.6 mg/h
Minitran (3M Pharm): 0.1, 0.2, 0.4, 0.6 mg/h
Deponit (Schwarz Pharma): 0.2, 0.4 mg/h
Nitrodisc (Roberts): 0.2, 0.3, 0.4 mg/h
Nitro-Dur (Key): 0.1, 0.2, 0.3, 0.4, 0.6, 0.8 mg/h

5. Pentaerythritol Tetranitrate (Pentaerythritol tetranitrate, Peritrate SA, Duotrate, Pentylan)

Indication

Angina pectoris prophylaxis

Dosage

Adults: *Regular tablets*: Give 10–20 mg four times daily, 30 min before or 1 h after meals and at bedtime; adjust to response. *Extended-release tablets:* Give up to 80 mg twice daily. *Extended-release capsules:* Give 30–80 mg twice daily. Take extended-release forms on empty stomach.

Elderly: May be more sensitive to adult dose.

Children: Dosage not established.

Note: Limit all forms to 160 mg/d.

Preparation

Pentylan (Lannett): 10, 20 mg tablets
Pentaerythritol tetranitrate tablets (generic): 10, 20, 80 mg tablets
Pentaerythritol tetranitrate extended-release tablets (generic; Peritrate SA): 80 mg extended-release tablets
Duotrate (Jones): 30, 45 mg extended-release capsules

6. Nitroprusside (Sodium Nitroprusside, Nitropress)

Indication

Hypertensive crisis (myocardial infarction adjunct therapy and congestive heart failure not included in U.S. product labeling; thus not all hypertensive crises are indicated)
Hypertension (treatment)
Malignant hypertension
Controlled hypotension during surgery to reduce bleeding into the surgical field

Dosage

Adults: For hypertension, the usual initial dose is 0.3 μg/kg/min (range, 0.1–0.5 μg/kg/min) intravenous infusion; can be adjusted slowly in increments of 0.5 μg/kg/min according to response. Usual dose is 3 μg/kg/min. Should not exceed 0.01 mg/ kg/min or a total dose of 3.5 mg/kg (0.5 mg/kg during short-term infusions such as in controlled hypotension during surgery). Infusion at the maximum dose rate (10 μg/kg/min) should never last more than 10 min. To keep the steady-state thiocyanate concentration below 1 mmol/L, the rate of a prolonged infusion should not exceed 3 μg/kg per minute (1 μg/kg per minute in anuric patients).

Note: After reconstitution with appropriate diluent, sodium nitroprusside injection is not suitable for direct injection. The reconstituted solution must be further diluted in the appropriate amount of sterile 5% dextrose injection before infusion. Sodium nitroprusside should not be infused through ordinary IV apparatus, regulated only by gravity and mechanical clamps. Only an infusion pump, preferably a volumetric pump, should be used (see product package insert for complete prescribing information).

Elderly: May be more sensitive to usual adult dose as a result of decreased renal function.

Children: Appropriate studies not performed. Initial dose should be 0.5 μg/kg/min in hypertension (maximum, 10 μg/kg/min).

Preparation

Sodium nitroprusside powder (generic); Nitropress (Abbott): 50 mg in 2 mL, and 5 mL vials

ANTIHYPERTENSIVE FIXED-DRUG COMBINATIONS

ACE INHIBITORS WITH THIAZIDE DIURETIC

1. Benazepril and Hydrochlorothiazide (Lotensin HCT)

Indication

Hypertension (This fixed combination drug is not indicated for the initial treatment of hypertension.)

Dosage

Adults: Benazepril, 20 mg, and HCTZ, 25 mg; benazepril, 20 mg, and HCTZ, 12.5 mg; benazepril, 10 mg, and HCTZ, 12.5 mg; benazepril, 5 mg, and HCTZ, 6.25 mg.

Elderly: Usually respond well; dose reduction generally not required.

Children: Safety and effectiveness not established.

Preparation

Lotensin HCT (CibaGeneva)

2. Captopril and Hydrochlorothiazide (Capozide)

Indication

Hypertension

Dosage

Adults: Captopril, 50 mg, and HCTZ, 25 mg; captopril, 25 mg, and HCTZ, 25 mg; captopril, 50 mg, and HCTZ, 15 mg; or captopril, 25 mg, and HCTZ, 15 mg. Adjust dosages to meet individual requirements of patient. Usual maintenance dose is one tablet 1–3 times daily.

Elderly: Dose should be kept as low as possible; in some patients half a tablet may be sufficient.

Children: Safety and effectiveness not established.

Preparation

Capozide (Bristol Myers Squibb)

3. Enalapril and Hydrochlorothiazide (Vaseretic)

Indication

Hypertension (This fixed combination drug is not indicated for the initial treatment of hypertension.)

Dosage

Adults: Enalapril, 5 mg and HCTZ, 12.5 mg, enalapril, 10 mg, and HCTZ, 25 mg. Usual adult dose is one tablet daily as determined by individual titration.

Elderly: May be more sensitive to the effects of the usual adult dose; keep dose as low as possible.

Children: Dosage not established.

Preparation

Vaseretic (Merck & Co.)

4. Lisinopril and Hydrochlorothiazide (Prinzide, Zestoretic)

Indication

Hypertension (This fixed combination drug is not indicated for the initial treatment of hypertension.)

Dosage

Adults: Lisinopril, 10 mg, and HCTZ, 12.5 mg, Lisinopril, 20 mg, and HCTZ, 12.5 mg; or lisinopril, 20 mg, and HCTZ, 25 mg. Usual adult dose is one tablet daily as determined by individual titration.

Elderly: Geriatric patients may be more sensitive to the effects of the usual adult dose; keep dose as low as possible.

Children: Dosage not established.

Preparation

Prinzide (Merck & Co.); Zestoretic (Zeneca)

ACE INHIBITOR WITH CALCIUM BLOCKER

1. Amlodipine and Benazepril HCl (Lotrel)

Indication

Hypertension (the fixed combination drug is not indicated for the initial therapy of hypertension).

Dosage

Capsules are given once daily for adults. No dosage adjustments are needed in elderly patients. Amlodipine, 2.5 mg, and benazepril HCl, 10 mg; amlodipine, 5 mg, and benazepril HCl, 10 mg; or amlodipine, 5 mg, and benazepril HCl, 20 mg. Amlodipine is an effective treatment of hypertension in once-daily doses of 2.5–10 mg, whereas benazepril is effective in doses of 10–80 mg. In clinical trials of amlodipine/benazepril combination therapy using amlodipine doses of 2.5–5 mg and benazepril doses of 10–20 mg, the antihypertensive effects increased with increasing dose of amlodipine in all patient groups, and the effects increased with increasing dose of benazepril in non-African American groups.

Elderly: Clinical experience has not identified differences in response between the elderly and younger patients, but greater sensitivity of some older individuals cannot be ruled out.

Children: Safety and effectiveness not established.

Preparation

Lotrel (CibaGeneva)

2. Enalapril Maleate and Diltiazem Malate Extended Release (Teczem)

Indication

Hypertension (This fixed combination drug is not indicated for the intial therapy of hypertension.)

Dosage

Tablets are usually given once daily for adults. The initial dose of enalapril maleate for hypertension in patients not receiving diuretics is 5 mg once daily. The usual dosage range of enalapril maleate for hypertension is 10–40 mg/d administered in a single dose or 2 divided doses. The usual dosage range of controlled-release formulations of diltiazem for hypertension is 120–540 mg once daily. In clinical trials of enalapril maleate–diltiazem malate controlled-release formulation, administered once daily, the antihypertensive effect of the combination generally increased as the dose of each ingredient was increased. In the combination trials, the doses studied were 12.5–20 mg of enalapril maleate and 60–360 mg of diltiazem malate.

Elderly: Clinical experience has not identified differences in response between the elderly and younger patients, but greater sensitivity of some older individuals cannot be ruled out.

Children: Safety and effectiveness have not been established.

Preparation

Teczem (Merck & Co.): 5/180 (5 mg enalapril maleate and 180 mg diltiazem malate extended-release) tablets

3. Felodipine extended release and Enalapril maleate (Lexxel)

Indication

Hypertension (This fixed combination drug is not indicated for the initial therapy of hypertension.)

Dosage

Usual adult dosage is one tablet daily. The recommended initial dose of enalapril maleate for hypertension in patients not receiving diuretics is 5 mg once daily. The usual dosage range of enalapril maleate for hypertension is 10–40 mg daily administered in a single dose or two divided doses. The recommended initial dose of felodipine extended release is 5 mg once daily with a usual dosage range of 2.5 mg–10 mg once daily. In clinical trials of enalapril-felodipine extended release combination therapy using enalapril doses of 5–20 mg once daily, the antihypertensive effects increased with increasing doses of each component in all patient groups.

Elderly: Patients over 65 years of age (or patients with impaired liver function) may have elevated plasma concentrations of felodipine; the recommended initial dose of felodipine is 2.5 mg.

Children: Safety and effectiveness not established.

Preparation

Lexxel (Astra Merck): 5–5 (5 mg of enalapril maleate and 5 mg of felodipine extended release) film-coated tablet.

4. Trandolapril/Verapamil hydrochloride extended release (Tarka)

Indication

Hypertension (This fixed combination drug is not indicated for the initial therapy of hypertension.)

Dosage

Tablets are given once daily with food for adults. The usual dosage range of trandolapril for hypertension is 1 to 4 mg per day administered in a single dose or two divided doses. The usual dosage range of verapamil extended release for hypertension is 120 to 480 mg per day administered in a single dose or two divided doses. Over the dose range of verapamil extended release 120 to 240 mg once daily and trandolapril 0.5 to 8 mg once daily, the effects of the combination increase with increasing doses of either component.

Elderly: Clinical experience has not identified differences in response between the elderly and younger patients, but greater sensitivity of some older individuals cannot be ruled out.

Children: Safety and effectiveness not established.

Preparation

Tarka (Knoll): 2/180 (2 mg trandolapril, 180 mg verapamil hydrochloride extended release), 1/240 (1 mg trandolapril, 240 mg verapamil hydrochloride extended release), 2/240 (2 mg trandolapril, 240 mg verapamil hydrochloride extended release), 4/240 (4 mg trandolapril, 240 mg verapamil hydrochloride extended release) tablets.

ANGIOTENSIN II RECEPTOR BLOCKER WITH THIAZIDE DIURETIC

1. Losartan Potassium and Hydrochlorothiazide (Hyzaar)

Indication

Hypertension (therapeutic)

Dosage

Tablets of losartan, 50 mg, and HCTZ, 12.5 mg. For maintenance, use 1 or 2 tablets once a day, as determined by individual titration with the component agents.

Note: Not indicated for initial therapy.

Children: Safety and efficacy not established.

Preparation

Hyzaar (Merck & Co.)

SYMPATHOLYTIC (β BLOCKER) WITH THIAZIDE DIURETIC

1. Atenolol and Chlorthalidone (Tenoretic)

Indication

Hypertension

Dosage

Adults: Atenolol, 100 mg, and chlorthalidone, 25 mg; or atenolol, 50 mg, and chlorthalidone, 25 mg. Usual adult dose is one or two tablets daily as a single dose or in divided doses as determined by individual patient titration.

Elderly: Use low-dose combination. Patients may have increased or decreased sensitivity to effects of usual adult dose.

Children: Safety and effectiveness not established.

Preparation

Atenolol and chlorthalidone (generic); Tenoretic (Zeneca)

2. Nadolol and Bendroflumethiazide (Corzide)

This combination provides increased acceptability and dosage flexibility for hypertensive patients receiving suboptimal control with single agent therapy.

Indication

Hypertension

Dosage

Adults: Nadolol, 40 mg, and bendroflumethiazide, 5 mg; or nadolol, 80 mg, and bendroflumethiazide, 5 mg. Usual adult dose one tablet once daily as determined by individual patient titration.

Elderly: Low dose advisable; may be sensitive to usual adult dose.

Children: Safety and effectiveness not established.

Preparation

Corzide (Bristol)

3. Metoprolol and Hydrochlorothiazide (Lopressor HCT)

Indication

Hypertension

Dosage

Adults: Metoprolol, 100 mg, and HCTZ, 50 mg; metoprolol, 100 mg, and HCTZ, 25 mg; or metoprolol, 50 mg, and HCTZ,

25 mg. Usual adult dose is one or two tablets daily as a single dose or in divided doses as determined by individual patient titration.

Preparation

Lopressor HCT (CibaGeneva)

4. Timolol and Hydrochlorothiazide (Timolide)

Indication

Hypertension

Dosage

Adults: Timolol, 10 mg, and HCTZ, 25 mg. Usual adult dose is one tablet twice daily.

Preparation

Timolide (Merck & Co.)

5. Propranolol and Hydrochlorothiazide (Inderide)

Indication

Hypertension

Dosage

Adults: Propranolol, 40 mg, and HCTZ, 25 mg; or propranolol, 80 mg, and HCTZ, 25 mg. Usual adult dose is one or two tablets twice daily.

Preparation

Propranolol and hydrochlorothiazide (generic); Inderide (Wyeth-Ayerst)

6. Propranolol and Hydrochlorothiazide Extended Release (Inderide LA)

Indication

Hypertension

Dosage

Adults: Propranolol extended release, 80 mg, and HCTZ, 50 mg; propranolol extended release, 120 mg, and HCTZ, 50 mg; or propranolol extended release, 160 mg, and HCTZ, 50 mg. Usual adult dose is one capsule daily. For detailed information regarding adverse effects, contraindications, and special precautions, refer to individual drug component profiles (see HCTZ). Usual adult dose for all of the above must be determined by individual titration with the component agents. Do not initiate therapy with any of the above combinations.

Preparation

Inderide LA (Wyeth-Ayerst)

Note: The preceding antihypertensive combinations have the following in common:

Elderly: Use low-dose combination.

Children: Not recommended; safety and efficacy not established.

VERY-LOW-DOSE β BLOCKER WITH THIAZIDE DIURETIC

1. Bisoprolol Fumarate and Hydrochlorothiazide (HCTZ) (Ziac)

Indication

Hypertension (can be considered first-line)

Dosage

Tablets: Bisoprolol, 2.5 mg, and HCTZ, 6.25 mg; bisoprolol, 5 mg, and HCTZ, 6.25 mg; or bisoprolol, 10 mg, and HCTZ 6.25 mg.

Adults: Initial dose is bisoprolol 2.5 mg/hydrochlorothiazide 6.25 mg tablet once daily. Titrate at 14 d intervals up to bisoprolol 20 mg/hydrochlorothiazide 12.5 mg (two 10 mg/6.25 mg tablets) until desired blood pressure levels are reached.

Elderly: No dosage adjustments necessary, unless significant renal or hepatic impairment is present.

Children: Safety and effectiveness not established.

Preparation

Ziac (Lederle)

SYMPATHOLYTIC (CENTRAL-ACTING AGENT) WITH THIAZIDE DIURETIC

1. Clonidine and Chlorthalidone (Combipres)

Indication

Hypertension

Dosage

Adults: Clonidine, 0.1 mg, and chlorthalidone, 15 mg; clonidine, 0.2 mg, and chlorthalidone, 15 mg; or clonidine, 0.3 mg, and chlorthalidone, 15 mg. Usual adult dose is one or two tablets once or twice daily (maximum daily dose of clonidine is 2.4 mg). Determine dose by individual patient titration.

Elderly: Lower-dose combinations are preferable; may be more sensitive to usual adult dose.

Children: Safety and effectiveness not established.

Preparation

Clonidine and chlorthalidone (generic); Combipres (Boehringer Ingelheim)

2. Methyldopa and Hydrochlorothiazide (Aldoril)

Indication

Hypertension

Dosage

Adults: Methyldopa, 250 mg, and HCTZ, 25 mg; methyldopa, 250 mg, and HCTZ, 15 mg; methyldopa, 500 mg, and HCTZ, 30 mg; or methyldopa, 500 mg, and HCTZ, 50 mg. Usual adult dose is two to four tablets a day in a single dose or in divided doses, as determined by individual patient titration.

Elderly: Initial dose should not exceed one tablet daily. The dose may then be increased slowly if required; may be more sensitive to usual adult dose.

Children: As determined by individual titration.

Preparation

Methyldopa and hydrochlorothiazide (generic); Aldoril (Merck & Co.)

3. Methyldopa and Chlorothiazide (Aldoclor)

Indication

Hypertension

Dosage

Adults: Methyldopa, 250 mg, and chlorothiazide, 250 mg; or methyldopa, 250 mg, and chlorothiazide, 150 mg. Usual adult dose is two to four tablets a day in a single or divided dose. Do not initiate therapy with this combination.

Elderly: May be more sensitive to the effects of the usual adult dose.

Children: Determined by individual patient titration.

Preparation

Methyldopa and chlorothiazide (generic); Aldoclor (Merck & Co.)

SYMPATHOLYTIC (PERIPHERAL-ACTING ADRENERGIC ANTAGONIST) WITH THIAZIDE DIURETIC

1. Reserpine and Chlorthalidone (Demi-Regroton, Regroton)

Indication

Hypertension

Dosage

Adults: Reserpine, 0.25 mg, and chlorthalidone, 50 mg; or reserpine, 0.125 mg, and chlorthalidone, 25 mg. Usual adult dose is one to two tablets once daily as determined by individual titration.

Elderly: May be more sensitive to usual adult dose.

Children: Safety and effectiveness not established.

Preparation

Regroton (Rhone-Poulenc Rorer): 0.25 mg reserpine and 50 mg chlorthalidone
Demi-Regroton (Rhone-Poulenc Rorer): 0.125 mg reserpine and 25 mg chlorthalidone

2. Reserpine and Hydroflumethiazide (Salutensin; Salutensin-Demi)

Indication

Hypertension

Dosage

Adults: Reserpine, 0.125 mg, and hydroflumethiazide, 25 mg; or reserpine, 0.125 mg, and hydroflumethiazide, 50 mg. Usual adult dose is one tablet once or twice daily.

Preparation

Salutensin-Demi (Roberts): 0.125 mg reserpine and 25 mg hydroflumethiazide
Salutensin (Roberts): 0.125 mg reserpine and 50 mg hydroflumethiazide

3. Reserpine and Methyclothiazide (Diutensen-R)

Indication

Hypertension

Dosage

Adults: Reserpine, 0.1 mg, and methyclothiazide, 2.5 mg. Usual adult dose is one to four tablets daily in single or divided doses.

Preparation

Diutensen-R (Wallace)

4. Reserpine and Chlorothiazide (Diupres)

Indication

Hypertension

Dosage

Adults: Reserpine, 0.125 mg, and chlorothiazide, 250 mg; or reserpine, 0.125 mg, and chlorothiazide, 500 mg. Usual adult dose is one to two tablets once or twice daily.

Preparation

Reserpine and chlorothiazide (generic); Diupres (Merck & Co.)

5. Reserpine and Polythiazide (Renese-R)

Indication

Hypertension

Dosage

Adults: Reserpine, 0.25 mg, and polythiazide, 2 mg. Usual adult dose is one-half to two tablets daily.

Preparation

Renese-R (Pfizer)

6. Rauwolfia Serpentina and Bendroflumethiazide (Rauzide)

Indication

Hypertension

Dosage

Adults: Rauwolfia serpentina, 50 mg, and bendroflumethiazide, 4 mg. Usual adult dose is one to four tablets daily.

Preparation

Rauwolfia serpentina plus bendroflumethiazide (generic); Rauzide (Apothecon)

7. Deserpidine and Methyclothiazide (Enduronyl, Enduronyl Forte)

Indication

Hypertension

Dosage

Adults: Deserpidine, 0.25 mg, and methyclothiazide, 5 mg; or deserpidine, 0.5 mg, and methyclothiazide, 5 mg. Usual adult dose is one-half to one tablet daily.

Preparation

Enduronyl Forte (Abbott): 0.5 mg deserpidine and 5 mg methyclothiazide
Enduronyl (Abbott): 0.25 mg deserpidine and 5 mg methyclothiazide

8. Guanethidine and Hydrochlorothiazide (Esimil)

Indication

Hypertension

Dosage

Adults: Guanethidine, 10 mg, and HCTZ, 25 mg. Usual adult dose is two tablets daily.

Children: Pediatric dose is determined by individual titration with the component agents.

Note: For detailed information regarding adverse effects, contraindications, and special precautions, refer to individual drug component profiles. Usual adult dose for all the above must be determined by individual titration with the component agents. Do not initiate therapy with any of the above combinations.

Preparation

Esimil (CibaGeneva)

Note: The preceding antihypertensive combinations have the following in common:

Elderly: May be more sensitive to the effects of the usual adult dose.

Children: Dosage has not been established (except for guanethidine and HCTZ).

SYMPATHOLYTIC (ALPHA-ADRENERGIC ANTAGONIST) WITH THIAZIDE DIURETIC

1. Prazosin and Polythiazide (Minizide)

Indication

Hypertension

Dosage

Adults: Prazosin, 1 mg, and polythiazide, 0.5 mg; prazosin, 2 mg, and polythiazide, 0.5 mg; or prazosin, 5 mg, and polythiazide, 0.5 mg. Usual adult dose is one capsule twice or thrice daily. Determine dose by individual titration.

Elderly: Reduced-dose combination preferred; patients may be more sensitive to adult dose.

Children: Dosage determined by individual titration.

Preparation

Minizide (Pfizer)

VASODILATOR WITH THIAZIDE DIURETIC

1. Hydralazine and Hydrochlorothiazide (Apresazide)

Indication

Hypertension

Dosage

Tablets: Hydralazine, 25 mg, and HCTZ, 25 mg (generic); hydralazine, 50 mg, and HCTZ, 50 mg (generic); or hydralazine, 100 mg, and HCTZ, 50 mg (generic). *Capsules*: Hydralazine, 25 mg, and HCTZ, 25 mg (generic, Apresazide); hydralazine, 50 mg, and HCTZ, 50 mg (generic, Apresazide); or hydralazine, 100 mg, and HCTZ, 50 mg (generic), Apresazide). Usual adult dose is one capsule or tablet twice daily as determined by individual titration of each component.

Elderly: May be more sensitive to usual adult dose.

Children: Safety and effectiveness not established.

Preparation

Hydralazine and hydrochlorothiazide (generic); Apresazide (CibaGeneva)

POTASSIUM-SPARING DIURETIC AND THIAZIDE DIURETIC

1. Amiloride Hydrochloride and Hydrochlorothiazide (Moduretic)

Indication

Hypertension
Mild congestive heart failure

Dosage

Adults: Amiloride hydrochloride, 5 mg, and HCTZ, 50 mg. Usual adult dose is one to two tablets daily in single or divided doses.

Elderly: Caution required because of susceptibility to electrolyte imbalance. Reduced dose preferred. Adjust according to renal function and clinical response.

Children: Safety and effectiveness not established.

Preparation

Amiloride hydrochloride and hydrochlorothiazide (generic); Moduretic (Merck)

2. Spironolactone and Hydrochlorothiazide (Aldactazide)

Indication

Hypertension
Edema

Dosage

Adults: Spironolactone, 25 mg, and HCTZ, 25 mg (generic; Aldactazide); or spironolactone, 50 mg, and HCTZ, 50 mg (Aldactazide). As a diuretic, give one to four tablets daily in single or divided doses. As an antihypertensive, two to four tablets daily in divided doses.

Pediatric dosing consists of orally administering 1.65 to 3.3 mg/kg body weight or 30 to 90 mg/m^2 body surface area a day as a single daily dose or in two to four divided doses; adjust after 5 d. Dosage may be increased to up to three times the initial dose.

Elderly: Increased sensitivity may occur with combinations; lower dose recommended.

Preparation

Spironolactone and hydrochlorothiazide (generic); Aldactazide (Searle)

3. Triamterene and Hydrochlorothiazide (Dyazide, Maxzide, Maxzide-25)

Indication

Hypertension
Edema

Dosage

Capsules: Triamterene, 37.5 mg, and HCTZ, 25 mg (Dyazide); triamterene, 50 mg, and HCTZ, 25 mg (generic); or triamterene, 75 mg, and HCTZ, 50 mg (generic). Adult dose is one to two capsules once daily (maximum, four capsules daily.) Dose determined by individual titration. *Tablets*: Triamterene, 37.5 mg, and HCTZ, 25 mg (Maxzide-25); or triamterene, 75 mg, and HCTZ, 50 mg (Maxzide, generic). Adult dose is one tablet daily, as determined by individual titration.

Elderly: Patients may be more sensitive to usual adult dose.

Children: Safety and effectiveness not established.

Preparation

Triamterene and hydrochlorothiazide (generic); Dyazide (Smith Kline Beecham)
Maxzide, Maxzide-25 (Lederle)

MISCELLANEOUS DRUG COMBINATIONS

1. Reserpine and Hydrochlorothiazide and Hydralazine (Ser-Ap-Es)

Indication

Hypertension

Dosage

Adults: Reserpine, 0.1 mg, and hydralazine, 25 mg, and HCTZ, 15 mg. Usual adult dose is determined by individual titration of component agents. For detailed information regarding adverse effects, special precautions, contraindications, and other details, refer to individual drug component profiles.

Note: The preceding miscellaneous combinations must be administered with great care. However, they have the following in common:

Elderly: More sensitive to usual adult dose. Very minimal dosing may be considered.

Children: Dosage not established.

Preparation

Reserpine and hydrochlorothiazide and hydralazine (generic); Ser-Ap-Es (CibaGeneva)

Appendix 3 Use of Cardiovascular Drugs in Special Populations

William H. Frishman and Angela Cheng

TABLE 1 Physiologic Changes With Aging Potentially Affecting Cardiovascular Drug Pharmacokinetics*

Process	Physiologic change	Result	Drugs affected
Absorption	Reduced gastric acid production	Reduced tablet dissolution and decreased solubility of basic drugs	
	Reduced gastric emptying rate	Decreased absorption for acidic drugs	
	Reduced GI mobility, GI blood flow, absorptive surface	Less opportunity for drug absorption	
Distribution	Decreased total body mass Increased proportion of body fat	Increased V_d of highly lipid-soluble drugs	↓ β blockers, central α agonists
	Decreased proportion of body water	Decreased V_d of hydrophilic drugs	Digoxin ↑ ACE inhibitors ↑
	Decreased plasma albumin, disease-related increased α_1-acid glycoprotein, altered relative tissue perfusion	Changed percentage of free drug, V_d, and measured levels of bound drugs	↑ disopyramide, lidocaine, propranolol, ↑ warfarin
Metabolism	Reduced liver mass, liver blood flow, and hepatic metabolic capacity	Accumulation of metabolized drugs	↑ propranolol, nitrates, lidocaine, diltiazem, warfarin, labetalol, verapamil, mexiletine
Excretion	Reduced glomerular filtration, renal tubular function, and renal blood flow	Accumulation of renal cleared drugs	Digoxin, ACE inhibitors, antiarrhythmic drugs, atenolol, sotalol, nadolol

*GI = gastrointestinal; ACE = angiotensin converting enzyme.

Source: Adapted from Hui KK: Gerontologic considerations in cardiovascular pharmacology and therapeutics, in Singh BN, Dzau VJ, Vanhoutte PM, Woosley RL (eds): *Cardiovascular Pharmacology and Therapeutics*. New York, Churchill-Livingstone, 1994, p 1130.

TABLE 2 Characteristics of the Elderly Relative to Drug Response*

Physiologic changes	Changes in response
Decreased cardiac reserve	Potential for heart failure
Decreased LV compliance due to thickened ventricular wall, increased blood viscosity, decreased aortic compliance, increased total and peripheral resistance	Decrease of cardiac output
Decreased baroreceptor sensitivity	Tendency to orthostatic hypotension
Diminished cardiac and vascular responsiveness to β agonists and antagonists	Decreased sensitivity to β agonists and antagonists
Suppressed renin-angiotensin-aldosterone system	Theoretically decreased response to ACE inhibitors, but not observed
Increased sensitivity to anti-coagulant agents	Increased effects of warfarin
Concurrent illnesses	Increased drug-disease interactions
Multiple drugs	Increased drug-drug interactions
Sinus and AV node dysfunction	Potential for heart block

*LV = left ventricular; ACE = angiotensin converting enzyme; AV = atrio-ventricular.

Source: Adapted from Hui KK: Gerontologic considerations in cardiovascular pharmacology and therapeutics, in Singh BN, Dzau VJ, Vanhoutte PM, Woosley RL (eds): *Cardiovascular Pharmacology and Therapeutics.* New York, Churchill-Livingstone, 1994, p 1130.

TABLE 3 Cardiovascular Drugs Regularly Detected as the Culprit in Some Common Disorders of the Elderly

Confusion states
β Blockers
Digoxin
Methyldopa and related drugs
Quinidine
Depression
β Blockers
Methyldopa
Reserpine
Falls
All drugs liable to produce postural hypotension
Glycerol trinitrates
Postural hypotension
All antihypertensives
Antianginal drugs
β Blockers
Diuretics
Constipation
Anticholinergics
Clonidine
Diltiazem
Diuretics
Verapamil
Urinary incontinence
β Blockers
Diuretics
Labetalol
Prazosin

Source: Adapted from Hui KK: Gerontologic considerations in cardiovascular pharmacology and therapeutics, in Singh BN, Dzau VJ, Vanhoutte PM, Woosley RL (eds): *Cardiovascular Pharmacology and Therapeutics*. New York, Churchill-Livingstone, 1994, p 1131.

TABLE 4 Important Drug-Disease Interactions in Geriatric Patients*

Underlying disease	Drugs	Adverse effect
Congestive heart failure	β blockers, verapamil	Acute cardiac decompensation
Cardiac conduction disorders	Tricyclic antidepressants	Heart block
Hypertension	NSAIDS	Increased blood pressure
Peripheral vascular disease	β blockers	Intermittent claudication
Chronic obstructive pulmonary disease	β blockers	Bronchoconstriction
Chronic renal impairment	NSAIDs, contrast agents, aminoglycosides	Acute renal failure
Diabetes mellitus	Diuretics	Hyperglycemia
Prostatic hypertrophy	Drugs with antimuscarinic side effects	Urinary retention
Depression	β blockers, centrally acting antihypertensives	Precipitation or exacerbation of depression
Hypokalemia	Digoxin	Cardiac arrhythmia
Peptic ulcer disease	Anticoagulants, salicylates	GI hemorrhage

*NSAIDS = nonsteroidal anti-inflammatory drugs; GI = gastrointestinal.
Source: Adapted from Cusack BJ: Polypharmacy and clinical pharmacology, in Beck JC (ed): *Geriatrics Review Syllabus: A Core Curriculum in Geriatric Medicine*. New York, Am Geriatr Society, 1989, pp 127–136.

TABLE 5 Dose Adjustment in Renal Failure

Drug class	Creatinine clearance, mL/min			Dialysis
	40–50	10–40	< 10	
Inotropic Agents				
Digoxin				
Loading	↓ by 25%	↓ by 25–50%	↓ by 50%	No
Maintenance	0.125 mg/d	0.125 mg/d	0.125 mg 2 to 4 times a week	
Digitoxin				
Loading	No change	No change	No change	No
Maintenance	No change	No change	Every other day	
Amrinone				
Loading	No change	No change	No change	Unknown
Maintenance	No change	↓ by 50%	↓ by 75%	
Milrinone				
Loading	No change	No change	No change	Unknown
Maintenance	No change	↓ by 50%	↓ by 75%	
Diuretics				
Loop diuretics				
Ethacrynic acid	No change	Give bid if at all	Try to avoid	No (useless to give)
Furosemide	No change	No change	No change	No (useless to give)
Bumetanide	No change	No change	No change	No (useless to give)
Torasemide	No change	No change	No change	No (useless to give)

Distal tubule diuretics: Thiazides and quinazolones				
Thiazides—hydrochlorothiazide	No change	No change	Ineffective	Useless to give
Quinazolones—chlorthalidone	No change	No change	Ineffective	Useless to give
Metolazone	No change	No change	No change	Useless to give
Potassium-sparing diuretics				
Amiloride	No change	↓ dose 50% if used at all	Dangerous (↑ K^+)	Useless to give
Triamterene	No change	Give once/day if used at all	Dangerous (↑ K^+)	Useless to give
Spironolactone	Give 2–3 times a day if at all	Give once/day if used at all	Dangerous (↑ K^+)	Useless to give
Carbonic anhydrase inhibitors				
Acetazolamide	No change	Give 2x/d if used at all	Try to avoid	Yes—HD, PD, but accumulates with repeat dose No diuretic effect
Antiarrhythmic agents (unclassified)				
Adenosine	No change	No change	No change	Unknown
Antiarrhythmics class I				
Moricizine	No change	No change	No change	Unknown
Antiarrhythmics class IA				
Quinidine				

(continued)

TABLE 5 (*continued*)

Drug class	Creatinine clearance, mL/min			Dialysis
	40–50	10–40	< 10	
Loading	No change	No change	No change	Yes—HD, PD
Maintenance	No change	No change	No change, but observe closely	Give 100–200 mg after HD
Procainamide[a]				
Loading	No change	No change	No change	Yes—HD
Maintenance	No change	q6–12h	q8–24h	Give 200 mg after HD
	Follow both procainamide and NAPA levels			
Disopyramide				
Loading	200 mg	150 mg	100 mg	Yes—HD
Maintenance	100–150 mg q6h	100–150 mg q8–12h	100–150 mg q24h	Give 50–100 mg after HD
Antiarrhythmics class IB				
Lidocaine				
Loading	No change	No change	No change	No
Maintenance	No change	No change	No change	
Mexiletine				
Loading	No change	No change	↓ by 25%	No
Maintenance	No change	No change	↓ by 25%	
Tocainide				
Loading	No change	No change	No change	Yes—HD
Maintenance	No change	May ↓ by 25%	↓ by 50%	Give $\frac{1}{4}$ dose after HD

Antiarrhythmics class IC				
Flecainide				
Loading	No change	↓ by 50% if $C_{cr} < 20$	↓ by 67–75%	No
Maintenance	No change	↓ by 50% if $C_{cr} < 20$	↓ by 67–75%	
Encainide				
Loading	No change	↓ by 50%	↓ by 50%	Probably No
Maintenance	No change	↓ by 50%	↓ by 50%	
Propafenone				
Loading	No change	No change	No change	No
Maintenance	No change	No change	No change	
Antiarrhythmics class II (β ***blockers****)*				
Propranolol[b]	No change	No change	No change	No
Metoprolol	No change	No change	No change	Yes—HD Give 50 mg after HD
Pindolol	No change	No change	No change	No
Timolol	No change	No change	No change	No
Nadolol	↓ by 50%	↓ by 50% or give q48h	↓ by 75% or give q48–60h	Yes—HD Give 40 mg after HD
Atenolol	No change	↓ by 50%	↓ by 75%	Yes—HD Give 25–50 mg after HD
Acebutolol	No change	↓ by 50%	↓ by 75%	No
Carteolol	Give q48h or ↓ by 50%	Give q48h or ↓ by 50–67%	Give q72h or ↓ by 75%	No

(continued)

TABLE 5 (*continued*)

Drug class	Creatinine clearance, mL/min			Dialysis
	40–50	10–40	< 10	
Carvedilol	No change	Start with lowest dose (3.125 mg) and tritrate up slowly	Start with lowest dose (3.125 mg) and titrate up slowly	No
Esmolol	No change	No change	No change	No
Sotalol	↓ by 50%	↓ by 67–70%	↓ by 85%	Yes—HD, PD Give 80 mg after HD
Penbutolol	No change	No change	No change	No
Labetalol	No change	No change	No change	No
Antiarrhythmics class III				
Amiodarone	No change	No change	No change	No
Bretylium				
Loading	↓ by 50%	↓ proportional to ↓ in C_{cr}	Try to avoid or ↓ by 90%	Yes—HD[c] Give $\frac{1}{4}$ dose after HD
Maintenance	↓ by 50%	↓ proportional to ↓ in C_{cr}	Try to avoid or ↓ by 90%	
Antiarrhythmics class IV (calcium channel blockers)				
Verapamil	No change	No change	No change	No
Nifedipine	No change	No change	No change	No
Diltiazem	No change	No change	No change	No
Amlodipine	No change	No change	No change	No
Felodipine	No change	No change	No change	No

Isradipine	No change	No change	No change	No
Mibefradil	No change	No change	No change	No
Nicardipine	No change	No change	No change	No
Nimodipine	No change	No change	No change	No
Nisoldipine	No change	No change	No change	No
Nitrendipine	No change	No change	No change	No
Angiotensin converting enzyme inhibitors				
Captopril	↓ by 50%	↓ proportional to ↓ in C_{cr}	↓ 75–90%	Yes—HD Give $\frac{1}{2}$ dose after HD
Enalapril	↓ by 50%	↓ by 75%	↓ by 80%	Yes—HD Give $\frac{1}{4}$ dose after HD
Lisinopril	No change	↓ by 50% if $C_{cr} < 30$	↓ by 75%	Yes—HD Give $\frac{1}{5}$ dose after HD
Benazepril	No change	↓ by 50% if $C_{cr} < 30$	↓ by 50%	Yes—HD Give $\frac{1}{4}$ dose after HD
Fosinopril	No change	No change	↓ by 25%	No
Moexipril	No change	↓ by 50%[d]	↓ by 50%[d]	Unknown
Quinapril	↓ by 50%	↓ by 50%	↓ by 75%	Yes—HD Give $\frac{1}{4}$ dose after HD
Ramipril	No change	↓ by 75%	↓ by 75%	Yes—HD Give $\frac{1}{4}$ dose after HD
Trandolapril	No change	↓ by 50% if $C_{cr} < 30$	↓ by 50% Start with 0.5 mg once daily and monitor patient closely	Yes—HD removes small amounts of trandolaprilat

(*continued*)

TABLE 5 (*continued*)

Drug class	Creatinine clearance, mL/min 40–50	10–40	< 10	Dialysis
Angiotensin receptor blockers				
Irbesartan[e]	No change	No change	No change	No
Losartan[e]	No change	No change	No change	No
Valsartan	No change	No change Use with caution	Use lower dose with caution	Unknown (probably no)
Antihypertensives				
Methyldopa	No change	↓ by 50% if $C_{cr} < 20$	↓ by 50%	Yes—HD Give ½ dose after HD
Clonidine	No change	No change	↓ starting dose by 50%	No
Hydralazine	No change	No change	Give q6–12h	No
Fenoldopam	No change	No change	No change	No—CAPD Unknown—HD
Minoxidil	No change	No change	No change	No
Prazosin	No change	No change	No change	No
Doxazosin	No change	No change	No change	No
Terazosin	No change	No change	No change	No
Nitroprusside	No change	No change	No change	Yes—titrate dose for BP during HD
Guanabenz	No change	No change	No change	Unknown
Guanfacine	No change	No change	No change	No

Nitrates	No change	No change	No change	No
Vasopressor (α_1 Agonist)				
Midodrine	Start with low doses (2.5 mg)	Start with low doses (2.5 mg)	Start with low doses (2.5 mg)	Unknown (probably yes)
Antithrombotic drugs				
Aspirin	No change up to 160 mg	No change up to 160 mg	No change up to 160 mg	Yes—HD Dose after HD
Ardeparin	No change	No change	No change, use with caution	No
Anagrelide	No change	May need to ↓ dose, monitor patient closely	May need to ↓ dose, monitor patient closely	Unknown
Heparin	No change	No change	No change	No
	Follow PTT, platelet count, and serum K^+			
Enoxaparin	No change	No change	No change, use with caution	No
Danaparoid	No change	Consider dose reduction when $C_{cr} < 20$, monitor patient closely	Consider dose reduction, monitor patient closely	Unknown
Ticlopidine	No change	No change	No change	Unknown
Warfarin	No change	No change	No change	Yes—HD Dose after HD

(continued)

TABLE 5 (*concluded*)

Drug class	Creatinine clearance, mL/min			Dialysis
	40–50	10–40	< 10	
Fibrinolytic agents				
Alteplase (tPA)	No change	No change	No change	Unknown
Reteplase	No change	No change	No change Monitor patient closely[f]	Unknown
Streptokinase	No change	No change	No change	Unknown
Lipid-lowering agents				
Atorvastatin	No change	No change	No change	No
Cerivastatin	↓ by 33%, start with 0.2 mg daily	↓ by 33%, start with 0.2 mg daily	Start with 0.2 mg daily and monitor patient closely	No
Clofibrate	Give q 12–18 h	Give q 18 h	Avoid	No
Gemfibrozil	No change	No change	No change	No
Lovastatin	No change	No change	No change	No
Simvastatin	No change	No change	No change	No
Niacin (nicotinic acid)	↓ by 50%	↓ by 50%	↓ by 75%	Unknown
Pravastatin	No change	No change	No change	No
Probucol	No change	No change	No change	No
Fluvastatin	No change	No change	No change	No

Cholestyramine	Not absorbed from GI tract—no change in dosage
Colestipol	Not absorbed from GI tract—no change in dosage

[a]Long-acting procainamide formulations should not be used in renal failure due to risk of drug accumulation.
[b]Propranolol may lower renal function and worsen existing kidney failure. Use propranolol with caution in patients with renal impairment.
[c]There is disagreement in the literature about whether bretylium is cleared by hemodialysis. A supplemental dose after dialysis should be given only if the patient's heart rhythm warrants it.
[d]Start moexipril with the lowest dose (3.75 mg once daily) and monitor patients with severe renal impairment closely.
[e]No dosage adjustment is necessary unless patient with renal impairment is also volume depleted.
[f]Although there is no specific recommendation for dosage reduction in patients with severe renal impairment, monitor patient closely for hemodynamic changes and signs of bleeding after the first bolus injection of reteplase.
CAPD = continuous ambulatory peritoneal dialysis; HD = hemodialysis
Adapted from: Feinfeld DA: Renal considerations in cardiovascular drug therapy. In Frishman WH, Sonnenblick EH (eds): *Cardiovascular Pharmacotherapeutics.* McGraw-Hill, NY 1997; 1283.

TABLE 6 Selected Cardiovascular Medications and Gender Issues

Drug	Evidence for efficacy in women	Considerations when treating women
Aspirin	*Primary prevention*: U.S. nurses cohort shows decreased risk of MI (A) Women's Health Study in progress (A) Women's Health Initiative in progress *Secondary prevention*: Decreases reinfarction (B) *Stroke Prevention*: Women's Health Study in progress (A)	Women have higher rate of hemorrhagic stroke than men Physician's Health Study showed increased risk of bleeding on aspirin Increased risk of bleeding at term in pregnancy and present in breast milk
ACE inhibitors	*Post-MI*: Decreased mortality (B) *CHF*: Decreased mortality (B)	Cough is 2–3 times greater in women Increased fetal abnormalities possible Present in breast milk
Angiotensin II inhibitors	Preliminary data shows efficacy for hypertension in women comparable to men	Cough is unusual
Beta blockers	*Hypertension*: Effective at preventing MI, CVA, death, in women (B) *Post-MI*: Decreases mortality (B)	Present in breast milk Blood levels of propranolol may be higher in men
Calcium channel blockers	Increased risk of MI in women? (B) Increased effect of amlodipine in women in reducing blood pressure (B)	Present in breast milk Verapamil clearance may be greater in women than in men.
Clonidine	No data looking at efficacy in women	Inability to achieve orgasm Possible decreased craving for tobacco in women greater than men (B)
Conjugated estrogens	Increased HDL-cholesterol decreases total cholesterol and lipoprotein (A)	Need for progestins in women with intact uterus to prevent endometrial abnormalities
Disopyramide	No data looking at efficacy in women	Complication of torsades de pointes more frequent in women (B)

Guanethidine		Orthostatic hypotension more common in women.
HMG-CoA reductase inhibitors		
Simvastatin	*Secondary prevention*: Possible efficacy for women (B)	
Lovastatin	Decreases cholesterol and slows plaque progression without respect to gender (A)	Estrogen has no effect GI side effects most common in women
Hypolipidemic agents		
Colestipol	No effect on primary prevention (B)	
Clofibrate	Effective in secondary prevention in women (B)	
Probucol	Effective in women	Greater tendency for prolongation of ECG QT interval in women
Hydralazine	Effective for hypertension in pregnancy and peripartum	Present in breast milk SLE more common in women than men
Methyldopa	Often preferred in pregnancy for treating hypertension	Painful breast enlargement, decreased libido
Nicotine preparations	Gum equally effective in women (B) Patch effective in women (B)	Gum may suppress weight gain, probably safe in pregnancy
Nitrates	Decreased mortality post-MI (B)	Potential for difference in metabolism in women
Procainamide	No gender-specific data available	Drug-induced SLE more common in women
Quinidine	No gender-specific data available	Torsades more common in women Clearance may be faster in women Present in breast milk

(*continued*)

TABLE 6 (*concluded*)

Drug	Evidence for efficacy in women	Considerations when treating women
Thrombolytics	Decreased mortality in MI (B)	Women had higher complication rate, but role of older age in women not clarified
Thiazide diuretics	Decreased CVA, MI, death (B)	Decreased urinary calcium excretion Increased bone density in women Less effect on lipid profile in women Women have greater increase in risk of gout Acute pulmonary edema and allergic interstitial pneumonitis is more common in women Excreted in breast milk

Note: A = studies of efficacy in women; B = studies of efficacy in both women and men, with analysis by gender; MI = myocardial infarction; CVA = cerebrovascular accident; GI = gastrointestinal; SLE = systemic lupus erythematosus.

Adapted from: Charney P, Meyer BR, Frishman WH, Ginsberg A, Eastwood B: Gender, race and genetic issues in cardiovascular pharmacotherapy. In Frishman WH, Sonnenblick EH (eds): *Cardiovascular Pharmacotherapeutics*. McGraw-Hill 1997:1347.

TABLE 7 Guide to Cardiovascular Drugs Used During Pregnancy

Drugs	Pregnancy	Lactation	Pregnancy Category
Inotropic Agents			
Digoxin	Relatively safe; weigh benefits vs. risks	Breast-feed with caution; excreted in breast milk	C
Digitoxin	Relatively safe; weigh benefits vs. risks	Breast-feed with caution; excretion in milk unknown	C
Amrinone	Weigh benefits vs. risks	Breast-feed with caution; excretion in milk unknown	C
Milrinone	Weigh benefits vs. risks	Breast-feed with caution; excretion in milk unknown	C
Antiarrhythmic Agents:			
Class IA:			
Quinidine	Relatively safe; weigh benefits vs. risks	Breast-feed with caution; excreted in breast milk	C
Procainamide	Weigh benefits vs. risks	Breast-feed with caution; excreted in breast milk	C
Disopyramide	Use with caution; weigh benefits vs. risks	Breast-feed with caution; excreted in breast milk	C
Class IB:			
Lidocaine	Weigh benefits vs. risks	Breast-feed with caution; excreted in breast milk	B
Mexiletine	Use with caution; weigh benefits vs. risks	Breast-feeding not recommended	C
Tocainide	Use with caution; only if necessary; little information available	Breast-feed with caution; excretion in milk unknown	C

(*continued*)

TABLE 7 (*continued*)

Drugs	Pregnancy	Lactation	Pregnancy Category
Class IC:			
Flecainide	Use with caution; weigh benefits vs. risks	Accumulates in milk; breast-feed with caution	C
Encainide	Use with caution; only if necessary; little information available	Breast-feed with caution; excreted in breast milk	C
Propafenone	Use with caution; weigh benefits vs. risks	Breast-feed with caution; excreted in breast milk	C
Class II (β blockers):			
Propranolol	Use with caution; weigh benefits vs. risks	Breast-feed with caution; excreted in breast milk	C
Metoprolol	Use with caution; weigh benefits vs. risks	Accumulates in milk; breast-feed with caution	C
Pindolol	Weigh benefits vs. risks	Breast-feed with caution; excreted in milk	B
Timolol	Use with caution; weigh benefits vs. risks	Breast-feed with caution; excreted in milk	C
Atenolol	Use with caution; weigh benefits vs. risks	Accumulates in milk; breast-feed with caution	D
Nadolol	Use with caution; weigh benefits vs. risks	Breast-feed with caution; excreted in milk	C
Acebutolol	Use only in third trimester if essential	Breast-feed with caution; excreted in milk	B
Esmolol	Use with caution; weigh benefits vs. risks	Breast-feed with caution	C

Sotalol	Use with caution; weigh benefits vs. risks	Accumulates in milk; breast-feed with caution	C
Carteolol	Use with caution; weigh benefits vs. risks	Breast-feeding not recommended; excretion in milk unknown	C
Betaxolol	Use with caution; weigh benefits vs. risks	Breast-feed with caution; excreted in milk	C
Bisoprolol	Use with caution; weigh benefits vs. risks	Breast-feeding not recommended; excretion in milk unknown	C
Penbutolol	Use with caution; only if necessary	Breast-feeding not recommended; excretion in milk unknown	C
Labetalol	Use with caution only in first trimester	Breast-feed with caution; excreted in milk	C
Carvedilol	Use with caution; weigh benefits vs. risks	Breast-feeding not recommended; excretion in milk unknown	C
Class III:			
Amiodarone	Contraindicated	Breast-feeding not recommended; excreted in breast milk	D
Bretylium	Use with caution; only if necessary; very little information available	Breast-feeding not recommended; excretion in milk unknown	C
Ibutilide	Use with caution; weigh benefits vs. risks	Breast-feeding not recommended; excretion in milk unknown	C
Class IV (Calcium channel blockers):			
Verapamil	Use with caution; weigh benefits vs. risks	Breast-feeding not recommended; excreted in milk	C
Diltiazem	Use with caution; only if necessary	Breast-feeding not recommended; excreted in milk	C

(continued)

TABLE 7 (*continued*)

Drugs	Pregnancy	Lactation	Pregnancy Category
Nifedipine	Use with caution; weigh benefits vs. risks	Breast-feeding not recommended; excreted in milk	C
Amlodipine	Contraindicated	Breast-feeding not recommended; excretion in milk unknown	C
Felodipine	Use with caution; weigh benefits vs. risks	Breast-feeding not recommended; excretion in milk unknown	C
Isradipine	Use with caution; only if necessary	Breast-feeding not recommended; excretion in milk unknown	C
Nicardipine	Use with caution; only if necessary	Breast-feeding not recommended; excretion in milk unknown	C
Nimodipine	Contraindicated	Breast-feeding not recommended; excretion in milk unknown	C
Nisoldipine	Use with caution; weigh benefits vs. risks	Breast-feeding not recommended; excretion in milk unknown	C
Nitrendipine	Contraindicated	Breast-feeding not recommended; excretion in milk unknown	C
Bepridil	Use with caution; weigh benefits vs. risks	Breast-feeding not recommended; excretion in milk unknown	C
Mibefradil	Use with caution; weight benefits vs. risks	Breast-feeding not recommended;	C
ACE Inhibitors:			
Captopril	Contraindicated	Breast-feeding not recommended; excreted in breast milk	C (1st trimester) D (2nd, 3rd trimesters)

Enalapril	Contraindicated	Breast-feeding not recommended; excretion in milk unknown	C (1st trimester) D (2nd, 3rd trimesters)
Lisinopril	Contraindicated	Breast-feeding not recommended; excretion in milk unknown	C (1st trimester) D (2nd, 3rd trimesters)
Benazepril	Contraindicated	Breast-feeding not recommended; excreted in breast milk	C (1st trimester) D (2nd, 3rd trimesters)
Fosinopril	Contraindicated	Breast-feeding not recommended; excreted in breast milk	C (1st trimester) D (2nd, 3rd trimesters)
Quinapril	Contraindicated	Breast-feeding not recommended; excretion in milk unknown	C (1st trimester) D (2nd, 3rd trimesters)
Ramipril	Contraindicated	Breast-feeding not recommended; excretion in milk unknown	C (1st trimester) D (2nd, 3rd trimesters)
Moexipril	Contraindicated	Breast-feeding not recommended; excretion in milk unknown	C (1st trimester) D (2nd, 3rd trimesters)
Trandolapril	Contraindicated	Breast-feeding not recommended; excretion in milk unknown	C (1st trimester) D (2nd, 3rd trimesters)
Angiotensin Receptor Blockers			
Irbesartan	Contraindicated	Breast-feeding not recommended; excretion in milk unknown.	C (first trimester) D (2nd, 3rd trimesters)
Losartan	Contraindicated	Breast-feeding not recommended; excretion in milk unknown	C (1st trimester) D (2nd, 3rd trimesters)
Valsartan	Contraindicated	Breast-feeding not recommended; excretion in milk unknown	C (first trimester) D (2nd, 3rd trimesters)
Lipid-Lowering Agents			
Clofibrate	Contraindicated	Breast-feeding not recommended; excreted in breast milk	C

(*continued*)

TABLE 7 (*continued*)

Drugs	Pregnancy	Lactation	Pregnancy Category
Gemfibrozil	Contraindicated	Breast-feeding not recommended; excretion in milk unknown	C
Atorvastatin	Contraindicated	Breast-feeding not recommended	X
Cerivastatin	Contraindicated	Breast feeding not recommended	X
Lovastatin	Contraindicated	Breast-feeding not recommended; excretiond in milk unknown	X
Simvastatin	Contraindicated	Breast-feeding not recommended; excretion in milk unknown	X
Pravastatin	Contraindicated	Breast-feeding not recommended; excreted in breast milk	X
Fluvastatin	Contraindicated	Breast-feeding not recommended; excreted in breast milk	X
Probucol	Use with caution; weigh benefits vs. risks	Breast-feeding not recommended; excretion in milk unknown	B
Niacin (nicotinic acid)	Use with caution; weigh benefits vs. risks	Breast-feed with caution; excretion in milk unknown	C
Cholestyramine	Use with caution; weigh benefits vs. risks	Breast-feed with caution; excretion in milk unknown	None mentioned
Colestipol	Use with caution; weigh benefits vs. risks	Breast-feed with caution; excretion in milk unknown	None mentioned
Antihypertensives			
Fenoldopam	Use with caution; only if necessary	Breast-feeding not recommended excretion in milk unknown.	B
Methyldopa	Use with caution; weigh benefits vs. risks	Breast-feed with caution; excreted in breast milk	B

Clonidine	Contraindicated in first trimester	Breast-feed with caution; excreted in breast milk	C
Hydralazine	Use with caution; weigh benefits vs. risks	Breast-feed with caution; excretion in milk unknown	C
Minoxidil	Contraindicated	Breast-feeding not recommended; excreted in breast milk	C
Prazosin	Use with caution; weigh benefits vs. risks	Breast-feed with caution; excreted in breast milk	C
Doxazosin	Use with caution; only if necessary; very little information available	Breast-feeding not recommended; excretion in milk unknown	C
Terazosin	Use with caution; only if necessary; very little information available	Breast-feeding not recommended; excretion in milk unknown	C
Nitroprusside	Contraindicated	Breast-feeding not recommended; excretion in milk unknown	C
Guanabenz	Contraindicated	Breast-feeding not recommended; excretion in milk unknown	C
Guanfacine	Contraindicated	Breast-feeding not recommended; excretion in milk unknown	B
Vasopressor (α_1 Agonist)			
Midodrine	Use with caution; weigh benefits vs. risks	Breast-feeding not recommended; excretion in milk unknown	C
Anticoagulants and Thombolytic Agents			
Heparin	Use with caution; weigh benefits vs. risks	Breast-feed with caution; not excreted in breast milk	C
Warfarin	Contraindicated	Breast-feeding not recommended; excreted in breast milk	C

(*continued*)

TABLE 7 (*continued*)

Drugs	Pregnancy	Lactation	Pregnancy Category
Aspirin	Use with caution; weigh benefits vs. risks	Breast-feed with caution; excreted in breast milk	C
Streptokinase	Use with caution; weigh benefits vs. risks	Breast-feeding not recommended; excretion in milk unknown	C
Urokinase	Use with caution; only if necessary	Breast-feeding not recommended; excretion in milk unknown	B
Alteplase (tPA)	Use with caution; only if necessary	Breast-feeding not recommended; excretion in milk unknown	C
Ticlopidine	Use with caution; weigh benefits vs. risks	Breast-feeding not recommended; excretion in milk unknown	B
Ardeparin	Use with caution; weigh benefits vs. risks	Breast-feeding not recommended; excretion in milk unknown	C
Anagrelide	Use with caution; weigh benefits vs. risks	Breast-feeding not recommended; excretion in milk unknown	C
Enoxaparin	Use with caution; only if necessary	Breast-feeding not recommended; excretion in milk unknown	B
Danaparoid	Use with caution; only if necessary	Breast-feeding not recommended; excretion in milk unknown	B
Reteplase	Use with caution; weigh benefits vs. risks	Breast-feeding not recommended; excretion in milk unknown	C
Nitrates	Use with caution; weigh benefits vs. risks	Breast-feeding not recommended; excretion in milk unknown	C

Diuretics			
Chlorothiazide	Use with caution; weigh benefits vs. risks	Breast-feed with caution; excreted in breast milk	B
Chlorthalidone	Use with caution; weigh benefits vs. risks	Breast-feed with caution; excreted in breast milk	B
Hydrochlorothiazide	Use with caution; weigh benefits vs. risks	Breast-feed with caution; excreted in breast milk	B
Metolazone	Use with caution; weigh benefits vs. risks	Breast-feeding not recommended; excreted in breast milk	B
Furosemide	Use with caution; weigh benefits vs. risks	Breast-feeding not recommended; excreted in breast milk	C
Ethacrynic acid	Use with caution; weigh benefits vs. risks	Breast-feeding not recommended; excreted in breast milk	B
Bumetanide	Use with caution; only if necessary	Breast-feeding not recommended; excreted in breast milk	C
Torsemide	Use with caution; weigh benefits vs. risks	Breast-feeding not recommended; excretion in milk unknown	B
Amiloride	Use with caution; weigh benefits vs. risks	Breast-feeding not recommended; excretion in milk unknown	B
Spironolactone	Use with caution; weigh benefits vs. risks	Breast-feed with caution; excreted in breast milk	none mentioned
Triamterene	Use with caution; weigh benefits vs. risks	Breast-feeding not recommended; excretion in milk unknown	B

(*continued*)

TABLE 7 (*continued*)

Pregnancy Category	Food & Drug Administration Pregnancy Risk Classification
A	No control studies in women demonstrate a risk to the fetus in the first trimester and there is no evidence of risk in the late trimesters. Possibility of danger to the fetus appears remote.
B	Either animal reproduction studies have not demonstrated a fetal risk or else they have not shown an adverse effect (other than a decrease in fertility). However, there are no controlled studies of pregnant women in the first trimester to confirm these findings and there is no evidence of risk in the later trimesters.
C	Either animal studies have revealed adverse effects (teratogenic or embryocidal) but there are no confirmatory studies in women, or studies in both animals and women are not available. Because of the potential risk to the fetus, drugs should be given only if justified by potentially greater benefits.
D	Evidence of human fetal risk is available. Despite the risk, benefits from use in pregnant women may be justifiable in select circumstances (e.g., if the drug is needed in a life-threatening situation, and/or no other safer acceptable drugs are effective). An appropriate "warnings" statement will appear on the labeling.
X	Studies in animals and humans have demonstrated fetal abnormalities, and/or there is evidence of fetal risk based on human experience. Thus, the risk of drug use and consequent fetal harm outweighs any potential benefit, and the drug is contraindicated in pregnant women. An appropriate "contraindicated" statement will appear on the labeling.

From: Ngo A, Frishman WH, Elkayam U: Cardiovascular pharmacotherapeutic considerations during pregnancy and lactation. In Frishman WH, Sonnenblick EH (eds): *Cardiovascular Parmacotherapeutics*. McGraw-Hill 1997: 1309.

Table 8 Hepatic Dysfunction

Drug	Cirrhosis	CHF
α_1-Selective Adrenergic Blockers		
Prazosin	Use lower dose	Reduce dose
Terazosin	Reduce dose; use caution	Dose reduction unnecessary
Doxazosin	Use caution	Use caution
Vasopressor (α_1 Agonist)		
Midodrine	Use caution; start with low doses (2.5 mg)	
ACE Inhibitors		
Benazepril	May need dose reduction	
Captopril	Dose reduction unnecessary	
Enalapril	May not need dose reduction	
Fosinopril	Dose reduction may be unnecessary; compensatory renal clearance	Dose reduction necessary
Lisinopril	Dose reduction unnecessary	Dose reduction unnecessary
Quinapril	Dose reduction unnecessary	
Ramipril	Use caution	Use caution
Moexipril	Use lower dose initially	
Trandolapril	Use lower dose; adjust according to therapeutic response	
Angiotensin II receptor antagonists		
Irbesartan	Dose reduction not necessary	
Losartan	Use lower starting dose	
Valsartan	Use caution	

(*continued*)

Table 8 (*continued*)

Drug	Cirrhosis	CHF
β-*Adrenergic Blockers*		
Nonselective		
Nadolol	Dose reduction unnecessary	
Propranolol	Use caution; low initial dose	Use caution
Sotalol	Dose reduction unnecessary	
Timolol	Use lower dose	
β_1-*Selective*		
Atenolol	Dose reduction unnecessary	
Betaxolol	Reduce dose in severe dysfunction	
Bisoprolol	Reduce dose in severe dysfunction	
Esmolol	Dose reduction unnecessary	
Metoprolol	Use caution; dose reduction may be necessary	
With ISA: Nonselective		
Carteolol	Dose reduction unnecessary	
Penbutolol	Dose reduction unnecessary	
Pindolol	Reduce dose or use alternative	
β_1-*Selective*		
Acebutolol	Dose reduction unnecessary	
Dual Acting		
Labetalol	Reduce dose	

Nonselective with α_1 Blocking Activity		
Carvedilol	Do not use in patients with clinically manifest hepatic impairment	
Calcium Channel Blockers		
Verapamil	Reduce dose	Use caution
Amlodipine	Reduce starting dose	
Felodipine	reduce dose initially	Start with lower dose
Isradipine	Reduce dose	
Nicardipine	Reduce starting dose	
Nifedipine	Reduce frequency of dose	May not need dose reduction; use caution
Nimodipine	Reduce dose	
Diltiazem	Reduce dose	Use caution
Bepridil	Use caution	
Mibefradil	Use caution	
Centrally Acting Antihypertensives		
Clonidine	Reduce dose	
Guanabenz	Reduce dose	
Guanfacine	Reduce dose	
Methyldopa	Reduce dose; contraindicated in active disease	
Neuronal and Ganglionic Blockers		
Guanadrel	Reduce dose	
Guanethidine	Reduce dose with severe impairment	
Reserpine	Reduce dose with severe impairment	

(*continued*)

Table 8 (*continued*)

Drug	Cirrhosis	CHF
Mecamylamine	Dose reduction unnecessary	
Trimethaphan	Reduce dose	
Vasodilators		
Fenoldopam	Dose reduction not necessary	
Cyclandelate	Unknown	
Diazoxide	Contraindicated	
Hydralazine	Reduce dose or prolong dosage interval	Increase dose for effectiveness
Isoxsuprine	Dose reduction unnecessary	
Nylidrin	Unknown	
Nitroglycerin	Use lower dose	May need dose reduction
Pentaerythriyol tetranitrate	Use caution	
Erythritol tetranitrate	Unknown	
Isosorbide dinitrate	Use lower dose; contraindicated in severe impairment	
Isosorbide mononitrate	Use caution with severe impairment	
Sodium Nitroprusside	Use lower dose	
Tolazoline	Unknown	
Diuretics		
Loop		
Bumetanide	May need dose reduction	Dose reduction may be unnecessary
Ethacrynic acid	Use caution; may disturb electrolytes balance; may precipitate death with advanced cirrhosis	

Furosemide	No adjustment necessary; use caution may disturb electrolytes	Dose reduction may be unnecessary
Torsemide	Use caution	Use caution
Thiazide		
Bendroflumethazide	Use caution; may disturb electrolytes	
Benthiazide	Use caution; may precipitate hepatic coma	
Chlorthiazide	Use caution; may disturb electrolytes	
Chlorthalidone	Use caution; may disturb electrolytes	
Cyclothiazide	Use caution; may disturb electrolytes and precipitate hepatic coma	
Hydrochlorothiazide	Use caution; may disturb electrolytes and precipitate hepatic coma	
Hydroflumethiazide	Use caution; may disturb electrolytes and precipitate hepatic coma	
Indapamide	Use caution; may disturb electrolytes and precipitate hepatic coma	
Methylclothiazide	Use caution; may disturb electrolytes and precipitate hepatic coma	
Metolazone	Use caution; may disturb electrolytes	
Polythiazide	Use caution; may disturb electrolytes and precipitate hepatic coma	
Quinethazone	Use caution; may disturb electrolytes and precipitate hepatic coma	
Trichlormethiazide	Use caution; may disturb electrolyes and precipitate hepatic coma	

(continued)

Table 8 (*continued*)

Drug	Cirrhosis	CHF
Potassium-Sparing		
Amiloride	Use caution; may distrub electrolytes; hepatic encephalopathy reported occasionally	
Spironolactone	Use caution	
Triamterene	Use caution	
Inotropic Agents		
Amrinone	Dose reduction may be required	
Milrinone		
Dopamine	Dose reduction unnecessary	
Dobutamine	Dose reduction unnecessary	
Norepinephrine		May need dose reduction
Digoxin	Dose reduction unnecessary	
Digitoxin	Reduce dose or use alternative	
Deslanoside	Dose reduction may not be required	
Antiarrythmics		
Quinidine	Reduce dose	Dose reduction necessary
Procainamide	Dose adjustments may be unnecessary	Dose reduction may be unnecessary
Disopyramide	Reduce dose 25%	
Moricizine	Use lower dose or alternative	
Lidocaine	Reduce dose 40–50%	Reduce dose 40–50%
Mexiletine	Reduce maintenance dose 25%	Dose reduction may be required; prolonged half-life
Tocainide	Reduce dose 50%	Adjustments may be necessary
Flecainide	Use lower dose or alternative	May need dose reduction; reduced clearance

Propafenone	Reduce initial dose 70–80%	
Amiodarone	Dose reduction unnecessary	Dose reduction unnecessary; use caution with severe impairment
Bretylium	Dose reduction unnecessary	
Atropine	Use caution half life increased; susceptible to adverse effects	
Adenosine	Adjustment unnecessary	
Lipid lowering		
Atorvastatin	Start at lowest dose and titrate cautiously; contraindicated in active liver disease or unexplained transaminase elevation	
Cerivastatin	Start at lowest dose and titrate cautiously; contraindicated in active liver disease or unexplained transaminase elevation	
Lovastatin Pravastatin Simvastatin	Start at lowest dose and titrate cautiously; contraindicated in active liver disease or unexplained transaminase elevation	
Nicotinic acid	Use caution; may aggravate gallstones and jaundice	
Clofibrate	Contraindicated	
Cholestyramine Colestipol	Ineffective with total biliary obstruction	
Gemfibrozil	Contraindicated	
Probucol	Avoid with severe impairment	

(*continued*)

Table 8 (*concluded*)

Drug	Cirrhosis	CHF
Anticoagulants		
Heparin	May reduce clearance; consider reduced dose	
Dicoumarol	Dose reduction may be required	
Anisindione	May need dose reduction	
Warfarin	Reduce dose	
Ardeparin	Use caution	
Enoxaparin	Use caution	
Danaparoid	Dose reduction unnecessary	
Antithrombotics		
Aspirin	May cause acute reversible hepatotoxicity	
Dipyridamole	Reduce dose with biliary obstruction	
Ticlopidine	May need dose reduction	
Anagrelide	Use caution; dosage adjustment may be necessary	Use caution; therapeutic doses of anagrelide may cause cardiovascular effects, including vasodilation, tachycardia, and CHF
Thrombolytics		
Alteplase Anistreplase Streptokinase Urokinase	Reduce dose with severe impairment	
Reteplase	Use caution	

CHF = congestive heart failure; ACE = angiotensin converting enzyme; ISA = intrinsic sympathomimetic activity

Adapted from: Frishman WH, Sokol SI: Cardiovascular drug therapy in patients with intrinsic hepatic disease and impaired hepatic function secondary to congestive heart failure. In Frishman WH, Sonnenblick EH (eds): *Cardiovascular Pharmacotherapeutics*. McGraw-Hill 1997:1561.

Index

Note: Page numbers followed by "*f*" indicate figures; page numbers followed by "*t*" indicate table.

A

Abbokinase. *See* Urokinase
Abciximab (ReoPro)
  elderly patients, 566
  pharmacokinetics, 507*t*
  therapeutic use, 565–566
Absolute bioavailability, 9
Absorption, drug, 8, 13
Accelerated hypertension
  ACE inhibitors, 122
Accupril. *See* Quinapril
ACE (angiotensin converting enzyme) inhibitors
  adverse effects
    ACE inhibitor cough, 116–117
    angioneurotic edema, 117
    dysgeusia, 117
    functional renal impairment, 115–116
    hematologic effects, 117–118
    hyperkalemia, 115
    hypotension, 114–115
    overview, 113–114, 114*t*, 119*t*
    skin rash, 117
    teratogenic effects, 118
  clinical uses
    cerebrovascular disease, 129–130
    congestive heart failure, 123–125
    diabetic nephropathy, 128–129
    hypertensive emergencies, 122
    left ventricular hypertrophy, 126
    mitral and aortic regurgitation, 126
    myocardial infarction, 125–126
    primary (essential) hypertension, 120–121
    primary hyperaldosteronism, 122–123, 123*t*
    renal insufficiency, 129
    renal parenchymal disease, 126–128
    renovascular hypertension, 121–122
  combination therapy with
    beta blockers, 131–132
    calcium entry antagonists, 132
    diuretics, 131, 395–396
  development of, 107–108
  diagnostic use
    primary hyperaldosteronism, 133–134
    renal artery stenosis, 132–133
  differences among, 134–135, 135*t*–136*t*, 137–138
    chemical class, 134–135
    inhibition of tissue ACE, 137
    pharmacokinetic properties, 137
    potency, 135
    prodrugs, 135

ACE inhibitors (*Cont.*):
drug-drug interactions, 491, 492*t*–493*t*
aspirin, 119, 503*t*
beta-adrenergic blocking drugs, 58*t*
diuretics, 118–119
lithium, 120
loop and thiazide diuretics, 490*t*
nonsteroidal anti-inflammatory agents, 119
potassium-sparing diuretics, 490*t*
elderly patients, 652*t*–653*t*
gender considerations, 666*t*
hepatic dysfunction, 679*t*
hypertensives, effects on
hemodynamic effects, 109–111, 110*t*
humoral effects of neurohumoral systems, 111–112
kallikrein-kinin system, 112
sympathetic nervous system, interactions with, 112
normotensives, effects on blood pressure of, 109
overview, 108–109, 123*t*, 135*t*–136*t*
pregnancy and lactation, 672*t*–673*t*
quality-of-life studies, 130–131
renal failure, dose adjustment in, 661*t*
structure-activity relationship, 134
therapeutic use, 541–547
Acebutolol (Sectral), 34
adverse effects, 267
antiarrhythmic effects, 267
drug-drug interactions, 267–268
barbiturates, 483*t*
cimetidine, 483*t*
phenytoin, 483*t*
rifampin, 483*t*
elderly patients, 582
electrophysiologic action, 266
hemodynamic effects, 267
hepatic dysfunction, 680*t*
indications and dosage, 268
pharmacodynamic properties and cardiac effects of, 35*t*, 43*t*
pharmacokinetics, 266–267, 507*t*
pharmacologic description, 266
pregnancy and lactation, 670*t*
renal failure, dose adjustment in, 659*t*
therapeutic use, 581–582
Acetaminophen
toxic metabolite of, 16–17
Acetazolamide, 153*t*, 156
renal failure, dose adjustment in, 657*t*
Acetylcholine, 69
epoprostenol, comparison to, 423
receptors, 65–66
Activase. *See* Alteplase
Activated partial thromboplastin time (APTT) test, 309–310
Acute myocardial infarction
aspirin, 296–297
heparin, 310–312
thrombolytic agents, 326, 328–337. *See also* Thrombolytic agents
Acute proximal deep vein thrombosis
low-molecular-weight heparins, 315
Acylation, 16
Adalat. *See* Nifedipine
Addison's disease, 447

Adenosine (Adenocard)
adverse effects, 284, 435
antiarrhythmic effects, 283–284
AV nodal reentrant tachycardia, 238
AV reentrant tachycardia (Wolff-Parkinson-White syndrome), 239
children, 558
dosage and administration, 434–435
drug-drug interactions, 284, 496–497
aminophylline, 284
benzodiazepines, 284
digitalis, 284
dipyridamole, 284
verapamil, 284
elderly patients, 558
electrophysiologic action, 283
epoprostenol, comparison to, 423
hemodynamic effects, 283
hepatic dysfunction, 685*t*
indications and dosage, 284–285
mechanism of action, 432–433
perfusion imaging with, 429*t*, 433–434
pharmacokinetics, 283, 507*t*
pharmacologic description, 283
renal failure, dose adjustment in, 657*t*
stress echocardiography, 434
therapeutic use, 558
vasovagal syncope, 451
Adenylcyclase-cyclic AMP system, 201
Adrenergic receptors, 23–25, 24*t*, 25, 412*t*
African-American patients. *See* Black patients
Aging. *See* Elderly patients
Aglycone, 191
Agrylin. *See* Anagrelide
Albumin, 12
Alcohol
beta-adrenergic blocking drugs, interaction with, 58*t*
in breast milk, 22
effects on drug metabolism, 19
Aldactazide (spironolactone and hydrochlorothiazide), therapeutic use of, 649
Aldactone. *See* Spironolactone
Aldoclor (methyldopa and chlorothiazide), therapeutic use of, 644
Aldomet. *See* Methyldopa
Aldoril (methyldopa and hydrochlorothiazide), therapeutic use of, 644
Aldosterone, 111–112
Aliphatic hydroxylation, 16
Allergic interstitial nephritis
adverse effect of diuretics, 173–174
Allopurinol
inhibitory effects on drug metabolism, 19
warfarin, interaction with, 503*t*
Alpha-adrenergic activity, of beta-adrenergic blocking drugs, 37–38
Alpha-adrenergic blocking drugs. *See also* $Alpha_1$-adrenergic blocking drugs; $Alpha_2$-adrenergic blocking drugs
adverse effects, 31–32
beta-adrenergic blocking drugs, interaction with, 58*t*
clinical pharmacology, 25–27, 26*t*
clinical use, 31–32
overview, 23, 24*t*, 25–26
receptors, 23–25, 24*t*

Alpha-adrenergic blocking drugs (*Cont.*):
therapeutic use, 540–541
use in cardiovascular disorders
congestive heart failure, 28–30
hypertension, 27–28
use in noncardiovascular disorders
arterioconstriction, 30–31
benign prostatic obstruction, 31
pheochromocytoma, 30
pulmonary hypertension, 30
shock, 30
vasovagal syncope, 451
$Alpha_1$-adrenergic blocking drugs
hepatic dysfunction, 678*t*
overview, 25–27
pharmacokinetics, 26*t*
receptors, 23, 24*t*, 25–26, 197, 198*t*–199*t*, 199–200
$Alpha_2$-adrenergic blocking drugs, 221–222. *See also* Clonidine; Guanabenz; Guanfacine
overview, 25–26, 28
receptors, 23, 24*t*, 25–26, 44, 197, 199*t*
Alpha-methyldopa, 222–223, 225, 226*t*
Altace. *See* Ramipril
Alteplase (Activase)
elderly patients, 570–571
hepatic dysfunction, 686*t*
pharmacokinetics, 508*t*
pregnancy and lactation, 676*t*
renal failure, dose adjustment in, 664*t*
therapeutic use, 569–571
Aluminim hydroxide gel
beta-adrenergic blocking drugs, interaction with, 58*t*
Amaurosis fugax
calcium channel blockers, 100–101
Amebonium, 70
Amiloride (Midamor), 153*t*
children, 608
digoxin, interaction with, 495*t*
elderly patients, 608
hepatic dysfunction, 684*t*
pharmacokinetics, 508*t*
pregnancy and lactation, 677*t*
renal failure, dose adjustment in, 657*t*
therapeutic use, 607–608
Aminoglycosides
elderly patients, 655*t*
Aminophylline, drug interactions with
adenosine, 284
beta-adrenergic blocking drugs, 58*t*
proarrhythmic drugs, 481*t*
Aminopyrine breath test, 21
Amiodarone (Cordarone), 26
adverse effects, 274
antiarrhythmic effects, 273–274
atrial fibrillation, 237
atrial flutter, 238
atrial tachycardia, 240
AV nodal reentrant tachycardia, 239
AV reentrant tachycardia (Wolff-Parkinson-White syndrome), 240
in breast milk, 22
children, 556–557
drug-drug interactions, 274
beta-adrenergic blocking drugs, 58*t*
digitalis, 287
digoxin, 274, 494, 495*t*
disopyramide, 499*t*, 501*t*
flecainide, 500*t*
phenothiazines, 501*t*
procainamide, 274, 501*t*

quinidine, 245, 274, 498*t*, 501*t*
sotalol, 501*t*
thiazide diuretics, 501*t*
tricyclic antidepressants, 501*t*
warfarin, 274, 503*t*
elderly patients, 556
electrophysiologic action, 272
hemodynamic effects, 273
hepatic dysfunction, 685*t*
indications and dosage, 274–275
pharmacokinetics, 273, 508*t*
pharmacologic description, 272
pregnancy and lactation, 671*t*
renal failure, dose adjustment in, 660*t*
therapeutic use, 556–557
ventricular fibrillation, 242
ventricular tachycardia, 241
Amitriptyline in breast milk, 21
Amlodipine (Norvasc)
adverse effects, 103*t*
chemical structure, 74
clinical applications
angina pectoris, 86–87
"silent" myocardial ischemia, 94
systemic hypertension, 86, 92
digoxin, interaction with, 487
elderly patients, 585
hepatic dysfunction, 681*t*
pharmacokinetics, 81*t*, 84*t*, 508*t*
pharmacologic effects, 76*t*, 77
pregnancy and lactation, 672*t*
renal failure, dose adjustment in, 660*t*
therapeutic use, 585
Amnioglycosides
infective endocarditis, 455
Ampicillin
beta-adrenergic blocking drugs, interaction with, 58*t*
Amrinone (Inocor), 201–202
drug-drug interactions
proarrhythmic drugs, 481*t*
thiazide diuretics, 495*t*
elderly patients, 610
hepatic dysfunction, 684*t*
pharmacokinetics, 509*t*
pregnancy and lactation, 669*t*
renal failure, dose adjustment in, 656*t*
therapeutic use, 609–610
Amyl nitrate, provocative testing with in cardiac ausculation, 427
Anagrelide (Agrylin)
children, 566
hepatic dysfunction, 686*t*
pharmacokinetics, 509*t*
pregnancy and lactation, 676*t*
renal failure, dose adjustment in, 663*t*
therapeutic use, 566
Angina pectoris
angina at rest
beta-adrenergic blocking drugs, 46–47
calcium channel blockers, 88
beta-adrenergic blocking drugs, 44–46
choice in patients with, 62*t*
combined with other antianginal therapies, 46
calcium channel blockers, 86–88, 86*t*, 89*t*
chronic stable angina
aspirin, 293–294
combination therapy
calcium channel blockers, nitrates, and/or beta blockers, 88, 89*t*

Angina pectoris (*Cont.*):
 diuretics, 169
 unstable angina
  aspirin, 294
  low-molecular-weight heparins, 314–315
Angioneurotic edema
 adverse effect of ACE inhibitors, 117
Angioplasty-induced restenosis
 probucol, 389
Angiotensin converting enzyme inhibitors. *See* ACE inhibitors
Angiotensin II receptor blockers
 angiotensin II receptors, 138–139, 139*f*
 beta-adrenergic blocking drugs, interaction with, 58*t*
 clinical applications
  cardiac hypertrophy, 144
  cerebrovascular and other neurologic diseases, 149
  congestive heart failure, 145–147
  myocardial infarction, 144–145
  oncogenesis, 149–150
  postangioplasty vascular restenosis, 147–148
  renal disease, 148
 development of, 107–108
 gender considerations, 666*t*
 hepatic dysfunction, 679*t*
 losartan. *See* Losartan
 therapeutic use, 547–548
 unresolved issues, 150
Angiotensin receptor blockers
 diuretics, combination therapy with, 396, 397*t*, 398
 pregnancy and lactation, 673*t*
 renal failure, dose adjustment in, 662*t*
Anisindione (Miradon)
 children, 559
 elderly patients, 559
 hepatic dysfunction, 686*t*
 pharmacokinetics, 509*t*
 therapeutic use, 559
Anistreplase (Eminase), 324, 327*t*
 elderly patients, 571
 hepatic dysfunction, 686*t*
 patency rates, 331*t*, 332*f*
 pharmacokinetics, 509*t*
 therapeutic use, 571
Antacids, interactions with
 digitalis, 287
 propranolol, 265
Anterior wall myocardial infarction
 thrombolytic agents, 333–334
Antiadrenergic drugs with central action
 classification and pharmacology, 220, 221*t*
  alpha-methyldopa, 222–223
  classic $alpha_2$-receptor agonists, 221–222
  reserpine, 223
 current and recommended use, 225, 226*t*
 effectiveness, 225
 overview, 220
Antianginal drugs
 drug-drug interactions, 486–487, 488*t*–489*t*
 elderly patients, disorders caused in, 654*t*
Antiarrhythmic drugs, 530–540
 class I
  beta-adrenergic blocking drugs, interaction with, 61*t*
  renal failure, dose adjustment in, 657*t*
 class IA, 243–250
  disopyramide. See Disopyramide
  pregnancy and lactation, 669*t*

procainamide. *See* Procainamide
quinidine. *See* Quinidine
renal failure, dose adjustment in, 657*t*–658*t*
class IB, 250–256
lidocaine. *See* Lidocaine
mexiletine. *See* Mexiletine
pregnancy and lactation, 669*t*
renal failure, dose adjustment in, 658*t*
tocainide. *See* Tocainide
class IC, 256–263
flecainide. *See* Flecainide
moricizine. *See* Moricizine
pregnancy and lactation, 670*t*
propafenone. *See* Propafenone
renal failure, dose adjustment in, 659*t*
classification, 234–236, 235*t*
class II, 263–270
acebutolol. *See* Acebutolol
esmolol. *See* Esmolol
pregnancy and lactation, 670*t*–671*t*
propranolol. *See* Propranolol
renal failure, dose adjustment in, 659*t*–660*t*
class III, 270–278
amiodarone. *See* Amiodarone
bretylium. *See* Bretylium
ibutilide. *See* Ibutilide
pregnancy and lactation, 671*t*
renal failure, dose adjustment in, 660*t*
sotalol. *See* Sotalol
class IV, 278–282
diltiazem. *See* Diltiazem
pregnancy and lactation, 671*t*–672*t*
renal failure, dose adjustment in, 660*t*–661*t*
verapamil. *See* Verapamil
drug-drug interactions, 496–497, 498*t*–501*t*
by hepatic mechanisms, 483*t*
genetic factors in metabolism, 17
hepatic dysfunction, 684*t*–685*t*
management
atrial fibrillation, 236–237
atrial flutter, 237–238
atrial tachycardia, 240
AV nodal reentrant tachycardia, 238–239
AV reentrant tachycardia (Wolff-Parkinson-White syndrome), 239–240
ventricular fibrillation, 242
ventricular tachycardia, 240–242
new agents in development, 282
overview, 234
renal failure, dose adjustment in, 657*t*–661*t*
unclassified agents, 283–290
adenosine. *See* Adenosine
digitalis. *See* Digitalis
electrolytes, 288
magnesium. *See* Magnesium as potential cardiovascular disease therapy
renal failure, dose adjustment in, 657*t*
Antibiotics, interactions with
digitalis, 287
quinidine, 498*t*
Anticholinergics
elderly patients, disorders caused in, 654*t*
Anticholinesterases, 68*t*, 69–70
quinidine, interaction with, 498*t*
Anticoagulants

Anticoagulants (*Cont.*):
elderly patients, 655*t*
hepatic dysfunction, 686*t*
pregnancy and lactation, 675*t*–676*t*
therapeutic use, 559–565
Antidiabetic drugs
beta-adrenergic blocking drugs, interaction with, 58*t*
Antihistamines
orthostatic hypotension, 450
Antihypertensives. *See also* Hypertension; Hypertension, combination therapy for
centrally acting agents
elderly patients, 655*t*
hepatic dysfunction, 681*t*
therapeutic use, 594–597
drug-drug interactions, 497
quinidine, 498*t*
elderly patients
disorders caused in, 654*t*
fixed drug combinations
angiotensin converting enzyme inhibitors with thiazide diuretic, 636–637
angiotensin converting enzyme inhibitor with calcium blocker, 638–640
angiotensin II receptor blocker with thiazide diuretic, 640
potassium-sparing diuretic and thiazide diuretic, 648–650
reserpine, hydrochlorothiazide, and hydralazine (Ser-Ap-Es), 650
sympatholytic (alpha-adrenergic antagonist) with thiazide diuretic, 647–648
sympatholytic (beta blocker) with thiazide diuretic, 640–643
sympatholytic (central-acting agent) with thiazide diuretic, 643–644
sympatholytic (peripheral-acting adrenergic antagonist) with thiazide diuretic, 644–647
vasodilator with thiazide diuretic, 648
very-low-dose beta blocker with thiazide diuretic, 643
pregnancy and lactation, 674*t*–675*t*
renal failure, dose adjustment in, 662*t*–663*t*
vasodilators. *See* Nonspecific antihypertensive vasodilators; Vasodilators
Antiobesity drugs, therapeutic use of, 559
Antiplatelet and antithrombotic drugs
aspirin. *See* Aspirin
clopidogrel, 302–303
danaparoid. *See* Danaparoid
dipyridamole. *See* Dipyridamole
drug-drug interactions, 497, 502, 503*t*
GP IIb/IIIa integrin glycoprotein receptor antagonists. *See* Glycoprotein IIb/IIIa receptor antagonists
heparin. *See* Heparin
hepatic dysfunction, 686*t*
overview, 292, 307–308
pregnancy and lactation, 675*t*–676*t*
renal failure, dose adjustment in, 663*t*
therapeutic use, 565–574
thrombolytic agents
therapeutic use, 550–555
ticlopidine. *See* Ticlopidine
warfarin. *See* Warfarin

Antipyrine
  propranolol, interaction with, 266
Antithrombotic drugs. *See* Antiplatelet and antithrombotic drugs
Aortic regurgitation
  ACE inhibitors, 126
Apoptosis, 51
Apresazide (hydralazine and hydrochlorothiazide), therapeutic use of, 648
Apresoline. *See* Hydralazine
APSAC (anisoylated plasminogen-streptokinase activator complex). *See* Anistreplase
APTT (activated partial thromboplastin time) test, 309–310
Ardeparin (Normiflo), 313*t*. *See also* Low-molecular-weight heparin
  hepatic dysfunction, 686*t*
  pharmacokinetics, 510*t*
  pregnancy and lactation, 676*t*
  renal failure, dose adjustment in, 663*t*
  therapeutic use, 562–563
Area under the curve (AUC), 10, 10*f*
Aromatic hydroxylation, 16
Arrhythmias. *See also* Antiarrhythmic drugs
  beta-adrenergic blocking drugs, 48, 49*t*
  calcium, 186
  calcium channel blockers, 89–92, 90*t*
  magnesium, 178–179
Arterioconstriction
  alpha-adrenergic blocking drugs, 30–31
Aspirin
  adjunctive antithrombotic therapy, 337–338
  adverse effects, 299–300
  atrial fibrillation, 299
  children, 568
  chronic stable angina, 293–294
  coronary artery bypass surgery, 298–299
  drug-drug interactions, 497, 503*t*
    ACE inhibitors, 119, 492*t*, 503*t*
    barbiturates, 503*t*
    phenytoin, 503*t*
    probenecid, 503*t*
    rifampin, 503*t*
    sulfinpyrazone, 503*t*
    thiazide diuretics, 503*t*
    warfarin, 503*t*
  elderly patients, 568
  gender considerations, 666*t*
  hepatic dysfunction, 686*t*
  myocardial infarction
    acute, 296–297
    primary prevention, 294–296
    secondary prevention, 296
  overview, 293
  percutaneous transluminal coronary angioplasty and arterial stenting, 297–298
  pharmacokinetics, 510*t*
  pregnancy and lactation, 676*t*
  renal failure, dose adjustment in, 663*t*
  therapeutic use, 566–568
  transient ischemia attack and stroke, 299
  unstable angina, 294
Asthma, beta-blocker choice in patients with, 62*t*
Atenolol (Tenormin), 39, 48, 50
  elderly patients, 578, 652*t*
  hepatic dysfunction, 680*t*
  pharmacodynamic properties and cardiac effects of, 35*t*, 43*t*
  pharmacokinetics, 510*t*
  pregnancy and lactation, 670*t*

Atenolol (Tenormin) (*Cont.*):
- renal failure, dose adjustment in, 659*t*
- therapeutic use, 577–578

Atherosclerosis
- calcium channel blockers, 101–102

Atorvastatin (Lipitor), 379
- children, 619
- elderly patients, 619
- hepatic dysfunction, 685*t*
- pharmacokinetics, 511*t*
- pregnancy and lactation, 674*t*
- renal failure, dose adjustment in, 664*t*
- therapeutic use, 619

Atrial fibrillation
- amiodarone, 237
- antiarrhythmic drugs, 236–237
- aspirin, 299
- calcium channel blockers, 89–90
- disopyramide, 237
- flecainide, 237
- ibutilide, 237
- procainamide, 237
- propafenone, 237
- quinidine, 237
- sotalol, 237
- warfarin, 322

Atrial flutter
- amiodarone, 238
- antiarrhythmic drugs, 237–238
- calcium channel blockers, 91

Atrial tachycardia
- amiodarone, 240
- antiarrhythmic drugs, 240
- flecainide, 240
- metoprolol, 240
- propafenone, 240
- propranolol, 240
- sotalol, 240
- verapamil, 240

Atrioventricular conduction defects, beta-blocker choice in patients with, 62*t*

Atromid-S. *See* Clofibrate

Atropine, 70–71, 71*t*
- in breast milk, 22
- children, 558
- elderly patients, 558
- hepatic dysfunction, 685*t*
- therapeutic use, 540, 558

AUC (area under the curve), 10, 10*f*

Avapro. *See* Irbesartan

AV conduction delay
- beta-adrenergic blocking drugs, 55

AV nodal reentrant tachycardia
- adenosine, 238
- amiodarone, 239
- antiarrhythmic drugs, 238–239
- beta-adrenergic receptor antagonists, 239
- digoxin, 239
- diltiazem, 239
- flecainide, 239
- propafenone, 239
- verapamil, 238–239

AV reentrant tachycardia (Wolff-Parkinson-White syndrome)
- adenosine, 239
- amiodarone, 240
- antiarrhythmic drugs, 239–240
- diltiazem, 239
- disopyramide, 240
- esmolol, 239
- flecainide, 240
- moricizine, 240
- procainamide, 239, 240
- propafenone, 240
- sotalol, 240
- verapamil, 91–92, 239

Azo reduction, 16

B

Barbiturates
- drug-drug interactions
  - acebutolol, 483*t*
  - aspirin, 503*t*

disopyramide, 499*t*
labetalol, 483*t*
metoprolol, 483*t*
mexiletine, 500*t*
propranolol, 483*t*
quinidine, 498*t*
timolol, 483*t*
BAS. *See* Bile acid sequestrants
Baycol. *See* Cerivastatin
Benazepril (Lotensin)
clinical applications, 136*t*
elderly patients, 541
hepatic dysfunction, 679*t*
pharmacokinetics, 511*t*
pregnancy and lactation, 673*t*
renal failure, dose adjustment in, 661*t*
therapeutic use, 541
Bendroflumethiazide (Naturetin), 153*t*
children, 601
elderly patients, 601
hepatic dysfunction, 683*t*
pharmacokinetics, 511*t*
therapeutic use, 601
Benthiazide, 153*t*
hepatic dysfunction, 683*t*
Benzafibrate, 362, 365
warfarin, interaction with, 504*t*
Benzodiazepines
adenosine, interaction with, 284
Benzthiazide (Exna)
children, 602
elderly patients, 602
therapeutic use, 601–602
Bepridil (Vascor)
adverse effects, 103*t*
angina pectoris, 86, 86*t*, 87
chemical structure, 74
elderly patients, 585–586
hepatic dysfunction, 681*t*
pharmacodynamics, 74
pharmacokinetics, 81*t*, 85*t*, 512*t*
pharmacologic effects, 76*t*, 77, 78
pregnancy and lactation, 672*t*
therapeutic use, 585–586
Beta-adrenergic blocking drugs. *See also* the names of specific drugs
ACE inhibitors, combination therapy with, 131–132
adverse effects
cardiac, related to beta-adrenoceptor blockade, 54–55
noncardiac, related to beta-adrenoceptor blockade, 55–57
unrelated to beta-adrenoceptor blockade, 57
basic pharmacologic differences among
alpha-adrenergic activity, 37–38
$beta_1$ selectivity, 35*t*, 36–37
direct vasodilator activity, 38
intrinsic sympathomimetic activity (partial agonist activity), 35*t*, 37
membrane-stabilizing activity, 35*t*, 36
pharmacokinetics, 38–39
potency, 35–36, 35*t*
relationship among dose, plasma level, and efficacy, 40
structure-activity relationships, 36
beta-adrenergic receptors, 23, 24*t*, 33–34, 36–37, 196–197, 198*t*–199*t*, 199–200
$beta_1$-selective, without intrinsic sympathomimetic activity
therapeutic use, 577–581

Beta-adrenergic blocking drugs (*Cont.*):
- choosing, 62, 62*t*–63*t*
- clinical effects and therapeutic applications
  - angina at rest, 46–47
  - angina pectoris, 44–46
  - AV nodal reentrant tachycardia, 239
  - central nervous system effect, 41
  - congestive cardiomyopathy, 51–52, 52*t*
  - differences in effects on plasma renin, 41
  - dissecting aneurysms, 53
  - electrophysiologic and antiarrhythmic effects, 47–48, 47*t*, 49*t*
  - elevated systemic blood pressure, 40–41, 42*t*–43*t*
  - hypertrophic cardiomyopathy, 50–51
  - mitral valve prolapse, 52
  - negative chronotropic and inotropic effects, 41
  - noncardiovascular applications, 54
  - overview, 40, 42*t*
  - peripheral resistance, 41–42, 44
  - prejunctional receptor effects, 44
  - QT-interval prolongation syndrome, 53
  - regression of left ventricular hypertrophy, 53
  - "silent" myocardial ischemia, 50
  - survivors of acute myocardial infarction, 48–50, 49*t*
  - syncope, 53–54
  - tetralogy of Fallot, 53
  - vasospastic angina, 46–47
- diuretics
  - combination therapy with, 398
- drug-drug interactions, 57, 58*t*–61*t*, 484, 485*t*, 486
  - ACE inhibitors, 58*t*
  - alcohol, 58*t*
  - alpha-adrenergic blocking drugs, 58*t*
  - aluminum hydroxide gel, 58*t*
  - aminophylline, 58*t*
  - amiodarone, 58*t*
  - ampicillin, 58*t*
  - angiotensin II receptor blockers, 58*t*
  - antiarrhythmics, type I, 61*t*
  - antidiabetic drugs, 58*t*
  - calcium, 58*t*
  - calcium antagonists, 58*t*, 485*t*
  - cimetidine, 59*t*
  - clonidine, 59*t*
  - diazepam, 59*t*
  - digitalis glycosides, 59*t*, 287
  - diltiazem, 485*t*, 489*t*
  - disopyramide, 499*t*, 500*t*
  - epinephrine, 59*t*
  - ergot alkaloids, 59*t*
  - flecainide, 485*t*
  - fluvoxamine, 59*t*
  - glucagon, 59*t*
  - halofenate, 59*t*
  - by hepatic mechanisms, 483*t*
  - hydralazine, 60*t*
  - ibuprofen, 60*t*
  - indomethacin, 60*t*
  - isoproterenol, 60*t*
  - levodopa, 60*t*
  - lidocaine, 60t, 500*t*
  - losartan, 58*t*
  - methyldopa, 60*t*
  - monoamine oxidase inhibitors, 60*t*
  - naproxen, 61*t*
  - nifedipine, 489*t*

nitrates, 60*t*
nonsteroidal antiinflammatory drugs (NSAIDs), 485*t*
omeprazole, 60*t*
phenobarbital, 60*t*
phenothiazines, 60*t*
phenylpropanolamine, 61*t*
phenytoin, 61*t*
quinidine, 498*t*
rantidine, 61*t*
reserpine, 61*t*
smoking, 61*t*
sulindac, 61*t*
tricyclic antidepressants, 61*t*
tubucuraine, 61*t*
verapamil, 485*t*, 488*t*
warfarin, 61*t*
dual-acting, therapeutic use of, 583–585
elderly patients, 652*t*, 655*t*
disorders caused in, 654*t*
gender considerations, 666*t*
hepatic dysfunction, 680*t*–681*t*
with intrinsic sympathomimetic activity
therapeutic use, 581–582
nonselective, without intrinsic sympathomimetic activity
therapeutic use, 574–577
overview, 23, 24*t*, 32–35, 35*t*, 62, 62*t*–63*t*
receptors, 23–25, 24*t*
renal failure, dose adjustment in, 659*t*–660*t*
therapeutic use, 574–585
withdrawal, 55
$Beta_1$-adrenergic receptors, 23, 24*t*, 36–37, 197, 198*t*–199*t*, 199–200
$Beta_2$-adrenergic receptors, 23, 24*t*, 36–37, 197, 198*t*–199*t*, 199–200
$Beta_3$-adrenergic receptors, 23, 24*t*
Beta-adrenergic stimulants
proarrhythmic drugs, interactions with, 481*t*
Beta and dopamine-receptor agonists, therapeutic use of, 610–613
Betapace. *See* Sotalol
Betaxolol (Kerlone), 34
elderly patients, 578
hepatic dysfunction, 680*t*
pharmacodynamic properties and cardiac effects of, 35*t*, 43*t*
pharmacokinetics, 512*t*
pregnancy and lactation, 671*t*
therapeutic use, 578
Bethanechol, 69
Bezold-Jarisch reflex, 53, 446*t*
Bile acid sequestrants (BAS)
adverse effects of resins, 358–359
chemistry, 353, 355
children, 353
clinical experience, 357
clinical use of resins, 357–358
drug-drug interactions, 356
warfarin, 504*t*
overview, 353
pharmacokinetics, 356–357
pharmacology, 355–356
therapeutic use, 616–617
Biliary excretion, 21
Bioavilability, drug, 9–10, 10*f*
Bisoprolol (Zebeta), 34
children, 579
elderly patients, 579
hepatic dysfunction, 680*t*
hydrochlorothiazide, combination therapy with, 398
pharmacodynamic properties and cardiac effects of, 35*t*, 43*t*
pharmacokinetics, 512*t*
pregnancy and lactation, 671*t*
therapeutic use, 579

Black patients
  ACE inhibitors, 109, 120
  beta blockers, 409
  calcium channel blockers and diuretics, combination therapy with, 398–399
  diuretics, 166–167, 395–396
  salt-sensitive hypertension, 162
Blocadren. *See* Timolol
Blood-brain barrier, 8
Blood pressure, systemic, elevated
  beta-adrenergic blocking drugs, 40–41, 42*t*–43*t*
Bradbury-Eggleston syndrome, 446*t*, 450
Bradycardia, beta-blocker choice in patients with, 62*t*
Braking phenomenon (thiazide diuretics), 155
Bretylium
  adolescents, 539
  adverse effects, 271
  antiarrhythmic effects, 271
  drug-drug interactions, 271–272
    protryptyline, 272
  elderly patients, 557
  electrophysiologic action, 270
  hemodynamic effects, 271
  hepatic dysfunction, 685*t*
  indications and dosage, 272
  pharmacokinetics, 270–271, 512*t*
  pharmacologic description, 270
  pregnancy and lactation, 671*t*
  renal failure, dose adjustment in, 660*t*
  therapeutic use, 557
  ventricular fibrillation, 242
  ventricular tachycardia, 241
Brevibloc. *See* Esmolol
Bromocriptine, 26
Bronchitis, chronic, beta-blocker choice in patients with, 62*t*
Bronchodilators
  proarrhythmic drugs, interactions with, 481*t*
Bucindolol, 34, 38
  pharmacodynamic properties and cardiac effects of, 35*t*, 43*t*
Bumetanide (Bumex), 153*t*, 154, 157
  children, 598
  elderly patients, 598
  hepatic dysfunction, 682*t*
  pharmacokinetics, 512*t*
  pregnancy and lactation, 677*t*
  renal failure, dose adjustment in, 656*t*
  therapeutic use, 597–598

C

Caffeine in breast milk, 21
Calan. *See* Verapamil
Calcium (as potential cardiovascular disease therapy)
  beta-adrenergic blocking drugs, interaction with, 58*t*
  cardiovascular effects
    arrhythmia, 186
    calcium supplements, 185
    cardiac arrest, 185–186
    renal excretion, 184–185
    systemic hypertension, 184
  clinical use, 186
  overview, 184, 187
Calcium antagonists
  ACE inhibitors, combination therapy with, 132
  adverse effects
    drug-drug interactions, 104–106
    drug overdose, 104, 105*t*
    drug withdrawal, 104
    overview, 102, 103*t*, 104
  cardiovascular effects

effects on coronary and peripehreal arterial blood vessels, 75
effects on muscular contraction, 75
effects on myocardial contractility, 75, 77
effects on nonvascular tissues, 78–79
effects on veins, 75
electrophysiologic effects, 77–78
overview, 76*t*
chemical structure, 74
clinical applications
amaurosis fugax, 100–101
angina pectoris, 86–88, 86*t*, 89*t*
arrhythmias, 89–92, 90*t*
atherosclerosis, 101–102
cerebral arterial spasm and stroke, 99–100
congestive heart failure, 97–98
dementia, 100
high-altitude pulmonary edema, 101
hypertensive emergencies and perioperative hypertension, 94
hypertrophic cardiomyopathy, 95–97
migraine, 100
myocardial infarction, 94–95
primary pulmonary hypertension, 99
Raynaud's phenomenon, 101
"silent" myocardial ischemia, 94
systemic hypertension, 92–94
combined with beta-adrenergic blocking drugs to treat angina pectoris, 46
diuretics
combination therapy with, 398–399, 400*f*
drug-drug interactions, 104–106, 486–487, 488*t*–489*t*
beta-adrenergic blocking drugs, 58*t*, 485*t*
digitalis, 287
by hepatic mechanisms, 483*t*
nitrates, 488*t*
gender considerations, 666*t*
hepatic dysfunction, 681*t*
overview, 73, 86, 106
pharmacodynamics, 74
pharmacokinetics, 79, 80*t*–85*t*
physiologic background, 73
renal failure, dose adjustment in, 660*t*–661*t*
therapeutic use, 585–594
Capozide (captopril and hydrochlorothiazide), therapeutic use of, 636–637
Captopril (Capoten), 108, 113, 117, 133
children, 542
clinical applications, 136*t*
drug-drug interactions
digoxin, 492*t*, 495*t*
furosemide, 487, 490*t*
hydralazine, 492*t*
immunosuppresive drugs, 492*t*
loop diuretics, 492*t*
probenecid, 492*t*
procainamide, 492*t*, 499*t*
elderly patients, 542
hepatic dysfunction, 679*t*
pharmacokinetics, 137, 513*t*
pregnancy and lactation, 672*t*
renal failure, dose adjustment in, 661*t*
therapeutic use, 542

Carbonic anhydrase inhibitors, 153*t*, 156. *See also* Diuretics
  renal failure, dose adjustment in, 657*t*
Cardene. *See* Nicardipine
Cardiac arrest
  calcium, 185–186
Cardiac ausculation, provocative testing in, 427
Cardiac hypertrophy
  angiotensin II receptor blockers, 144
  losartan, 144
Cardilate. *See* Erythrityl tetranitrate
Cardiogenic shock
  thrombolytic agents, 335–336
Cardioquin. *See* Quinidine
Cardizem. *See* Diltiazem
Cardura. *See* Doxazosin
Carteolol (Cartrol), 34
  elderly patients, 582
  hepatic dysfunction, 680*t*
  pharmacodynamic properties and cardiac effects of, 35*t*, 43*t*
  pharmacokinetics, 513*t*
  pregnancy and lactation, 671*t*
  renal failure, dose adjustment in, 659*t*
  therapeutic use, 582
Carvedilol (Coreg), 26, 34, 36, 38–39
  elderly patients, 584
  hepatic dysfunction, 681*t*
  pharmacodynamic properties and cardiac effects of, 35*t*, 43*t*
  pharmacokinetics, 513*t*
  pregnancy and lactation, 671*t*
  renal failure, dose adjustment in, 660*t*
  therapeutic use, 583–584
Catapres. *See* Clonidine
Catecholamines and similar inotropic agents, 23–25, 51, 196–201, 198*t*–199*t*
Ceiling effect (thiazide diuretics), 155
Cell membranes, passage of drugs across, 7–8
Centrally acting antihypertensives
  therapeutic use, 594–597
Cerebral arterial spasm
  calcium channel blockers, 99–100
Cerebrovascular disease
  ACE inhibitors, 129–130
  angiotensin II receptor blockers, 149
  losartan, 149
Cerivastatin (Baycol), 379
  elderly patients, 620
  hepatic dysfunction, 685*t*
  pharmacokinetics, 514*t*
  pregnancy and lactation, 674*t*
  renal failure, dose adjustment in, 664*t*
  therapeutic use, 619–620
Certroparin (Sandoparin), 313*t*. *See also* Low-molecular-weight heparin
Children. *See* "children" subentries under individual drug names in the index and in Appendix 2
Chloramphenicol
  inhibitory effects on drug metabolism, 19
Chlorothiazide (Diuril), 153*t*
  bile acid sequestrants, interaction with, 356
  children, 602
  elderly patients, 602
  hepatic dysfunction, 683*t*
  pharmacokinetics, 510*t*
  pregnancy and lactation, 677*t*
  therapeutic use, 602–603

Chlorpromazine, 26
in breast milk, 22
Chlorthalidone (Hygroton, Thalitone), 153*t*
children, 603
elderly patients, 603
hepatic dysfunction, 683*t*
pharmacokinetics, 514*t*
pregnancy and lactation, 677*t*
renal failure, dose adjustment in, 657*t*
therapeutic use, 603
Cholesterol
HDL. *See* HDL cholesterol
LDL. *See* LDL cholesterol
lowering. *See* Lipid-lowering drugs
total. *See* Total cholesterol
VLDL. *See* VLDL cholesterol
Cholestipol (Colestid), 355–359
Cholestyramine (Questran), 353, 355–359. *See also* Bile acid sequestrants
drug-drug interactions
colestipol, 504*t*
digoxin, 496
warfarin, 503*t*, 504*t*
elderly patients, 597
hepatic dysfunction, 685*t*
pregnancy and lactation, 674*t*
renal failure, dose adjustment in, 665*t*
therapeutic use, 596–597
Choline esters, 69
Chronic stable angina
aspirin, 293–294
Chronotropic effects of beta blockers, 41
Cimetidine
in breast milk, 22
drug-drug interactions
acebutolol, 483*t*
beta-adrenergic blocking drugs, 59*t*
diltiazem, 489*t*
disopyramide, 499*t*
flecainide, 501*t*
labetalol, 483*t*, 485*t*
lidocaine, 252, 483*t*, 500*t*
metoprolol, 483*t*, 485*t*
mexiletine, 256
nifedipine, 483*t*, 489*t*
procainamide, 247, 483*t*, 499*t*
propafenone, 263
propranolol, 266, 483*t*, 485*t*
quinidine, 245, 483*t*, 498*t*
timolol, 483*t*
tocainide, 254
verapamil, 483*t*, 488*t*
warfarin, 503*t*
inhibitory effects on drug metabolism, 19
Cin-Quin. *See* Quinidine
Ciprofibrate, 362
Clearance, drug, 13–14, 13*f*, 15*f*
Clinical pharmacology. *See* Pharmacology, basic principles of
Clivarine (Reviparin), 313*t*. *See also* Low-molecular-weight heparin
Clofibrate (Atromid-S), 362
elderly patients, 617
gender considerations, 667*t*
hepatic dysfunction, 685*t*
pharmacokinetics, 514*t*
pregnancy and lactation, 673*t*
renal failure, dose adjustment in, 664*t*
therapeutic use, 617–618
warfarin, interaction with, 360
Clonidine (Catapres), 9, 222, 226*t*
beta-adrenergic blocking drugs
choice in patients using, 63*t*
interaction with, 59*t*
elderly patients, 595
disorders caused in, 654*t*
gender considerations, 666*t*
hepatic dysfunction, 681*t*
orthostatic hypotension, 450
pharmacokinetics, 514*t*

Clonidine (Catapres) (*Cont.*):
pregnancy and lactation, 675*t*
renal failure, dose adjustment in, 662*t*
therapeutic use, 595–596
Clonidine hydrochloride (Duraclon)
children, 596
therapeutic use, 595–596
Clopidogrel (Plavix), 302–303
therapeutic use, 568
Cocaine in breast milk, 21–22
Colestipol (Colestid). *See also* Bile acid sequestrants
elderly patients, 617
gender considerations, 667*t*
hepatic dysfunction, 685*t*
pregnancy and lactation, 674*t*
renal failure, dose adjustment in, 665*t*
therapeutic use, 617
warfarin, interaction with, 503*t*
Combipres (clonidine and chlorthalidone), therapeutic use of, 643
Competitive inhibition, 4
Congestive cardiomyopathy
beta-adrenergic blocking drugs, 51–52, 52*t*
Congestive heart failure
ACE inhibitors, 123–125
alpha-adrenergic blocking drugs, 28–30
angiotensin II receptor blockers, 145–147
beta-adrenergic blocking drugs, 54, 62*t*
calcium channel blockers, 97–98
digoxin, 193–195
losartan, 145–147
magnesium, 177–178
nitrates, 210
Conjugated estrogens
gender considerations, 666*t*
Conjugation pathways, 16
Contrast agents
elderly patients, 655*t*
Cordarone. *See* Amiodarone
Coreg. *See* Carvedilol
Corgard. *See* Nadolol
Corlopam. *See* Fenoldopam
Coronary artery bypass surgery
aspirin, 298–299
Coronary artery disease
dobutamine, detection using, 438
nicotinic acid, 3813–383
patients with idiopathic dilated cardiomyopathy, detection of using dobutamine, 439
Corticosteroids
digitalis, interaction with, 287
Corvert. *See* Ibutilide
Corzide (nadolol and bendroflumethiazide), therapeutic use of, 641
Cough, adverse effect of ACE inhibitors, 116–117
Coumadin. *See* Warfarin
Covera. *See* Verapamil
Cozaar. *See* Losartan
Crystodigin. *See* Digitoxin
Cutaneous reactions to diuretics, 174
Cyclandelate (Cyclospasmol)
elderly patients, 624
hepatic dysfunction, 682*t*
therapeutic use, 624
Cyclosporine
in breast milk, 22
drug-drug interactions
diltiazem, 489*t*
HMG-CoA reductase inhibitors, 504*t*
nicardipine, 489*t*
Cyclothiazide, 153*t*
hepatic dysfunction, 683*t*
Cytochrome P450 system, 16, 482

D

Dalteparin (Fragmin), 313*t*. *See also* Low-molecular-weight heparin
  pharmacokinetics, 515*t*
  therapeutic use, 563–564
Danaparoid (Orgaran), 315–316
  hepatic dysfunction, 686*t*
  pharmacokinetics, 515*t*
  pregnancy and lactation, 676*t*
  renal failure, dose adjustment in, 663*t*
  therapeutic use, 563–564
Debrisoquin
  genetic factors in metabolism, 17
Deep vein thrombosis
  low-molecular-weight heparins, 315
Demadex. *See* Torsemide
Dementia
  calcium channel blockers, 100
Demi-Regroton (reserpine and chlorthalidone), therapeutic use of, 644–645
Deponit. *See* Nitroglycerin
Depression, beta-blocker choice in patients with, 62*t*
Deslanoside
  hepatic dysfunction, 684*t*
Dexfenfluramine (Redux)
  pharmacokinetics, 515*t*
  therapeutic use, 559
Dextromethorphan
  genetic factors in metabolism, 17
Diabetes mellitus, 446*t*
  beta-blocker choice in patients with, 62*t*
  diabetic nephropathy
    ACE inhibitors, 128–129
  magnesium, 177–178
Diazepam
  beta-adrenergic blocking drugs, interaction with, 59*t*
Diazoxide (Hyperstat, Proglycem), 230–232. *See also* Nonspecific antihypertensive vasodilators
  children, 625
  elderly patients, 625
  hepatic dysfunction, 682*t*
  therapeutic use, 624–625
Dibenzyline. *See* Phenoxybenzamine
Dicoumarol
  children, 560
  elderly patients, 560
  hepatic dysfunction, 686*t*
  pharmacokinetics, 516*t*
  therapeutic use, 559–560
Digibind. *See* Digoxin immune fab
Digitalis
  discussion, indications, and therapeutic use guidelines. *See* Digitalis preparations and other inotropic agents
  drug-drug interactions, 481*t*, 494, 495*t*, 496
    adenosine, 284
    amiodarone, 287
    antacids, 287
    antibiotics, 287
    beta-adrenergic blocking drugs, 59*t*, 287
    bile acid sequestrants, 356
    calcium channel antagonists, 287
    corticosteroids, 287
    digitalis toxicity, 494, 499*t*
    diuretics, 287
    flecainide, 287
    phenobarbital, 287
    phenytoin, 287
    propafenone, 287
    quinidine, 287
    verapamil, 287, 488*t*

Digitalis preparations and other inotropic agents
  beta and dopamine receptor agonists, therapeutic use of, 610–613
  catecholamines and similar inotropic agents, 23–25, 51, 196–201, 198*t*–199*t*
  digitalis glycosides
    adverse effects, 286–287
    antiarrhythmic effects, 286
    clinical use, 192–193
    congestive heart failure, 193–195
    digitoxin. *See* Digitoxin
    digoxin. *See* Digoxin
    drug-drug interactions. *See* Digitalis, drug-drug interactions
    electrophysiologic action, 285
    hemodynamic effects, 286
    history of, 188
    indications and dosage, 288
    pharmacology, 188–191, 285
    structure, pharmacokinetics, and metabolism, 191–192, 285–286
    therapeutic use, 613–616
    toxicity, 195–196
  hepatic dysfunction, 684*t*
  PDE (phosphodiesterase) inhibitors, 201–202
    clinical use of noncatecholamine inotropes, 202
    proarrhythmic drugs, interaction with, 481*t*
    therapeutic use, 609–613
  pregnancy and lactation, 669t
  renal failure, dose adjustment in, 656*t*
  therapeutic use, 609–616
Digitoxin (Crystodigin), 191–192. *See also* Digitalis preparations and other inotropic agents
  children, 613
  drug-drug interactions
    quinidine, 245
    verapamil, 495*t*
  elderly patients, 613
  hepatic dysfunction, 684*t*
  pharmacokinetics, 516*t*
  pregnancy and lactation, 669*t*
  renal failure, dose adjustment in, 656*t*
  therapeutic use, 613–614
Digoxin (Lanoxicaps, Lanoxin), 191–192. *See also* Digitalis preparations and other inotropic agents
  adolescents, 615–616
  AV nodal reentrant tachycardia, 239
  in breast milk, 21
  children, 614, 616
  congestive heart failure, 193–195
  drug-drug interactions
    amiloride, 495*t*
    amiodarone, 274, 494, 495*t*
    amlodipine, 487
    captopril, 492*t*, 495*t*
    diltiazem, 489*t*, 495*t*
    disopyramide, 496, 500*t*
    diuretics, 495*t*
    encainide, 496
    erythromycin, 496
    flecainide, 260, 501*t*
    hydralazine, 493*t*
    kaolin pectate, 496
    lidocaine, 496
    mexiletine, 496
    moricizine, 258
    nicardipine, 489*t*
    nifedipine, 489*t*, 495*t*
    nitrendipine, 487, 495*t*
    phenytoin, 496
    prazosin, 495*t*

proarrhythmic drugs, 481*t*
procainamide, 496
propafenone, 263, 495*t*, 501*t*
quinidine, 245, 494, 495*t*, 498*t*
quinine, 495*t*
sotalol, 496
spironolactone, 495*t*
tetracycline, 496
triamterene, 495*t*
verapamil, 280, 488*t*, 494, 495*t*
elderly patients, 652*t*, 655*t*
disorders caused in, 654*t*
esmolol, combination therapy with, 269
hepatic dysfunction, 684*t*
pharmacokinetics, 516*t*
pregnancy and lactation, 669*t*
renal failure, dose adjustment in, 656*t*
therapeutic use, 614–616
Digoxin immune fab (ovine) (Digibind)
adolescents, 615–616
children, 616
elderly patients, 616
therapeutic use, 615–616
Dihydroxyphenylserine
orthostatic hypotension, 450
Dilacor. *See* Diltiazem
Dilatrate. *See* Isosorbide dinitrate
Diltiazem (Cardizem, Dilacor, Tiazac)
adverse effects, 103, 281–282
antiarrhythmic effects, 281
AV nodal reentrant tachycardia, 239
AV reentrant tachycardia (Wolff-Parkinson-White syndrome), 239
clinical applications
angina pectoris, 86, 86*t*, 87
angioplasty patients, 102
cardioplegia solution component, 102
heart transplant recipients, 102
Raynaud's phenomenon, 101
renal transplant patients, 102
"silent" myocardial ischemia, 94
supraventricular arrhythmias, 86, 89–92, 90*t*
systemic hypertension, 86, 92–93
drug-drug interactions, 282
beta-adrenergic blocking drugs, 485*t*, 489*t*
cimetidine, 489*t*
cyclosporine, 489*t*
digoxin, 489*t*, 495*t*
flecainide, 489*t*
nifedipine, 483*t*
quinidine, 498*t*
elderly patients, 586, 652*t*
disorders caused in, 654*t*
electrophysiologic action, 281
hemodynamic effects, 281
hepatic dysfunction, 681*t*
hydrochlorothiazide, combination therapy with, 399, 400*f*
indications and dosage, 282
pharmacokinetics, 79, 80*t*, 82*t*, 281, 516*t*
pharmacology, 76*t*, 77, 78, 281
pregnancy and lactation, 671*t*
renal failure, dose adjustment in, 660*t*
therapeutic use, 586–588
Diovan. *See* Valsartan
Dipyridamole (Persantine), 300–301
adenosine, interaction with, 284
adverse effects, 301
aspirin, combination therapy with, 301
children, 569

Dipyridamole (Persantine) (*Cont.*):
clinical studies, 300–301
elderly patients, 569
hepatic dysfunction, 686*t*
mechanism of action, 428, 430
perfusion imaging with, 429*t*
accuracy of test, 430–431
adverse effects, 432
echocardiography, 431–432
limited exercise stress, 432
procedure, 430
test developmnt, 430
pharmacokinetics, 516*t*
therapeutic use, 568–569
Disease states and drug metabolism, 18
Disopyramide (Norpace)
adverse effects, 249
antiarrhythmic effects, 249
atrial fibrillation, 237
AV reentrant tachycardia (Wolff-Parkinson-White syndrome), 240
children, 549
drug-drug interactions, 249–250
amiodarone, 499*t*, 501*t*
barbiturates, 499*t*
beta-adrenergic blocking drugs, 61*t*, 499*t*, 500*t*
cimetidine, 499*t*
digitalis toxicity, 499*t*
digoxin, 496, 500*t*
erythromycin, 249
methyldopa, 500*t*
phenobarbital, 249
phenytoin, 249, 499*t*
propranolol, 265
pyridostigmine, 500*t*
quinidine, 498*t*, 499*t*, 500*t*
rifampin, 499*t*
sotalol, 499*t*
verapamil, 280, 488*t*
elderly patients, 549, 652*t*
electrophysiologic action, 248
gender considerations, 666*t*
hemodynamic effects, 249
indications and dosage, 250
pharmacokinetics, 248, 517*t*
pharmacologic description, 248
pregnancy and lactation, 669*t*
renal failure, dose adjustment in, 658*t*
therapeutic use, 548–549
vasovagal syncope, 451
ventricular tachycardia, 241
Dissecting aneurysms
beta-adrenergic blocking drugs, 53
Distal tubule diuretics
renal failure, dose adjustment in, 657*t*
Distribution, drug. *See* Pharmacology, basic principles of
Diucardin. *See* Hydroflumethiazide
Diupres (reserpine and chlorothiazide), therapeutic use of, 645–646
Diuretics
adverse effects
allergic interstitial nephritis, 173–174
cutaneous reactions, 174
glucose intolerance, 171–172
gout, 173
hypokalemia, 169–170
hypomagnesemia, 170–171
hyponatremia, 171
lipid metabolism, 172
ototoxicity, 173
postural hypotension, 172–173
angina pectoris, 169
beta blockers, comparison to, 164
classes of
carbonic anhydrase

inhibitors. *See* Carbonic anhydrase inhibitors
loop diuretics. *See* Loop diuretics
osmotic diuretics. *See* Osmotic diuretics
potassium-sparing diuretics. *See* Potassium-sparing diuretics
thiazides. *See* Thiazide diuretics
combination therapy with, 159, 395–401
ACE inhibitors, 131, 395–396
angiotensin receptor antagonists, 396, 397*t*, 398
beta blockers, 398
calcium channel blockers, 398–399, 400*f*
sympatholytics, 399
two diuretics, 401
drug-drug interactions
ACE inhibitors, 118–119, 492*t*
digitalis, 287
digoxin, 495*t*
proarrhythmic drugs, 481*t*
quinidine, 498*t*
sotalol, 501*t*
elderly patients, 164–166, 655*t*
disorders caused in, 654*t*
factors influencing diuretic efficacy in heart failure
altered pharmacodynamics, 159
altered pharmacokinetics, 156–158
other pharmacologic approaches to diuresis
angiotensin converting enzyme inhibitors, 161–162
dopamine, 159–161
overview, 152, 153*t*
pregnancy and lactation, 677*t*
renal failure, dose adjustment in, 656*t*–657*t*
systemic hypertension
black patients, 166–167
clinical trials, 163–164
combination therapy with other antihypertensives, 168–169
elderly patients, 164–166
mechanisms by which diuretics lower blood pressure, 163
regression of cardiac hypertrophy and diuretic therapy, 168
salt-sensitive hypertension, 162–163
women, 167–168
therapeutic use, 597–609
Diuril. *See* Chlorothiazide
Diutensen-R (reserpine and methyclothiazide), therapeutic use of, 645
Dobutamine (Dobutrex), 200
adverse effects, 440
drug-drug interactions
proarrhythmic drugs, 481*t*
thiazide diuretics, 495*t*
hepatic dysfunction, 684*t*
pharmacokinetics, 517*t*
stress echocardiography with, 429*t*, 435–440
accuracy, 438–440
coronary artery disease, detection of, 438
coronary artery disease in patients with idiopathic dilated cardiomyopathy, detection of, 439
development, 436
early postymocardial infarction risk stratification, 438–439
hibernating myocardium, detection of, 439–440

Dobutamine (Dobutrex) (*Cont.*):
myocardial viability, assessment of, 439
preoperative assessment before noncardiac surgery, 438
procedure, 436–438
stunned myocardium, detection of, 439
therapeutic use, 610–611
Dobutrex. *See* Dobutamine
Dopamine, 159–160, 197
diuresis, 159–161
elderly patients, 612
hepatic dysfunction, 684*t*
pharmacokinetics, 517*t*
proarrhythmic drugs, interaction with, 481*t*
therapeutic use, 611–612
Dopamine receptors, 199, 411, 412*f*, 412*t*, 414–415
agonists. *See* Fenoldopam
Dose-response curves, 4, 5*f*, 7*f*
Doxazosin (Cardura), 25, 27–29, 31, 32
drug-drug interactions
nifedipine, 493*t*
nitrates, 493*t*
verapamil, 493*t*
elderly patients, 540
hepatic dysfunction, 679*t*
metoprolol, combination therapy with, 29
pharmacokinetics, 26*t*, 517*t*
pregnancy and lactation, 675*t*
renal failure, dose adjustment in, 662*t*
therapeutic use, 540
Doxorubicin in breast milk, 22
D-propranolol, 45, 48
pharmacodynamic properties and cardiac effects of, 35*t*, 43*t*
Drug interactions. *See also* "drug- drug interactions" and similar subentries under individual drug names
aging, effects of, 484
angiotensin converting enzyme inhibitors, 491, 492*t*–493*t*
antianginal vasodilators and calcium channel antagonists, 486–487, 488*t*–489*t*
antiarrhythmic drugs, 496–497, 498*t*–501*t*
adenosine, 496–497
antihypertensive drugs, 497
antithrombotic drugs, 497, 502
aspirin, 497, 503*t*
heparin, 502
warfarin, 497, 502, 503*t*
beta-adrenergic blocking drugs, 484, 485*t*, 486
digoxin and positive inotropic agents, 494, 495*t*, 496
diuretics
loop diuretics, 487, 490*t*, 491
potassium-retaining diuretics, 491
thiazide diuretics, 491
heart as site for
intraventricular conduction system, 480
myocardial contractile mechanism, 480
proarrhythmic drug interactions, 480, 481*t*
sinoatrial and atrioventricular nodes, 479–480
hepatic interactions, 483*t*
pharmacodynamic, 482, 484
pharmacokinetic, 482
hydralazine, 494

lipid-lowering agents, 502, 504*t*, 505
nitroprusside, 494
plasma protein binding as site for, 484
prazosin, 494
renal interactions, 484
vascular smooth muscle as site for, 480, 482
Drug metabolism. *See* Pharmacology, basic principles of
Drug receptors. *See* Receptors
Duraclon. *See* Clonidine hydrochloride
Duteplase, 325
Dyazide (triamterene and hydrochlorothiazide), therapeutic use of, 393, 401, 649–650
DynaCirc. *See* Isradipine
Dyrenium. *See* Triamterene
Dysgeusia, adverse effect of ACE inhibitors, 117

E

Ecainide
genetic factors in metabolism, 17
Echocardiography. *See also* Noninvasive cardiovascular diagnosis, use of pharmaceuticals in
adenosine, 434
dipyridamole, 431–432
dobutamine. *See* Dobutamine, stress echocardiography with
ergonine, 440–441
prosthetic valve endocarditis, 475
transesophageal echocardiography (TEE), 464, 475
transthoracic echocardiography (TTE), 475
ultrasonic contrast agents, 441–442
Edecrin, *See* Ethacrynic acid
Efficacy, 6
Elderly patients. *See also* "elderly patients" subentries under individual drug names in index; and "elderly" therapeutic use information under drug names in Appendix 2
age and drug metabolism, 17
calcium channel blockers and diuretics, combination therapy with, 398–399
diuretics, 164–166, 395
effects of aging on drug interactions, 484
orthostatic hypotension and vasovagal syncope, 444
pharmacokinetics, 652*t*–655*t*
absorption, 652*t*
distribution, 652*t*
excretion, 652*t*
metabolism, 652*t*
salt-sensitive hypertension, 162
systolic hypertension
calcium channel blockers, 93
thrombolytic agents, 335–337
Eminase. *See* Anistreplase
Enalaprilat
clinical applications, 136*t*
Enalapril (Vasotec)
clinical applications, 136*t*
elderly patients, 543
hepatic dysfunction, 679*t*
pharmacokinetics, 518*t*
pregnancy and lactation, 673*t*
renal failure, dose adjustment in, 661*t*

Enalapril (Vasotec) (*Cont.*):
  therapeutic use, 542–543
Encainide
  drug-drug interactions
    digoxin, 496
    quinidine, 245
  pharmacokinetics, 518*t*
  pregnancy and lactation, 670*t*
  renal failure, dose adjustment in, 659*t*
Endocarditis, infective. *See* Infective endocarditis
Endrophonium, 69–70
Enduron. *See* Methyclothiazide
Enduronyl (deserpidine and methyclothiazide), therapeutic use of, 646–647
Enoxaparin (Lovenox), 313*t*. *See also* Low-molecular-weight heparin
  hepatic dysfunction, 686*t*
  pharmacokinetics, 518*t*
  pregnancy and lactation, 676*t*
  renal failure, dose adjustment in, 663*t*
  therapeutic use, 564
Enoximone
  proarrhythmic drugs, interactions with, 481*t*
Enterococcal streptococcal endocarditis, 461–462
Enterohepatic circulation, 19
Enzymes, 1
Epinephrine
  beta-adrenergic blocking drugs, interaction with, 59*t*
  proarrhythmic drugs, interactions with, 481*t*
Epoprostenol
  adverse effects, 420*t*–421*t*
  clinical use, 420, 422
  overview, 419–420
  primary pulmonary hypertension, 422–426, 425*f*, 426*t*
Ergonine echocardiography, 440–441
Ergot alkaloids
  beta-adrenergic blocking drugs, interaction with, 59*t*
Ergotamine, 8
  orthostatic hypotension, 450
Erythrityl tetranitrate (Cardilate)
  elderly patients, 630
  hepatic dysfunction, 682*t*
  therapeutic use, 630
Erythromycin, interaction with
  digoxin, 496
  disopyramide, 249
  HMG-CoA reductase inhibitors, 504*t*
  terfenadine, 19
Erythropoietin
  orthostatic hypotension and vasovagal syncope, 450
Esidrex. *See* Hydrochlorothiazide
Esimil (guanethidine and hydrochlorothiazide), therapeutic use of, 647
Esmolol (Brevibloc), 34, 39, 48
  adverse effects, 269
  antiarrhythmic effects, 269
  AV reentrant tachycardia (Wolff-Parkinson-White syndrome), 239
  digoxin, combination therapy with, 269
  drug-drug interactions, 269
    morphine, 269
  elderly patients, 580
  electrophysiologic action, 268
  hemodynamic effects, 269
  hepatic dysfunction, 680*t*
  indications and dosage, 269–270

pharmacodynamic properties and cardiac effects of, 35*t*, 43*t*
pharmacokinetics, 268, 519*t*
pharmacologic description, 268
pregnancy and lactation, 670*t*
renal failure, dose adjustment in, 660*t*
therapeutic use, 579–580
ventricular fibrillation, 242
Estradiol, 9
Ethacrynic acid (Edecrin), 153*t*
children, 598–599
elderly patients, 598–599
hepatic dysfunction, 682*t*
pharmacokinetics, 519*t*
pregnancy and lactation, 677*t*
renal failure, dose adjustment in, 656*t*
therapeutic use, 598–599
Ethmozine. *See* Moricizine
Ethosuximide
in breast milk, 21
Excretion, drug, 20–22
biliary, 21
kidney, 20–21
lungs, 21
milk, 21–22
saliva, 22
Exna. *See* Benzthiazide
Exogenous endothelium-derived relaxing factor (ERDF), 208–209
Extraction ratio, 8–9

F

FAD (fibric acid derivatives). *See* Gemfibrozil and other fibric acid derivatives
Felodipine (Plendil)
adverse effects, 103*t*
chemical structure, 74
clinical applications
Raynaud's phenomenon, 101
systemic hypertension, 86, 92
elderly patients, 588
hepatic dysfunction, 681*t*
pharmacokinetics, 79, 81*t*, 85*t*, 519*t*
pharmacologic effects, 76*t*
pregnancy and lactation, 672*t*
renal failure, dose adjustment in, 660*t*
therapeutic use, 588
Fenofibrate, 362–363, 365
warfarin, interaction with, 504*t*
Fenoldopam (Corlopam), 411–417, 416*t*
chemical structure, 415*f*
dopamine receptors, 411, 412*f*, 412*t*, 414–415
elderly patients, 626
hepatic dysfunction, 682*t*
pharmacokinetics, 519*t*
pregnancy and lactation, 674*t*
renal failure, dose adjustment in, 662*t*
therapeutic use, 625–626
Fibrates
HMG-CoA reductase inhibitors, interaction with, 504*t*
Fibric acid derivatives. *See* Gemfibrozil and other fibric acid derivatives
Fibrinolytic agents
renal failure, dose adjustment in, 664*t*
Fibrinolytic system, 325*f*
First messenger, 23
Flecainide (Tambocor)
adverse effects, 260
antiarrhythmic effects, 260
atrial fibrillation, 237

Flecainide (Tambocor) (*Cont.*):
- atrial tachycardia, 240
- AV nodal reentrant tachycardia, 239
- AV reentrant tachycardia (Wolff-Parkinson-White syndrome), 240
- drug-drug interactions, 260–261
  - amiodarone, 500*t*
  - beta-adrenergic blocking drugs, 485*t*
  - cimetidine, 501*t*
  - digitalis, 287
  - digoxin, 260, 501*t*
  - diltiazem, 489*t*
  - propranolol, 260
  - verapamil, 280, 488*t*
- elderly patients, 549
- electrophysiologic action, 259
- genetic factors in metabolism, 17
- hemodynamics, 260
- hepatic dysfunction, 684*t*
- indications and dosage, 261
- pharmacokinetics, 259–260, 520*t*
- pharmacologic description, 259
- pregnancy and lactation, 670*t*
- renal failure, dose adjustment in, 659*t*
- therapeutic use, 549–550
- ventricular tachycardia, 241

Fludrocortisone
- orthostatic hypotension and vasovagal syncope, 448–449, 451

Fluoxetine
- vasovagal syncope, 451

Fluvastatin (Lescol)
- clinical use, 378
- coronary artery disease, 378
- elderly patients, 620
- overview, 378
- pharmacokinetics, 520*t*
- pregnancy and lactation, 674*t*
- renal failure, dose adjustment in, 664*t*
- therapeutic use, 620

Fluvoxamine
- beta-adrenergic blocking drugs, interaction with, 59*t*

Fosinopril (Monopril)
- clinical applications, 136*t*
- elderly patients, 543
- hepatic dysfunction, 679*t*
- pharmacokinetics, 520*t*
- pregnancy and lactation, 673*t*
- renal failure, dose adjustment in, 661*t*
- therapeutic use, 543–544

Fragmin. *See* Dalteparin

Fraxiparine (naroparin), 313*t*. *See also* Low-molecular-weight heparin

Furosemide (Lasix), 152–154, 153*t*, 156–159
- captopril, interaction with, 487, 490*t*
- children, 599–600
- elderly patients, 599–600
- hepatic dysfunction, 683*t*
- pharmacokinetics, 521*t*
- pregnancy and lactation, 677*t*
- renal failure, dose adjustment in, 656*t*
- therapeutic use, 599–600

G

Ganglionic blocking agents, 220, 223–224
- effectiveness, 225
- hepatic dysfunction, 681*t*–682*t*
- lipid lowering, 602–603

therapeutic use, 225, 226*t*, 622–623
Gated channels, 1
Gemfibrozil (Lopid) and other fibric acid derivatives (FADs), 364
adverse effects, 364–365
clinical experience and use, 363–364
combination drug therapy, 363–364
elderly patients, 617–618
hepatic dysfunction, 685*t*
mechanism of action, 360–363
overview, 360
pharmacokinetics, 360, 521*t*
pregnancy and lactation, 674*t*
renal failure, dose adjustment in, 664*t*
therapeutic use, 617–618
warfarin, interaction with, 360, 504*t*
Gender and cardiovascular pharmacotherapeutics
calcium channel blockers, 93
diuretics, 167–168
efficacy of selected medications, 666*t*–668*t*
pregnancy and lactation. *See* Pregnancy and lactation
salt-sensitive hypertension, 162
Genetic factors and drug metabolism, 17, 18*f*
Gentamicin
infective endocarditis, 456*t*–457*t*, 459*t*, 461–463
Glucagon
beta-adrenergic blocking drugs, interaction with, 59*t*
Glucose intolerance, adverse effect of diuretics, 171–172
Glucuronide formation, 16
Glutathione conjugate formation, 16
Glycerin, 153*t*, 156
Glycerol trinitrates
elderly patients, disorders caused in, 654*t*
Glycoprotein IIb/IIIa receptor antagonists, 303–308
as antiplatelet agents, 304–305
murine monoclonal antibodies, 305–307
synthetic peptide and nonpeptide antagonists, 307
Gout, adverse effect of diuretics, 173
GP (glycoprotein). *See* Glycoprotein IIb/IIIa receptor antagonists
G proteins, 1, 3*f*
Guanabenz (Wytensin), 226*t*
elderly patients, 596
hepatic dysfunction, 681*t*
pharmacokinetics, 521*t*
pregnancy and lactation, 675*t*
renal failure, dose adjustment in, 662*t*
therapeutic use, 596
Guanadrel (Hylorel), 224, 226*t*
elderly patients, 622
hepatic dysfunction, 681*t*
pharmacokinetics, 521*t*
therapeutic use, 622
Guanethidine (Ismelin), 224, 226*t*
children, 622
elderly patients, 622
gender considerations, 667*t*
hepatic dysfunction, 681*t*
pharmacokinetics, 522*t*
therapeutic use, 622
Guanfacine (Tenex), 226*t*
elderly patients, 596
hepatic dysfunction, 681*t*
pharmacokinetics, 522*t*
pregnancy and lactation, 675*t*
renal failure, dose adjustment in, 662*t*
therapeutic use, 596

Guillain-Barré syndrome, 446*t*

H

Half-life ($t_{1/2}$), drug, 13–14, 13*f*, 15*f*
Halofenate
  beta-adrenergic blocking drugs, interaction with, 59*t*
Haloperidol, 26
Halothane
  lidocaine, interaction with, 253, 500*t*
HDL (high-density lipoprotein) cholesterol, 346, 348, 349*f*, 350, 352, 355*t*
  acyl coenzyme A transferase inhibitors
  bile acid sequestrants, 358
  fibric acid derivatives, 360, 362, 364
  HDL_2, 362, 369
  HDL_3, 369
  lovastatin, 368–369
  low, treatment of, 350, 352, 355*t*
  nicotinic acid, 380, 382–386
  pravastatin, 375
  probucol, 387–390
  simvastatin, 371
Heart as site for drug interactions, 479–480, 481*t*
Heparin
  adjunctive antithrombotic therapy, 338–339
  adverse effects, 312–313
  children, 561–562
  clinical use
    acute myocardial infarction, 310–312
    orthopedic and general surgery, 310
    venous thrombosis, 310
  dosing, 312
  drug-drug interactions, 502
  elderly patients, 562, 564
  hepatic dysfunction, 686*t*
  low-molecular-weight heparins
    acute proximal deep vein thrombosis, 315
    background, 313–314, 313*t*
    clinical trials, 310, 314
    therapeutic use, 562–564
    unstable angina, 314–315
  mechanisms of action, 308, 309*f*
  pharmacodynamics, 309–310
  pharmacokinetics, 308–309, 522*t*
  pregnancy and lactation, 675*t*
  renal failure, dose adjustment in, 663*t*
  therapeutic use, 560–564
Hepatic disease, cardiovascular drug therapy in
  ACE inhibitors
    benazepril, 679*t*
    captopril, 679*t*
    enalapril, 679*t*
    fosinopril, 679*t*
    lisinopril, 679*t*
    moexipril, 679*t*
    quinapril, 679*t*
    ramipril, 679*t*
    trandolapril, 679*t*
  $alpha_1$-selective adrenergic blockers
    doxazosin, 679*t*
    prazosin, 679*t*
    terazosin, 679*t*
  antiarrythmics
    adenosine, 685*t*
    amiodarone, 685*t*
    atropine, 685*t*
    bretylium, 685*t*
    disopyramide, 684*t*
    flecainide, 684*t*
    lidocaine, 684*t*
    mexiletine, 684*t*
    moricizine, 684*t*
    procainamide, 684*t*

- propafenone, 685*t*
- quinidine, 684*t*
- tocainide, 684*t*
- anticoagulants
  - anisindione, 686*t*
  - ardeparin, 686*t*
  - danaparoid, 686*t*
  - dicoumarol, 686*t*
  - enoxaparin, 686*t*
  - heparin, 686*t*
  - warfarin, 686*t*
- antiotensin receptor antagonists
  - irbesartan, 679*t*
  - losartan, 679*t*
  - valsartan, 679*t*
- antithrombotics
  - anagrelide, 686*t*
  - aspirin, 686*t*
  - dipyridamole, 686*t*
  - ticlodipine, 686*t*
- beta-adrenergic blockers
  - acebutolol, 680*t*
  - atenolol, 680*t*
  - betaxolol, 680*t*
  - bisoprolol, 680*t*
  - carteolol, 680*t*
  - carvedilol, 681*t*
  - esmolol, 680*t*
  - labetalol, 680*t*
  - metoprolol, 680*t*
  - nadolol, 680*t*
  - penbutolol, 680*t*
  - pindolol, 680*t*
  - propranolol, 680*t*
  - sotalol, 680*t*
  - timolol, 680*t*
- calcium channel blockers
  - amlodipine, 681*t*
  - bepridil, 681*t*
  - diltiazem, 681*t*
  - felodipine, 681*t*
  - isradipine, 681*t*
  - mibefradil, 681*t*
  - nicardipine, 681*t*
  - nifedipine, 681*t*
  - nimodipine, 681*t*
  - verapamil, 681*t*
- centrally acting antihypertensives
  - clonidine, 681*t*
  - guanabenz, 681*t*
  - guanfacine, 681*t*
  - methyldopa, 681*t*
- inotropic agents
  - amrinone, 684*t*
  - deslanoside, 684*t*
  - digitoxin, 684*t*
  - digoxin, 684*t*
  - dobutamine, 684*t*
  - dopamine, 684*t*
  - milrinone, 684*t*
  - norepinephrine, 684*t*
- lipid-lowering agents
  - atorvastatin, 685*t*
  - cerivastatin, 685*t*
  - cholestyramine, 685*t*
  - clofibrate, 685*t*
  - colestipol, 685*t*
  - gemfibrozil, 685*t*
  - lovastatin, 685*t*
  - nicotinic acid, 685*t*
  - pravastatin, 685*t*
  - probucol, 685*t*
  - simvastatin, 685*t*
- loop diuretics
  - bumetanide, 682*t*
  - ethacrynic acid, 682*t*
  - furosemide, 683*t*
  - torsemide, 683*t*
- neuronal and ganglionic blockers
  - guanadrel, 681*t*
  - guanethidine, 681*t*
  - mecamylamine, 682*t*
  - reserpine, 681*t*
  - trimethaphan, 682*t*
- potassium-sparing diuretics
  - amiloride, 684*t*
  - spironolactone, 684*t*
  - triamterene, 684*t*
- thiazide diuretics

Hepatic disease, cardiovascular drug therapy in
thiazide diuretics (*Cont.*):
bendroflumethazide, 683*t*
benthiazide, 683*t*
chlorthalidone, 683*t*
chlorthiazide, 683*t*
cyclothiazide, 683*t*
hydrochlorothiazide, 683*t*
hydroflumethiazide, 683*t*
indapamide, 683*t*
methylclothiazide, 683*t*
metolazone, 683*t*
polythiazide, 683*t*
quinethazone, 683*t*
trichlormethiazide, 683*t*
thrombolytics
alteplase, 686
anistreplase, 686*t*
reteplase, 686*t*
streptokinase, 686*t*
urokinase, 686*t*
vasodilators
cyclandelate, 682*t*
diazoxide, 682*t*
erythritol tetranitrate, 682*t*
fenoldopam, 682*t*
hydralazine, 682*t*
isosorbide dinitrate, 682*t*
isosorbide mononitrate, 682*t*
isoxsuprine, 682*t*
nitroglycerin, 682*t*
nylidrin, 682*t*
pentaerythriyol tetranitate, 682*t*
sodium nitroprusside, 682*t*
tolazoline, 682*t*
vasporessor
midodrine, 679*t*
Hepatic drug interactions, 482, 483*t*, 484
Hexamethonium, 224
Hibernating myocardium, detecting with dobutamine, 439–440
High-altitude pulmonary edema
calcium channel blockers, 101
High-density lipoprotein cholesterol. *See* HDL cholesterol
HMG-CoA reductase inhibitors
drug-drug interactions
cyclosporine, 504*t*
erythromycin, 504*t*
fibrates, 504*t*
nicotinic acid, 504*t*
gender considerations, 667*t*
lovastatin. *See* Lovastatin
overview, 366
therapeutic use, 619–621
Hormonal receptors, 23–25
Hydralazine (Apresoline), 228–230, 231*f*. *See also* Nonspecific antihypertensive vasodilators
in breast milk, 21
children, 626–627
combination therapy with, 401
drug-drug interactions, 494
beta-adrenergic blocking drugs, 60*t*
captopril, 492*t*
digoxin, 493*t*
nonsteroidal antiinflammatory drugs (NSAIDs), 493*t*
elderly patients, 626
gender considerations, 667*t*
genetic factors in metabolism, 17
hepatic dysfunction, 682*t*
pharmacokinetics, 522*t*
pregnancy and lactation, 675*t*
renal failure, dose adjustment in, 662*t*
therapeutic use, 626–627
Hydrochlorothiazide (Esidrex, Hydrodiuril, Oretic), 153*t*, 155
children, 604
combination therapy with
bisoprolol, 398

diltiazem, 399, 400*f*
losartan, 396, 397*t*, 398
elderly patients, 604
hepatic dysfunction, 683*t*
pharmacokinetics, 523*t*
pregnancy and lactation, 677*t*
renal failure, dose adjustment in, 657*t*
therapeutic use, 603–604
Hydrodiuril. *See* Hydrochlorothiazide
Hydroflumethiazide (Diucardin, Saluron), 153*t*
children, 604
elderly patients, 604
hepatic dysfunction, 683*t*
pharmacokinetics, 523*t*
therapeutic use, 604
Hydromox. *See* Quinethazone
Hygroton. *See* Chlorthalidone
Hylorel. *See* Guanadrel
Hyperaldosteronism, primary
ACE inhibitors, 122–123, 123*t*
Hypercholesterolemia treatment, 348, 349*f*, 350, 351*f*–352*f*, 351*t*, 354*f*
Hyperglycemia
beta-adrenergic blocking drugs, 56
Hyperkalemia, adverse effect of ACE inhibitors, 115
Hyperlipidemia
beta-blocker choice in patients with, 63*t*
screening, 348
Hyperstat. *See* Diazoxide
Hypertension. *See also* Antihypertensives; Systemic hypertension
ACE inhibitors, 109–112, 110*t*
alpha-adrenergic blocking drugs, 27–28
combination therapy. *See* Hypertension, combination therapy for
emergencies
ACE inhibitors, 122
calcium channel blockers, 94
magnesium, 179
primary (essential)
ACE inhibitors, 120–121
renovascular
ACE inhibitors, 121–122
salt-sensitive
diuretics, 162–163
Hypertension, combination therapy for
additive vasculoprotective actions, 408
adverse effects, reduction in, 403–406
low-dose strategy, 404–405, 404*t*
pharmacologic interactions, 405–406, 405*t*
combinations with a diuretic, 395–401
ACE inhibitors, 395–396
angiotensin receptor antagonists, 396, 397*t*, 398
beta blockers, 398
calcium channel blockers, 398–399, 400*f*
sympatholytics, 399
two diuretics, 401
combinations without a diuretic, 401–403
convenience and inconvenience, 406–407
definition, 393
dual-acting molecules, 409
duration of action, effects on, 407–408
efficacy, 395
evolution of care, 391–392
overview, 391
rationale, 393–394, 394*t*
Hypertensive emergencies
ACE inhibitors, 122
calcium channel blockers, 94
Hypertriglyceridemia treatment, 350

Hypertrophic cardiomyopathy
beta-adrenergic blocking drugs, 50–51
calcium channel blockers, 95–97
propranolol, 95–96
Hypoglycemia
beta-adrenergic blocking drugs, 56–57
Hypokalemia, 182
adverse effect of diuretics, 169–170
Hypomagnesemia, adverse effect of diuretics, 170–171
Hyponatremia, adverse effect of diuretics, 171
Hypotension
adverse effect of ACE inhibitors, 114–115
orthostatic. *See* Orthostatic hypotension and vasovagal syncope, drug treatment of
Hytrin. *See* Terazosin
Hyzaar (losartan potassium and hydrochlorothiazide), therapeutic use of, 639

I

Ibuprofen
beta-adrenergic blocking drugs, interaction with, 60*t*
Ibutilide (Corvert)
adverse effects, 278
antiarrhythmic effects, 277–278
atrial fibrillation, 237
drug-drug interactions, 278
elderly patients, 550
electrophysiologic action, 277
hemodynamic effects, 277
indications and dosage, 278
pharmacokinetics, 277, 523*t*
pharmacologic description, 277
pregnancy and lactation, 671*t*
therapeutic use, 550
IE. *See* Infective endocarditis
Imdur. *See* Isosorbide mononitrate
Immunosuppressive drugs
captopril, interaction with, 492*t*
Implantable cardioverter defibrillators, 242
Indapamide (Lozol), 153*t*
elderly patients, 605
hepatic dysfunction, 683*t*
pharmacokinetics, 523*t*
therapeutic use, 604–605
Inderal. *See* Propranolol
Inderide (propranolol and hydrochlorothiazide), therapeutic use of, 642
Indomethacin
drug-drug interactions
beta-adrenergic blocking drugs, 60*t*, 485*t*
loop and thiazide diuretics, 490*t*
orthostatic hypotension, 450
Indoramin, 25
Induction, 18–19, 20*f*
Infective endocarditis (IE)
overview, 453
therapy
anticoagulation and, 464–466
endocarditis caused by *Staphylococcus aureus*, 463–464
enterococcal endocarditis, 461–462
nonenterococcal streptococcal endocarditis, 455, 461
overview, 453–455, 456*t*–460*t*
prophylaxis, 466, 467*f*, 468*t*–471*t*, 472

    prosthetic valve endocarditis, 472–473, 475–476, 477*t*
    rheumatic fever, 472, 473*t*–475*t*
    surgery, indication for, 464

Inferior wall myocardial infarction
  thrombolytic agents, 334

Inhibition of drug metabolism, 4, 19

Injected drugs, 9

Inocor. *See* Amrinone

Inotropic agents. *See* Digitalis preparations and other inotropic agents

Insulin
  beta-blocker choice in patients using, 63*t*

Interactions, drug. *See* Drug interactions

Intermittent claudication
  beta-blocker choice in patients with, 62*t*

Intestinal microorganisms, drug metabolism and, 19

Intramuscular drug administration, 9

Intravenous drug administration, 9

Intrinsic sympathomimetic activity, beta-adrenergic blocking drugs, 35*t*, 37

Inversine. *See* Mecamylamine

Irbesartan (Avapro)
  elderly patients, 547
  hepatic dysfunction, 679*t*
  pharmacokinetics, 524*t*
  pregnancy and lactation, 673*t*
  therapeutic use, 547

Ischemic heart disease
  magnesium, 176–177

Ischemic stroke
  thrombolytic agents, 344

Ismelin. *See* Guanethidine

Ismo. *See* Isosorbide mononitrate

Isoniazid
  genetic factors in metabolism, 17, 18*f*

Isoproterenol
  beta-adrenergic blocking drugs, interaction with, 60*t*

Isoptin. *See* Verapamil

Isordil. *See* Isosorbide dinitrate

Isosorbide dinitrate (Dilatrate, Isordil, Sorbitrate), 211–212, 212*t*. *See also* Nitrates
  hepatic dysfunction, 682*t*
  pharmacokinetics, 524*t*
  therapeutic use, 630–631

Isosorbide mononitrate (Imdur, Ismo, Monoket), 212, 212*t*. *See also* Nitrates
  elderly patients, 631
  hepatic dysfunction, 682*t*
  pharmacokinetics, 513*t*
  therapeutic use, 631

Isoxsuprine (Vasodilan)
  children, 627
  elderly patients, 627
  hepatic dysfunction, 682*t*
  pharmacokinetics, 524*t*
  therapeutic use, 627

Isradipine (DynaCirc)
  adverse effects, 103*t*
  chemical structure, 74
  clinical applications
    Raynaud's phenomenon, 101
    systemic hypertension, 86, 92
  elderly patients, 589
  hepatic dysfunction, 681*t*
  pharmacokinetics, 81*t*, 84*t*, 524*t*
  pharmacologic effects, 76*t*
  pregnancy and lactation, 672*t*
  renal failure, dose adjustment in, 661*t*
  therapeutic use, 588–589

J

Joint National Committee on Detection, Evaluation and Treatment of High Blood Pressure, 40

K

Kabinkinase. *See* Streptokinase
Kallikrein-kinin system, 112
Kaolin pectate
  digoxin, interaction with, 496
Kerlone. *See* Betaxolol
Ketanserin, 26
Ketoconazole
  terfenadine, interaction with, 19
Kidney, drug excretion by, 20–21

L

Labetalol (Normodyne, Trandate), 26, 34, 36–38, 409
  drug-drug interactions
    barbiturates, 483*t*
    cimetidine, 483*t*, 485*t*
    phenytoin, 483*t*
    rifampin, 483*t*
  elderly patients, 585, 652*t*
    disorders caused in, 654*t*
  hepatic dysfunction, 680*t*
  pharmacodynamic properties and cardiac effects of, 35*t*, 43*t*
  pharmacokinetics, 525*t*
  pregnancy and lactation, 671*t*
  renal failure, dose adjustment in, 660*t*
  therapeutic use, 584–585
Lactation. *See* Pregnancy and lactation
Lanoxicaps. *See* Digoxin
Lanoxin. *See* Digoxin
Laplace's law, 44
Lasix. *See* Furosemide
L-channel, 74–75
LDL (low-density lipoprotein) cholesterol, 346–348, 350, 351*f*–352*f*, 353*t*, 354*f*
  atorvastatin, 379
  bile acid sequestrants, 353, 356–358
  fibric acid derivatives, 360–364
  fluvastatin, 378
  lovastatin, 367–369
  nicotinic acid, 380, 382–386
  pravastatin, 374–375, 377
  probucol, 387–390
  simvastatin, 371
Left bundle branch block myocardial infarction
  thrombolytic agents, 335
Left ventricular hypertrophy
  ACE inhibitors, 126
  regression of
    beta-adrenergic blocking drugs, 53
Lescol. *See* Fluvastatin
Levatol. *See* Penbutolol
Levodopa
  beta-adrenergic blocking drugs, interaction with, 60*t*
Levophed. *See* Norepinephrine
Lexxel (felodipine extended release and enalapril maleate), 393, 402, 639
Lidocaine (Xylocaine)
  adverse effects, 251–252
  antiarrhythmic effects, 251
  children, 550–551
  drug-drug interactions, 252
    beta-adrenergic blocking drugs, 60*t*, 500*t*
    cimetidine, 252, 483*t*, 500*t*
    digoxin, 496
    halothane, 252, 500*t*
    metoprolol, 252
    propranolol, 252, 266, 485*t*, 500*t*
    verapamil, 500*t*

elderly patients, 550, 652*t*
electrophysiologic action, 250
hemodynamic effects, 251
hepatic dysfunction, 684*t*
indications and dosage, 252
pharmacokinetics, 251, 525*t*
pharmacologic description, 250
pregnancy and lactation, 669*t*
renal failure, dose adjustment in, 658*t*
therapeutic use, 550–552
ventricular fibrillation, 242
ventricular tachycardia, 241

Lipid-lowering drugs
atorvastatin. *See* Atorvastatin
bile acid sequestrants. *See* Bile acid sequestrants
cerivastatin. *See* Cerivastatin
drug-drug interactions, 504*t*, 505
fluvastatin. *See* Fluvastatin
gemfibrozil. *See* Gemfibrozil and other fibric acid derivatives
gender considerations, 667*t*
hepatic dysfunction, 685*t*
HMG-CoA reductase inhibitors. *See* HMG-CoA reductase inhibitors
hypercholesterolemia treatment, 348, 349*f*, 350, 351*f*–352*f*, 351*t*, 354*f*
hyperlipidemia screening, 348
hypertriglyceridemia treatment, 350
low serum HDL cholesterol, 350, 352, 355*t*
nicotinic acid. *See* Nicotinic acid
overview, 346, 347*f*, 349*f*
pravastatin. *See* Pravastatin
pregnancy and lactation, 673*t*–674*t*
probucol. *See* Probucol
rationale for, 346–348
renal failure, dose adjustment in, 664*t*–665*t*
risk assessment, 348, 349*f*, 350
simvastatin. *See* Simvastatin
therapeutic use, 616–621

Lipid metabolism
diuretics and, 172

Lipoprotein lipase (LPL), 360–361, 363

Lisinopril (Prinivil, Zestril)
clinical applications, 136*t*
elderly patients, 544
hepatic dysfunction, 679*t*
pharmacokinetics, 525*t*
pregnancy and lactation, 673*t*
renal failure, dose adjustment in, 661*t*
therapeutic use, 544

Lithium
ACE inhibitors, interaction with, 120
in breast milk, 22

Logimax, 402

Logiparin (Tinzaparin), 313*t*. *See also* Low-molecular-weight heparin

Loniten. *See* Minoxidil

Loop diuretics, 152–154, 153*t*. *See also* Diuretics
children, 598
continuous IV infusion, 158
drug-drug interactions, 487, 490*t*, 491
captopril, 492*t*
proarrhythmic drugs, 481*t*
elderly patients, 598
hepatic dysfunction, 681*t*–682*t*
high-dose, 157–158
renal failure, dose adjustment in, 656*t*
therapeutic use, 597–598

Lopid. *See* Gemfibrozil and other fibric acid derivatives

Lopressor. *See* Metoprolol

Lopressor HCT (metoprolol and hyrdochlorothiazide), therapeutic use of, 641

Losartan (Cozaar), 139–141
beta-adrenergic blocking drugs, interaction with, 58*t*
clinical applications, 142–144
cardiac hypertrophy, 144
cerebrovascular and other neurologic diseases, 149
congestive heart failure, 145–147
hypertension, 141–142
myocardial infarction, 144–145
oncogenesis, 149–150
postangioplasty vascular restenosis, 147–148
renal disease, 148
unresolved issues, 150
elderly patients, 548
hepatic dysfunction, 679*t*
hydrochlorothiazide, combination therapy with, 396, 397*t*, 398
pharmacokinetics, 141, 526*t*
pregnancy and lactation, 673*t*
renal failure, dose adjustment in, 662*t*
therapeutic use, 547–548
Lotensin. *See* Benazepril
Lotensin HCT (benazepril and hydrochlorothiazide), therapeutic use of, 636
Lotrel (amlodipine and benazepril HCl), 393, 402, 406
therapeutic use, 638
Lovastatin (Mevacor, Mevinolin)
adverse effcts, 370–371
chemistry, 366
clinical experience, 367–369
combination therapy, 367
coronary and carotid artery disease progression, 368–369
triglycerides, HDL, and other lipoproteins, 369
clinical use, 369–370
drug-drug interactions
cyclosporine, 504*t*
erythromycin, 504*t*
fibrates, 504*t*
nicotinic acid, 504*t*
elderly patients, 620
gender considerations, 667*t*
hepatic dysfunction, 685*t*
pharmacokinetics, 366–367, 526*t*
pharmacology, 366
pregnancy and lactation, 674*t*
renal failure, dose adjustment in, 664*t*
therapeutic use, 620–621
Lovenox. *See* Enoxaparin
Low-density lipoprotein cholesterol. *See* LDL cholesterol
Low-molecular-weight heparin
acute proximal deep vein thrombosis, 315
background, 313–314, 313*t*
clinical trials, 310, 314
therapeutic use, 562–564
unstable angina, 314–315
Lozol. *See* Indapamide
Lp(a) elevation
nicotinic acid, 383
LPL (lipoprotein lipase), 360–361, 363
L-propranolol, 45
Lungs, drug excretion by, 21

M

Magnesium as potential cardiovascular disease therapy. *See also* Antiarrhythmic drugs
adverse effects, 290
antiarrhythmic effects, 290
cardiovascular effects, 175–179
arrhythmias, 178–179
congestive heart failure, 177–178

diabetes, 177–178
hypertension, 179
ischemic heart disease, 176–177
myocardial infarction, 176–177
clinical use, 179–180, 180*t*
electrophysiologic action, 289
hemodynamic effects, 289–290
indications and dosage, 290
overview, 175
pharmacokinetics, 289
pharmacologic description, 288–289
Malignant hypertension
ACE inhibitors, 122
Mannitol, 153*t*, 156
Marfan syndrome, 53
Mavik. *See* Trandolapril
Maxzide (triamterene and hydrochlorothiazide), 393, 401
therapeutic use of, 649–650
Mecamylamine (Inversine), 224, 226*t*
elderly patients, 623
hepatic dysfunction, 682*t*
pharmacokinetics, 526*t*
therapeutic use, 623
Medroxyprogesterone in breast milk, 21
Medullary thick ascending limb of Henle (mTAL), 152
Membranes, cell, passage of drugs across, 7–8
Membrane-stabilizing activity, beta-adrenergic blocking drugs, 35*t*, 36
Metahydrin. *See* Trichlormethiazide
Methacholine, 69
Methicillin
infective endocarditis, 455, 457*t*–458*t*
Methoxamine, provocative testing with in cardiac ausculation, 427
Methyclothiazide (Enduron), 153*t*
children, 605
elderly patients, 605
hepatic dysfunction, 683*t*
therapeutic use, 605
Methyldopa (Aldomet)
children, 597
drug-drug interactions
beta-adrenergic blocking drugs, 60*t*
disopyramide, 500*t*
elderly patients, 597
disorders caused in, 654*t*
gender considerations, 667*t*
hepatic dysfunction, 681*t*
pharmacokinetics, 526*t*
pregnancy and lactation, 674*t*
renal failure, dose adjustment in, 662*t*
therapeutic use, 597
Metolazone (Mykrox, Zaroxolyn), 153*t*, 155, 159
children, 606
elderly patients, 605
hepatic dysfunction, 683*t*
pharmacokinetics, 527*t*
pregnancy and lactation, 677*t*
renal failure, dose adjustment in, 657*t*
therapeutic use, 605–606
Metoprolol (Lopressor, Toprol), 29, 38–39, 41, 48, 50
atrial tachycardia, 240
doxazosin, combination therapy with, 29
drug-drug interactions
barbiturates, 483*t*
cimetidine, 483*t*, 485*t*
lidocaine, 252
phenytoin, 483*t*

Metoprolol (Lopressor, Toprol)
drug-drug interactions (*Cont.*):
rifampin, 483*t*
verapamil, 280, 483*t*, 485*t*
elderly patients, 581
hepatic dysfunction, 680*t*
pharmacodynamic properties and cardiac effects of, 35*t*, 43*t*
pharmacokinetics, 527*t*
pregnancy and lactation, 670*t*
renal failure, dose adjustment in, 659*t*
therapeutic use, 580–581
vasovagal syncope, 451
ventricular fibrillation, 242
Metronidazole in breast milk, 21
Mevacor. *See* Lovastatin
Mevinolin. *See* Lovastatin
Mexiletine (Mexitil)
adverse effects, 256
antiarrhythmic effects, 255
drug-drug interactions, 256
barbiturates, 500*t*
cimetidine, 256
digoxin, 496
phenobarbital, 256
phenytoin, 256, 500*t*
rifampin, 500*t*
elderly patients, 552, 652*t*
electrophysiologic action, 254–255
genetic factors in metabolism, 17
hemodynamic effects, 255
hepatic dysfunction, 684*t*
indications and dosage, 256
pharmacokinetics, 255, 527*t*
pharmacologic description, 254
pregnancy and lactation, 669*t*
renal failure, dose adjustment in, 658*t*
therapeutic use, 552
ventricular tachycardia, 241
Mexitil. *See* Mexiletine
MI. *See* Myocardial infarction
Mibefradil
adverse effects, 103*t*
chemical structure, 74
clinical applications
angina pectoris, 86, 86*t*, 87
systemic hypertension, 86
elderly patients, 589
hepatic dysfunction, 681*t*
pharmacodynamics, 74
pharmacokinetics, 85*t*, 528*t*
pharmacologic effects, 76*t*, 77, 78, 81*t*
pregnancy and lactation, 672*t*
renal failure, dose adjustment in, 661*t*
therapeutic use, 589
Midamor. *See* Amiloride
Midodrine (ProAmantine)
hepatic dysfunction, 679*t*
orthostatic hypotension, 449
pharmacokinetics, 528*t*
pregnancy and lactation, 675*t*
renal failure, dose adjustment in, 663*t*
therapeutic use, 613
Migraine
calcium channel blockers, 100
Milk, drug excretion by, 21–22
Milrinone (Primacor), 201–202
drug-drug interactions
proarrhythmic drugs, 481*t*
thiazide diuretics, 495*t*
elderly patients, 610
hepatic dysfunction, 684*t*
pharmacokinetics, 528*t*
pregnancy and lactation, 669*t*
renal failure, dose adjustment in, 656*t*
therapeutic use, 610
Minipress. *See* Prazosin
Minitran. *See* Nitroglycerin
Minizide (prazosin and polythiazide), therapeutic use of, 647–648

Minoxidil (Loniten, Rogaine), 230–232. *See also* Nonspecific antihypertensive vasodilators
children, 627
elderly patients, 627
pharmacokinetics, 528*t*
pregnancy and lactation, 675*t*
renal failure, dose adjustment in, 662*t*
therapeutic use, 627–628
Miradon. *See* Anisindione
Mitral regurgitation
ACE inhibitors, 126
Mitral valve prolapse
beta-adrenergic blocking drugs, 52
Moduretic (amiloride hydrochloride and hydrochlorothiazide), therapeutic use of, 648–649
Moexipril (Univasc)
clinical applications, 136*t*
elderly patients, 544
hepatic dysfunction, 679*t*
pharmacokinetics, 529*t*
pregnancy and lactation, 673*t*
renal failure, dose adjustment in, 661*t*
therapeutic use, 544–545
Monoamine oxidase inhibitors
beta-adrenergic blocking drugs, interaction with, 60*t*
inhibitory effects on drug metabolism, 19
Monoket. *See* Isosorbide mononitrate
Monopril. *See* Fosinopril
Moricizine (Ethmozine)
adverse effects, 258
antiarrhythmic effects, 258
AV reentrant tachycardia (Wolff-Parkinson-White syndrome), 240
digoxin, interaction with, 258
elderly patients, 553
electrophysiologic action, 257
hemodynamic effects, 258
hepatic dysfunction, 684*t*
indications and dosage, 258–259
pharmacokinetics, 257, 529*t*
pharmacologic description, 257
renal failure, dose adjustment in, 657*t*
therapeutic use, 552–553
ventricular tachycardia, 241
Morphine
in breast milk, 22
esmolol, interaction with, 269
mTAL (medullary thick ascending limb of Henle), 152
Muscarinic activity, 66
parasympathetic drugs that diminish, 70–71*t*
parasympathetic drugs that enhance, 68*t*, 69–70
receptors, 66, 67*t*–68*t*
Mykrox. *See* Metolazone
Myocardial infarction (MI)
ACE inhibitors, 125–126
acute
aspirin, 296–297
thrombolytic agents, 326, 328–337. *See also* Thrombolytic agents
angiotensin II receptor blockers, 144–145
aspirin, 294–297
calcium channel blockers, 94–95
losartan, 144–145
magnesium, 176–177
primary prevention
aspirin, 294–296
secondary prevention
aspirin, 296

Myocardial infarction (MI) (*Cont.*):
  survivors
    beta-adrenergic blocking drugs, 48–50, 49*t*
    early postmyocardial infarction risk stratification, 438–439
  warfarin, 321
Myocardial viabililty, assessing with dobutamine, 439

N

Nadolol (Corgard), 39, 48
  elderly patients, 574, 652*t*
  hepatic dysfunction, 680*t*
  pharmacodynamic properties and cardiac effects of, 35*t*, 43*t*
  pharmacokinetics, 529*t*
  pregnancy and lactation, 670*t*
  renal failure, dose adjustment in, 659*t*
  therapeutic use, 574
Naproxen
  beta-adrenergic blocking drugs, interaction with, 61*t*
Naqua. *See* Trichlormethiazide
Narcotics in breast milk, 21
Naroparin (Fraxiparine), 313*t*. *See also* Low-molecular-weight heparin
National Cholesterol Education Program (NCEP), 346–347
Naturetin. *See* Bendroflumethiazide
N dealkylation, 16
Neonates, drug metabolism in, 17
Neostigmine, 70
Neurologic disease
  angiotensin II receptor blockers, 149
  losartan, 149
Neuronal and ganglionic blockers, 220, 223–224
  effectiveness, 225
  hepatic dysfunction, 681*t*–682*t*
  lipid lowering, 602–603
  therapeutic use, 225, 226*t*, 622–623
Neuron depletors. *See* Peripheral neuron depletors
N hydroxylation, 16
Niacin. *See* Nicotinic acid
Niacor. *See* Nicotinic acid
Nicardipine (Cardene)
  adverse effects, 103*t*
  chemical structure, 74
  clinical applications
    angina pectoris, 86–87
    cerebral arterial spasm and stroke, 99
    hypertensive emergencies, 86
    perioperative hypertension, 86
    systemic hypertension, 86
  drug-drug interactions
    cyclosporine, 489*t*
    digoxin, 489*t*
  elderly patients, 590
  hepatic dysfunction, 681*t*
  pharmacokinetics, 79, 81*t*, 83*t*–84*t*, 529*t*
  pharmacologic effects, 76*t*
  pregnancy and lactation, 672*t*
  renal failure, dose adjustment in, 661*t*
  therapeutic use, 590–591
Nicobid. *See* Nicotinic acid
Nicolar. *See* Nicotinic acid
Nicotine in breast milk, 21
Nicotinex. *See* Nicotinic acid
Nicotinic acetylcholine receptor, 1, 3*f*
Nicotinic acid (NA, niacin)
  adverse effects, 386–387
  clinical experience, 381–383
    coronary heart disease, 381–383
    Lp(a) elevation, 383
  clinical use

combination therapy, 385–386
single-drug therapy, 384–385
elderly patients, 618
gender considerations, 667*t*
hepatic dysfunction, 685*t*
HMG-CoA reductase inhibitors, interaction with, 504*t*
overview, 380
pharmacokinetics, 380, 530*t*
pharmacologic action, 380–381
pregnancy and lactation, 674*t*
renal failure, dose adjustment in, 664*t*
therapeutic use, 618–619
Nicotinic receptors, 1, 3*f*, 223
Nifedipine (Adalat, Procardia)
adverse effects, 103*t*
chemical structure, 74
clinical applications
amaurosis fugax, 101
angina pectoris, 86, 86*t*, 87–88
congestive heart failure, 97
high-altitude pulmonary edema, 101
migraine, 100
Raynaud's phenomenon, 101
"silent" myocardial ischemia, 94
systemic hypertension, 92–93
drug-drug interactions
beta-adrenergic blocking drugs, 485*t*, 489*t*
cimetidine, 483*t*, 489*t*
digoxin, 489*t*, 495*t*
diltiazem, 483*t*
doxazosin, 493*t*
prazosin, 489*t*, 493*t*
propranolol, 489*t*
quinidine, 489*t*, 499*t*
terazosin, 493*t*
elderly patients, 591
epoprostenol, comparison to, 423
hepatic dysfunction, 681*t*
pharmacokinetics, 79, 80*t*, 83*t*, 530*t*
pharmacologic effects, 4, 76*t*, 77
pregnancy and lactation, 672*t*
renal failure, dose adjustment in, 660*t*
therapeutic use, 591–592
Nimodipine (Nimotop)
adverse effects, 103*t*
chemical structure
clinical applications
cerebral arterial spasm and stroke, 99–100
subarachnoid hemorrhage, 86
elderly patients, 592
hepatic dysfunction, 681*t*
pharmacokinetics, 81*t*, 84*t*, 530*t*
pharmacologic effects, 76*t*, 77
pregnancy and lactation, 672*t*
renal failure, dose adjustment in, 661*t*
therapeutic use, 592
Nimotop. *See* Nimodipine
Nisoldipine
adverse effects, 103*t*
chemical structure, 74
pharmacokinetics, 79, 81*t*, 84*t*, 530*t*
pharmacologic effects, 76*t*
pregnancy and lactation, 672*t*
renal failure, dose adjustment in, 661*t*
systemic hypertension, 86, 92
Nitrates
adverse effects, 213
clinical indications, 208*t*, 209–210
combined with beta-adrenergic blocking drugs to treat angina pectoris, 46

Nitrates (*Cont.*):
- dosing suggestions, 212–213
- drug-drug interactions
  - beta-adrenergic blocking drugs, 60*t*
  - calcium antagonists, 488*t*
  - doxazosin, 493*t*
  - prazosin, 488*t*, 493*t*
  - terazosin, 493*t*
- elderly patients, 652*t*
- formulations and pharmacokinetics, 205*t*, 210–213, 211*t*–212*t*
- gender considerations, 667*t*
- hemodynamic correlates of clinical nitrate efficacy, 207–208, 208*t*
- isosorbide dinitrate. *See* Isosorbide dinitrate
- isosorbide mononitrate. *See* Isosorbide mononitrate
- mechanisms of action
  - cellular, 204–205, 204*f*
  - nitrate tolerance, 203, 205, 211*t*, 213–214, 214*t*
- nitrate effects on regional circulation, 206–207, 206*f*
- nitroglycerin. *See* Nitroglycerin
- overview, 203, 204*f*, 205*t*, 218
- pregnancy and lactation, 676*t*
- renal failure, dose adjustment in, 663*t*
- therapeutic use, 630–636

Nitrendipine, 93
- digoxin, interaction with, 487, 495*t*
- pregnancy and lactation, 672*t*
- renal failure, dose adjustment in, 661*t*

Nitric oxide
- epoprostenol, comparison to, 423
- vasovagal syncope, 451

Nitrites, therapeutic use of, 630–636

Nitro-bid. *See* Nitroglycerin

Nitrodisc. *See* Nitroglycerin

Nitrofurantoin in breast milk, 22

Nitrogard. *See* Nitroglycerin

Nitroglycerin (NTG), 8, 203, 208–211. *See also* Nitrates
- children, 612
- elderly patients, 612
- hepatic dysfunction, 682*t*
- pharmacokinetics, 205*t*, 210–211, 530*t*
- special formulations, 612–614
- therapeutic use, 631–634

Nitroglyn. *See* Nitroglycerin

Nitrolingual. *See* Nitroglycerin

Nitroprusside (Nitropress), 203, 214–218. *See also* Nonspecific antihypertensive vasodilators
- children, 616, 636
- dosage, 217–218
- drug-drug interactions, 494
- elderly patients, 635
- indications, 215–217, 216*f*, 217*t*
- pregnancy and lactation, 675*t*
- renal failure, dose adjustment in, 662*t*
- therapeutic use, 635–636

Nitro reduction, 16

Nitrostat. *See* Nitroglycerin

Nitrovasodilators. *See* Nitrates; Nitroprusside

Nonenterococcal streptococcal endocarditis, 455, 461

Noninvasive cardiovascular diagnosis, use of pharmaceuticals in
- arbutamine stress testing, 440
- dobutamine stress echocardiography. *See* Dobutamine, stress echocardiography with
- ergonine echocardiography, 440–441

overview, 427, 429*t*
provocative testing in cardiac ausculation
amyl nitrate, 427
methoxamine, 427
phenylephrine, 427
radionuclide testing and stress electrocardiography for detecting myocardial ischemia, 428–435
adenosine. *See* Adenosine
dipyridamole. *See* Dipyridamole
ultrasonic contrast agents during pharmacologic stress echocardiography, 441–442
Non-Q-wave myocardial infarction
thrombolytic agents, 334
Nonspecific antihypertensive vasodilators
effectiveness and current use, 232–233
overview, 228, 232–233
pharmacology and classification
ATP-K$^+$ channel openers, 230–232
hydralazine. *See* Hydralazine
nitroprusside. *See* Nitroprusside
Nonsteroidal antiinflammatory drugs (NSAIDs)
drug-drug interactions
ACE inhibitors, 119, 492*t*
beta-adrenergic blocking drugs, 485*t*
hydralazine, 493*t*
loop and thiazide diuretics, 490*t*
elderly patients, 655*t*
Norepinephrine (Levophed), 30–31, 44
children, 612–613
hepatic dysfunction, 684*t*
proarrhythmic drugs, interaction with, 481*t*
therapeutic use, 612–613
Normiflo. *See* Ardeparin
Normodyne. *See* Labetalol
Norpace. *See* Disopyramide
Norvasc. *See* Amlodipine
NSAIDs. *See* Nonsteroidal antiinflammatory drugs
NTG. *See* Nitroglycerin
Nutrition and drug metabolism, 18
Nylidin
hepatic dysfunction, 682*t*

O

Obesity, pharmacologic approach to, 559
Obstructive mechanical prosthetic valve
thrombolytic agents, 343
Octreotide
orthostatic hypotension, 450
Oculomucocutaneous syndrome
beta-adrenergic blocking drug choice in patients with, 63*t*
beta-adrenergic blocking drugs, adverse effect of, 57
O dealkylation, 16
Omeprazole
beta-adrenergic blocking drugs, interaction with, 60*t*
O methylation, 16
Oncogenesis
angiotensin II receptor blockers, 149–150
losartan, 149–150
Oral drug administration, 8–9
Oretic. *See* Hydrochlorothiazide
Organic nitrates and nitroprusside. *See* Nitrates; Nitroprusside

Orgaran. *See* Danaparoid
Orthopedic surgry
  heparin, 310
Orthostatic hypotension and vasovagal syncope, drug treatment of
  beta-adrenergic blocking drugs, 53–54
  differential diagnosis, 445, 446*t*, 447
  erythropoietin, 450
  fludrocortisone, 448–449
  miscellaneous agents, 450
  overview, 443–444, 447, 448*t*
  physiology and pathophysiology, 444–445
  sympathomimetic agents
    agonists, 449
    antagonists, 449–450
  vasovagal syncope, pharmacologic treatment, 451–452, 451*t*
Osmotic diuretics, 153*t*, 156. *See also* Diuretics
Ototoxicity, adverse effect of diuretics, 173
Oxprenolol, 34
  pharmacodynamic properties and cardiac effects of, 35*t*, 43*t*

P

Parasympathetic drugs
  drugs that diminish muscarinic activity (muscanarinic receptor antagonists), 70–71, 71*t*
  drugs that enhance muscarinic activity
    anticholinesterase agents, 68*t*, 69–70
    choline esters, 69
  overview, 65–66, 67*t*–68*t*
Parasympathetic nervous system, 65
Parnaparin (Flaxum), 313*t*. *See also* Low-molecular-weight heparin
Paroxysmal supraventricular tachycardia
  calcium channel blockers, 90–91
Partial agonist activity, beta-adrenergic blocking drugs, 35*t*, 37
PDE inhibitors. *See* Phosphodiesterase inhibitors
Pediatric population. *See* "children" subentries under individual drug names in the index and in Appendix 2
Penbutolol (Levatol), 34, 36
  elderly patients, 583
  hepatic dysfunction, 680*t*
  pharmacodynamic properties and cardiac effects of, 35*t*, 43*t*
  pharmacokinetics, 531*t*
  pregnancy and lactation, 671*t*
  renal failure, dose adjustment in, 660*t*
  therapeutic use, 583
Penicillin
  bile acid sequestrants, interaction with, 356
  infective endocarditis, 455, 456*t*–459*t*, 461–463
  penicillinase-resistant
    infective endocarditis, 455, 456*t*–459*t*, 461–463
Pentaerythritol tetranitrate (Duotrate, Pentylan, Peritrate), 203
  elderly patients, 634
  hepatic dysfunction, 682*t*
  therapeutic use, 634–635
Pentolinium, 224
Pentoxifylline (Trental)
  elderly patients, 628

pharmacokinetics, 531*t*
therapeutic use, 628
Penylephrine, provocative testing with in cardiac auscultation, 427
Percutaneous transluminal coronary angioplasty and arterial stenting
aspirin, 297–298
Perioperative hypertension
calcium channel blockers, 94
Peripheral neuron depletors, 220, 224–225
current and recommended use, 225, 226*t*
effectiveness, 225
Peripheral resistance, effects of beta blockers on, 41–42, 44
Persantine. *See* Dipyridamole
Pharmacokinetic properties of cardiovascular drugs, 507–539. *See also* "pharmacokinetics" under entries for individual drug names
Pharmacology, basic principles of
drug disposition and pharmacokinetics
absorption, 8
bioavailability, 9–10, 10*f*
half-life and clearance, 13–14, 13*f*, 15*f*
passage of drugs across cell membranes, 7–8
plasma proteins, binding to, 11–12
routes of drug administration, 8–9
steady-state kinetics, 14–16
tissue distribution, 10–11
volume of distribution, 12
drug metabolism
age and, 17
disease states and, 18
enterohepatic circulation, 19
genetic factors and, 17, 18*f*
induction, 18–19, 20*f*
inhibition, 19
by intestinal microorganisms, 19
mechanisms and pathways, 16–17
nutrition and, 18
species, 17
excretion, 20–22
biliary, 21
kidney, 20–21
lungs, 21
milk, 21–22
saliva, 22
receptors. *See also* Receptors
description of, 1–2, 3*f*
kinetics of drug-receptor interactions, 2, 4
quantitative considerations, 4–6, 5*f*, 7*f*
Pharmacology, cardiovascular
basic principles. *See* Pharmacology, basic principles of
drug interactions. *See* Drug interactions
Phenformin
genetic factors in metabolism, 17
Phenindione in breast milk, 22
Phenobarbital, interactions with
beta-adrenergic blocking drugs, 60*t*
bile acid sequestrants, 356
digitalis, 287
disopyramide, 249
mexiletine, 256
propranolol, 265
quinidine, 245
Phenothiazines, interactions with
amiodarone, 501*t*
beta-adrenergic blocking drugs, 60*t*
Phenoxybenzamine (Dibenzyline), 25, 31
children, 628

Phenoxybenzamine (Dibenzyline) (*Cont.*)
  elderly patients, 628
  therapeutic use, 628
Phentolamine (Regitine), 25, 31
  children, 629
  elderly patients, 629
  therapeutic use, 629
Phenylbutazone
  bile acid sequestrants, interaction with, 356
Phenylproanolamine
  beta-adrenergic blocking drugs, interaction with, 61*t*
Phenytoin
  in breast milk, 22
  drug-drug interactions
    acebutolol, 483*t*
    aspirin, 503*t*
    beta-adrenergic blocking drugs, 61*t*
    digitalis, 287
    digoxin, 496
    disopyramide, 249, 499*t*
    labetalol, 483*t*
    metoprolol, 483*t*
    mexiletine, 256, 500*t*
    propranolol, 265, 483*t*
    quinidine, 245, 498*t*
    timolol, 483*t*
Pheochromocytoma
  alpha-adrenergic blocking drugs, 30
  beta-blocker choice in patients with, 62*t*
Phosphodiesterase (PDE) inhibitors, 201–202
  proarrhythmic drugs, interactions with, 481*t*
  therapeutic use, 609–613
Physostigmine, 70
Pindolol (Visken), 4, 34, 48
  elderly patients, 583
  hepatic dysfunction, 680*t*
  orthostatic hypotension, 450
  pharmacodynamic properties and cardiac effects of, 35*t*, 43*t*
  pharmacokinetics, 531*t*
  pregnancy and lactation, 670*t*
  renal failure, dose adjustment in, 659*t*
  therapeutic use, 583
Plasma protein binding, 11–12
  as site for drug interactions, 484
Plasma renin, effects of beta blockers on, 41
Plateau effect, 14, 15*f*
Plavix. *See* Clopidogrel
Plendil. *See* Felodipine
Polythiazide (Renese), 153*t*
  children, 606
  elderly patients, 606
  hepatic dysfunction, 683*t*
  pharmacokinetics, 531*t*
  therapeutic use, 606
Postangioplasty vascular restenosis
  angiotensin II receptor blockers, 147–148
  losartan, 147–148
Postdiuretic sodium retention, 157
Postural hypotension, adverse effect of diuretics, 172–173
Potassium as potential cardiovascular disease therapy
  cardiovascular effects
    systemic hypertension, 180–182, 181*t*
  electrophysiologic effects
    hypokalemia, 182
  overview, 180, 183
  potassium supplementation, 182–183
    IV therapy, 183
    oral therapy, 182–183, 183*t*

Potassium-sparing diuretics, 153*t*, 155–156. *See also* Diuretics
drug-drug interactions, 491
ACE inhibitors, 492*t*
hepatic dysfunction, 684*t*
renal failure, dose adjustment in, 657*t*
therapeutic use, 607–609
Potency, 6
Pravastatin (Pravachol)
adverse effects, 377
clinical use, 377
coronary and cerebral artery disease, 374–377, 376*f*
drug-drug interactions
cyclosporine, 504*t*
erythromycin, 504*t*
fibrates, 504*t*
nicotinic acid, 504*t*
elderly patients, 621
hepatic dysfunction, 685*t*
overview, 374
pharmacokinetics, 531*t*
pregnancy and lactation, 674*t*
renal failure, dose adjustment in, 664*t*
therapeutic use, 621
Prazosin (Minipress), 25, 27–29, 31–32
children, 540–541
drug-drug interactions, 494
digoxin, 495*t*
nifedipine, 489*t*, 493*t*
nitrates, 488*t*, 493*t*
verapamil, 488*t*, 493*t*
elderly patients, 540
disorders caused in, 654*t*
hepatic dysfunction, 679*t*
pharmacokinetics, 26*t*, 532*t*
pregnancy and lactation, 675*t*
renal failure, dose adjustment in, 662*t*
therapeutic use, 540–541
Preexcitation
calcium channel blockers, 91–92
Pregnancy and lactation
ACE inhibitors
benazepril, 673*t*
captopril, 672*t*
enalapril, 673*t*
fosinopril, 673*t*
lisinopril, 673*t*
moexipril, 673*t*
quinapril, 673*t*
ramipril, 673*t*
trandolapril, 673*t*
alcohol, 22
amitriptyline, 21
angiotensin-receptor blockers
irbesartan, 673*t*
losartan, 673*t*
valsartan, 673*t*
anticoagulants and thrombolytics
alteplase, 676*t*
anagrelide, 676*t*
ardeparin, 676*t*
aspirin, 676*t*
danaparoid, 676*t*
enoxaparin, 676*t*
heparin, 675*t*
reteplase, 676*t*
streptokinase, 676*t*
ticlodipine, 676*t*
urokinase, 676*t*
warfarin, 675*t*
antihypertensives
clonidine, 675*t*
doxazosin, 675*t*
fenoldopam, 674*t*
guanabenz, 675*t*
guanfacine, 675*t*
hydralazine, 21, 675*t*
methyldopa, 674*t*
minoxidil, 675*t*
nitroprusside, 675*t*
prazosin, 675*t*
terazosin, 675*t*

Pregnancy and lactation (*Cont.*):
atropine, 22
bile acid sequestrants, 353
caffeine, 21
chlorpromazine, 22
cimetidine, 22
class IA antiarrhythmics
disopyramide, 669*t*
procainamide, 669*t*
quinidine, 669*t*
class IB antiarrhythmics
lidocaine, 669*t*
mexiletine, 669*t*
tocainide, 669*t*
class IC antiarrhythmics
encainide, 670*t*
flecainide, 670*t*
propafenone, 670*t*
class II antiarrhythmics
acebutolol, 670*t*
atenolol, 670*t*
betaxolol, 671*t*
bisoprolol, 671*t*
carteolol, 671*t*
carvedilol, 671*t*
esmolol, 670*t*
labetalol, 671*t*
metoprolol, 670*t*
nadolol, 670*t*
penbutolol, 671*t*
pindolol, 670*t*
propranolol, 670*t*
sotalol, 671*t*
timolol, 670*t*
class III antiarrhythmics
amiodarone, 22, 671*t*
bretylium, 671*t*
ibutilide, 671*t*
class IV antiarrhythmics
amlodipine, 672*t*
bepridil, 672*t*
diltiazem, 671*t*
felodipine, 672*t*
isradipine, 672*t*
mibefradil, 672*t*
nicardipine, 672*t*
nifedipine, 672*t*
nimodipine, 672*t*
nisoldipine, 672*t*
nitrendipine, 672*t*
verapamil, 671*t*
cocaine, 21–22
cyclosporine, 22
diuretics
amiloride, 677*t*
bumetanide, 677*t*
chlorthalidone, 677*t*
chlorthiazide, 677*t*
ethacrynic acid, 677*t*
furosemide, 677*t*
hydrochlorothiazide, 677*t*
metolazone, 677*t*
spironolactone, 677*t*
torsemide, 677*t*
triamterene, 677*t*
doxorubicin, 22
ethosuximide, 21
inotropic agents
amrinone, 669*t*
digitoxin, 669*t*
digoxin, 21, 669*t*
milrinone, 669*t*
lipid-lowering agents
atorvastatin, 674*t*
cerivastatin, 674*t*
cholestyramine, 674*t*
clofibrate, 673*t*
colestipol, 674*t*
fluvastatin, 674*t*
gemfibrozil, 674*t*
lovastatin, 674*t*
niacin (nicotinic acid), 674*t*
pravastatin, 674*t*
probucol, 674*t*
simvastatin, 674*t*
lithium, 22
medroxyprogesterone, 21
metronidazole, 21
midodrine, 675*t*
morphine, 22
narcotics, 21

nicotine, 21
nitrates, 676*t*
nitrofurantoin, 22
orthostatic hypertension, 446*t*, 447
phenindione, 22
phenytoin, 22
primadone, 21
salicylates, 22
tetracycline, 22
tinidazole, 22
Primacor. *See* Milrinone
Primadone in breast milk, 21
Primary (essential) hypertension
ACE inhibitors, 120–121
Primary hyperaldosteronism
ACE inhibitors, 122–123, 123*t*, 133–134
Primary prevention, myocardial infarction
aspirin, 294–296
Primary pulmonary hypertension
calcium channel blockers, 99
Prinivil. *See* Lisinopril
Prinzide (lisinopril and hydrochlorothiazide), therapeutic use of, 637
Priscoline. *See* Tolazoline
ProAmantine. *See* Midodrine
Probenecid, interactions with
aspirin, 503*t*
captopril, 492*t*
loop and thiazide diuretics, 490*t*
Probucol
adverse effects, 389
chemistry, 388
clinical experience
combination therapy, 389
monotherapy, 388–389
preventing angioplasty-induced restenosis, 389
clinical use, 389–390
gender considerations, 667*t*
hepatic dysfunction, 685*t*
mechanisms of action, 388
overview, 387
pharmacokinetics, 388, 532*t*
pregnancy and lactation, 674*t*
renal failure, dose adjustment in, 664*t*
thiazides, interaction with, 504*t*
Procainamide (Procanbid, Pronestyl)
adverse effects, 247
antiarrhythmic effects, 246–247
atrial fibrillation, 237
AV reentrant tachycardia (Wolff-Parkinson-White syndrome), 239–240
children, 554
drug-drug interactions, 247
amiodarone, 274, 501*t*
captopril, 492*t*, 499*t*
cimetidine, 247, 483*t*, 499*t*
digoxin, 496
trimethoprim, 247
elderly patients, 553
electrophysiologic action, 245–246
gender considerations, 667*t*
genetic factors in metabolism, 17
hemodynamic effects, 246
hepatic dysfunction, 684*t*
indications and dosage, 247
pharmacokinetics, 246, 532*t*
pharmacologic description, 245
pregnancy and lactation, 669*t*
renal failure, dose adjustment in, 658*t*
therapeutic use, 553–554
ventricular fibrillation, 242
ventricular tachycardia, 241
Procanbid. *See* Procainamide
Procardia. *See* Nifedipine
Prodrugs, 11
Proglycem. *See* Diazoxide
Programmed cell death, 51

Pronestyl. *See* Procainamide
Propafenone (Rythmol)
  adverse effects, 262–263
  antiarrhythmic effects, 262
  atrial fibrillation, 237
  atrial tachycardia, 240
  AV nodal reentrant tachycardia, 239
  AV reentrant tachycardia (Wolff-Parkinson-White syndrome), 240
  drug-drug interactions, 263
    beta-adrenergic blocking drugs, 61*t*
    cimetidine, 263
    digitalis, 287
    digoxin, 263, 495*t*, 501*t*
    quinidine, 245, 263
    warfarin, 263
  elderly patients, 554
  electrophysiologic action, 261
  genetic factors in metabolism, 17
  hemodynamic effects, 262
  hepatic dysfunction, 685*t*
  indications and dosage, 263
  pharmacokinetics, 261–262, 532*t*
  pharmacologic description, 261
  pregnancy and lactation, 670*t*
  renal failure, dose adjustment in, 659*t*
  therapeutic use, 554
  ventricular tachycardia, 241
Propranolol (Inderal), 34, 38, 39, 41, 45, 53
  adverse effects, 265
  angina at rest
    verapamil, comparison to, 88
  antiarrhythmic effects, 265
  atrial tachycardia, 240
  children, 576
  depression, contraindicated in, 62*t*
  drug-drug interactions, 265–266
    antacids, 265
    antipyrine, 266
    barbiturates, 483*t*
    bile acid sequestrants, 356
    cimetidine, 266, 483*t*, 485*t*
    disopyramide, 265
    flecainide, 260
    lidocaine, 252, 266, 485*t*, 500*t*
    nifedipine, 489*t*
    phenobarbital, 265
    phenytoin, 265, 483*t*
    rifampin, 265, 483*t*
    theophylline, 266
    tubucuraine, 61*t*
    verapamil, 265
  elderly patients, 575–576, 652*t*
  electrophysiologic action, 264
  hemodynamic effects, 264
  hepatic dysfunction, 680*t*
  hypertrophic cardiomyopathy, 95–96
  indications and dosage, 266
  pharmacodynamic properties and cardiac effects of, 35*t*, 43*t*
  pharmacokinetics, 264, 533*t*
  pharmacologic description, 264
  pregnancy and lactation, 670*t*
  renal failure, dose adjustment in, 659*t*
  therapeutic use, 575–576
  ventricular fibrillation, 242
Prostacyclin
  epoprostenol. *See* Epoprostenol
  overview, 419
Prostatic obstruction, benign
  alpha-adrenergic blocking drugs, 31
Prosthetic valves
  endocarditis, 472–473, 475–476, 477*t*
  warfarin, 321–322

Protryptyline
  bretylium, interaction with, 272
Provocative testing in cardiac ausculation, 427
Pulmonary drug administration, 9
Pulmonary embolism
  thrombolytic agents, 343–344
Pulmonary hypertension
  alpha-adrenergic blocking drugs, 30
  epoprostenol, 422–426, 425*f*, 426*t*
Pyridostigmine, 70
  disopyramide, interaction with, 500*t*

Q

QT-interval prolongation syndrome
  beta-adrenergic blocking drugs, 53
Quality-of-life studies
  ACE inhibitors, 130–131
Questran. *See* Cholestyramine
Quinaglute. *See* Quinidine
Quinapril (Accupril)
  clinical applications, 136*t*
  elderly patients, 545
  hepatic dysfunction, 679*t*
  pharmacokinetics, 533*t*
  pregnancy and lactation, 673*t*
  renal failure, dose adjustment in, 661*t*
  therapeutic use, 545
Quinazolones
  renal failure, dose adjustment in, 657*t*
Quinethalone, 153*t*
Quinethazone (Hydromox)
  elderly patients, 607
  hepatic dysfunction, 683*t*
  therapeutic use, 606–607
Quinidex. *See* Quinidine
Quinidine (Cardioquin, Cin-Quin, Quinaglute, Quinidex)
  adverse effects, 244–245
  antiarrhythmic effects, 244
  atrial fibrillation, 237
  drug-drug interactions, 245
    amiodarone, 245, 274, 498*t*, 501*t*
    antibiotics, 498*t*
    anticholinesterases, 498*t*
    antihypertensive agents, 498*t*
    barbiturates, 498*t*
    beta-adrenergic blocking drugs, 61*t*, 498*t*
    cimetidine, 245, 483*t*, 498*t*
    digitalis, 287
    digitoxin, 245
    digoxin, 245, 494, 495*t*, 498*t*
    diltiazem, 498*t*
    disopyramide, 498*t*, 499*t*, 500*t*
    diuretics, 498*t*
    encainide, 245
    nifedipine, 489*t*, 499*t*
    phenobarbital, 245
    phenytoin, 245, 498*t*
    propafenone, 245, 263
    rifampin, 245, 498*t*
    sotalol, 499*t*
    verapamil, 280, 488*t*, 499*t*
    warfarin, 499*t*, 503*t*
  elderly patients, 555
    disorders caused in, 654*t*
  electrophysiologic action, 243
  gender considerations, 667*t*
  hemodynamic effects, 244
  hepatic dysfunction, 684*t*
  indications and dosage, 245
  pharmacokinetics, 243–244, 533*t*
  pharmacologic description, 26, 243
  pregnancy and lactation, 669*t*
  renal failure, dose adjustment in, 657*t*–658*t*
  therapeutic use, 554–555
  ventricular tachycardia, 241
Quinine
  digoxin, interaction with, 495*t*

R

Radioligand techniques, 33
Radionuclide testing and stress electrocardiography, 428–435
  adenosine. *See* Adenosine
  dipyridamole. *See* Dipyridamole
Ramipril (Altace)
  clinical applications, 136*t*
  elderly patients, 546
  hepatic dysfunction, 679*t*
  pharmacokinetics, 533*t*
  pregnancy and lactation, 673*t*
  renal failure, dose adjustment in, 661*t*
  therapeutic use, 545–546
Ranitidine
  beta-adrenergic blocking drugs, interaction with, 61*t*
Rauzide (rauwolfia serpentina and bendroflumethiazide), therapeutic use of, 646
Raynaud's phenomenon
  beta-adrenergic blocking drugs, side effect of, 56
  beta-blocker choice in patients with, 62*t*
  calcium channel blockers, 101
Receptors, 23, 24*t*, 25
  acetylcholine, 65–66
  adrenergic, 23, 24*t*, 25, 412*t*
  alpha-adrenergic, 23–25, 24*t*
    $alpha_1$-adrenergic, 23, 24*t*, 25–26, 197, 198*t*–199*t*, 199–200
    $alpha_2$-adrenergic, 23, 24*t*, 25–26, 44, 197, 199*t*
  angiotensin II, 138–139, 139*t*
  beta-adrenergic, 1–2, 3*f*, 33–34, 196–197
    $beta_1$-adrenergic, 23, 24*t*, 36–37, 197, 198*t*–199*t*, 199–200
    $beta_2$-adrenergic, 23, 24*t*, 36–37, 197, 198*t*–199*t*, 199–200
    $beta_3$-adrenergic, 23, 24*t*
  dopamine, 199, 411, 412*f*, 412*t*, 414–415
  hormonal, 23–25
  kinetics of drug-receptor interactions, 2, 4
  muscarinic, 66, 67*t*–68*t*
  nicotinic, 1, 3*f*, 223
  quantitative considerations, 4–6, 5*f*, 7*f*
Rectal drug administration, 9
Redux. *See* Dexfenfluramine
Regitine. *See* Phentolamine
Regroton (reserpine and chlorthalidone), therapeutic use of, 644–645
Regulatory proteins, 1
Relative bioavilability, 9
Renal artery stenosis
  ACE inhibitors, 132–133
Renal disease
  angiotensin II receptor blockers, 148
  losartan, 148
Renal drug interactions, 484
Renal failure
  beta-blocker choice in patients with, 63*t*
  drug adjustment in, 656*t*–665*t*
Renal impairment
  adverse effect of ACE inhibitors, 115–116
Renal insufficiency
  ACE inhibitors, 129
Renal parenchymal disease
  ACE inhibitors, 126–128
Renese. *See* Polythiazide
Renese-R (reserpine and polythiazide), therapeutic use of, 646
Renin-angiotensin system, pharmacologic inhibition of

ACE inhibitors. *See* ACE inhibitors
angiotensin II receptor antagonists. *See* Angiotensin II receptor blockers
Renovascular hypertension
ACE inhibitors, 1212–122
Reocclusion and reinfarction, 331–332
ReoPro. *See* Abciximab
Reperfusion, 332–333
Reserpine, 223, 225, 226*t*
beta-adrenergic blocking drugs, interaction with, 61*t*
children, 623
elderly patients, 623
disorders caused in, 654*t*
hepatic dysfunction, 681*t*
pharmacokinetics, 534*t*
therapeutic use, 623
Reteplase (Retavase), 326, 327*t*
hepatic dysfunction, 686*t*
pharmacokinetics, 534*t*
pregnancy and lactation, 676*t*
renal failure, dose adjustment in, 664*t*
therapeutic use, 571–572
Reviparin (Clivarine), 313*t*. *See also* Low-molecular-weight heparin
Rheumatic fever, 472, 473*t*–475*t*
Rifampin
drug-drug interactions
acebutolol, 483*t*
aspirin, 503*t*
disopyramide, 499*t*
labetalol, 483*t*
metoprolol, 483*t*
mexiletine, 500*t*
propranolol, 265, 483*t*
quinidine, 245, 498*t*
timolol, 483*t*
tocainide, 254
infective endocarditis, 458*t*–459*t*, 463–464
Riley-Day syndrome, 446*t*
Rogaine. *See* Minoxidil
Routes of drug administration, 8–9
Rythmol. *See* Propafenone

S
Salicylates
in breast milk, 22
elderly patients, 655*t*
Saliva, drug excretion by, 22
Salt-sensitive hypertension
diuretics, 162–163
Saluron. *See* Hydroflumethiazide
Salutensin (reserpine and hydroflumethiazide), therapeutic use of, 645
Sandoparin (certroparin), 313*t*. *See also* Low-molecular-weight heparin
Saralasin, 107
Scleroderma
ACE inhibitors, 122
Scopolamine, 9
Secondary prevention, myocardial infarction
aspirin, 296–297
Second messenger systems, 2, 3*f*
Sectral. *See* Acebutolol
Seldane. *See* Terfenadine
Ser-Ap-Es (reserpine, hydrochlorothiazide, and hydralazine), 401
therapeutic use, 650
Shock
alpha-adrenergic blocking drugs, 30
Shy-Drager syndrome, 446*t*, 450
"Silent" myocardial ischemia
beta-adrenergic blocking drugs, 50
calcium channel blockers, 94
Simvastatin (Zocor)
adverse effects, 373–374
clinical use, 373
coronary artery disease, 371–373, 372*f*–373*f*

Simvastatin (Zocor) (*Cont.*):
  drug-drug interactions
    cyclosporine, 504*t*
    erythromycin, 504*t*
    fibrates, 504*t*
    nicotinic acid, 504*t*
  elderly patients, 621
  gender considerations, 667*t*
  hepatic dysfunction, 685*t*
  overview, 371
  pharmacokinetics, 534*t*
  pregnancy and lactation, 674*t*
  renal failure, dose adjustment in, 664*t*
  therapeutic use, 621
Single photon emission computed tomography (SPECT)
  stress electrocardiography, 428, 430
Sinus node dysfunction
  beta-adrenergic blocking drugs, 55
Skin rash, adverse effect of ACE inhibitors, 117
Slo-Niacin. *See* Nicotinic acid
Slow channels, 74
Smoking
  beta-adrenergic blocking drugs, interaction with, 61*t*
Sodium nitroprusside
  hepatic dysfunction, 682*t*
  pharmacokinetics, 534*t*
Somatostatin
  orthostatic hypotension, 450
Sorbitrate. *See* Isosorbide dinitrate
Sotalol (Betapace), 34, 36, 48
  adverse effects, 276
  antiarrhythmic effects, 276
  atrial fibrillation, 237
  atrial tachycardia, 240
  AV reentrant tachycardia (Wolff-Parkinson-White syndrome), 240
  drug-drug interactions, 276
    amiodarone, 501*t*
    digoxin, 496
    disopyramide, 499*t*
    diuretics, 501*t*
    quinidine, 499*t*
    tricyclic antidepressants, 61*t*
  elderly patients, 577, 652*t*
  electrophysiologic action, 275
  hemodynamic effects, 275–276
  hepatic dysfunction, 680*t*
  indications and dosage, 276–277
  pharmacodynamic properties and cardiac effects of, 35*t*, 43*t*
  pharmacokinetics, 275, 534*t*
  pharmacologic description, 275
  pregnancy and lactation, 671*t*
  renal failure, dose adjustment in, 660*t*
  therapeutic use, 576–577
  ventricular fibrillation, 242
  ventricular tachycardia, 241
Species, drug metabolism and, 17
SPECT (single photon emission computed tomography)
  stress electrocardiography, 428, 430
Spironolactone (Aldactone), 153*t*, 155
  children, 608
  digoxin, interaction with, 495*t*
  elderly patients, 608
  hepatic dysfunction, 684*t*
  pharmacokinetics, 535*t*
  pregnancy and lactation, 677*t*
  renal failure, dose adjustment in, 657*t*
  therapeutic use, 608–609
Stable angina pectoris
  calcium channel blockers, 87
Staphylococcus aureus-caused endocarditis, 463–464

Steady-state kinetics, 14–16
Stepped-care approach (to hypertension treatment), 391
Streptokinase (Kabinkinase, Streptase), 324, 327*t*
  children, 573
  elderly patients, 573
  hepatic dysfunction, 686*t*
  patency rates, 331, 331*t*, 332*f*
  pharmacokinetics, 535*t*
  pregnancy and lactation, 676*t*
  renal failure, dose adjustment in, 664*t*
  therapeutic use, 572–573
Stress electrocardiography
  radionuclide testing and, 428–435
    adenosine. *See* Adenosine
    dipyridamole. *See* Dipyridamole
Stroke
  calcium channel blockers, 99–100
Structural proteins, 1
Stunned myocardium, detecting with dobutamine, 439
Subcutaneous drug administration, 9
Sublingual drug administration, 8
Sulfasalazine
  genetic factors in metabolism, 17
Sulfate formation, 16
Sulfinpyrazone, interaction with
  aspirin, 503*t*
  warfarin, 503*t*
Sulfonylurea, beta-blocker choice in patients using, 63*t*
Sulfoxidation, 16
Sulindac
  beta-adrenergic blocking drugs, interaction with, 61*t*
Supraventricular arrhythmias
  beta-adrenergic blocking drugs, 48, 49*t*
Surgery
  noncardiac
    preoperative assessment with dobutamine before, 438
  orthopedic and general
    heparin, 310
Sympatholytics
  diuretics, combination therapy with, 399
Sympathomimetic drugs
  orthostatic hypotension and vasovagal syncope, 449–450
Syncope, vasovagal. *See* Orthostatic hypotension and vasovagal syncope, drug treatment of
Systemic blood pressure, elevated
  beta-adrenergic blocking drugs, 40–41, 42*t*–43*t*
Systemic hypertension. *See also* Hypertension
  calcium and, 184
  calcium channel blockers, 92–94
  diuretics, 162–169. *See also* Diuretics
  potassium and, 180–182, 181*t*

T

Tambocor. *See* Flecainide
Tamsulosin, 31
Tarka (trandolapril/verapamil hydrochloride extended release), 402
  therapeutic use, 639–640
Teczem (enalapril maleate and diltiazem malate extended release), 393, 402
  therapeutic use, 638–639
TEE (transesophageal echocardiography), 464, 475

Tenex. *See* Guanfacine
Tenoretic (atenolol and chlorthalidone), therapeutic use of, 640–641
Tenormin. *See* Atenolol
Terazosin (Hytrin), 25, 27–28, 31–32
  drug-drug interactions
    nifedipine, 493*t*
    nitrates, 493*t*
    verapamil, 493*t*
  elderly patients, 541
  hepatic dysfunction, 679*t*
  pharmacokinetics, 26, 535*t*
  pregnancy and lactation, 675*t*
  renal failure, dose adjustment in, 662*t*
  therapeutic use, 541
Terfenadine (Seldane), interaction with
  erythromycin, 19
  ketoconazole, 19
Testosterone, 8
Tetracycline
  in breast milk, 22
  drug-drug interactions
    bile acid sequestrants, 356
    digoxin, 496
Tetralogy of Fallot
  beta-adrenergic blocking drugs, 53
Thalitone. *See* Chlorthalidone
Theophylline
  drug-drug interactions
    proarrhythmic drugs, 481*t*
    propranolol 266
    verapamil, 488*t*
  vasovagal syncope, 451
Therapeutic use of cardiovascular drugs, 540–650. *See also* "therapeutic use," and similar subentries, under entries for individual drug names
alpha-adrenergic blockers, 540–541
angiotensin converting enzyme inhibitors, 541–547
angiotensin II receptor blockers, 547–548
antiarrhythmic agents, 548–559
antihypertensive fixed drug combinations
  angiotensin converting enzyme inhibitors with thiazide diuretic, 636–637
  angiotensin converting enzyme inhibitor with calcium blocker, 638–640
  antiotensin II receptor blocker with thiazide diuretic, 640
  potassium-sparing diuretic and thiazide diuretic, 648–650
  reserpine, hydrochlorothiazide, and hydralazine (Ser-Ap-Es), 650
  sympatholytic (alpha-adrenergic antagonist) with thiazide diuretic, 647–648
  sympatholytic (beta blocker) with thiazide diuretic, 640–643
  sympatholytic (central-acting agent) with thiazide diuretic, 643–644
  sympatholytic (peripheral-acting adrenergic antagonist) with thiazide diuretic, 644–647
  vasodilator with thiazide diuretic, 648
  very-low-dose beta blocker with thiazide diuretic, 643

antiobesity drug, 559
antithrombotic therapy
anticoagulants, 559–565
antiplatelet agents, 565–569
thrombolytic agents, 569–574
beta-adrenergic blockers
beta$_1$-selective, without intrinsic sympathomimetic activity, 577–581
dual-acting, 583–585
with intrinsic sympathomimetic activity, 581–583
nonselective, without intrinsic sympathomimetic activity, 574–577
calcium antagonists, 585–594
centrally acting antihypertensive agents, 595–597
diuretics
loop diuretics, 597–601
potassium-sparing diuretics, 607–609
thiazide-type diuretics, 601–607
inotropic agents
beta and dopamine-receptor agonists, 610–613
digitalis, 613–616
phosphodiesterase inhibitors, 609–610
lipid-lowering drugs
bile-acid sequestrants, 616–617
fibric acid derivatives, 617–618
HMG-CoA reductase inhibitors, 619–621
neuronal and ganglionic blockers, 622–623
nicotinic acid, 618–619
vasodilators, 624–636
nitrates and nitrites, 630–636
Thiazide diuretics, 153*t*, 155. *See also* diuretics
drug-drug interactions, 491
amiodarone, 501*t*
amrinone, 495*t*
aspirin, 503*t*
dobutamine, 495*t*
milrinone, 495*t*
proarrhythmic drugs, 481*t*
probucol, 504*t*
gender considerations, 668*t*
hepatic dysfunction, 682*t*
renal failure, dose adjustment in, 657*t*
therapeutic use, 601–607
Thrombolytic agents
acute myocardial infarction, 326, 328–337
anterior wall myocardial infarction, 333–334
cardiogenic shock, 335–336
comparison of thrombolytic agents, 329, 329*t*
effect on mortality, 328–329, 328*t*
elderly patients, 336–337
importance of time on efficacy, 329–330
inferior wall myocardial infarction, 334
left bundle branch block, 335
non-Q-wave myocardial infarction, 334
patency, 330–331, 331*t*, 332*f*
reocclusion and reinfarction, 331–332
reperfusion, completeness of, 332–333
adjunctive antithrombotic therapy, 337–339
aspirin and other antiplatelet drugs, 337–338

Thrombolytic agents
  adjunctive antithrombotic therapy (*Cont.*):
    heparin and other antithrombin drugs, 338–339
  anistreplase. *See* Anistreplase
  complications
    cardiac rupture, 341
    intracranial hemorrhage, 339–340, 339*t*
    noncererbral hemorrhage, 341
    treatment of bleeding with thrombolysis, 341
  gender considerations, 668*t*
  hepatic dysfunction, 686*t*
  indications and contraindications to thrombolysis, 342, 342*t*
  ischemic stroke, 344
  obstructive mechanical prosthetic valve, 343
  overview, 324, 325*f*, 327*t*
  pulmonary embolism, 343–344
  streptokinase. *See* Streptokinase
  thrombotic arterial occlusion, 344
  tissue plasminogen activator. *See* Tissue plasminogen activator
  urokinase. *See* Urokinase
Thrombotic arterial occlusion
  thrombolytic agents, 344
Thromboxane, 337
Thyroid preparations
  bile acid sequestrants, interaction with, 356
Thyrotoxicosis
  beta-blocker choice in patients with, 62*t*
Thyroxine preparations
  bile acid sequestrants, interaction with, 356
Tiazac. *See* Diltiazem
Ticlopidine (Ticlid), 338, 3013–302
  adverse effects, 302
  cardiovascular disease, 302
  cerebrovascular and peripheral vascular disease, 301–302
  children, 569
  elderly patients, 569
  hepatic dysfunction, 686*t*
  pharmacokinetics, 535*t*
  pregnancy and lactation, 676*t*
  renal failure, dose adjustment in, 663*t*
  therapeutic use, 569
Timolide (timolol and hydrochlorothiazide), therapeutic use of, 641–642
Timolol (Blocadren, Timoptic), 34, 36, 39
  drug-drug interactions
    barbiturates, 483*t*
    cimetidine, 483*t*
    phenytoin, 483*t*
    rifampin, 483*t*
  elderly patients, 577
  hepatic dysfunction, 680*t*
  pharmacodynamic properties and cardiac effects of, 35*t*, 43*t*
  pharmacokinetics, 536*t*
  pregnancy and lactation, 670*t*
  renal failure, dose adjustment in, 659*t*
  therapeutic use, 577
Timoptic. *See* Timolol
Tinidazole in breast milk, 22
Tinzaparin (Logiparin), 313*t*. *See also* Low-molecular-weight heparin
Tissue distribution, drug, 10–11
Tissue plasminogen activator, 325–326, 327*t*
  patency rates, 331, 331*t*, 332*f*
Tocainide (Tonocard)
  adverse effects, 254

antiarrhythmic effects, 253
drug-drug interactions, 254
cimetidine, 254
rifampin, 254
elderly patients, 556
electrophysiologic action, 252–253
hemodynamic effects, 253
hepatic dysfunction, 684*t*
indications and dosage, 254
pharmacokinetics, 253, 536*t*
pharmacologic description, 252
pregnancy and lactation, 669*t*
renal failure, dose adjustment in, 658*t*
therapeutic use, 555–556
Tolazoline (Priscoline)
hepatic dysfunction, 682*t*
pharmacokinetics, 536*t*
therapeutic use, 629
Tonocard. *See* Tocainide
Toprol. *See* Metoprolol
Torsemide (Demadex), 153*t*, 154
elderly patients, 600
hepatic dysfunction, 683*t*
pharmacokinetics, 536*t*
pregnancy and lactation, 677*t*
renal failure, dose adjustment in, 656*t*
therapeutic use, 600–601
Total cholesterol, 349*f*, 350, 357, 371–372, 378–382
cerivastatin, 379
Trandate. *See* Labetalol
Trandolapril (Mavik)
clinical applications, 136*t*
elderly patients, 546
hepatic dysfunction, 679*t*
pharmacokinetics, 537*t*
pregnancy and lactation, 673*t*
renal failure, dose adjustment in, 661*t*
therapeutic use, 546
Transdermal drug administration, 9
Transderm-Nitro. *See* Nitroglycerin
Transesophageal echocardiography (TEE), 464, 475
Transient ischemic attack and stroke
aspirin, 299
Transmembranal enzymes, 2
Transport proteins, 1
Transthoracic echocardiography (TTE), 475
Trental. *See* Pentoxifylline
Triamterene (Dyrenium), 153*t*
children, 609
digoxin, interaction with, 495*t*
elderly patients, 609
hepatic dysfunction, 684*t*
pharmacokinetics, 537*t*
pregnancy and lactation, 677*t*
renal failure, dose adjustment in, 657*t*
therapeutic use, 609
Trichlormethiazide (Metahydrin, Naqua), 153*t*
children, 607
elderly patients, 607
hepatic dysfunction, 683*t*
pharmacokinetics, 537*t*
therapeutic use, 607
Tricyclic antidepressants
drug-drug interactions
amiodarone, 501*t*
beta-adrenergic blocking drugs, 61*t*
elderly patients, 655*t*
genetic factors in metabolism, 17
Triglycerides
hypertriglyceridemia treatment, 350
lovastatin, 239
Trimazosin, 25, 28
Trimethaphan, 224, 226*t*
hepatic dysfunction, 682*t*

Trimethoprim
procainamide, interaction with, 247
TTE (transthoracic echocardiography), 475
T-type channel, 74
Tubucuraine
beta-adrenergic blocking drugs, interaction with, 61*t*

U

Ultrasonic contrast agents during pharmacologic stress echocardiography, 441–442
Univasc. *See* Moexipril
Unstable angina
aspirin, 294
low-molecular-weight heparins, 314–315
Urapadil, 26
Urea, 153*t*, 156
Urokinase (Abbokinase), 324–325, 327*t*
elderly patients, 574
hepatic dysfunction, 686*t*
patency rates, 331*t*, 332*f*
pharmacokinetics, 538*t*
pregnancy and lactation, 676*t*
therapeutic use, 573–574

V

Valsartan (Diovan)
elderly patients, 548
hepatic dysfunction, 679*t*
pharmacokinetics, 538*t*
pregnancy and lactation, 673*t*
renal failure, dose adjustment in, 662*t*
therapeutic use, 548
Vancomycin
infective endocarditis, 455, 456*t*–459*t*, 462–464
Van der Waals bond, 4
Vascor. *See* Bepridil
Vascular smooth muscle as site for drug interactions, 480, 482
Vaseretic (enalapril and hydrochlorothiazide), therapeutic use of, 637
Vasoconstriction-volume analysis model, 163
Vasodilan. *See* Isoxsuprine
Vasodilators
beta-adrenergic blocking drugs, 38
drug-drug interactions, 493*t*
nitrates and nitrites
therapeutic use, 630–636
nonspecific. *See* Nonspecific antihypertensive vasodilators
therapeutic use, 624–636
Vasopressors
hepatic dysfunction, 678*t*
Vasospastic angina
beta-adrenergic blocking drugs, 46–47
Vasotec. *See* Enalapril
Vasovagal syncope. *See* Orthostatic hypotension and vasovagal syncope, drug treatment of
Vaughn Williams classification of antiarrhythmic drugs, 234, 235*t*
Vd (volume of distribution), 12
Venous thrombosis
heparin, 310
Ventricular arrhythmias
beta-adrenergic blocking drugs, 48, 49*t*
calcium channel blockers, 92
Ventricular fibrillation
amiodarone, 242
antiarrhythmic drugs, 242
bretylium, 242
esmolol, 242

lidocaine, 242
metoprolol, 242
procainamide, 242
propranolol, 242
sotalol, 242
Ventricular tachycardia
amiodarone, 241
antiarrhythmic drugs, 240–242
bretylium, 241
disopyramide, 241
flecainide, 241
lidocaine, 241
mexiletine, 241
moricizine, 241
procainamide, 241
propafenone, 241
quinidine, 241
sotalol, 241
verapamil, 242
Verapamil (Calan, Covera, Isoptin, Verelan), 4, 26, 73
adolescents, 593
adverse effects, 103*t*, 280
antiarrhythmic effects, 279–280
atrial tachycardia, 240
AV nodal reentrant tachycardia, 238–239
chemical structure, 74
children, 593–594
clinical applications
amaurosis fugax, 101
angina pectoris, 86, 86*t*, 87–88
migraine, 100
renal transplant patients, 102
"silent" myocardial ischemia, 94
supraventricular arrhythmias, 86, 89–92, 90*t*
systemic hypertension, 86, 92–93
drug-drug interactions, 280
adenosine, 284
beta-adrenergic blocking drugs, 485*t*, 488*t*
cimetidine, 483*t*, 488*t*
digitalis, 287, 488*t*
digitoxin, 495*t*
digoxin, 280, 488*t*, 494, 495*t*
disopyramide, 280, 488*t*
doxazosin, 493*t*
flecainide, 280, 488*t*
lidocaine, 500*t*
metoprolol, 280, 483*t*, 485*t*
prazosin, 488*t*, 493*t*
propranolol, 265
quinidine, 280, 488*t*, 499*t*
terazosin, 493*t*
theophylline, 488*t*
elderly patients, 593–594, 652*t*, 655*t*
disorders caused in, 654*t*
electrophysiologic action, 278
hemodynamic effects, 279
hepatic dysfunction, 681*t*
hypertrophic cardiomyopathy, 96
indications and dosage, 280
pharmacokinetics, 79, 80*t*, 82*t*–83*t*, 279, 538*t*
pharmacology, 76*t*, 77, 78, 278
pregnancy and lactation, 671*t*
renal failure, dose adjustment in, 660*t*
therapeutic use, 593–594
vasovagal syncope, 451
ventricular tachycardia, 242
Verelan. *See* Verapamil
Visken. *See* Pindolol
VLDL (very low-density lipoprotein) cholesterol, 352. *See also* Lipid-lowering drugs
atorvastatin, 379
bile acid sequestrants, 356–357
fibric acid derivatives, 360–362
nicotinic acid, 380, 384–386
probucol, 388

Volume of distribution (Vd), 12

W

Warfarin (Coumadin)
- adverse effects, 322–323
- children, 565
- clinical use
  - atrial fibrillation, 322
  - myocardial infarction, 321
  - prosthetic valves, 321–322
- dosage, 318–320, 319*f*
- drug-drug interactions, 497, 502, 503*t*
  - allopurinol, 503*t*
  - amiodarone, 274, 503*t*
  - aspirin, 503*t*
  - beta-adrenergic blocking drugs, 61*t*
  - bile acid sequestrants, 356, 504*t*
  - cholestyramine, 503*t*
  - cimetidine, 503*t*
  - clofibrate, 360
  - colestipol, 503*t*
  - fibric acids, 504*t*
  - gembifrozil, 360
  - propafenone, 263
  - quinidine, 499*t*, 503*t*
  - sulfinpyrazone, 503*t*
- elderly patients, 565, 652*t*–653*t*
- hepatic dysfunction, 686*t*
- laboratory monitoring, 317–318, 318*f*
- mechanism of action, 316
- pharmacokinetics, 316–317, 539*t*
- pregnancy and lactation, 675*t*
- renal failure, dose adjustment in, 663*t*
- therapeutic use, 564–565

Wolff-Parkinson-White syndrome (AV reentrant tachycardia)
- adenosine, 239
- amiodarone, 240
- antiarrhythmic drugs, 239–240
- diltiazem, 239
- disopyramide, 240
- esmolol, 239
- flecainide, 240
- moricizine, 240
- procainamide, 239, 240
- propafenone, 240
- sotalol, 240
- verapamil, 91–92, 239

Women
- calcium channel blockers, 93
- diuretics, 167–168
- efficacy of selected medications, 666*t*–668*t*
- pregnancy and lactation. *See* Pregnancy and lactation
- salt-sensitive hypertension, 162

Wytensin. *See* Guanabenz

X

Xylocaine. *See* Lidocaine

Y

Yohimbine, 26, 32
- orthostatic hypotension, 449–450

Z

Zaroxolyn. *See* Metolazone
Zebeta. *See* Bisoprolol
Zestoretic (lisinopril and hydrochlorothiazide), therapeutic use of, 637
Zestril. *See* Lisinopril
Ziac (bisoprolol fumarate and hydrochlorothiazide), 393, 404
- therapeutic use, 643

Zocor. *See* Simvastatin

ISBN 0-07-022488-9
90000
9 780070 224889